Cardiac Arrhythmias 2005

Cardiac Arrhythmias 2005

Edited by
Antonio Raviele

Proceedings of the
9th International Workshop
on Cardiac Arrhythmias

(Venice, 2-5 October 2005)

Springer

Antonio Raviele, MD
Divisione di Cardiologia
Ospedale Umberto I
Via Circonvallazione 50
I-30174 Venezia Mestre

Library of Congress Control Number: 2005933282

ISBN-10 88-470-0370-9 Springer Milan Berlin Heidelberg New York
ISBN-13 978-88-470-0370-5 Springer Milan Berlin Heidelberg New York

Springer is a part of Springer Science + Business Media

springeronline.com

Printed in Italy

Cover design: Simona Colombo, Milan
Typesetting: Graphostudio, Milan
Printing and binding: Grafiche Porpora, Cernusco sul Naviglio (MI)

Preface

The year 1988 marked the beginning of the International Workshop on Cardiac Arrhythmias. This biannual series of meetings was initiated with the following goals: (1) to present technological advances in the field of cardiac arrhythmias, (2) to publicise the results of current research, and (3) to assess the impact of new diagnostic and therapeutic approaches. In addition, by bringing together experts in this field, controversial aspects in the diagnosis and treatment of cardiac arrhythmias could be discussed, allowing a consensus to be reached regarding the evaluation and management of specific disease conditions. The success achieved in reaching these goals and the utility of the workshops have been confirmed by their increasing recognition and level of attendance.

The Proceedings of the Ninth Edition of the Workshop is a compilation of the topics presented at the most recent meeting, which was held in Venice at the Fondazione Giorgio Cini from the 2nd to the 5th of October 2005. The book is divided into eight sections, each addressing a different aspect of cardiac arrhythmia: Supraventricular Arrhythmia and Atrial Flutter; Atrial Fibrillation: Pathophysiology, Clinical and Therapeutic Aspects; Atrial Fibrillation: Catheter Ablation and Other Non-pharmacological Therapies; Hereditary Arrhythmogenic Syndromes; Sudden Death: Prediction and Prevention; Cardiac Resynchronisation Therapy: Indications and Results; Cardiac Pacing: Technical and Clinical Aspects; Syncope: Evaluation and Therapies.

By presenting a comprehensive and up-to-date overview of all pertinent aspects of cardiac arrhythmias, this book provides a highly valuable source of information for general cardiologists, internists, and medical students, as well for researchers involved in all aspects of the field of cardiology. The knowledge and expertise offered by the various contributors will improve our understanding of cardiac arrhythmias and motivate further developments in the field.

This volume is the result of the efforts of several authors, each of whom deserves recognition and thanks. In addition, I thank Springer and its staff, in particular Donatella Rizza, Executive Editor, for their highly professional editorial efforts. I am especially grateful to Rita Reggiani, Project Manager of Adria Congrex, for her exceptional skills and enthusiasm in preparing the workshop. I would also like to thank my colleagues at Umberto I Hospital, Drs. Bonso, Gasparini, Themistoclakis, Giada, Rossillo, Corrado, Rigo, De Piccoli, Di Pede, both for their help and support in organising the meeting and for their continuous scientific and clinical collaboration.

The personal engagement and invaluable assistance of Susanna Orbolato, Stefania Damiani, and other members of the secretarial and nurse staff at my institution are gratefully acknowledged. I also extend my gratitude to Professor Piccolo, whose example and advice have provided a continual source of guidance and inspiration. Finally, I sincerely thank my wife Carmen and my children, Francesca and Michele. Their encouragement and support were essential to the successful preparation and completion of both the meeting and this book.

Antonio Raviele

Table of Contents

List of Contributors

SUPRAVENTRICULAR ARRHYTHMIA AND ATRIAL FLUTTER

Right and Left Atrial Flutter: How To Differentiate Them on the Basis of Surface Electrocardiogram?

G. Inama, C. Pedrinazzi, O. Durin, P. Gazzaniga, P. Agricola

Introduction

Atrial flutter is a common arrhythmia that may cause significant symptoms, including palpitations, dyspnoea, chest pain, and even syncope. For five decades, the mechanism of atrial flutter remained controversial, with protagonists and antagonists of theories proposing circus movement versus ectopic focus. The development of clinical electrophysiology in the 1970s and the observations made by many investigators in various canine heart models supported the concept that flutter is a macro-reentrant arrhythmia, often determined by a reentrant circuit confined to the right atrium [1–3].

The atrial rhythm during atrial flutter is regular (250–350 beats/min), with little or no isoelectric interval on ECG. The surface 12-leads ECG is helpful in establishing a diagnosis of atrial flutter for the common form due to counterclockwise reentry in the right atrium and for the uncommon form with reverse activation sequence [4–6].

In 2001, the European Society of Cardiology and the North American Society of Pacing and Electrophysiology [7] published a new atrial flutter nomenclature. More recently, Scheinman et al. [8] provided an updated classification and nomenclature (Table 1).

It is frequently possible to diagnose atrial flutter with 12-lead surface ECG, looking for distinctive waves in leads II, III, aVF, and V1. When flutter waves are not clearly visible, slowing AV nodal conduction through vagal stimulation manoeuvres or using drugs, such as Verapamil, to increase AV conduction block makes their recognition easier.

Cardiology Department, Maggiore Hospital, Crema, (Cremona), Italy

Table 1. Classification of the electrophysiological mechanisms of atrial flutter (modified from [8])

1. Right atrial CTI-dependent flutter
-Counterclockwise flutter (common)
-Clockwise flutter (uncommon)
-Double-wave reentry
-Lower loop reentry
-Intra-isthmus reentry
2. Right atrial non-CTI-dependent flutter
-Scar-related flutter
-Upper loop flutter
3. Left atrial flutter
-Mitral annulus flutter
-Scar and pulmonary vein-related flutter
-Coronary sinus flutter
-Left septal flutter

Right Atrial CTI-Dependent Flutter

Counterclockwise Flutter (Common Form)

The ECG is very helpful in establishing a diagnosis of right atrial cavotricuspid isthmus (CTI)-dependent flutter, mainly the common form due to counterclockwise reentry in the right atrium. This is the most common type of atrial flutter and accounts for about 90% of clinical cases. It is sustained by macroreentrant circuit in the right atrium and supported by endocardial structures, such as the crista terminalis, eustachian ridge/valve (posteriorly), and tricuspid annulus (anteriorly). The activation wave front proceeds in a cranial direction over the right atrial septum, reaches the top of the right atrium, then descends on the right atrial free wall in a caudal direction, and finally reaches the space located between the lower part of the right atrium and the atrial septum. The CTI, which forms the inferior area, is the critical link in the circuit and is the target of the radiofrequency (RF) catheter ablation procedure. Several investigators reported that RF energy applied in the isthmus between the inferior vena cava and tricuspid valve isthmus is effective in eliminating atrial flutter.The creation of a line of block with RF application in the isthmus between the inferior vena cava (IVC) and the tricuspid valve annulus (TA), with documentation of bidirectional block during pacing in coronary sinus, is actually considered to be the success index of RF ablation of right atrial CTI-dependent counterclockwise flutter and the electrophysiological end-point of the procedure [9–17].

In right atrial CTI-dependent counterclockwise flutter, an inverted F wave with a sawtooth pattern is observed in the inferior leads II, III, and aVF, with low-amplitude biphasic F waves in leads I and aVL, an upright F wave in lead V1, and transition to an inverted F wave in lead V6 (Fig. 1). Diagnosis made with the 12-lead ECG can be confirmed by an electrophysiological study with mapping and entrainment to demonstrate the counterclockwise sequence in the right atrium (Fig. 2) [18].

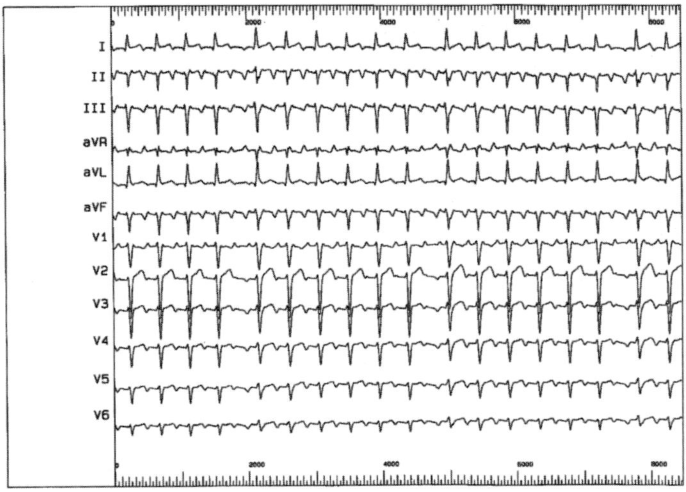

Fig. 1. 12-lead ECG recorded from a patient with counterclockwise (CTI)-dependent flutter (common type). Note the typical saw-toothed pattern of inverted F waves in the inferior leads II, III, and aVF. Counterclockwise right atrial flutter is also characterised by flat to biphasic F waves in I and aVL, an upright F wave in V1, and an inverted F in V6

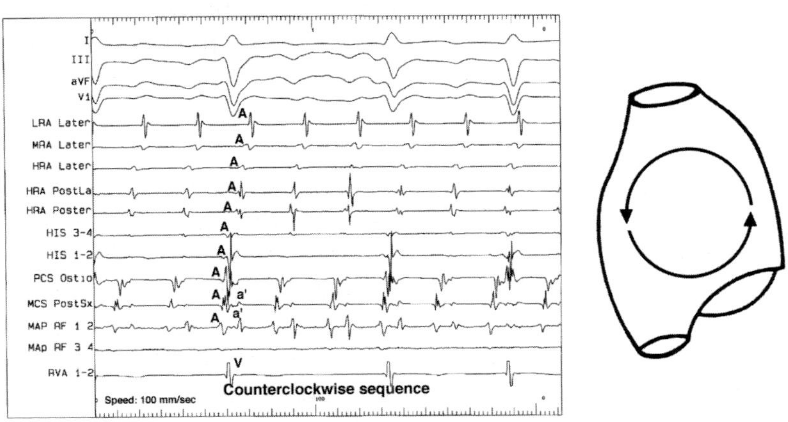

Fig. 2. Endocardial electrograms and surface ECG leads I, III, aVF, and V1 during RF ablation in the same patient as in Fig. 1. The recordings from the ablation catheter, coronary sinus, His bundle, and Halo catheters demonstrate a counterclockwise sequence of activation in the right atrium

Clockwise Flutter (Uncommon Form)

In the uncommon form of right atrial CTI-dependent flutter, the F wave pattern on 12-lead ECG is less specific and variable. Figure 3 shows another episode of right atrial CTI-dependent flutter in the same patient as in Figs. 1 and 2 during a RF ablation procedure [6]. The activation sequence of this 'reverse' version of flutter proceeds superiorly over the right atrial anterior and lateral walls and inferiorly over the right atrial posterior and septal walls (Fig. 4).

Clockwise flutter accounts for about 10% of clinical cases and has ECG findings that include positive F waves in the inferior leads II, III, and aVF, and negative deflection in V1. During electrophysiological study, the diagnosis of common or uncommon form of right atrial CTI-dependent flutter is suggested by observing a counterclockwise or clockwise activation pattern in the right atrium and around the tricuspid valve annulus.

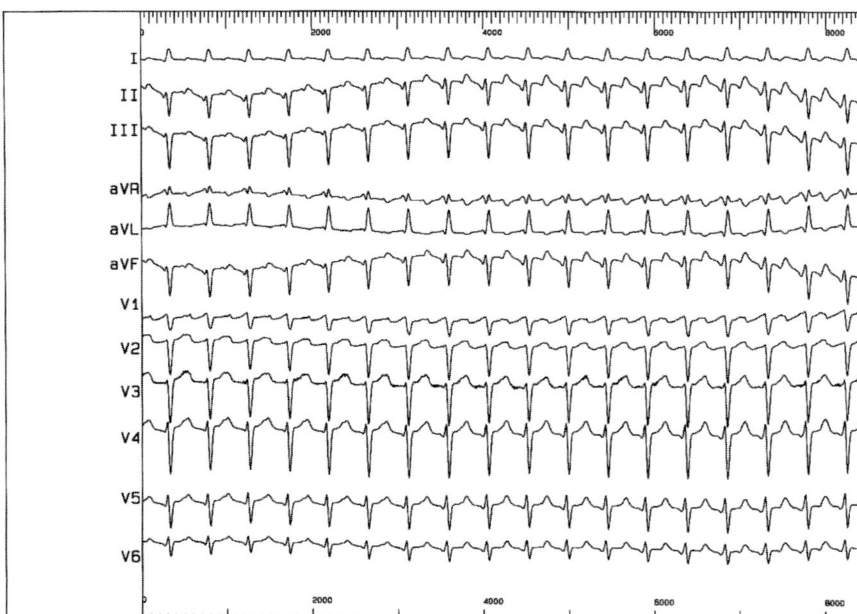

Fig. 3. 12-lead ECG recorded, during RF ablation in the same patient as in Figs. 1 and 2, now with the clockwise (CTI)-dependent form of flutter (uncommon type). The F wave in this reverse form may manifest as the mirror image of the CTI form, with positive F waves in the inferior leads II, III, and aVF, biphasic in leads I and aVL, negative deflection in V1, and an inverted F in V6

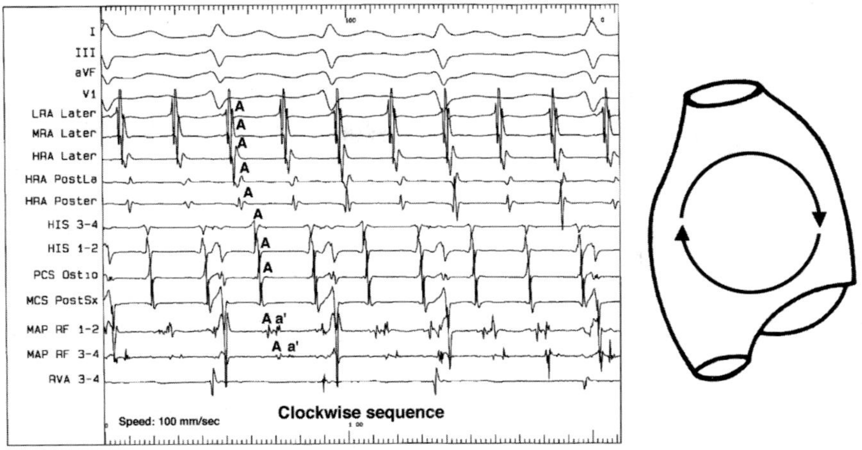

Fig. 4. Endocardial electrograms and surface ECG leads I, III, aVF, and V1 recorded during the clockwise form of flutter in the same patient. The recording from the ablation catheter, coronary sinus, His bundle, and Halo catheters demonstrate a clockwise sequence around the right atrium and tricuspid valve annulus, with cranial to caudal activation in the interatrial septum and caudal to cranial activation in the right atrial free wall, the opposite sequence of that seen in counterclockwise right atrial CTI-dependent flutter (Fig. 2)

The uncommon form of right atrial CTI-dependent flutter is diagnosed electrophysiologically by demonstrating a clockwise activation sequence around the right atrium and tricuspid valve annulus, with cranial to caudal activation in the interatrial septum and caudal to cranial activation in the right atrial free wall, the opposite sequence of that seen in counterclockwise right atrial CTI-dependent flutter. Confirmation that the reentry circuit involves the inferior isthmus requires the demonstration, for the common and uncommon forms, of the classic criteria for entrainment, including concealed entrainment with tachycardia acceleration to the pacing cycle length without a change in the F wave pattern on surface 12-lead ECG [19, 20].

Lower-Loop Reentry

Lower-loop reentry is a CTI-dependent flutter circuit that localises in the lower right atrium. Several endocavitary studies, using the electroanatomic mapping CARTO system, documented that the circuit rotates around the inferior vena cava, either in a counterclockwise or clockwise sequence, or around both the inferior vena cava and the tricuspid valve annulus, resulting in a figure of eight double-loop configuration [21–23]. The surface 12-lead ECG findings are similar to those of counterclockwise or clockwise atrial flutter.

Right Atrial Non-CTI-Dependent Flutter

Scar-related flutter and upper-loop reentry flutter are macro-reentrant circuits due to anatomic obstacles located outside the CTI.

Surgical atrial scars, especially due to cardiac surgery in the treatment of congenital heart disease, are the anatomopathological substrate of scar-related circuits in right atrial non-CTI-dependent flutter [12, 24–26]. Nakagawa et al. [26] reported that areas of slow conduction in narrow channels within islands of scar set up reentrant circuits in the right atrial free wall. RF catheter ablation of the critical corridors can eliminate the tachycardia.

Upper-loop flutter is characterised by a critical circuit confined to the superior portion of the right atrium, and this circuit is non-CTI-dependent [24, 28]. The diagnosis is possible only during an electrophysiological mapping study. The direction of rotation can be either counterclockwise, with descending sequence in the free wall anterior to the crista terminalis, or clockwise with ascending sequence in the free wall anterior to the crista. Surface 12-leads ECG shows no difference from the ECG obtained in counterclockwise or clockwise flutter.

Left Atrial Flutter

The incidence of left atrial flutter in an unselected patient population is unknown. A structural heart disease in the left heart is frequently present in patients with this condition. In addition, surface 12-lead ECG findings of left atrial flutter are often not specific to one particular tachycardia mechanism, making the analysis of atrial flutter based only on ECG problematic. Electrically silent areas are frequently identified in the left atrium by conventional and electroanatomic 3D mapping techniques during left atrial flutter, and similar areas in the posterior and anterior wall of the left atrium have been also found during sinus rhythm. Several studies have demonstrated that in most patients there is a fractionated atrial activation before the onset of stable atrial flutter, and it is usual to observe right atrial non-CTI-dependent flutter or left atrial flutter in patients with untreated atrial fibrillation and with periodic transition between the two arrhythmias. Frequently, patients without structural heart disease and a history suggestive of paroxysmal atrial fibrillation may have evidence of atrial flutter triggering fibrillation episodes. The atrial flutter circuit is postulated to play a critical role in the initiation and maintenance of atrial fibrillation in some patients [29, 30].

CARTO electroanatomic 3D mapping provides important information to completely map and characterise left atrial flutter. It also allows precise localisation of the ablation catheter and graphical presentation of the ablation line.

Mitral Annulus Flutter

This form is sustained by macroreentrant circuit in the left atrium that rotates around the mitral annulus either in a counterclockwise or clockwise direction, supported by endocardial structures, such as the mitral annulus anteriorly and low-voltage areas or scars posteriorly [18, 31–33]. Surface 12-lead ECG findings of mitral annulus flutter are low amplitude flutter waves in the inferior leads II, III, and aVF, and positive waves in V1 and V2 (Fig. 5).

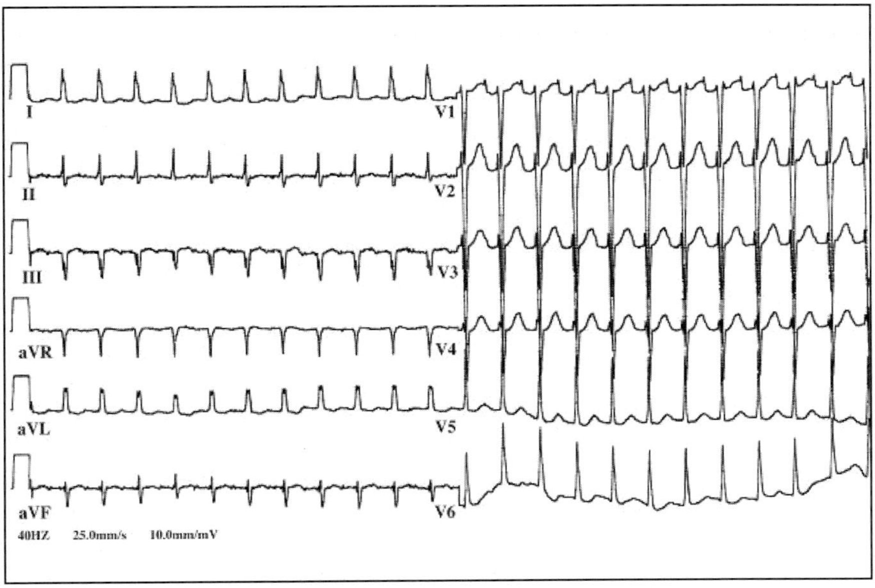

Fig. 5. 12-lead ECG recorded in a patient with atrial flutter. The ECG findings of low-amplitude flutter waves in the inferior leads II, III, and aVF, and positive waves in V1 and V2, suggest the diagnosis of mitral valve flutter sustained by a macroreentrant circuit in the left atrium that rotates around the mitral annulus

Scar and Pulmonary-Vein-Related Flutter

The reentry circuit in this form involves one or more pulmonary veins in the posterior wall of the left atrium, especially in patients with mitral valve disease and sometimes after RF ablation in the left atrium to cure atrial fibrillation. These circuits can have multiple loops and are related to regions with low voltage or scar areas. RF catheter ablation is complex and requires a 3D electroanatomic mapping approach to demonstrate the circuit and to guide the ablation, with several RF applications from a pulmonary vein to the mitral annulus or to the opposite pulmonary vein. Surface 12-lead ECG shows low amplitude of the flutter waves in inferior leads and a positive wave in lead I.

Left Septal Flutter

Recently, several authors [18, 34, 35] reported a different form of left atrial flutter, with circuits rotating around the fossa ovalis in a counterclockwise or clockwise sequence.

The critical isthmus is located on the septum between the fossa ovalis and the pulmonary vein or the mitral annulus. Surface 12-lead ECG findings show prominent positive flutter waves only in V1 or V2 and diminished amplitude of atrial waves in the other leads. The use of 3D mapping systems can improve correct diagnosis of the flutter and may provide precise localisation of the circuit to guide ablation.

Conclusions

Resetting responses and response to entrainment have confirmed the reentrant nature of flutter and established the presence of a fully excitable gap in the majority of patients. During atrial flutter, the use of 3D electroanatomic mapping studies and the entrainment pacing technique have aided in defining the mechanism of the arrhythmia with the activation sequence, providing information regarding the timing of intra-atrial events with respect to the surface electrocardiogram, especially for the non-CTI-dependent form and for left flutter.

Further study will be needed, however, to definite the precise boundaries of flutter and to better identify correlations between the location of the different electrophysiologic types of reentrant circuits and their electrocardiographic characteristics.

References

1. Disertori M, Inama G, Vergara G et al (1983) Evidence of a reentry circuit in the common type of atrial flutter in man. Circulation 67:434–440
2. Waldo AL, Mackall JA, Biblo LA (1997) Mechanisms and medical management of patients with atrial flutter. Cardiol Clin 15:661–676
3. Scheinman MM, Yang Y (2004) Atrial flutter: historical notes – Part 1. Pacing Clin Electrophysiol 27:379–381
4. Halligan SC, Gersh BJ, Brown RD Jr et al (2004) The natural history of lone atrial flutter. Ann Intern Med 140:265–268
5. Calkins H, Leon AR, Deam AG et al (1994) Catheter ablation of atrial flutter using radiofrequency energy. Am J Cardiol 73:353–356
6. Saoudi N, Nair M, Abdelazziz A et al (1996) Electrocardiographic patterns and

results of radiofrequency catheter ablation of clockwise type I atrial flutter. J Cardiovasc Electrophysiol 7:931–942

7. Saoudi N, Cosio F, Waldo A et al (2001) A classification of atrial flutter and regular atrial tachycardia according to electrophysiological mechanisms and anatomical bases; a Statement from a Joint Expert Group from The Working Group of Arrhythmias of the European Society of Cardiology and the North American Society of Pacing and Electrophysiology. Eur Heart J 22:1162–1182
8. Scheinman MM, Yang Y, Cheng J (2004) Atrial flutter: Part II. Nomenclature. Pacing Clin Electrophysiol 27:504–506
9. Kalman JM, Olgin JE, Saxon LA et al (1996) Activation and entrainment mapping defines the tricuspid annulus as the anterior barrier in typical atrial flutter. Circulation 94:398–406
10. Nakagawa H, Lazzara R, Khastgir T et al (1996) Role of the tricuspid annulus and the eustachian valve/ridge on atrial flutter. Relevance to catheter ablation of the septal isthmus and a new technique for rapid identification of ablation success. Circulation 94:407–424
11. Arribas F, Lopez-Gil M, Cosio FG et al (1997) The upper link of human common atrial flutter circuit: definition by multiple endocardial recordings during entrainment. Pacing Clin Electrophysiol 20:2924–2929
12. Kalman JM, Olgin JE, Saxon LA et al (1997) Electrocardiographic and electrophysiologic characterization of atypical atrial flutter in man: use of activation and entrainment mapping and implications for catheter ablation. J Cardiovasc Electrophysiol 8:121–144
13. Milliez P, Richardson AW, Obioha-Ngwu O et al (2002) Variable electrocardiographic characteristics of isthmus-dependent atrial flutter. J Am Coll Cardiol 40:1125–1132
14. Chan DP, Van Hare GF, Mackall JA et al (2000) Importance of atrial flutter isthmus in postoperative intra-atrial reentrant tachycardia. Circulation 102:1283–1289
15. Tsuchiya T, Okumura K, Tabuchi T et al (1996) The upper turnover site in the reentry circuit of common atrial flutter. Am J Cardiol 78:1439–1442
16. Inama G, Gramegna L, Pessano P et al (1998) Una esperienza italiana sull'ablazione transcatetere con radiofrequenza nel flutter atriale tipo I°: risultati e follow-up. G Ital Cardiol 28:666–677
17. Inama G, Gramegna L, Pessano P et al (1998) Long-term results in radiofrequency catheter ablation of type 1 atrial flutter. G Ital Cardiol 28(Suppl 1): 371–374
18. Bochoeyer A, Yang Y, Cheng J et al (2003) Surface electrocardiographic characteristics of right and left atrial flutter. Circulation 108:60–66
19. Frame LH (1987) Double reentry: a mechanism of overdrive acceleration of reentrant tachycardias. Circulation 76(Suppl IV):430
20. Frame LH, Rhee EK, Bernstein RC et al (1996) Reversal of reentry and acceleration due to double-wave reentry: two mechanisms for failure to terminate tachycardias by rapid pacing. J Am Coll Cardiol 28:137–145
21. Cheng J, Cabeen JWR, Scheinman MM (1999) Right atrial flutter due to lower loop reentry: mechanisms and anatomic substrates. Circulation 99:1700–1705
22. Zhang S, Younis G, Hariharan R et al (2004) Lower loop reentry as a mechanism of clockwise right atrial flutter. Circulation 109:1630–1635
23. Cheng J, Scheinman MM (1998) Acceleration of typical atrial flutter due to double-wave reentry induced by programmed electrical stimulation. Circulation 97:1589–1596
24. Yang Y, Cheng J, Bochoeyer A et al (2001) Atypical right atrial flutter patterns.

Circulation 103:3092–3098
25. Kall J, Rubenstein DS, Kopp DE et al (2000) Atypical atrial flutter originating in the right atrial free wall. Circulation 101:270–279
26. Nakagawa H, Shah N, Matsudaira K et al (2001) Characterization of reentrant circuit in macroreentrant right atrial tachycardia after surgical repair of congenital heart disease: isolated channels between scars allow 'focal' ablation. Circulation 103:699–709
27. Feld GK, Shahandeh-Rad F (1992) Activation patterns in experimental canine atrial flutter produced by right atrial crush injury. J Am Coll Cardiol 20:441–451
28. Tai CT, Huang JL, Lin YK et al (2002) Noncontact three-dimensional mapping and ablation of upper loop re-entry originating in the right atrium. J Am Coll Cardiol 40:746–753
29. Lelorier P, Humphries KH, Krahn A et al (2004) Prognostic differences between atrial fibrillation and atrial flutter. Am J Cardiol 93:647–649
30. Vidaillet H, Granada JF, Chyou PH et al (2002) A population based study of mortality among patients with atrial fibrillation or flutter. Am J Med 113:365–370
31. Jaïs P, Shah DC, Haïssaguerre M et al (2000) Mapping and ablation of left atrial flutters. Circulation 101:2928–2934
32. Ouyang F, Ernst S, Vogtmann T et al (2002) Characterization of reentrant circuits in left atrial macroreentrant tachycardia: critical isthmus block can prevent atrial tachycardia recurrence. Circulation 105:1934–1942
33. Cosio FG, Martin-Penato A, Pastor A et al (2003) Atypical flutter: a review. Pacing Clin Electrophysiol 26:2157–2169
34. Olgin JE, Jayachandran JV, Engesstein E et al (1998) Atrial macroreentry involving the myocardium of the coronary sinus: a unique mechanism for atypical flutter. J Cardiovasc Electrophysiol 9:1094–1099
35. Marrouche NF, Natale A, Wazni OM et al (2004) Left septal atrial flutter: electrophysiology, anatomy, and results of ablation. Circulation 109:2440–2447

Atypical Atrial Flutter: How to Diagnose, Locate, and Ablate It

Y. Yang, M.M. Scheinman

Atrial flutter (AFL) is defined as a rapid macro-reentrant atrial tachycardia characterised by little or no isoelectric interval between flutter (F) waves on ECG. Typical AFL refers to cavotricuspid isthmus (CTI)-dependent flutter with its reentrant circuit propagating around the tricuspid annulus in clockwise (CW) or counterclockwise (CCW) form (left anterior oblique projection) [1–7]. Typically, CCW flutter is characterised by negative F waves in the inferior leads (II, III, aVF) and positive waves in V1, while CW flutter is manifest by positive F waves in the inferior leads and negative waves in V1 [8, 9]. Entrainment pacing during typical AFL helps define the reentrant circuit, and typical AFLs show concealed entrainment when pacing from the CTI. The typical AFLs are cured by ablative lesions transecting the CTI [10–13].

So-called atypical AFL includes a wide variety of non-CTI-dependent flutter. In order to better understand different flutter circuits and provide an ablation strategy for them, we have proposed an updated classification and nomenclature of known flutter circuits [14]. Table 1 shows a brief classification of the atypical AFL.

CTI-dependent AFLs may have atypical surface ECG patterns [15] and vice versa [16]. For example, the surface ECG of upper loop reentry (ULR) can mimic typical CW flutter [16]. Compared to the CTI-dependent AFLs, the surface ECGs of these atypical flutters are less specific for predicting the reentrant circuit. Hence, it highlights the importance of entrainment and electroanatomic mapping in these cases. However, prior distinguishing between right and left AFLs from the surface ECG helps determine the mapping techniques. Although left AFLs showed more inhomogeneous patterns [17], our

Department of Medicine – Cardiac Electrophysiology Section, University of California, San Francisco, CA, USA

Table 1. Classification of atypical atrial flutter

Right atrial atypical flutter	Upper loop reentry Scar-related macroreentrant tachycardia
Left atrial atypical flutter	Mitral annular atrial flutter Scar and pulmonary-vein-related atrial flutter Left septal atrial flutter
Bi-atrial atypical flutter	Coronary sinus atrial flutter

study suggested that they are often associated with lower amplitude or flat F waves and greater isoelectric intervals (due to the higher incidence of left atrial abnormalities), and a predominant F wave in V1 in most cases [16].

Right Atrial Non-Isthmus-Dependent Flutter

Atypical flutter from right atrium includes those of ULR and scar-related macroreentrant tachycardia.

Upper Loop Reentry

In 2001, we first described ULR as a non-CTI dependent reentrant circuit involving the upper portion of the right atrium, with breakthrough over the lateral tricuspid annulus [18]. Later, Tai et al. verified this circuit by noncontact 3D mapping [19]. They found that gap(s) along the CT acted as the isthmus for this circuit, and the wave front within the circuit rotated either in a CW or CCW fashion using the CT as a functional obstacle. They also showed that linear ablation sealing the crystal gap terminated the tachycardia.

Right Atrial Scar-Related Macroreentrant Tachycardia

Various forms of macroreentrant circuits most commonly occur in patients with congenital heart disease or patients who have had surgical correction for their congenital cardiac defects. Using both entrainment and electroanatomic mapping can help define such circuits and its critical isthmus for guiding the ablation. In such patients, Nakagawa et al. used 3D electroanatomic mapping to show that one or more reentrant circuits used channels between the scar areas, and ablation of these channels proved to be successful for flutter termination [20]. Scar-related macroreentrant tachycardia is also found in patients without prior atriotomy. Our study showed that those patients had low-voltage (< 0.25 mV) or scarred areas along the posterior or lateral right atrium (Fig. 1) [18].

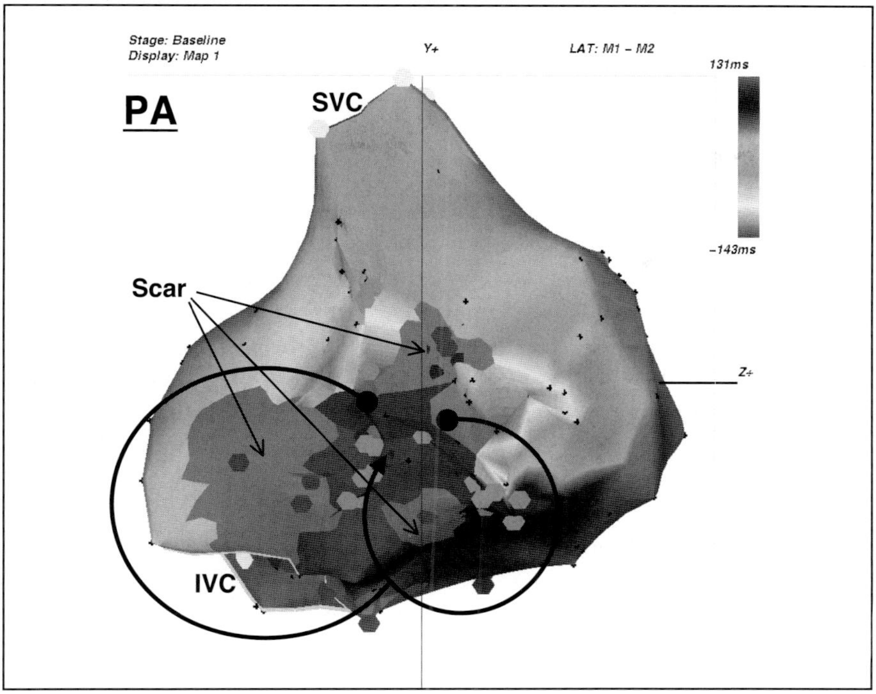

Fig. 1. A 3D electroanatomic (CARTO) map, under the posteroanterior (*PA*) projection, in a patient with right atrial scar-related macroreentrant tachycardia. The right atrial map showed several scarred areas (indicated by *thin arrows*) along the posterior wall, although the patient had no structural heart disease. The activation map showed a figure-8 type of reentrant circuit using the channel between the two lower scars as its common pathway, one looped around the inferior vena cava (*IVC*) and the other around the lateral scar. The wave front propagated through the channels between the scars (*bold arrow*), and concealed entrainment was demonstrated during pacing from the channel between the lower scars (the common pathway). A radiofrequency (RF) lesion that sealed these channels abolished the tachycardia. *SVC* Superior vena cava

Left Atrial Flutter

Left atrial flutters are less common than CTI-dependent right AFLs. Most of these arrhythmias are associated with structural abnormalities in the left atrium. In a study by Jaïs et al. [17], about 77% of patients with left AFL had underlying heart disease. Most of these left atrial circuits are associated with the low-voltage/scar area(s) in the posterior left atrium [16, 17, 21]. The 12-lead surface ECGs of left AFL can be variable. Some of them are compatible with typical CCW or CW flutter, but most show flat or low-amplitude flutter waves and isoelectric intervals between the flutter waves on ECG due to the left atrium abnormality [16, 17].

Mitral Annular Atrial Flutter

The most common form of left AFL is the reentrant circuit around the mitral annulus (MA), with the latter as its anterior boundary and the posterior low-voltage/scar area(s) as its posterior boundary. The wave front can propagate around the MA in either a CCW or CW fashion. It can also join the reentrant circuit around other anatomic barrier(s), such as the ostium of pulmonary veins, and/or low-voltage/scar area(s) to form double loop reentry [22]. Ablation of MA–AFL can be accomplished by a radiofrequency (RF) lesion transecting the mitral isthmus, which is from the MA to the left lower pulmonary vein; or, in the case of double loop reentry, tachycardia can be cured by a linear lesion extending from the MA to another anatomic structure (e.g., scar, or other PVs).

Scar and Pulmonary Vein-Related AFL

Having the low-voltage area(s) or scar(s), or functional zone of block within the left atrium allows for macro-reentrant circuits. These circuits often include these obstacles alone or they occur in association with one or more pulmonary veins [16, 17, 21]. Such AFL circuits can be single loop reentry, but more often present as figure-8-type, double loop reentry, or multiple loops (Fig. 2). Using 3D electroanatomic mapping can help to define these complex circuits and assist ablation. The type of ablation line depends on the anatomy of the circuit. For eliminating the tachycardia, appropriate ablation lines are required to join the scars, or from scar to the MA, or from a pulmonary vein to the MA.

Left Septal AFL

We recently described a left AFL circuit confined to the left atrial septum [23]. By using entrainment and electroanatomic mapping, the flutter circuit was found to rotate around the left septum primum, with the fossa ovalis acting as a central obstacle, the right pulmonary veins as its posterior boundary, and the MA as the anterior boundary. The critical isthmus of the reentrant circuit was located between the septum primum and pulmonary veins posteriorly and/or the MA anteriorly by the demonstration of concealed entrainment at these sites. A linear lesion extending from the septum primum to either the MA or the right inferior pulmonary vein resulted in tachycardia elimination.

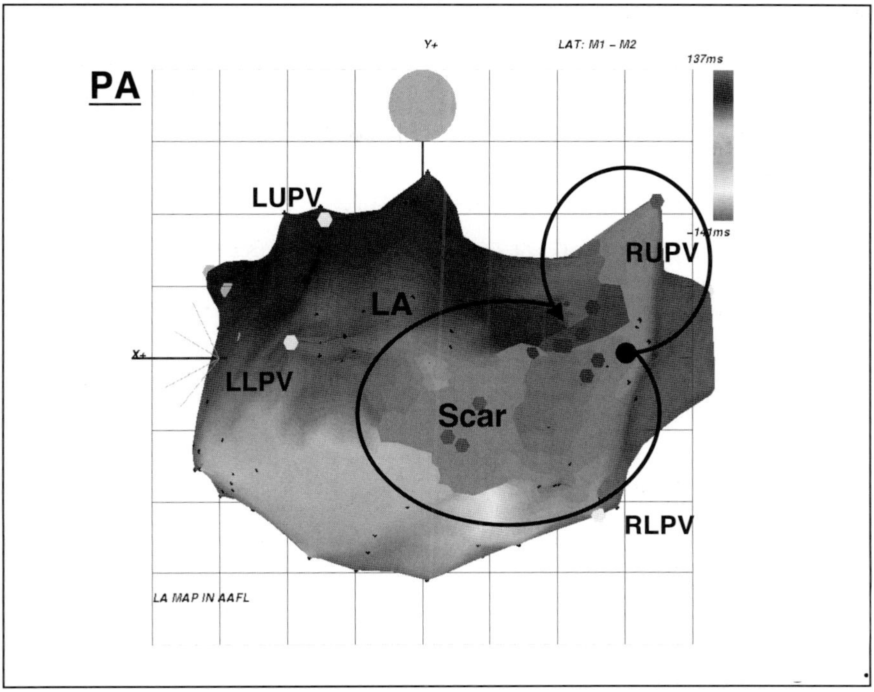

Fig. 2. A CARTO map, under the posteroanterior (*PA*) projection, in a patient with left atrial (*LA*) scar and pulmonary-vein-related flutter. The activation map demonstrated a figure-8 reentrant circuit around the right upper pulmonary vein (*RUPV*) and the scar in the posterior wall (*bold arrow*). Entrainment pacing from the channel between the scar and the RUPV showed the in-circuit response. Linear ablation across this gap terminated the flutter. *LUPV* left upper pulmonary vein, *LLPV* left lower pulmonary vein, *RLPV* right lower pulmonary vein

Bi-atrial AFL

To our knowledge, there is only one reported case of an AFL circuit involving both the left and the right atrium. Olgin et al. reported an atypical AFL circuit involving the myocardium of the coronary sinus (CS), left atrium, and interatrial septum [24]. In this type of circuit, the CS muscle conduction could be dissociated from the left atrial myocardium, as demonstrated by double potentials along the CS with disparate activation sequences. The wave front propagated through the myocardium of the CS and exited in the lateral left atrium, travelled down the interatrial septum and back to the CS. Circumferential ablation within the CS with bi-directional conduction block across the lesion resulted in the termination of tachycardia and no inducibility.

References

1. Wells JL Jr, MacLean WAH, James TN et al (1979) Characteristics of atrial flutter: studies in man after open heart surgery using fixed atrial electrodes. Circulation 60:665–673
2. Waldo AL, MacLean WAH, Karp RB et al (1977) Entrainment and interruption of atrial flutter with atrial pacing: studies in man following open heart surgery. Circulation 56:737–745
3. Lewis T, Drury A, Iliescu C (1921) A demonstration of circus movement in clinical flutter of the auricles. Heart 8:341–357
4. Klein G, Guiraudon G, Sharma A et al (1986) Demonstration of macroreentry and feasibility of operative therapy in the common type of atrial flutter. Am J Cardiol 57:587–591
5. Olgin JE, Kalman JM, Fitzpatrick AP et al (1995) Role of right atrial endocardial structures as barriers to conduction during human type I atrial flutter: activation and entrainment mapping guided by intracardiac echocardiography. Circulation 92:1839–1848
6. Kalman JM, Olgin JE, Lee RJ et al (1995) The anterior barrier in human atrial flutter: role of the tricuspid annulus. Circulation 92(suppl I):I-406 (abs)
7. Cosio FG, Goicolea A, Lopez-Gil M et al (1990) Atrial endocardial mapping in the rare form of atrial flutter. Am J Cardiol 66:715–720
8. Saoudi N, Nair M, Abdelazziz A et al (1996) Electrocardiographic patterns and results of radiofrequency catheter ablation of clockwise type I atrial flutter. J Cardiovasc Electrophysiol 7:931–942
9. Saoudi N, Cosio F, Waldo A et al (2001) A classification of atrial flutter and regular atrial tachycardia according to electrophysiological mechanisms and anatomical bases; a Statement from a Joint Expert Group from The Working Group of Arrhythmias of the European Society of Cardiology and the North American Society of Pacing and Electrophysiology. Eur Heart J 22:1162–1182
10. Saoudi N, Derumeaux G, Cribier A et al (1991) The role of catheter ablation techniques in the treatment of classic (type I) atrial flutter. Pacing Clin Electrophysiol 11:2022–2027
11. Feld GK, Fleck RP, Chen PS et al (1992) Radiofrequency catheter ablation for the treatment of human type 1 atrial flutter: identification of a critical zone in the reentrant circuit by endocardial mapping techniques. Circulation 86:1233–1240
12. Cosio FG, Lopez-Gil M, Goicolea A et al (1993) Radiofrequency ablation of the inferior vena cava-tricuspid valve isthmus in common atrial flutter. Am J Cardiol 71:705–709
13. Nakagawa H, Lazzara R, Khastgir T et al (1996) Role of the tricuspid annulus and the eustachian valve/ridge on atrial flutter: relevance to catheter ablation of the septal isthmus and a new technique for rapid identification of ablation success. Circulation 94:407–424
14. Scheinman MM, Yang Y, Cheng J (2004) Atrial flutter: Part II Nomenclature. Pacing Clin Electrophysiol 27:504–506
15. Milliez P, Richardson AW et al (2002) Variable electrocardiographic characteristics of isthmus-dependent atrial flutter. J Am Coll Cardiol 40:1125–1132
16. Bochoeyer A, Yang Y, Cheng J et al (2003) Surface electrocardiographic characteristics of right and left atrial flutter. Circulation 108:60–66
17. Jais P, Shah DC, Haissaguerre M et al (2000) Mapping and ablation of left atrial flutters. Circulation 101:2928–2934

18. Yang Y, Cheng J, Bochoeyer A et al (2001) Atypical right atrial flutter patterns. Circulation103:3092–3098
19. Tai CT, Huang JL, Lin YK et al (2002) Noncontact three-dimensional mapping and ablation of upper loop re-entry originating in the right atrium. J Am Coll Cardiol 40:746–753
20. Nakagawa H, Shah N, Matsudaira K et al (2001) Characterization of reentrant circuit in macroreentrant right atrial tachycardia after surgical repair of congenital heart disease: isolated channels between scars allow 'focal' ablation. Circulation103:699–709
21. Ouyang F, Ernst S, Vogtmann T et al (2002) Characterization of reentrant circuits in left atrial macroreentrant tachycardia: critical isthmus block can prevent atrial tachycardia recurrence. Circulation 105:1934–1942
22. Cosio FG, Martin-Penato A, Pastor A et al (2003) Atypical flutter: a review. Pacing Clin Electrophysiol 26:2157–2169
23. Marrouche NF, Natale A, Wazni OM et al (2004) Left septal atrial flutter: electrophysiology, anatomy, and results of ablation. Circulation 109:2440–2447
24. Olgin JE, Jayachandran JV, Engesstein E et al (1998) Atrial macroreentry involving the myocardium of the coronary sinus: a unique mechanism for atypical flutter. J Cardiovasc Electrophysiol 9:1094–1099

Catheter Ablation of Typical Atrial Flutter. What Are the Long-Term Results and Predictors of Recurrences?

P. DELISE, N. SITTA, L. CORO', L. SCIARRA, E. MARRAS, M. BOCCHINO, G. BERTON

Introduction

Catheter ablation of typical atrial flutter, targeting the cavo-tricuspid (CT) isthmus, is an effective treatment that is frequently used in clinical settings [1–7]. In fact, due to recent technical improvements (e.g. 8-mm catheters, irrigated-tip catheters), the short-term success rate of this approach exceeds 90% with low recurrence rates (no more than 5–10% of cases). However, a major problem in patients with atrial flutter is the possible coexistence of atrial fibrillation (AF). In fact, at least 10–35% of patients with clinically predominant atrial flutter also suffer from AF [8–10] and 5–22% of patients with AF also have atrial flutter, particularly those who are on antiarrhythmic therapy [10–14]. Therefore, there is reasonable risk that ablation of flutter, despite the elimination of arrhythmia, may not resolve the clinical problem owing to the recurrence of AF.

Electrophysiologic Relationships Between Atrial Fibrillation and Atrial Flutter

The presence of AF and flutter in the same patient is related to multiple mechanisms. First, the same atrial anatomic substrate can facilitate both multiple wavelet re-entry of AF and right atrial macro re-entry of atrial flutter. Second, AF can trigger atrial flutter [8–14]. In fact, frequently during AF the wave front originating from the left atrium tends to proceed in the right atrium along its anatomic barriers (crista terminalis, inferior vena cava,

Operative Unit of Cardiology, Hospital of Conegliano (Treviso), Italy etc.), which constitute the anatomic circuit of atrial flutter. Consequently, in many cases, as AF extinguishes, atrial flutter initiates. Third, atrial flutter, like other supraventricular arrhythmias [15–18], can trigger AF, a phenomenon that was described by Pristowsky [19] as 'tachycardia-induced tachycardia.' Finally, the two arrhythmias may have a common trigger, represented by automatic foci of pulmonary veins [18].

Antiarrhythmic drugs may have opposite effects on AF and atrial flutter. More precisely, many drugs (propafenone, flecainide, amiodarone) are able to prevent AF but they have little effect on, or may even facilitate atrial flutter. This observation has been made by several investigators, who demonstrated the occurrence of atrial flutter in 5–22% of patients with AF after treatment with class1 C drugs or amiodarone [10–14]. This phenomenon has been attributed to the slowing of conduction in the potential circuit of flutter.

Factors Influencing Recurrence of Flutter After Radiofrequency Ablation

The most important feature which avoids the recurrence of flutter is the creation of a stable and complete block of isthmus conduction [2–7]. In fact when the validation of block was not made in the first '90s the recurrence rate of flutter ablation was very high (30% or more) [1].

The validation of block may be reached documenting a clockwise activation of the right atrium stimulating from the inferolateral wall and, respectively, a counterclockwise activation stimulating from the ostium of the coronary sinus. This demontration can be obtained by multielectrode mapping of lateral and septal walls of the right atrium (for example with a Halo catheter) or by non fluoroscopic mapping (CARTO system) or by non contact mapping.

In some cases however an incomplete isthmus block with a marked conduction delay can mimick a complete block, thus facilitating the recurrence of the arrhythmia. The differential diagnosis can be obtained using the following additional criteria [5–7]:

1. The demonstration of double potential along the whole line of block
2. Change of unipolar electrograms in the right atrium opposite the pacing site after ablation
3. Maximum delay in the activation of the atrium opposite to the line of block obtained when stimulating close to the lesion in respect to a stimulation 1–2 cm more distant
4. Wider double potentials recorded along the ablation line when stimulating close to the lesion when compared to a stimulation a 1–2 cm more distantThe second factor influencing the possibility of a recurrent atrial flutter, is the resumption of isthmus conduction after a successful block. It

is important to know that 97% of conduction recovery occurs within 15 minutes [4].

In conclusion after obtaining a complete isthmus block and waiting for at least 15 minutes to confirm the stability of the lesion, the recurrence rate may be less than 5% [2].

Effects of Cavo-Tricuspid Isthmus Ablation of Atrial Fibrillation. Brief- and Mid-Term Results

At mid-term follow-up, the occurrence of AF in patients who were treated with isthmus ablation for documented atrial flutter is rare: less than 15% of patients, in the absence of antiarrhythmic therapy. In contrast, in patients with both atrial flutter and AF before ablation, the recurrence rate of AF is high (35–74% of patients), despite the use of antiarrhythmic drugs [7, 20–22].

Nevertheless, for the latter group of patients, many authors have recommended CT-isthmus ablation together with antiarrhythmic drugs (hybrid therapy), as this strategy has been shown to eliminate atrial flutter and to prevent or at least significantly reduce AF episodes in 73–90% of patients [13, 14, 21–25], thus significantly improving the quality of life for most patients.

For example, Schumacher et al. [13], who performed CT-isthmus ablation in patients with both arrhythmias, observed that during 11 ± 4 months of follow-up 37% of patients remained free from all arrhythmias, and an additional 42% of patients had significantly lower AF recurrence, while only 15% had no clinical benefit.

Nabar et al. [24] in another observational study covering a mean follow-up of 4 months, observed a clinical benefit in 85% of patients (70% disappearance of AF and flutter and 15% less AF recurrence).

Lee et al. [26] compared the effect of CT-isthmus ablation on quality of life in two groups of patients, one with only documented atrial flutter and the other with atrial flutter and AF, who had discontinued and continued drug therapy, respectively, after ablation. Quality of life significantly improved in both groups, although the improvement was greater in patients with only atrial flutter before ablation.

Finally our group, in a previous study [22] that included a follow-up after CT-isthmus ablation of about 18 months, observed a 13% recurrence rate of AF in patients with only atrial flutter compared to 38% (despite antiarrhythmic prophylaxis) in patients with both atrial flutter and AF before ablation. Two thirds of the latter group, however, had an improvement in quality of life, which was correlated with a significant reduction in the number of episodes of AF.

Long-Term Results of Atrial Flutter Ablation with Respect to Atrial Fibrillation Recurrence: Personal Experience

Methods

We studied 141 patients (114 males, 27 females, mean age 63 ± 10) with common atrial flutter who underwent successful CT-isthmus ablation, defined on the basis of short-term electrophysiologic validation at the end of the procedure [5, 27] and on the absence of clinical recurrence of atrial flutter during the first year of follow-up. These strict inclusion criteria were chosen to avoid the possibility that recurrence of atrial flutter played a role in the recurrence of AF.

Patients were divided into two groups on the basis of their characteristics before ablation. Group A included 48 patients with only documented common atrial flutter; group B included 93 patients who had both documented atrial flutter and AF.

In group A, 40/48 patients consumed 1.5 ± 1 antiarrhythmic drugs, while in group B all patients consumed 2.5 ± 1.2 antiarrhythmic drugs before ablation. The last antiarrhythmic therapy before ablation is reported in Table 1.

In group B, 31 patients had only atrial flutter during their last antiarrhythmic therapy (group B1), while 62 patients (group B2) continued to present with atrial flutter and AF during their last antiarrhythmic therapy. Among the latter, the ratio between documented episodes of AF and atrial flutter was about 1 (1 ± 0.1) in 20% of patients, > 1.1 in 60% of patients, and < 0.9 in 20% of patients.

After ablation, all group A patients discontinued any antiarrhythmic therapy, while group B patients continued their last (group B1) or best (group B2) antiarrhythmic drug therapy: amiodarone, flecainide, propafenone, or sotalol. Patients at risk of thromboembolic events continued anticoagulant therapy after discharge. Clinical characteristics were similar in both groups, except for the duration of symptoms, which was longer in group B (Table 1).

In all patients, CT-isthmus ablation was performed according to standard criteria [2–13]. Electrophysiologic success was defined when a bidirectional isthmus block was obtained, as demonstrated by coronary sinus and right low lateral atrium stimulation [14].

Quality of life was evaluated in the basal state and during follow-up by administering a Specific Symptom Scale (SSS) evaluation, which consisted of six questions concerning symptoms: palpitations, rest and effort dyspnoea, effort intolerance, asthenia, and angina. The SSS is scored from 0 (well) to 10 (unwell).

Table 1. Characteristics of patients. Group A (atrial flutter alone) and B (atrial flutter and AF)

	Group A (n = 48)	Group B (n = 93)	*P*
M/F	41/7	73/20	NS
Age	64 ± 10	63 ± 10	NS
Heart disease:	31 (64%)	54 (58%)	NS
HHD	18 (38%)	35 (37%)	NS
DCM	7 (14%)	9 (9%)	NS
CAD	6 (12%)	6 (6%)	NS
VHD		4 (4%)	NS
Last AATx :	n = 29	n = 87	
Amiodarone	17	32	
Flecainide	5	26	
Propaphenon	4	27	
Sotalol	3	2	
ACT	26 (54%)	70 (75%)	
LA	44 ± 10	44 ± 10	NS
EF	56 ± 10	57 ± 10	NS
Mean AFL	3.4 ± 2.4	3.2 ± 1.8	NS
Mean AF		5 ± 4.5	

HHD Hypertensive heart disease, *DCM* dilated cardiomyopathy, *CAD* coronary artery disease, *VHD* valvular heart disease, AATx antiarrhythmic therapy, *ACT* anticoagulant therapy, *LA* left atrium, *EF* ejection fraction, *AFL* atrial flutter, *AF* atrial fibrillation, *NS* not significant

On discharge, patients were instructed to promptly return to hospital in the event of sustained palpitations or of sustained symptoms possibly related to arrhythmia relapse, in order to undergo electrocardiography. In the case of unsustained symptoms, patients underwent one or more 24-h Holter monitorings. In any case, patients were asked to keep a diary of the number and duration of episodes of recurrent palpitations.

Patients were called back 3 months after ablation and at the end of follow-up (44 ± 20 months). During follow-up examinations, an interview focusing particularly on arrhythmia relapses, a clinical evaluation, and an electrocardiogram were carried out. AF recurrence was defined when AF was documented in the standard ECG or in the Holter (> 1 min). For the purposes of this report, the last SSS questionnaire was considered.

Results

During follow-up, no patient had recurrent typical atrial flutter. However, 13/48 (27%) of group A and 57/93 (61%) of group B patients had documented recurrent AF ($P< 0.001$). Within the latter group, AF recurred in 16/31 (51%) of group B1 and in 41/62 (66%) of group B2 patients (B1 vs B2, P=NS).

A comparison of the event-free survival curves (Fig. 1) shows that the three curves (groups A, B1, and B2, respectively) diverge from each other just during the first few months. Subsequently, the B1 and B2 curves tend to furother diverge and overlap with prolonged follow-up.

Permanent AF occurred in 3/48 (6%) of group A, in 1/31 (3%) of group B1, and in 13/62 (21%) of group B2 (A vs B1 P = NS, A and B1 vs B2 $P < 0.01$) .

Between patients with heart disease and those without, there was no difference either in the incidence of paroxysmal/persistent AF in groups A (26% vs 18%), B1 (46% vs 50%), and B2 (50% vs 42%) or in the incidence of permanent AF in groups A (7% vs 6%) and B1 (0% vs 5%). In contrast, there was a significant difference in the incidence of permanent AF in group B2 between patients without heart disease (4%) and those with heart disease (33%, $P < 0.01$) (Table 2).

Before ablation, 31/48 (64%) of group A, 18/31 (58%) of group B1, and 36/62 (58%) of group B2 had at least one electrical cardioversion (mean 1.35,

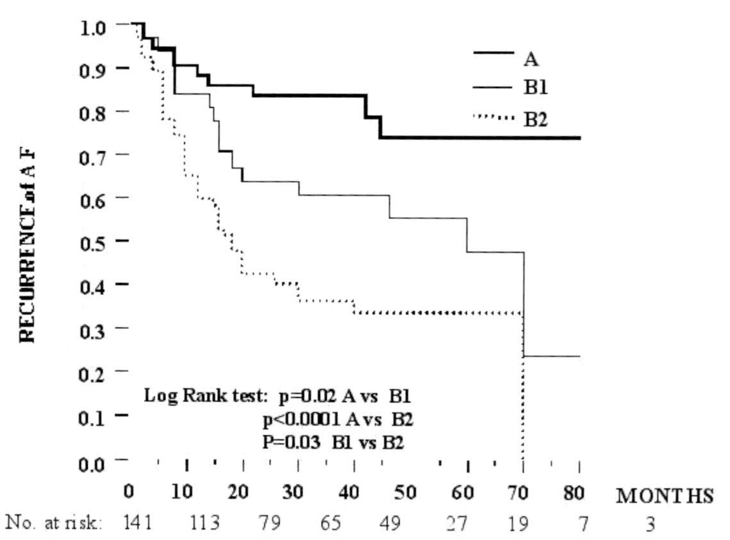

Fig. 1. Event-free survival curves for recurrent atrial fibrillation in groups A (atrial flutter only before ablation), B1, and B2 (both atrial flutter and AF before ablation)

Table 2. Comparison of recurrence rates of atrial fibrillation in the various patient groups according to the absence or presence of heart disease

	Group A ($n = 48$)	Group B1 ($n = 31$)	Group B2 ($n = 62$)
Recurrent AF	13 (27%)	16 (51%)	41 (66%)
Par/Pers AF	10 (21%)	15 (48%)	28 (45%)
-Absence of HD	4/15 (26%)	6/33 (18%)	13/26 50%)
-Presence of HD	6/13 (46%)	9/18 (50%)	15/36 (42%)
P (Absence vs presence of HD)	*NS*	*NS*	*NS*
Permanent AF	3 (6%)	1 (3%)	13 (21%)
-Absence of HD	1/15 (7%)	0/13 (0%)	1/26 (4%)
-Presence of HD	2/33 (6%)	1/18 (5%)	12/36 (33%)
P (Absence vs presence of HD)	NS	NS	< 0.01

Par Paroxysmal, *pers* persistent, *HD* heart disease

1.03, and 1.37 per patient, respectively). After CT-isthmus ablation 5/48 (10%) of group A, 2/31 (6%) of group B1, and 14/62 (22%) of group B2 had at least one electrical cardioversion (mean 0.12, 0.06, 0.27 per patient, respectively) (groups A, B1, and B2 before ablation vs after ablation $P < 0.001$ the difference remrined higlity significant also), excluding patients who developed permanent AF (Table 3).

Table 3. Electrical cardioversions before and after ablation

	PRE RF n.	PRE RF mean	AFTER RF n.	AFTER RF mean	*P* (mean)
All patients					
Group A (48)	31 (65%)	1.35	5 (10%)	0.12	< 0.0001
Group B1 (31)	18 (58%)	1.03	1 (3%)	0.03	< 0.0001
Group B2 (62)	36 (58%)	1.37	14 (22%)	0.27	< 0.0001
Permanent AF excluded					
Group A (45)	29 (64%)	1.3	3 (6.6%)	0.06	< 0.0001
Group B1 (30)	18 (60%)	1.04	1 (3%)	0.03	< 0.0001
Group B2 (49)	26 (53%)	1.28	8 (16%)	0.18	< 0.0001

Before ablation, SSS scores were similar in groups A and B. After ablation, at the end of follow-up, SSS scores decreased in all groups: In group A, from 16 ± 5 to 1.2 ± 1 ($P < 0.001$); in group B1, from 21 ± 10 to 7.8 ± 7 ($P < 0.001$); in group B2, from 21.3 ± 5 to 10.8 ± 8 ($P < 0.001$). The improvement in SSS score, however, was significantly higher in group A than in groups B1 and B2 (Table 4).

Table 4. Specific symptom scale (SSS) score. Group A post-ablation vs group B1 post-ablation, $P < 0.001$; group A post-ablation vs group B2 post-ablation, $P < 0.001$; group B1 post-ablation vs group B2 post-ablation, $P = 0.09$

	Before ablation	After ablation	*P*
Group A	16 ± 5	1.2 ± 1	< 0.0001
Group B1	21 ± 10	7.8 ± 7	< 0.0001
Group B2	21.3 ± 9.4	10.8 ± 8.5	< 0.001

Conclusions and Practical Considerations

Atrial flutter and AF have different electrophysiological mechanisms. While the two arrhythmias may coexist in the same patient, in most cases, during long-term follow-up, they have different natural courses.

In patients with documented atrial flutter only, isthmus ablation is usually curative. In some patients (less than 30% of cases), despite the elimination of atrial flutter, AF occurs, probably as a result of the previous existence of a non-documented form of this arrhythmia.

According to other investigators [28], in patients with both atrial flutter and AF, CT-isthmus ablation (despite the use of antiarrhythmic therapy) prevents AF in less than 40% of patients. In the remaining patients, AF relapses. According to another study (13), group B1 patients (with so-called IC/amiodarone atrial flutter) have a better outcome than group B2 patients (with both atrial flutter and AF during antiarrhythmic therapy). However, longer follow-up showed a tendency of similar recurrence rates compared to group B2 patients.

This pattern is not surprising, as it is well-known that the efficacy of antiarrhythmic therapy in preventing AF is inversely proportional to the duration of follow-up.

Permanent AF was very rare in group A (6%) while it occurred in about 20% of group B patients. Notably, AF rarely occurred (3%) in the B1 subgroup of patients, whereas there was a particularly high rate of permanent

AF (33%) in group B2 patients with heart disease.

On the basis of our results, CT-isthmus ablation seems mainly indicated in patients with atrial flutter alone. However, it can also be proposed as first-line therapy in symptomatic patients with both atrial flutter and AF, particularly if they have no heart disease and/or if they have only atrial flutter during antiarrhythmic drugs. In fact in such patients, quality of life frequently improves, probably as a result of the abolition of flutter and of the lower number of symptomatic episodes of AF, in particular those needing treatment by electrical cardioversion.

CT-isthmus ablation is a questionable form of therapy in patients with heart disease, particularly if they continue to present with AF during antiarrhythmic drug treatment.

In patients in whom therapy is unsuccessful (frequent AF relapses and/or compromised quality of life,) pulmonary-vein isolation or an ablate and pace strategy should be proposed only as a second-line therapy. Our opinion derives from the observation that pulmonary-vein isolation, although potentially curative in patients with AF, is a complex and risky procedure, while an ablate and pace strategy is an irreversibly destructive therapy. By contrast, CT-isthmus ablation is simple and safe and provides significant clinical benefit in most patients.

References

1. Cosio FG, Lopez-Gil M, Giocolea A et al (1993) Radiofrequency ablation of the inferior vena cava-tricuspid valve isthmus in common atrial flutter. Am J Cardiol 71:705–709
2. Poty H, Saoudi N, Nair M et al (1996) Radiofrequency catheter ablation of atrial flutter: further insights into the various types of isthmus block : applications to ablation during sinus rhythm. Circulation 94:3204–3213
3. Jaïs P, Haïssaguerre M, Shah D et al (1998) Successful irrigated-tip catheter ablation of atrial flutter resistant to conventional radiofrequency ablation. Circulation 98:835–838
4. Nabar A, Rodriguez LM, Timmermans C et al (1999) Isoproterenol to evaluate resumption of conduction after right atrial isthmus ablation in type I atrial flutter. Circulation 99:3286–3291
5. Chen J, de Chillou C, Basiouny T et al (1999) Cavotricuspid isthmus mapping to assess bidirectional block during common atrial flutter radiofrequency ablation. Circulation 100:2507–2513
6. Shah DC, Haïssaguerre M, Takahashi A et al (2000) Differential pacing for distiguishing block from persistent conduction through an ablation line. Circulation; 102:1517–1522
7. Villacastin J, Almendral J, Arenal A et al (2000) Usefulness of unipolar electrograms to detect isthmus block after radiofrequency ablation of typical atrial flutter. Circulation 102:3080–3085

8. Rothinger FX, Karch MR, Steiner PR et al (1997) Relationship between atrial fibrillation and typical atrial flutter in humans. Activation sequence changes during spontaneous conversion. Circulation 96:3484–3491
9. Kalman JM, Olgin JE, Saxon LA et al (1997) Electrocardiographic and electrophysiologic characterization of atypical atrial flutter in man. Use of activation and entrainment mapping and implications for catheter ablation. J Cardiovasc Electrophysiol 8:121–144
10. Levy S, Breithrd G, Campbell WF et al (1998) Atrial fibrillation: current knowledge and recommendations for management. Eur Heart J 19:1294–1320
11. Bianconi L, Mennuni M, Lukic V et al (1996) Effect of oral propafenone administered before electrical cardioversion of chronic atrial fibrillation: a placebo-controlled study. J Am Coll Cardiol 28:700–706
12. Riva S, Tondo C, Carbucicchio C et al (1999) Incidence and clinical significance of trasformation of atrial fibrillation to atrial flutter in patients undergoing long-term antiarrhythmic drug treatment. Europace 1:242–247
13. Schumaker B, Jung W, Lewalter T et al (1999) Radiofrequency ablation of atrial flutter due to administration of class 1 C antiarrhythmic drugs for atrial fibrillation, Am J Cardiol 83:710–713
14. Natale A, Tomassoni F, Fanelli R et al (1997) Occurrence of atrial flutter after initiation of amiodarone therapy of paroxysmal atrial fibrillation. Circulation 96:I–385
15. Sung RJ, Castellanos A, Mallon SM et al (1977) Mechanisms of spontaneous alternation between reciprocating tachycardia and atrial flutter–fibrillation in the Wolff–Parkinson–White syndrome. Circulation 56:409–416
16. Roark S, McCarthy E, Pritchet E (1986) Observations on the occurrence of atrial fibrillation in paroxysmal supraventricular tachycardia. Am J Cardiol 57:571–575
17. Delise P, Gianfranchi L, Paparella N et al (1997) Clinical usefulness of slow pathway ablation in patients with both paroxysmal AV nodal reentrant tachycardia and atrial fibrillation. Am J Cardiol 79:1421–1423
18. Jaïs P, Haïssaguerre M, Shah DC et al (1997) A focal source of atrial fibrillation treated by discrete radiofrequency ablation. Circulation 95:572–576
19. Pristowsky EN (1995) Tachycardia–induced tachycardia: a mechanism of initiation of atrial fibrillation. In: Di Marco JP, Prystowsky EN (eds) Atrial arrhhythmias: State of the art. NY, Futura Publishing Company, Armonk, pp 81–95
20. Paydak H, Kall J, Burke MC et al (1998) Atrial fibrillation after radiofrequency ablation of type I atrial flutter. Time of onset, determinants and clinical course. Circulation 98:315–322
21. Delise P, Sitta N, Coro' L et al (2002) Clinical usefulness of hybrid therapy in patients with both atrial futter and fibrillation. G Ital Aritm Cardiostim 5:266–269
22. Delise P, Sitta N, Coro' L et al (2004) Atrial flutter induced by calss IC Drugs/amiodarone: what are the long term results of cavo–tricuspidal isthmus ablation? In: Raviele A (ed) Cardiac Arrhythmias 2004, Springer Verlag Italia, Milan, pp 263–270
23. Huang DT, Monaham KM, Zimetbaum P et al (1998) Hybrid pharmacological and ablative therapy: a novel and effective approach for the management of atrial fibrillation. J Cardiovasc Electrophysiol 9:462–469
24. Nabar A, Rodriguez LM, Timmermans C et al (2001) Class I C antiarrhythmic drug–induced atrial flutter: electrocardiographic and electrophysiologic findings and their importance for long–term outcome after right atrial isthmus ablation. Heart 85:424–429
25. Bonso A, Rossillo A, Zoppo F et al (2002) Class IC or amiodarone induced atrial flutter during chronic treatment of atrial fibrillation. Long term follow up of

hybrid pharmacological and ablative therapy. PACE 24:614
26. Lee H, Tai CT, Yu WC et al (1999) Effects of radiofrequency catheter ablation on quality of life in patients with atrial flutter. Am J Cardiol 84:278–283
27. Shah D, Haïssaguerre M, Takahashi A et al (2000) Differential pacing for distiguishing block from persistent conduction through an ablation line. Circulation 102:1517–1522
28. Bertaglia E, Bonso A, Zoppo F et al (2004) Different clinical courses and predictors of atrial fibrillationoccurrence after transisthmic ablation in patients with preablation lone atrial flutter, coexistence atrial fibrillation and drug induced atrial fibrillation. Pacing Clin Electrophysiol 27:1507–1512

Atrial Fibrillation After Ablation of Atrial Flutter: Who Is at Risk?

E. Bertaglia

Radiofrequency catheter ablation targeting the isthmus between the tricuspid anulus and the inferior vena cava is an established therapy for typical atrial flutter (AFL). It is successful in more than 90% of patients [1–7]. However, in the clinical setting, AFL and atrial fibrillation (AF) often coexist, and the follow-up of patients successfully treated with transisthmus ablation is complicated by the occurrence of AF in 10–47% of patients [2, 5, 8–15]. Indeed, although caused by different electrophysiological mechanisms, AFL and AF may share the same arrhythmogenic substrate [12, 16, 17]. Identifying patients at higher risk of post-ablation AF occurrence after ablation was a major issue until the introduction of transisthmus catheter ablation.

Occurrence of Atrial Fibrillation After Transisthmus Ablation

As reported in several papers, AF frequently occurs after transisthmus ablation of AFL: its occurrence ranges from 12% to 54% [8–15, 18–23]. In the study that enrolled the largest cohort, AF was observed in 42% of patients after a mean of 20.5 months from ablation of AFL [23]. The occurrence of AF increased progressively as time passed (Fig. 1): at 4 years, the cumulative probability of AF occurrence rose to 62%. The progression of AF behaved differently in patients with and patients without AF before ablation (Fig. 2). While in the former group almost all of the recurrences of AF appeared during the first 2 years (66%), in patients without pre-ablation AF the rate of AF occurrence was quite low during the first 2 years (12%), and increased significantly later (52% at 4 years).

Dipartimento di Cardiologia, Ospedale Civile, Mirano (Venice), Italy

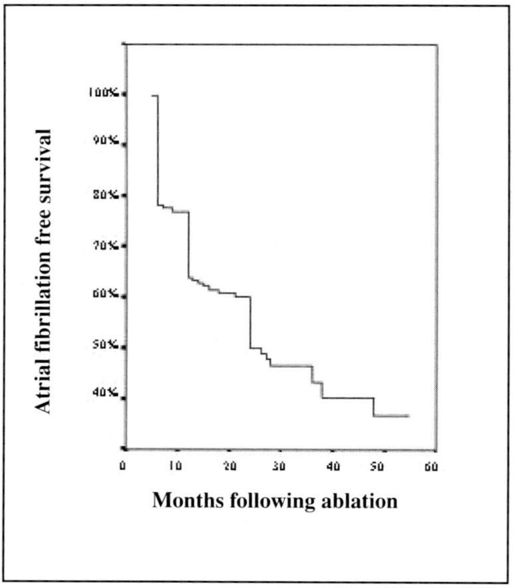

Fig. 1. Kaplan–Meier estimate of the time to atrial fibrillation occurrence in the general population after atrial flutter ablation. From [23], with permission

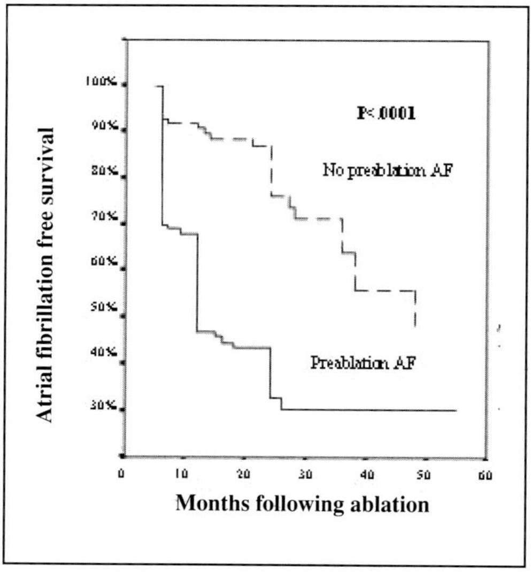

Fig. 2. Kaplan–Meier estimates of the time to occurrence of atrial fibrillation after atrial flutter ablation in patients without pre-ablation atrial fibrillation (*dashed line*) and in patients with pre-ablation atrial fibrillation (*unbroken line*). From [23], with permission

However, not all patients with pre-ablation AF present the same risk of post-ablation AF. Some authors have already suggested that patients with drug-induced AFL [those with paroxysmal or persistent AF in whom persistent or paroxysmal AFL appeared only after the beginning of treatment with class IC drugs (so-called IC-AFL) or only after the beginning of treatment with amiodarone (so-called amio-AFL)] present an incidence of post-ablation AF occurrence as low as the incidence in patients with pre-ablation lone AFL [14, 20, 24]. More recently, we directly compared the long-term outcome of four subgroups of patients after transisthmus ablation: patients with AFL in whom AF had never been documented prior to transisthmus ablation; patients with AFL in whom AF had been documented prior to transisthmus ablation; patients with IC-AFL; and patients with amio-AFL [25].

The clinical courses after transisthmus ablation were significantly different among the four subgroups of patients (Fig. 3). In the patients with amio-AFL the cumulative probability of post-ablation AF occurrence was significantly lower than in the patients with pre-ablation coexistent AF, and similar to that seen in the patients with pre-ablation lone AFL. By contrast, a similar cumulative probability of post-ablation AF to that recorded among patients with pre-ablation coexistent AF was observed in the patients with IC-AFL. Thus, a significant difference emerges between class IC anti-arrhythmic drugs and amiodarone in respect of the possibility of preventing AF relapses after transisthmus ablation [25]. The protective effect of amiodarone on AF recurrences could be related to the great reduction in intra-atrial conduction velocity exerted by this drug [20]. In this way, amiodarone prevents the simultaneous occurrence of the reentrant circuits which might trigger and perpetuate AF despite the block of the cavo-tricuspid isthmus.

Some interesting differences can also be observed regarding the time of onset of AF recurrences after transisthmus ablation (Fig. 3). Post-ablation AF began later in the patients without pre-ablation AF than in patients with pre-ablation AF. At least in some patients, AFL, rather than triggering AF, seems to be a different clinical expression of the same electrical disease, which is able, as time passes, to induce AF once the preferential route through the flutter circuit is blocked.

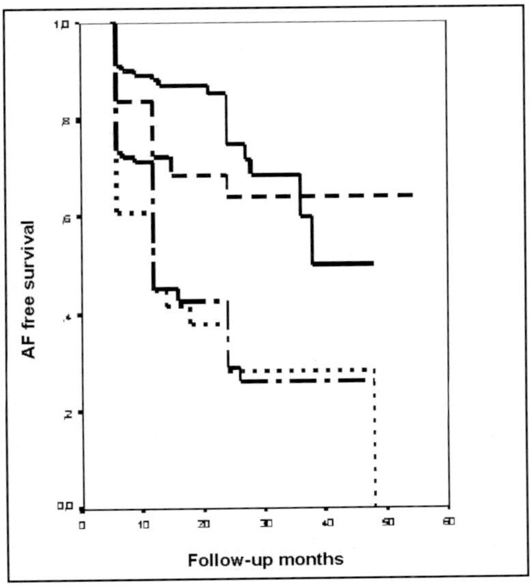

Fig. 3. Kaplan–Meier estimates of the time to occurrence of atrial fibrillation in patients with lone atrial flutter (*unbroken line*), with pre-ablation coexistent atrial fibrillation (*dashed and dotted line*), with class IC drug-induced atrial flutter (*dotted line*), and with amiodarone-induced flutter (*dashed line*). From [25], with permission

Predictors of Atrial Fibrillation Occurrence

Predictors of post-ablation AF are: pre-ablation AF, left atrial size, left ventricular ejection fraction, inducibility of sustained AF after transisthmus ablation, and age [8, 10–12, 14–16, 21–23, 26, 27].

Left atrial size is closely correlated with AF: this arrhythmia is likely to occur in a more diseased, and thus enlarged, atrium [10]. Patients with low left ventricular ejection fraction are more prone to develop AF [8, 11, 12, 15, 21]. AF inducibility to programmed electrical stimulation is associated with high spatial atrial refractoriness and with the development of AF before and after the ablation [27]. A surprising result is the inverse correlation of age with occurrence of post-ablation AF [23]. According to our knowledge about the prevalence of AF in the general population [28], it would be expected that post-ablation AF would occur more frequently in the elderly. On the contrary, however, it was found that patients younger than 65 years experienced post-ablation AF more frequently than patients aged over 65 years despite similar rates of pre-ablation AF, predominant pre-ablation AF, and of anti-arrhythmic drug use [23].

A pre-ablation history of AF remains the most common predictor of post-ablation AF occurrence [8, 11, 12, 15, 16, 22, 23, 26, 27]. Pre-ablation AF identifies patients in whom there is a structural and electrophysiological substrate that allows multiple reentrant circuits favouring AF [11, 12, 27]. However, among patients with pre-ablation AF different variables predict the occurrence of AF after transisthmus ablation in different subgroups of patients [25]. In patients with pre-ablation AF and not drug-induced AFL, post-ablation AF relapses correlated significantly with an enlarged left atrium. In contrast to this, among patients with IC-AFL, the presence of structural heart disease correlated significantly with post-ablation AF recurrences. Treatment with class IC anti-arrhythmic drugs is not the first choice for patients with structural heart disease. Treatment of patients with structural heart disease with a class IC anti-arrhythmic drug generally stems from failure of other anti-arrhythmic drugs. Patients with structural heart disease receiving treatment with a class IC anti-arrhythmic drug are therefore at very high risk of AF occurrence [25].

Clinical Implications

AF occurs frequently after ablation, and its occurrence increases during the follow-up period. This is true both for patients with AF before the ablation and for those without. After 4 years, the probability of post-ablation AF was 68% for patients with pre-ablation AF and 52% for patients without pre-ablation AF. This means that even patients with pre-ablation lone AFL are at high risk of developing AF as time passes. Hence, they must be advised of the risk of recurrent symptoms and late AF, and closely followed up even if transisthmus ablation was successful. ECG Holter monitoring must be advised too, because up to 34% of AF episodes are asymptomatic.

Patients with pre-ablation AF and not drug-induced AFL with an enlarged left atrium, and patients with IC-AFL with structural heart disease, are at high risk of developing AF despite continuation of anti-arrhythmic drug treatment, and anticoagulation therapy should be continued during the follow-up due to the risk of stroke.

Patients with AFL induced by amiodarone run a significantly lower risk of post-ablation AF than patients with spontaneous AFL and those with IC-AFL.

References

1. Cosio FG, Lopez-Gil M, Giocolea A et al (1993) Radiofrequency ablation of the inferior cava–tricuspid valve isthmus in common atrial flutter. Am J Cardiol 71:705–709
2. Fischer B, Haïssaguerre M, Garrigues S et al (1995) Radiofrequency catheter ablation of common atrial flutter in 80 patients. J Am Coll Cardiol 25:1365–1372
3. Lee SH, Tai CT, Yu WC et al (1999) Effects of radiofrequency catheter ablation on quality of life in patients with atrial flutter. Am J Cardiol 84:278–283
4. Natale A, Newby KH, Pisanò E et al (2000) Prospective randomized comparison of antiarrhythmic therapy versus first-line radiofrequency ablation in patients with atrial flutter. J Am Coll Cardiol 35:1898–1904
5. Poty H, Saoudi N, Aziz AA et al (1995) Radiofrequency catheter ablation of type 1 atrial flutter: prediction of late success by electrophysiological criteria. Circulation 92:1389–1392
6. Shah DC, Takahashi A, Jaïs P et al (1999) Local electrogram-based criteria of cavotricuspid isthmus block. J Cardiovasc Electrophysiol 10:662–669
7. Anselme F, Savouré A, Cribier A et al (2001) Catheter ablation of typical atrial flutter. A randomized comparison of 2 methods for determining complete bidirectional isthmus block. Circulation 103:1434–1439
8. Philippon F, Plumbe VJ, Epstein A et al (1995) The risk of atrial fibrillation following radiofrequency catheter ablation of common atrial flutter. Circulation 92:430–435
9. Saxon LA, Kalman JM, Olgin JE et al (1996) Results of radiofrequency catheter ablation for atrial flutter. Am J Cardiol 77:1014–1016
10. Frey B, Kreiner B, Binder T et al (1997) Relation between left atrial size and secondary atrial arrhythmias after successful catheter ablation of common atrial flutter. Pacing Clin Electrophysiol 20:2936–2942
11. Tai CT, Chen SA, Chiang CE et al (1998) Long term outcome of radiofrequency catheter ablation for typical atrial flutter: risk prediction of recurrent arrhythmias. J Cardiovasc Electrophysiol 9:115–121
12. Paydak H, Kall JG, Burke MC et al (1998) Atrial fibrillation after radiofrequency

ablation of type I atrial flutter: time to onset, determinants and clinical course. Circulation 98:315–322
13. Anselme F, Saoudi N, Poty H et al (1999) Radiofrequency catheter ablation of common atrial flutter: significance of palpitations and quality of life evaluation in patients with proven isthmus block. Circulation 99:534–540
14. Nabar A, Rodriguez LM, Timmermans C et al (1999) Effect of right atrial isthmus ablation on the occurrence of atrial fibrillation. Observations in four patient groups having type I atrial flutter with or without associated atrial fibrillation. Circulation 99:1441–1445
15. Da Costa A, Romeyer C, Mourot S et al (2002) Factors associated with early atrial fibrillation after ablation of common atrial flutter. A single centre prospective study. Eur Heart J 23:498–506
16. Hsieh MH, Tai CT, Tsai CF et al (2001) Mechanism of spontaneous transition from typical atrial flutter to atrial fibrillation. Pacing Clin Electrophysiol 24:46–52
17. Roithinger FX, Lesh MD (1999) What is the relationship of atrial flutter and fibrillation? Pacing Clin Electrophysiol 22[Pt I]:643–654
18. Huang DT, Monahan KM, Papageorgiou P et al (1998) Hybrid pharmacologic and ablative therapy: a novel and effective approach for the management of atrial fibrillation. J Cardiovasc Electrophysiol 9:462–469
19. Schumacher B, Jung W, Lewalter T et al (1999) Radiofrequency ablation of atrial flutter due to administration of class IC antiarrhythmic drugs for atrial fibrillation. Am J Cardiol 83:710–713
20. Reithmann C, Hoffmann E, Spitzberger G et al (2000) Catheter ablation of atrial flutter due to amiodarone therapy for paroxysmal atrial fibrillation. Eur Heart J 21:565–572
21. Hsieh MH, Tai CT, Chiang CE et al (2002) Recurrent atrial flutter and atrial fibrillation after catheter ablation of the cavotricuspid isthmus: a very long-term follow-up of 333 patients. J Interv Card Electrophysiol 7:225–231
22. Bottoni N, Donateo P, Quartieri F (2004) Outcome after cavo-tricuspid isthmus ablation in patients with recurrent atrial fibrillation and drug related typical atrial flutter. Am J Cardiol 94:504–508
23. Bertaglia E, Zoppo F, Bonso A et al (2004) Long term follow up of radiofrequency catheter ablation of atrial flutter: clinical course and predictors of atrial fibrillation occurrence. Heart 90:59–63
24. Reithmann C, Dorwarth U, Dugas M et al (2003) Risk factors for recurrence of atrial fibrillation in patients undergoing hybrid therapy for antiarrhythmic drug-induced atrial flutter. Eur Heart J 24:1264–1272
25. Bertaglia E, Bonso A, Zoppo F et al (2005) Different clinical courses and predictors of atrial fibrillation occurrence after transisthmic ablation in patients with preablation lone atrial flutter, coexistent atrial fibrillation, and drug-induced atrial flutter. Pacing Clin Electrophysiol 27:1507–1512
26. Schmieder S, Ndrepepa G, Dong J et al (2003) Acute and long-term results of radiofrequency ablation of common atrial flutter and the influence of right atrial isthmus ablation on the occurrence of atrial fibrillation. Eur Heart J 24:956–962
27. Ramanna H, De Bakker JMT, Hauer RNW (2005) Mechanism of propensity to atrial fibrillation in patients undergoing isthmus ablation for typical atrial flutter. J Cardiovasc Electrophysiol 16:167–172
28. Onundarson PT, Thorgeirsson G, Jonmundsson E et al (1987) Chronic atrial fibrillation: epidemiologic features and 14 years follow-up: a case-control study. Eur Heart J 8:521–527

Electroanatomic Mapping to Support Ablation of Complex Supraventricular Arrhythmias: Does It Matter?

R. De Ponti[1], R. Verlato[2], G. Pelargonio[3], F. Drago[4], A. Fusco[5], J.A. Salerno-Uriarte[1] on behalf of the Investigators of the Project of ElectroAnatomic mapping for Complex arrhythmia Evaluation (PEACE)*

Introduction

Over the last 15 years, experience in catheter ablation of cardiac arrhythmias has greatly increased. This has gone hand in hand with technical improvements and the development of new approaches. Currently, catheter ablation is considered the first-line therapy for arrhythmia exhibiting a 'stereotyped' substrate, such as typical atrial flutter, atrioventricular nodal reentrant tachycardia, and tachycardias mediated by an accessory pathway [1, 2]. For these supraventricular arrhythmias, a high success rate with minimal procedural risks can be obtained by experienced operators in a relatively short-lasting procedure. Conversely, in atypical atrial flutter and, generally, in postsurgical supraventricular arrhythmias, clear definition of the arrhythmia mechanism, extensive mapping, and precise localisation of the target area are required to provide a tailored ablation strategy. Especially in patients with prior surgery for complex congenital heart disease and in the presence of multiple clinical arrhythmias, the ablation procedure may be prolonged, have limited procedural and long-term success, and be associated with a higher risk of complications. In fact, the results of catheter ablation previously reported in this subset of patients and based on conventional mapping were promising but still suboptimal [3–6], considering also that in these patients arrhythmia-related morbidity and mortality are increased compared to the general population with supraventricular arrhythmias.

[1]Department of Cardiovascular Sciences, Ospedale di Circolo e Fondazione Macchi, University of Insubria, Varese; [2]Electrophysiology Laboratory, Ospedale Civile of Camposampiero, Camposampiero (Padua); [3]Institute of Cardiology, Department of Cardiovascular Medicine, Catholic University of the Sacred Heart, Rome; [4]Department of Pediatric Cardiology, Ospedale Bambino Gesù, Rome; [5]Electrophysiology Laboratory, Pederzoli Hospital, Peschiera del Garda (Verona), Italy; *See the Appendix for the list of the other Investigators of the project

Moreover, in some patients, 12-lead ECG can be of very limited help in understanding the arrhythmia mechanism and in orienting the ablation strategy (Fig. 1).

Non-conventional mapping systems have been extensively introduced in the electrophysiology laboratory, especially to assist in diagnosing patients with complex forms of disease and to provide essential information for planning the ablation strategy in patients with a non-stereotyped arrhythmogenic substrate. Recently, single-centre experiences involving a limited number of patients have been reported regarding the use of electroanatomic mapping to support ablation of right or left atypical atrial flutter, and in patients with atrial tachycardias after surgery for congenital and acquired heart disease [7–12]. In these patients, electroanatomic mapping has proved useful to identify the critical area of the tachycardia, especially in double-loop reentry and multiple wavefront collision, providing a road map for ablation of unconventional isthmuses in reentrant arrhythmias [11]. This rationalised approach in patients with complex arrhythmias is expected to lead to optimised short- and long-term results, reducing significantly the procedural difficulties and duration.

To better assess the contribution of electroanatomic mapping to ablative treatment of complex arrhythmias in a larger and multicentre experience, the Project of Electro-Anatomic mapping for Complex Arrhythmia Evaluation (PEACE) was organised in 2003 and coordinated by our University. In this project, roughly a dozen Italian electrophysiology laboratories (see Appendix) with different profiles, but similarly willing to share the experi-

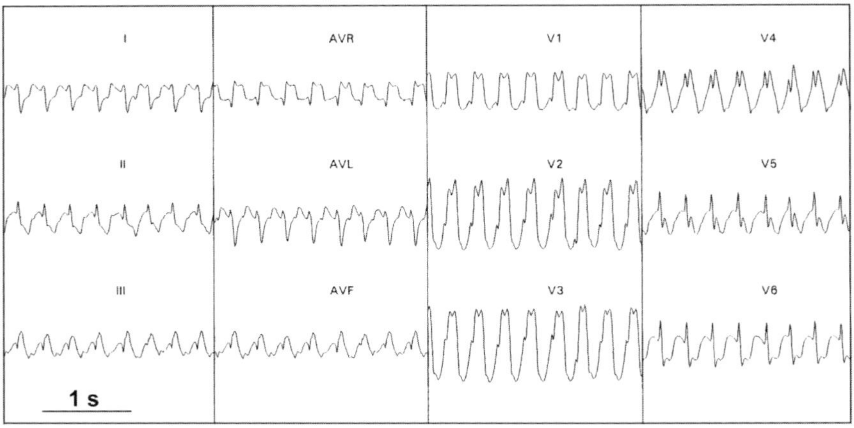

Fig. 1. Clinical atrial tachycardia of the first presented case, showing a cycle length of 290 ms. The wide QRS complex (superimposible to the one on sinus rhythm) does not allow clear visualisation of the surface P wave

ence of approaching complex arrhythmias by electroanatomic mapping, were involved. Over this time period, 41 patients were studied for macro-reentrant or focal atrial arrhythmias with or without prior cardiac surgery or for complex forms (incessant or nonsustained/noninducible) of ventricular tachycardias. In these patients, after their histories were evaluated and pre-procedure diagnostics were obtained, electrophysiologic and extensive electroanatomic evaluations were carried out to plan a rationale for ablation, which was successful in the vast majority of the patients. The following is a presentation of four typical cases involving study patients with postsurgical or postablation focal or macro-reentrant atrial tachycardia/flutter.

Postsurgical Focal Atrial Tachycardia

Focal atrial tachycardia has been reported occasionally as an accompanying arrhythmia in patients with macro-reentrant atrial tachycardia after cardiac surgery [8, 11, 13–17]. In these reports, the overall number of focal atrial tachycardia morphologies was 19 and, with two exception [15, 16], they accounted for less than 10% of the total number of atrial tachycardia morphologies in these series of postsurgical patients. Interestingly, in the majority of the cases (14/19 morphologies), the tachycardia focus was located in the anterolateral wall of the right atrium. In the following, two cases of focal atrial tachycardia in patients previously operated on for congenital heart disease are described.

The first case involves a 43-year-old male patient, who at the age of 15 underwent surgery for tetralogy of Fallot. Ten years later, he began complaining of palpitations, which became more frequent in recurrence and drug refractory. As a result, in 1999, he underwent the first electrophysiology procedure in our institution. Clinical atrial tachycardia at a cycle length of 440 ms was reproducibly inducible and was diagnosed as an intraatrial macro-reentrant tachycardia with the critical isthmus of slow conduction located between the coronary sinus os and the inferior vena cava. Limited radiofrequency energy delivery in that region suppressed the tachycardia, and no other tachycardia was inducible thereafter. Of interest, conventional mapping during sinus rhythm showed two vertical lines of double potentials along the septum and the anterolateral right atrium, likely related to surgical incisions/sutures. Moreover, during programmed atrial stimulation, conduction delay over the anterolateral right atrial wall was observed, with preserved voltage amplitude. The patient remained asymptomatic for the next few years, up to February 2004, when he had palpitation recurrence documented at ECG as the arrhythmia shown in Fig. 1. Since the QRS complex was superimposible on the sinus rhythm, its supraventricular origin was clear; but the wide QRS complex did not allow analysis of the P-wave morphology. Adenosine injection reproducibly terminated the tachycardia, such that surface ECG did not contribute to orienting the site of origin of the tachycardia. During the same hospital admission, the patient experienced multiple drug-refractory arrhythmia recurrences and therefore underwent electrophysiologic evaluation. At baseline, a nonsustained form of the same tachycardia with 1:1 atrioventricular conduction was present and became sustained with a cycle length of 290 ms during isoprenalin infusion. Electroanatomic mapping was performed during sinus rhythm and atrial tachycardia, with a coronary sinus atriogram as reference signal. Surprisingly, during mapping, a complete absence of electrical activity in a wide right atrial area, which included the anterolateral wall, the cavotricuspid isthmus and a part of the posterior wall, became evident early on (Fig. 2A). A line of double potentials was still recorded along the atrial septum (Fig. 2B). During tachycardia, right atrial activation lasted 148 ms, equal to 51% of the tachycardia cycle length, with a centrifugally spreading activation pattern from the earliest site, located on the crest of the right appendage. Bipolar recording at this site preceded the coronary sinus atriogram by 252 ms and the initial unipolar deflection was completely negative. Even in the absence of identification of the P-wave onset, this finding favoured a focal origin from this site. As also shown in Fig. 2B, later activation of the atrial septum and of the expected site of Bachmann's bundle insertion in the right atrium excluded left-to-right atrial propagation due to a left-sided arrhythmia. In this case, the late diastolic activation of the coronary sinus reflected very delayed inter-atrial propagation, rather than being a consequence of a reentrant left atrial circuit. Analysis of the voltage mapping of the tachycardia (Fig. 2C) and comparison with the map of sinus rhythm (Fig. 2D) evidenced that the tachycardia focus was located in a low-voltage (< 0.6 mV), but still viable area at the border zone of the scar tissue at a distance of 16 mm from the sinus node area. Radiofrequency energy delivery at the earliest activated site by cool-tip catheter (40 Watts) for 45 s produced early and sudden tachycardia termination, with no sign of damage to the sinus node. Two other applications, on sinus rhythm, were then delivered just superiorly and inferiorly to the tachycardia focus. Afterwards, the tachycardia was no longer inducible even at the maximal infusion rate of isoprenalin, and no other arrhythmia was observed. During follow-up on the previously ineffective antiarrhythmic agent (sotalol), the patient has been symptom-free. Interestingly, analysis of the first 15 ms of the propagation map in sinus rhythm and during tachycardia showed a wider activated area in sinus rhythm than on tachycardia, suggesting a more complex anatomic substrate for the sinus node than for the focal atrial tachycardia, which, in this case, required a relatively small amount of energy to be abolished.

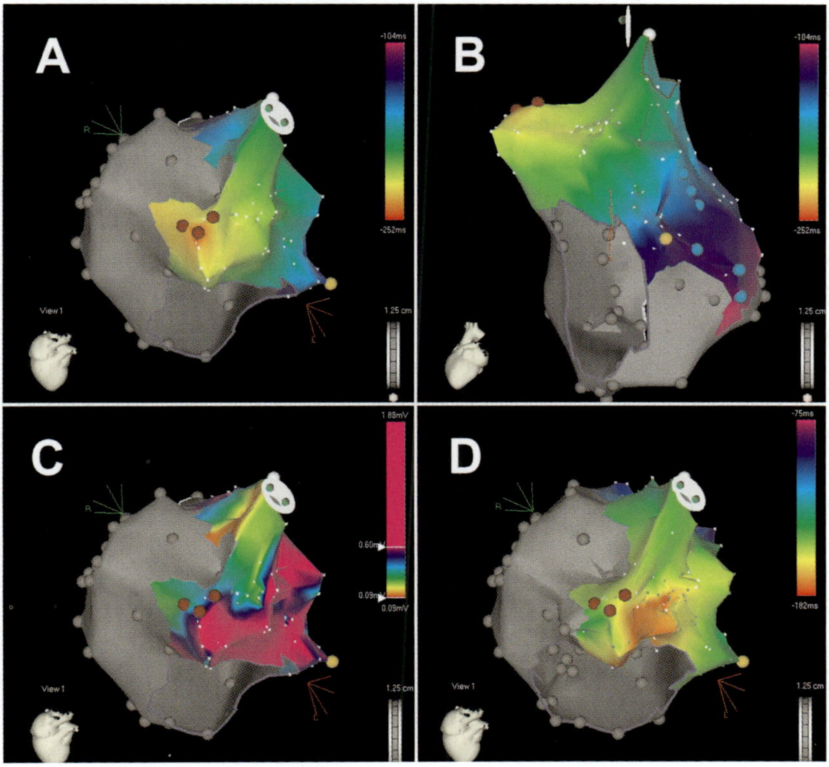

Fig.2. Electroanatomic mapping of the right atrium of the first presented case, during clinical atrial tachycardia (**A–C**) and sinus rhythm (**D**). **A, C, D** Cranial left anterior oblique projection; **B** left lateral view. the extension of the scar tissue (in grey) is well evident in all of the maps. **A, B** Activation mapping in tachycardia, with the earliest activated site (*in red*) in the crest of the right appendage, where ablation is performed (central red dot corresponds to the effective application; the other two dots are bonus applications on sinus rhythm). Moreover, in **B**, the prior atriotomy is evident as a vertical line of double potentials (*blue dots*) along the atrial septum. **C** Bipolar voltage mapping: areas with voltage > 0.60 mV are identified in *purple.* **D** Distance from the ablation site and the extension of the sinus node area (*in red*). See text for further explanation

In this patient, electroanatomic mapping provided very useful data for practical use and for gaining further insight into the patient's arrythmia. In the presence of complex anatomy and in the absence of information provided by P-wave morphology, mapping identified the tachycardia mechanism, excluded involvement of the left atrium, located precisely the arrhythmia focus, and determined its distance from the sinus node to guide ablation successfully and safely. In addition, the progressive and extensive loss of atrial electrical activity, the location of the arrhythmia focus at the border with the scar tissue, together with its different activation pattern as compared to the sinus node posed interesting questions for further study.

The second case involved a 39-year-old female patient with transposition of the great vessels and ventricular septal defect. At the age of 5, she underwent Rastelli's operation at the Mayo Clinic, with external homograft conduit between the right ventricle and the pulmonary artery. Seven years later, she underwent another operation to substitute the conduit. At the age of 35, the patient started developing signs and symptoms of congestive heart failure, with enlargement of both the right atrium and ventricle. Despite optimal medical therapy, she complained of palpitations due to atrial tachycardia and atrial fibrillation. Due to coexistence of life-threatening ventricular arrhythmias, a dual-chamber ICD was implanted. In the months before the procedure, despite therapy with amiodarone and beta-blockers, she developed atrial tachycardia at 400-ms cycle length with 1:1 atrioventricular conduction with periods of incessant-iterative presentation. These were responsible for severe functional limitations and a worsening of heart failure. Similar to the previous case, a wide QRS complex due to right bundle-branch block and 1:1 atrioventricular conduction during tachycardia rendered analysis of the P-wave morphology, especially of its initial deflection, very difficult. During electrophysiologic evaluation, at baseline, under general anaesthesia, the patient was stably on sinus rhythm with right bundle-branch block. Atrioventricular conduction was normal and only antegrade. By S2S3 programmed atrial stimulation during isoprenalin infusion, the clinical atrial tachycardia at a cycle length of 420 ms was reproducibly induced with a 1:1 atrioventricular conduction ratio. The coronary sinus atriogram served as a reference, which allowed initiation of electroanatomic mapping of the right atrium, using a long sheath to support the mapping catheter for the enlarged chamber size. Despite optimal catheter-to-tissue contact, the right atrium lacked atrial electrical activity over a vast area of the anterolateral and posterior walls, which, therefore, were tagged as scar tissue. At the beginning of mapping, the earliest activated site was the medial upper right atrium, where a bipolar signal with an amplitude of 0.61 mV preceded the reference signal by 120 ms. In the same site, a fast negative initial unipolar deflection was recorded. Any attempt to stably change the 1:1 atrioventricular conduction ratio during tachycardia, in order to evaluate P-wave onset and the interval between it and the local bipolar electrogram, was unsuccessful or terminated the tachycardia. Although the local signal and the centrifugally spreading propagation pattern suggested focal atrial tachycardia originating from that site, it was decided to continue mapping, since the geometry of the chamber appeared incomplete in its anterosuperior area. During further mapping, a more anterior site showed an earlier activation (-28 ms compared to the previous site) with a similar unipolar pattern and a bipolar amplitude of 0.87 mV. From there, a channel of low bipolar signals between two areas of scar tissue (Fig. 3A) was identified, leading to the earliest activated site, which preceded the reference signal by 195 ms (Fig. 3B). In this site, the unipolar deflection could not be evaluated, since it was superimposed on one of the previous ventricular beats. Nonetheless, the atrial origin of the bipolar signal was validated by a single ventricular extrastimulus, which dissociated this signal from the ventricular activity. Based on this evidence and considering the remote position of the sinus node, previously assessed (Fig. 3C), radiofrequency energy at 30 Watts was delivered by cool-tip catheter. This led to early termination and complete suppression of the tachycardia. Subsequently, a second atrial tachycardia with a 500-ms cycle length and negative P wave in the inferior lead was reproducibly induced and then was targeted and successfully ablated as a second focal atrial tachycardia originating in the central part of the cavotricuspid isthmus. During follow-up, the patients had relevant clinical improvement with persistent suppression of the treated forms and only rare nonsustained runs of slow, well-tolerated atrial tachycardia. Interestingly, the analysis of the voltage map of clinical atrial tachycardia (Fig. 3D) showed very low voltage (0.07–0.15 mV) along the channel leading to the tachycardia focus, located also in this case at the border zone between viable and scar tissue, whereas relatively preserved bipolar voltage (> 0.5 mV) was observed at the channel exit. It is not clear why the unipolar signal was negative at sites different and even remote from the site of tachycardia origin. The most likely explanation is that activation of the very low voltage channel was not detected by unipolar recording at the site of exit from the channel. Therefore, the wavefront propagating from this site to the atria was read as negative from the unipolar recording, although remote from the site of origin of the tachycardia.

Thus, also in this case of postsurgical atrial tachycardia, electroanatomic mapping was very useful to search for and localise the tachycardia focus in a very low voltage area at the border with a wide zone of scar tissue in the presence of discordant conventional criteria and of a very distorted atrial anatomy. Similar to the previous case, it could be speculated that the origin of postsurgical focal atrial tachycardia was in the upper right atrium, at the border between the scar and the still viable tissue, which is often not easy to define. Here a progressive process may be responsible for the creation of tachycardia foci, even years after surgery. Due to the unique environment where this form of tachycardia develops, the conventional criteria to identify the tachycardia focus might not be invariably reliable. Moreover, intra-atrial or inter-atrial (as in the previous case) delayed propagation during tachycardia may represent a complexity in clarifying the arrhythmia mechanism (focal vs re-entry). At the same time, it may be responsible for the exception to the rule that during a focal rhythm the atria are activated for a limited part (usually < 50%) of the atrial cycle. Finally, the evidence obtained from voltage mapping of large areas of scar tissue and/or low voltage could give an

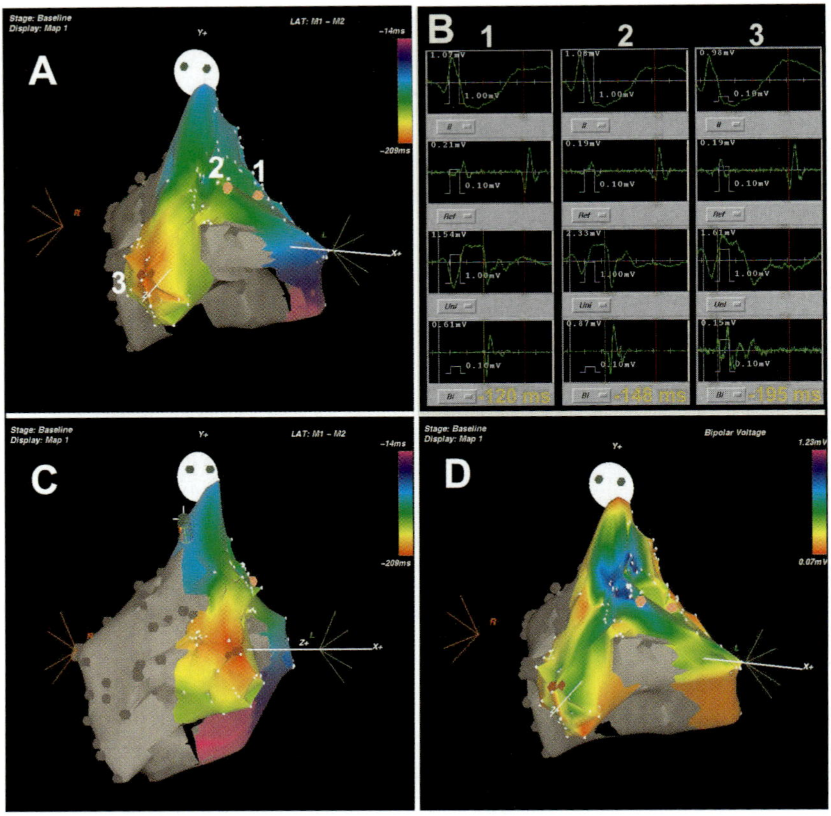

Fig. 3A–D. Electroanatomic mapping of the cranial part of the right atrium during tachycardia in the second presented case. **A, D** Cranial left anterior oblique view; **C** right anterior oblique view. **A** Activation mapping during tachycardia, with the earliest activated site (*in red*) in the antero-ateral area of the superior right atrium, between two areas of scar tissue (*in grey*). The site of successful ablation is marked by *red dots.* **B** From top to bottom, lead II, the reference coronary sinus atriogram (Ref), the unipolar (Uni) and bipolar (Bi) deflections recorded at sites marked as 1, 2 and 3 in the previous panel are shown. Numbers at the bottom express how much earlier the bipolar recording at each site is, as compared to the reference signal. **C** Another view of the activation mapping during tachycardia, which better shows the ablation site and its distance from the sinus node area, where the catheter icon is positioned. **D** Distribution of the bipolar voltage: low voltage (0.07–0.15 mV) is identified by red-to-green colours in the channel between the two scars, where the tachycardia focus is located. See text for further explanation

idea of both the poor haemodynamic contribution of these atria and the prognosis in these patients, especially in term of recurrences and of possible sinus node dysfunction.

Postsurgical/Postablation Macrore-entrant Atrial Tachycardia/Flutter

As already mentioned, surgical atrial incisions may create an isthmus of slow conduction, responsible for re-entrant tachycardia occurring after a variable time interval from surgery. On the other hand, left atrial flutter may occur also after pulmonary vein isolation for atrial fibrillation by percutaneous technique, endangering the long-term success of the procedure [18–21]. Although rare, left atrial flutter may be less tolerated and less responsive to antiarrhythmic drugs than atrial fibrillation. Whether it is due to a focal mechanism [18], a re-entry related to gaps in a linear lesion previously deployed [19], or a combination of the two mechanisms in different patient subsets [20] is still debated. The two cases presented below show how electroanatomic mapping may contribute to an in-depth understanding of the arrhythmogenic substrate in patients with postsurgical/postablation macrore-entrant arrhythmias.

The third case involves a 61-year-old male patient affected by hypertension with only mild dilatation of the left atrium. The patient underwent ablation for typical atrial flutter with complete bidirectional block of the cavotricuspid isthmus conduction at the age of 54. Three years later, he underwent elsewhere electrophysiologically guided pulmonary vein isolation for recurrent atrial fibrillation refractory to multiple antiarrhythmic drugs. During the same hospital stay, he underwent three ablation procedures. Afterwards, he had episodes of palpitation, with ECG documenting atrial tachycardia with a stable cycle length of 260 ms and flat P-wave morphology separated by isoelectric lines in all leads, except for V1, showing a distinct positive P wave. Six months before the procedure, the arrhythmia became persistent and was poorly tolerated. During the procedure, at baseline, the patient exhibited clinical arrhythmia with a variable ratio of atrioventricular conduction. In order to map the expected macrore-entry, the window of interest was set to start in mid-diastole on surface ECG, spanning 95% of the cycle length, as described elsewhere [22]. Electroanatomic mapping in the right atrium did not show a head-meets-tail pattern, entrainment had a return cycle markedly longer than the tachycardia cycle length, and the propagation pattern favoured a left atrial origin. After trans-septal puncture, the left atrium was extensively mapped, which showed an absence of electrical activity in a large area around the oses of the four pulmonary veins and in the posterior left atrium. In the remaining part of the left atrium, between the scar tissue and the mitral ring, the electroanatomic activation map showed electrical activity spanning the entire tachycardia cycle length with a single-loop clockwise re-entry around the mitral annulus (Fig. 4A). Having set the window of interest from mid-diastole to the next mid-diastole, the mid-diastolically activated area was identified as the interface between the red and the purple area in the activation map. As shown in Fig. 4A, this area was located between the scar tissue around the os of the right pulmonary veins and another small scar at 11 o'clock of the mitral ring. This was possibly a gap in an incomplete linear lesion previously attempted between the mitral ring and the right superior pulmonary vein. In the area identified as critical at the electroanatomic mapping, concealed entrainment with a postpacing interval equalling the tachycardia cycle length was obtained. The bipolar voltage map (Fig. 4B) showed an extensive low voltage (< 0.10 mV) in the critical area, suggesting a relatively easy substrate to ablate. Higher voltage (> 4 mV) was observed in the left atrial appendage. Radiofrequency energy delivery (cool-tip catheter; 35 Watts) in the area identified as critical, where an isolated mid-diastolic potential was recorded, terminated the tachycardia early during the application. Ablation was then continued in the area identified by the interface between the head and the tail of the circuit, in the conducting gap between the two scars, to minimise recurrences. This further ablation produced complete disappearance of electrical activity in this area. Subsequently, no arrhythmia was inducible by aggressive atrial pacing and the patient remained asymptomatic in the follow-up.

This case is paradigmatic of how electroanatomic mapping can reconstruct the re-entrant loop(s), identifying a head-meets-tail pattern and the critical area of mid-diastolic activation. Moreover, the extension and the

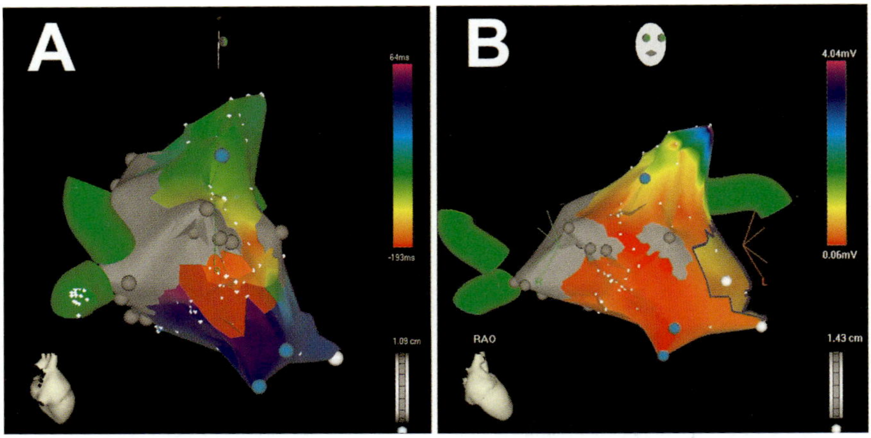

Fig. 4 A, B. Electroanatomic mapping of the left atrium during atrial tachycardia in the third presented case. **A** Right lateral view of the activation mapping with an 'early-meets-late' pattern in the upper left aspect of the atrial septum. **B** Bipolar voltage mapping is displayed in right anterior oblique view with evident low voltage (0.06 mV) around the incomplete line (*in grey*) from the medial mitral annulus to the right superior pulmonary vein. Of interest, the extension of scar tissue (*in grey*) after segmental pulmonary vein ablation. See text for further explanation

voltage of the critical area may be indicative of how difficult the ablation is expected to be. All these elements are essential to rationalise the approach to every single case, in order to plan a successful and safe ablation strategy. As a speculative aspect, this case addresses also the problems related to macroreentrant tachycardias around the peri-pulmonary lesions or involving a conduction gap of an incomplete linear lesion, which may occur even late after ablation in the left atrium for atrial fibrillation, possibly affecting the long-term benefit of the procedure. For atrial fibrillation ablation, a tailored approach for each patient, based on conventional and non-conventional data, should identify and target the arrhythmogenic substrate, thus avoiding overtreatment and its long-term electrical and, possibly, haemodynamic consequences.

The last case is a 21-year-old male patient with complex congenital heart disease, which included single ventricle, transposition of the great vessels, pulmonary valve stenosis, and persistence of the left superior vena cava. At the age of four, he underwent a Fontan operation with insertion of the left superior vena cava in the left pulmonary artery, of the right superior vena cava in the right pulmonary artery with direct closure of its orifice in the right atrium, which, in turn, was connected through a conduit to the pulmonary artery. In the same intervention, the tricuspid orifice was closed by a prosthetic patch, to separate venous from arterial blood flow. Six months before the procedure, the patient had episodes of what completely resembled a typical common atrial flutter on surface ECG, with 285-ms cycle length and 2:1 atrioventricular conduction ratio. In spite of therapy with amiodarone, the arrhythmia recurred and was responsible for syncope. Before the procedure, since the coronary sinus had not been visualised or cannulated in the past, a bipolar catheter was positioned in the oesophagus to stably record a left atrial electrogram, serving as reference. Afterwards, the right atrium was electroanatomically mapped with a long sheath to support the roving catheter on spontaneous rhythm at a cycle length of 920 ms, which was found to originate close to the os of the coronary sinus. On this rhythm, the chamber volume was 265 ml. The clinical arrhythmia was then reproducibly induced by programmed right atrial stimulation. After having set the window of interest as in the previous case, high density electroanatomic mapping was performed. As shown in Fig. 5A, activation in the right atrium covered the entire length of the flutter cycle with a mid-diastolically activated area located in the low lateral right atrium. From this area, the activation proceeded simultaneously anterior and posterior to the inferior vena cava and then started a single counter-clockwise loop, resembling the one of typical common atrial flutter. Interestingly, the pathway of diastolic activation had apparently no anatomic or acquired boundaries, and scar tissue was observed in a very limited area, not strictly in relation with the diastolic pathway. Moreover, at the analysis of the bipolar voltage map on tachycardia (Fig. 5B), the diastolic pathway was clearly evident as a channel of very low voltage (0.05 mV), limited anteriorly and posteriorly by areas of preserved/normal voltage (0.5–5 mV). A plausible explanation of the presence of a re-entrant circuit without an anatomically protected isthmus could be as follows. At flutter cycle, functional conduction block occurred linearly in the transitional areas between low and preserved voltage, and these lines served as anterior and posterior boundaries to the diastolic pathway, thus allowing and stabilising re-entry. Of interest, the anterior right atrium, where the prosthetic patch was positioned on the tricuspid orifice, showed a relatively preserved voltage, suggesting a possible neogenesis of atrial tissue on the patch, positioned early during patient life. Entrainment mapping in the diastolic pathway was not possible due to lack of capture even at the maximum output. Radiofrequency energy (cool-tip catheter, maximum output 40 Watts) was delivered in the area identified as critical by electroanatomic mapping in order to transect completely, from posterior to anterior, the diastolic pathway. This resulted in termination of the tachycardia after prolonging the cycle length and producing a line of double potentials. Afterwards, the clinical flutter was no longer inducible even by very aggressive atrial stimulation. This induced a non-clinical atrial flutter with positive P wave in the inferior leads and a shorter cycle length (265 ms). High density electroanatomic mapping showed that right atrial activation was equal to the tachycardia cycle length, with a mid-diastolically activated area corresponding to the entire vertical length of the crista terminalis and a single loop re-entry rotating around the complete perimeter of the right atrium (Fig. 5C, D). Possibly, in this very enlarged atrial chamber, even transverse conduction over the crista terminalis may serve as slow conduction pathway of a re-entrant circuit in the right atrium. Since this arrhythmia was not clinical, the creation of a vertical and complete line of bidirectional block, was thought to be challenging and possibly proarrhythmic if incomplete, it was decided not to target this second arrhythmia morphology. On the same previously ineffective antiarrhythmic drug, the patient has been asymptomatic in the follow-up.

The experience acquired from this case also shows how electroanatomic mapping can provide all the necessary data for a tailored and evidence-based approach to ablation of complex re-entrant arrhythmias. Moreover, the information gathered can increase our knowledge on peculiar phenomena occurring in particular cases.

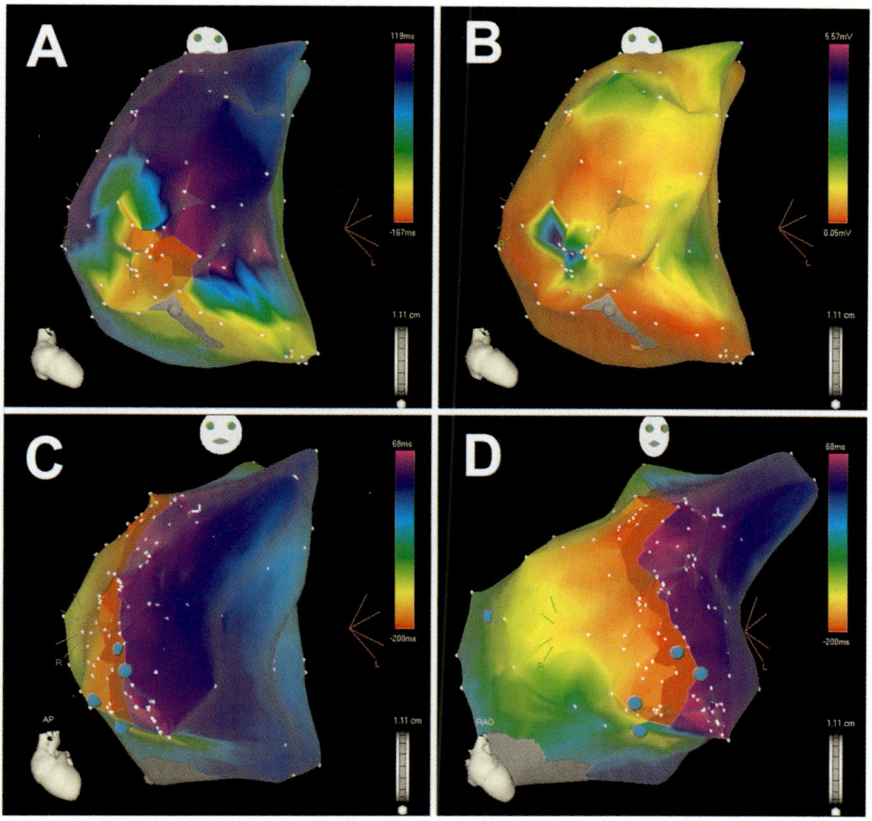

Fig. 5. Electroanatomic mapping of the right atrium during the clinical (**A, B**) and non-clinical (**C, D**) atrial flutter in the last presented case. **A, B** Caudal right anterior oblique view; **C, D** Antero-posterior and right anterior oblique projection, respectively. **A** Activation mapping with an 'early-meets-late' pattern and a diastolically activated isthmus in the lateral low right atrium, where the 'latest' activated area (*in purple*) encounters the 'earliest' activated area (*in red*). **B** Bipolar voltage mapping with a clear difference in voltage between the isthmus (0.05 mV) and the surrounding anterior and posterior areas (0.5–5 mV). **C, D** Activation mapping during the non-clinical atrial flutter, with a clear 'head-meets-tail' pattern in the crista terminalis, which in this morphology serves as slow pathway for re-entry. See text for further explanation

Summary and Future Perspectives

These samples of the experience gathered in our project support the hypothesis that electroanatomic mapping has an essential role in the approach to complex focal or re-entrant arrhythmias. In fact, a detailed analysis of the arrhythmogenic substrate, other than being the core for a successful ablation strategy, may be a key issue in 'learning before burning' and it may anticipate when ablation could be particularly difficult and failure expected. Moreover, increased experience in electroanatomic mapping, together with technology improvements, such as imaging integration, should lead to the simplification of complex procedures, with an expected reduction in the procedure fluoroscopy time and an increased success rate. Whether this will expand the indication for ablation in complex cases remains to be demonstrated by further studies.

Appendix

The following is the list of the investigators participating in the Project of Electro-Anatomic mapping for Complex arrhythmia Evaluation (PEACE):

Roberto Verlato, Pietro Turrini, Unità di Elettrofisiologia Diagnostica ed Interventistica, Ospedale Civile di Camposampiero, Camposampiero (Padua); Raffaele Luise, Dipartimento di Cardiologia-Elettrofisiologia, Clinica Villa Pini d'Abruzzo, Chieti; Luigi Sciarra, Leonardo Coro', Unità Operativa di Cardiologia, Ospedale di Conegliano (Treviso); Emanuele Bertaglia, Francesca Zerbo, Dipartimento di Cardiologia, Ospedale Civile di Mirano (Venice); Antonio Fusco, Alfredo Vicentini, Laboratorio di Elettrofisiologia, C.C. dott.Pederzoli, Presidio Ospedaliero ULSS22-Regione Veneto, Peschiera del Garda (Verona); Maria Grazia Bongiorni, Giuseppe Arena, Unità di Aritmologia, Dipartimento Cardiotoracico, Azienda Ospedaliera Universitaria Pisana, Pisa; Nicola Bottoni, Fabio Quartieri, Unità Operativa di Cardiologia Interventistica, Dipartimento di Cardiologia, Azienda Ospedaliera S.Maria Nuova, Reggio Emilia; Gemma Pelargonio, Antonio Dello Russo, Laboratorio di Elettrofisiologia, Istituto di Cardiologia, Dipartimento di Medicina Cardiovascolare, Università Cattolica del Sacro Cuore, Rome; Fabrizio Drago, Massimo Silvetti, Dipartimento Medico-Chirurgico di Cardiologia Pediatrica, Ospedale Bambino Gesù, Rome; Andrea Avella, Francesco Laurenzi, Sezione Elettrofisiologia-Elettrostimolazione, II Unità Operativa di Cardiologia, Ospedale S.Camillo, Rome; Maurizio Del Greco, Massimiliano Marini, Laboratorio di Elettrofisiologia U.O. di Cardiologia, Ospedale S.Chiara, Trento; Raffaella Marazzi, Fabrizio Caravati, Laboratorio di Elettrofisiologia, Dipartimento di Scienze Cardiovascolari, Ospedale di Circolo e Fondazione Macchi-Università dell'Insubria, Varese.

References

1. Natale A, Newby KH, Pisanò E et al (2000) Prospective randomized comparison of antiarrhythmic therapy versus first-line radiofrequency ablation in patients with atrial flutter. J Am Coll Cardiol 35:1898–1904
2. Cheng CHF, Sanders GD, Hlatky MA et al (2000) Cost-effectiveness of radiofrequency ablation for supraventricular tachycardia. Ann Intern Med 133:864–876

3. Kalman JM, VanHare GF, Olgin JE et al (1996) Ablation of 'incisional' reentrant atrial tachycardia complicating surgery for congenital heart disease: use of entrainment to define a critical isthmus of conduction. Circulation 93:502–512
4. Baker BM, Lindsay BD, Bromberg BI et al (1996) Catheter ablation of clinical intraatrial reentrant tachycardias resulting from previous atrial surgery: localizing and transecting the critical isthmus. J Am Coll Cardiol 28:411–417
5. Triedman JK, Bergau DM, Saul JP et al (1997) Efficacy of radiofrequency ablation for control of intraarial reentrant tachycardia in patients with congenital heart disease. J Am Coll Cardiol 30:1032–1038
6. Della Bella P, Fraticelli A, Tondo C et al (2002) Atypical atrial flutter: clinical features, electrophysiological characteristics and response to radiofrequency catheter ablation. Europace 4:241–253
7. Jaïs P, Shah DC, Haïssaguerre M et al (2000) Mapping and ablation of left atrial flutters. Circulation 101:2928–2934
8. Shah D, Jaïs P, Haïssaguerre M (2002) Electrophysiologic evaluation and ablation of atypical right atrial flutter. Card Electrophysiol Rev 6:365–370
9. Ouyang F, Ernst S, Vogtmann T et al (2002) Characterization of reentrant circuits in left atrial macroreentrant tachycardia: critical isthmus block can prevent atrial tachycardia recurrence. Circulation 105:1934–1942
10. Heist EK, Doshi SK, Singh JP et al (2004) Catheter ablation of atrial flutter after orthotopic heart transplantation. J Cardiovasc Electrophysiol 15:1366–1370
11. Nabar A, Timmermans C, Medeiros A et al (2005) Radiofrequency ablation of atrial arrhythmias after previous open-heart surgery. Europace 7:40–49
12. Lukac P, Pedersen AK, Mortensen PT et al (2005) Ablation of atrial tachycardia after surgery for congenital and acquired heart disease using an electroanatomic mapping system: which circuit to expect in which substrate? Heart Rhythm 2:64–72
13. Ott P, Kelly PA, Mann DE et al (1995) Tachycardia-induced cardiomyopathy in a cardiac transplant recipient: treatment with radiofrequency catheter ablation. J Cardiovasc Electrophysiol 6:391–395
14. De Ponti R, Zardini M, Tritto M et al (1999) Sistema non fluoroscopico per mappaggio cardiaco elettroanatomico tridimensionale (CARTO). Cardiologia: 44 (Suppl I):387–390
15. Leonelli FM, Tomassoni G, Richey M et al (2001) Ablation of incisional atrial tachycardias using a three-dimensional nonfluoroscopic mapping system. Pacing Clin Electrophysiol 24:1653–1659
16. Markowitz SM, Brodman RF, Stein KM et al (2002) Lesional tachycardias related to mitral valve surgery. J Am Coll Cardiol 39:1973–1983
17. Magnin-Poull I, De Chillou C, Miljoen H et al (2005) Mechanism of right atrial tachycardia occuring late after surgical closure of atrial septal defects. J Cardiovasc Electrophysiol 16:681-687
18. Gerstenfeld EP, Callans DJ, Dixit S et al (2004) Mechanisms of organized left atrial tachycardias occuring after pulmonary vein isolation. Circulation 110:1351–1357
19. Kobza R, Hindricks G, Tanner H et al (2004) Late recurrent arrhythmias after ablation of atrial fibrillation: incidence, mechanisms, and treatment. Heart Rhythm 1:676–683
20. Cummings JE, Schweikert R, Saliba W et al (2005) Left atrial flutter following pulmonary vein antrum isolation with radiofrequency energy: linear lesions or repeated isolation. J Cardiovasc Electrophysiol 16:293–297
21. Kilicaslan F, Verma A, Yamaji H et al (2005) The need for atrial flutter ablation fol-

lowing pulmonary vein antrum isolation in patients with and without previous cardiac surgery. J Am Coll Cardiol 45:690–696

22. De Ponti R, Avella A, Bertaglia E et al (2004) Standardized setting of the window of interest in the electroanatomic mapping of reentrant tachycardias to identify the critical area: a multicentric Italian evaluation. Eur Hear J 25:280 (abs)

ATRIAL FIBRILLATION: PATHOPHYSIOLOGY, CLINICAL AND THERAPEUTIC ASPECTS

Idiopathic Atrial Fibrillation: Which Electrophysiological Substrate?

R.N.W. Hauer

Introduction

Atrial fibrillation (AF) frequently occurs in the setting of structural heart disease. Fibrosis and dilatation of the atria related to hypertension, cardiomyopathy, valvular heart disease, and other causes of haemodynamic overload are important contributors to the development of AF. However, AF may also occur in apparently structurally normal hearts. Several studies have shown shortening of atrial refractoriness after long-lasting periods of atrial tachyarrhythmias, also known as electrical remodelling [1–7]. At a later stage, this electrical remodelling is followed by structural remodelling, which includes dedifferentiation of atrial cardiomyocytes [4]. Thus, this form of structural disease is due to long-lasting AF itself. In contrast, the development of AF in the very early stages cannot be explained by a substrate due to remodelling. In these early stages, triggers, very often single or multiple premature complexes originating from the pulmonary veins [8], are important. Multiple premature complexes may occur as short-lasting atrial tachycardia episodes with a high rate and the appearance of AF in the surface electrocardiogram. However, after termination of the firing of the focus, the tachyarrhythmia is interrupted as well. In this situation isolation of the trigger is a logical therapeutic approach and indeed is often very successful. In addition, an initiating electrophysiologic substrate in the atrium may enhance susceptibility to the occurrence of long-lasting AF episodes. In the presence of such a substrate, the above-mentioned trigger is still necessary for the onset of the AF episode. However, after termination of the focal trigger activity, the tachyarrhythmia will continue and contribute to a more sus-

Department of Cardiology, Heart Lung Center Utrecht, University Medical Center, Utrecht, The Netherlands

tained pattern. In previous studies we found that patients with rare episodes of idiopathic AF (AF in the absence of structural heart disease) had enhanced spatial dispersion of refractoriness unrelated to electrical remodelling [9, 10]. This initiating electrophysiologic substrate will favour reentrant mechanisms because of unidirectional block and activation delays at multiple sites. This is supported by the facilitation of AF induction by programmed electrical stimulation.

Human and animal studies have demonstrated that the gap-junction protein connexin40 (Cx40) is expressed mainly in the atrium and conduction system. Lack of Cx40 has been reported to result in increased atrial vulnerability and propensity to arrhythmias in the mouse [11]. In addition, it has been described that changes in the expression levels and distribution pattern of Cx40 may act as a substrate promoting AF susceptibility [12]. A previous study found that a linked polymorphism at nucleotides –44(G?A) and +71(A?G) in regulatory regions of the Cx40 gene, combined with a mutation in the cardiac sodium channel gene SCN5A, was associated with familial atrial standstill [13]. The described polymorphism in the Cx40 gene occurs in about 7% of the general population. In a recent study, we found that this rare, linked Cx40 polymorphism is related to enhanced spatial dispersion of refractoriness and susceptibility to reentry and AF [14].

Methods

Thirty patients with Wolff-Parkinson-White syndrome were studied. Of these, 14 had prior documented sporadic episodes of AF (AF group) and 16 had no evidence of AF (control group). The mean number of AF episodes in the AF group was 1 (range 1–5), medium duration 1 h (range 15 min to 3 h). The mean asymptomatic interval prior to the electrophysiologic study was 148 days. Electrocardiographic telemetric monitoring was carried out for at least 24 h immediately before the electrophysiologic study. None of the patients had AF episodes during the telemetric observation period. Structural heart disease and conditions with potential effect on haemodynamic or electrophysiologic functions were carefully excluded. None of the patients were on antiarrhythmic drugs.

During the electrophysiologic study, a decapolar catheter was positioned at the right atrial free wall and a quadripolar catheter was placed in the right atrial appendage. Twelve unipolar electrograms were recorded. AF was induced with a progressively aggressive stimulation protocol. Fibrillation intervals were measured at all recording sites. The mean of all fibrillatory intervals at a single site was used as an index for the local refractory period. The averages and SD for these indices were calculated. Spatial dispersion of refractoriness was determined by calculating the coefficient of dispersion (CD), defined as the standard deviation of all local mean fibrillatory intervals expressed as a percentage of the overall mean fibrillatory interval. Based on the previous study [9], a CD value of 3.0 or less was considered normal.

Cx40 polymorphisms were detected by direct DNA sequencing [13].

Results

In the control group, AF was induced by burst pacing in the large majority of patients, whereas in the AF group burst pacing was required in only one out of 14 patients. Most patients were inducible to AF with only a single extra stimulus in the AF group. Mean CD in control group was 1.59 ± 0.18 and in the AF group 5.96 ± 0.70. In the AF group, 13 out of 14 patients had enhanced CD (> 3.0), whereas in the control group all patients had a normal CD. This difference was significant ($P < 0.001$). Since mean fibrillatory intervals were not different in the two groups, the occurrence of remodelling was very unlikely.

Through molecular genetic analyses, three groups could be distinguished: (1) –44AA/+71GG, (2) –44GG/+71AA, and (3) the heterozygous group –44GA/+71GA. AF was induced more easily with a single extra stimulus in patients with the –44AA genotype (the rare genotype) than in those with the –44GG genotype (86% vs 29%, $P = 0.042$). Carriers of the –44AA genotype had a significantly higher CD than those with the –44GG genotype (6.37 1.21 vs 2.38 ± 0.39, $P = 0.018$). Heterozygotes had intermediate values.

Conclusions

Both triggers and an atrial electrophysiologic substrate contribute to the development of AF episodes. In the absence of structural heart disease, AF itself promotes a substrate due to electrical remodeling by shortening of refractoriness. However, before this remodeling susceptibility to AF is due to an initiating substrate. This substrate facilitates reentrant mechanisms and appeared to be due to enhanced spatial dispersion of refractoriness. The initiating substrate is associated with a minor form of Cx40 polymorphism in selected patients. Further studies are needed to confirm this relationship in other patient categories and to assess causation.

References

1. Wijffels MC, Kirchhof CJ, Dorland R et al (1995) Atrial fibrillation begets atrial fibrillation. A study in awake chronically instrumented goats. Circulation 92(7):1954–1968
2. Elvan A, Wylie K, Zipes DP (1996) Pacing-induced chronic atrial fibrillation impairs sinus node function in dogs. Electrophysiological remodeling. Circulation 94(11):2953–2960
3. Elvan A, Huang XD, Pressler ML et al (1997) Radiofrequency catheter ablation of the atria eliminates pacing-induced sustained atrial fibrillation and reduces connexin 43 in dogs. Circulation 96(5):1675–1685
4. Ausma J, Wijffels M, van Eys G et al (1997) Dedifferentiation of atrial cardiomyocytes as a result of chronic atrial fibrillation. Am J Pathol 151(4):985–997
5. Yue L, Feng J, Gaspo R et al (1997) Ionic remodeling underlying action potential changes in a canine model of atrial fibrillation. Circ Res 81(4):512–525
6. Gaspo R, Bosch RF, Talajic M et al (1997) Functional mechanisms underlying tachycardia-induced sustained atrial fibrillation in a chronic dog model. Circulation 96(11):4027–4035
7. Fareh S, Villemare C, Nattel S (1998) Importance of refractoriness heterogeneity in the enhanced vulnerability to atrial fibrillation induction caused by tachycardia-induced atrial electrical remodeling. Circulation 98(20):2202–2209
8. Haïssaguerre M, Jaïs P, Shah DC et al (1998) Spontaneous initiation of atrial fibrillation by ectopic beats originating in the pulmonary veins. N Engl J Med 339(10):659–666
9. Ramanna H, Hauer RN, Wittkampf FH et al (2000) Identification of the substrate of atrial vulnerability in patients with idiopathic atrial fibrillation. Circulation 101(9):995–1001
10. Ramanna H, de Bakker JM, Elvan A et al (2004) On the atrial response to focal discharges in man. J Cardiovasc Electrophysiol 15(6):629–636
11. Hagendorff A, Schumacher B, Kirchhoff S et al (1999) Conduction disturbances and increased atrial vulnerability in Connexin40-deficient mice analyzed by transesophageal stimulation. Circulation 99:1508–1515
12. Van der Velden HM, Ausma J, Rook MB et al (2000) Gap junctional remodeling in relation to stabilization of atrial fibrillation in the goat. Cardiovasc Res 46:476–486
13. Groenewegen WA, Firouzi M, Bezzina CR et al (2003) A cardiac sodium channel mutation cosegregates with a rare connexin40 genotype in familial atrial standstill. Circ Res 92:14–22
14. Firouzi M, Ramanna H, Kok B et al (2004) Association of human connexin40 gene polymorphisms with atrial vulnerability as a risk factor for idiopathic atrial fibrillation. Circ Res 95(4):29–33

Inflammation and Infection: Underestimated Causes of Atrial Fibrillation?

A.S. Montenero

Atrial fibrillation (AF) is the most common arrhythmia seen in clinical practice and exacts a huge social and economic cost [1, 2]. Mortality in patients with AF has been reported to be twice as high as that in controls and stroke is the most important cause of death, occurring in up to 30% of patients age 80–89 and in up to 15% patients age 50–59 [3]. Even in the absence of a clinically apparent stroke, patients with AF, including those with lone AF, have a high incidence of silent cerebral infarction on computed tomography scan [4].

Recent advances raise the hope of effective pharmacological and non-pharmacological treatments of AF, and a better understanding of the pathophysiological mechanisms involved in the initiation and persistence of the arrhythmia. AF was initially defined as paroxysmal and chronic, but chronic has been subdivided more recently into persistent and permanent [5]. Thus, AF is 'paroxysmal' when it terminates spontaneously, 'persistent' when it requires pharmacological or electrical cardioversion to terminate, and 'permanent' when all attempts to restore sinus rhythm fail. Specific management of AF depends on clinical presentation, symptoms status, and the presence of comorbidity. AF is associated with several medical and cardiac conditions including ischaemic heart disease, hypertension, diabetes, hyperthyroidism, rheumatic valvular disease, and congenital heart disease. In a sizable minority of patients, no medical or cardiac disease is present, prompting the designation of 'lone AF' (2.7–11.4%) [6].

Inflammatory changes in atrial structure have been demonstrated after cardiac surgery [7], but also in patients with non-postoperative AF. Atrial

Department of Cardiology and Cardiac Arrhythmia Centre, Policlinico MultiMedica, Sesto S. Giovanni (Milan), Italy histological abnormalities have been shown to be present in lone AF but not in Wolff-Parkinson-White (WPW) syndrome. In the 66% of patients with lone AF, the biopsies were compatible with myocarditis [8].

Recently, the level of C reactive protein (CRP), a sensitive marker of systemic inflammation as shown in multiple prospective epidemiological studies, was found to be twice as high in AF patients than in a control group with no history of atrial arrhythmia [9]. Therefore, CRP elevation in patients with AF might be an expression of chronic infection.

Chronic gastritis due to chronic *Helicobacter pylori* (*H. pylori*) infection has been suggested as a potential non-cardiovascular disease that predisposes to AF. *H. pylori* infects a large portion of the general population and the infection is generally acquired in the childhood, progress long-life unless treated and causes chronic gastric inflammation. Furthermore, some studies reported that low-grade chronic systemic inflammation is associated with *H. pylori* infection [10]. Thus, Montenero et al. [11] recently hypothesised that *H. pylori* might be both a trigger and a substrate of chronic atrial inflammation, resulting in paroxysmal or persistent AF. They confirmed previously reported data on higher levels of CRP in patients with AF and assessed the possible association between *H. pylori* infection and AF in patients without demonstrable structural heart disease [12].

That case-control study enrolled 60 consecutive patients (mean age 64.28 ± 12.69) who were admitted to our Cardiology Department for AF, either paroxysmal or persistent, and 23 patients with accessory pathways (WPW) (mean age 45.75 ± 17.94). The control group, included 45 apparently healthy volunteers (mean age 38.36 ± 12.95) with no history of atrial arrhythmias and no concomitant acute or chronic disease. The case group included patients suffering from AF but without structural heart disease; some patients with hypertension but without structural heart disease were also included. Exclusion criteria were: myocardial infarction, cardiothoracic surgery, ischaemic heart disease, valvular disease, thyroid dysfunction, congenital heart disease, diabetes, and acute or chronic infections.

All patients underwent physical examination, ECG, echocardiography, electrophysiological study, routine laboratory tests, including blood cell count, erythrocyte sedimentation rate, serum electrolytes, transaminase, urea, creatinaemia, glycaemia, cholesterol and triglycerides levels, thyroid function tests, serological test for *H. pylori,* and CRP determination. Stress test and coronary artery angiogram were also done when coronary artery disease was suspected.

This study was planned after a prolonged clinical observation by Montenero and colleagues, that a great number patients admitted to the Cardiology Department of Policlinico MultiMedica for paroxysmal or persistent AF also had gastric complaints. In particular, a 51-year-old man, who underwent several failed attempts to restore sinus rhythm with electrical cardioversion and pulmonary-vein ablation, was admitted to the Internal Medicine Department for chronic gastritis and *H. pylori* infection. He was examined in the out-patients clinic after complete eradication of *H. pylori* infection, at which time he was in sinus rhythm without antiarrhythmic therapy.

As a result of this experience, Montenero et al. introduced the routine determination of antibodies against *H. pylori* in laboratory tests and noticed an association between AF and infection with the bacterium. Recent studies have shown that false-negative, but not false positive results occur with the serum antibody assay [12]. To the best of our knowledge, this was the first study that demonstrated a highly significant correlation between AF and *H. pylori* infection. In particular, the association between AF and infection was very strong in patients with persistent AF, who demonstrated higher antibody seropositivity [median, 100 (72.6–100.00) UI/ml]. Moreover, the high levels of CRP confirmed the presence of systemic inflammation, perhaps due to *H. pylori* infection, in patients with AF.

In the past, many studies were aimed at identifying the triggers and the substrate that sustain AF in the absence of structural heart disease ('lone AF'). Triggers may be sympathetic or parasympathetic stimulation, the presence of an accessory AV pathways, atrial stretch, and, more recently, atrial beats originating from ectopic foci within pulmonary veins or the vena cava [13]. The persistence of AF was considered as resulting from electrical and structural remodelling, characterised by atrial dilatation and shortening of the atrial effective refractory period, which promoted multiple reentrant wavelets [14]. A chronic increase of haemodynamic load, such as happens in hypertension, mitral valve disease, and heart failure, is often accompanied by changes in myocardial segment length, causing extrasystoles in the stretch region that can lead to AF [15]. Stress and strain activate stretch-activated channel (SACs), resulting in channel opening, and modify the activities of receptors and enzymes [16–17]. In addition, the presence of advanced fibrosis in the atrial region can perpetuate AF, because it produces slow electrical conduction causing reentrant circuits [18].

Chung et al. were the first to document that an inflammatory state was present in AF patients. In fact, CPR levels were higher in arrhythmia patients than in controls, and particularly in persistent AF patients. The data of Montenero's group confirmed these preliminary results.

Thus, the persistence of AF may be induced by structural changes in the atria promoted by inflammation, and recently reported results have supported the hypothesis that an inflammatory process may modify the atrial substrate, leading to AF [9].

Moreover, the occasional observation of complete disappearance of AF episodes after total eradication of *H. pylori* in the first very symptomatic patient led to the idea that the bacterium could have been associated with the inflammatory process. Therefore, this study supported a link between *H. pylori* seropositivity and the presence of AF, with infection acting as the trigger and substrate of the inflammation sustaining AF.

In industrialised countries, the prevalence of *H. pylori* infection in middle age is 20–50%, and is mainly transmitted within families by oral ingestion, saliva, and faeces [19]. *H. pylori* is a very aggressive bacterium that is able to cross the gastric mucosa and attach to epithelial cells, evading the immune response. *H. pylori* infection stimulates an important systemic and mucosal humoral response, but the antibodies do not eradicate infection and may contribute to tissue damage [20].

In the past, several studies have described a connection between *H. pylori* infection and chronic disease, such as peptic ulcer, severe gastritis, gastric cancer, and, more recently, atherosclerosis [21–23]. Infection has been shown to increase the levels of lipid [24], fibrinogen [25], heat shock protein 65 [26], all of which are risk factors of atherosclerosis, and antibodies to the *H. pylori* antigen CagA cross-react with antigens of both normal and atherosclerosis blood vessels. Moreover CagA-positive strains of *H. pylori* were found not only in patients with coronary disease but also in those with ischaemic stroke [27].

The study of Montenero et al. was the first to develop a correlation between *H. pylori* and AF. Although all species of *H. pylori* are able to produce local inflammation, is likely that only certain strains induce the expression of host genes encoding potent pro-inflammatory agents, such as interleukin-8 [28]. Evidence of this effect in patients with AF is currently lacking, and, as recently demonstrated, it can change according to the host genetics for cytokine production [29].

An interesting hypothesis is that some *H. pylori* strains are able to gain access to the systemic circulation and have a peculiar tropism for the pulmonary veins and other veins, such as the vena cava or coronary sinus. However, the bacterium has yet to be detected in the blood, and it is therefore conceptually difficult to explain how it could reach the target vessel.

Moreover, some HP patients have autoantibodies against the H^+/K^+ ATP-ase of gastric parietal cells; these antibodies have been found to cause corpus atrophy [31]. Considering that there is a perfect similitude between the H+/K+ ATP-ase, proton pump of gastric cells and the Na^+/K^+ ATP-ase pump of cardiac cells, it may be that these autoantibodies against H^+/K^+ ATP-ase also target the Na^+/K^+ ATP-ase, causing atrial damage. In fact, cardiac Na^+/K^+ ATP-ase and H^+/K^+ ATP-ase have a similar 35-kDa glycoprotein necessary for catalytic activity. The role of these pumps is to maintain ionic homeostasis by ATP hydrolysis; therefore, loss of this balance may be a trigger for AF by inducing abnormal automaticity or an activity that causes delayed after-depolarisations, leading to very rapid, premature atrial contractions. Moreover, *H. pylori* may be the cause of epithelial cell damage resulting from reactive oxygen or nitrogen species produced by activated neutrophils [32], which lead to chronic inflammation and thus a substrate for persistent form of AF.

While the current data point to an association between AF and *H. pylori* infection, more data will be necessary to understand how this infection can influence the pathogenesis of AF.

References

1. Bialy D, Lehmann MH, Schumacher DN et al (1992) Hospitalization for arrhythmias in the United States: importance of atrial fibrillation. J Am Coll Cardiol 19:41A
2. Wolff PA, Mitchell JB, Baker CS et al (1995) Mortality and hospital cost associated with atrial fibrillation. Circulation 92:I–140
3. Wolff PA, Dawber TR, Thomas HE jr, et al (1978) Epidemiological assessment of chronic atrial fibrillation and risk of stroke: the Framingham study. Neurology 28:973–977
4. Petersen P, Madesn EB, Brun B et al Silent cerebral infarction in chronic atrial fibrillation. Stroke 1987:18:1098–1100
5. Gallagher JJ, Camm AJ (1998) Classification of atrial fibrillation. Am J Cardiol 82:18N–28N
6. Brand FN, Abbot RD, Kannel WB, Wolf PA (1985) Characteristic and prognosis of lone atrial fibrillation: 30 years follow–up in the Framingham study. JAMA 254:3449–3453
7. Bruins P, te Velthuis H, YazdanbakhshAP et al (1997) Activation of the complement system during and after cardiopulmunary by–pass surgery: post-surgery activation involves C–reactive protein and is associated with postoperative arrhythmia. Circulation 96:3542–3548
8. Frustaci A, Chimenti C, Bellocci F et al (1997) Histotogical substrate of atrial biopsies in Patients with Lone Atrail Fibrillation. Circulation 96:1180–1184
9. Chung MN, Martin OM, Sprecher D et al (2001) C–Reactive protein elevation in patients with atrial arrhythmias. Inflammatory mechanism and persistence of atrial fibrillation. Circulation 104:2886–2891
10. Danesh J, Peto R (1998) Risk factor for coronary artery disease and infections with Helicobacter pylori: meta-analyses of prospective studies. JAMA 279:1477–1482
11. Montenero AS, Mollichelli N, Antonelli A et al (2005) Atrial fibrillation and Helicobacter pylori: a possible pathogenic link. Heart 91:960–961
12. Miwa H, Kikuchi S, Ohtaka K et al (2000) Insufficient diagnostic accurancy of imported serological kits for Helicobacter pylori infection in Japanese population. Diagn Microbiol Infect Dis 36:95–99
13. Haïssaguerre M, Jaïs P, Shah DC et al (2000) Spontaneous initiation of atrial fibrillation by ectopic beats originating in the pulmonary venous foci. Circulation 101:1409–1417
14. Hobbs WJ, Van Gelder IC, Fitzpatrick AP et al (1999) The role of atrial electrical

remodeling in the progression of focal atrial ectopy to persistent atrial fibrillation. J Cardiovascular Electrophysiol 10:866–870
15. Franz MR (2000) Mechano-electrical feedback. Cardiovasc res 45:263–266
16. Hu H, Sachs F (1997) Stretch-activated ion channels in the heart. J Mol Cell Cardiol 29:1511–1523
17. Satoh T, Zipes DP (1996) Unequal atrial stretch in dogs increases dispersion of refractoriness conducive to developing atrial fibrillation. J Cardiovasc Electrophysiol 7:833–842
18. Kucera JP, Kleber AG, Rohr S (1998) Slow conduction in cardiac tissue, II: effects of brunching tissue geometry. Circ Res 83:795–805
19. Parsonnet J, Shmuely H, Haggerty T (1999) Fecal and oral shedding of H Pylori from healthy infected adults. JAMA 282:2240–2245
20. Suerbaum S, Michetti P (2002) Helicobacter pilori infection. N Engl J Med 347:1175–1186
21. Pasceri V, Cammarota G, Patti G et al (1998) Association of virulent Helicobacter pilori strains with ischemic heart disease. Circulation 97:1675–1679
22. Mendall MA,Goggin PM, Molineaux N et al (1994) Relation of Helicobacter pilori infection and coronary heart disease. BR Heart J 71:437–439
23. Rathbone B, Martin D, Stephen J et al (1996) Helicobacter pylori seropositivity in subjects with acute myocardial infarction. Hearts 76:308–311
24. Laurila A, Bloigu A, Nayha S et al (1999) Association of Helicobacter pilori infection with elevated serum lipids. Atherosclerosis 142:207–210
25. Torgano G, Cosentini R, Mandelli C et al (1999) Treatment of Helicobacter pilori and Chlamydia pneumonite infections decreases fibrinogen plasma level in patients with ischemic heart disease. Circulation 99:1555–1559
26. Birnie DH, Holme ER, McKay IC et al (1998) Association between antibodies to heat shock protein and other bacterial infections in increasing cardiovascular risk. Eur Heart J 19:387–394
27. Franceschi F, Sepulveda AR, Gasbarrini A et al (2002) Cross-reactivity of anti-CagA antibodies with vascular wall antigens. Possible pathogenic link between Helicobacter pylori infection and atherosclerosis. Circulation 106:430–434
28. Yamaoka Y, Kita M, Kodama T et al (1996) Helicobacter Pylori Cag A gene and expression of cytokine messenger RNA in gastric mucosa. Gastroenterology 110:1744–1752
29. Petrogiusti A, Topa S, Luzzi I et al (2002) Resistance to peptic ulcer disease in CagA-H. pylori infected subjects is associated with IL-1 genes polymorphisms. Gastroenterology 112:A425 (abs)
30. Pietrogiusti A, Diomedi M, Silvestrini M et al (2002) Cytotoxin-associated gene A-positive Helicobacter pilori strains are associated with atherosclerosis stroke. Circulation 106:580–584
31. Negrini R, Savio A, Appelmelk BJ (1997) Autoantibodies to gastric mucosa in Helicobacter pylori infection. Helicobacter 2(Suppl 1):S13–S16
32. Zhang QB, Nakashabendi IM, Mokhashi MS et al (199) Association of cytotoxin production and neutrophils activation by strains of Helicobacter Pylori isolated from patients with peptic ulceration and chronic gastritis. Gut 38:841–845

Atrial Remodelling: What Have We Learned in the Last Decade?

G.V. Naccarelli[1], M.A. Allessie[2]

Atrial Fibrillation Begets Atrial Fibrillation

Atrial fibrillation often progresses from its paroxysmal form to a more persistent and permanent form. The evolution of this disease over time can be partially explained by atrial remodelling, which may occur sooner rather than later depending on whether atrial fibrillation is allowed to continue, with progression of the structural heart disease. Three kinds of atrial remodelling have been proposed: electrical, structural, and contractile [1, 2].

In the instrumented goat model, Wijffels et al. documented that 'atrial fibrillation begets atrial fibrillation' [3]. In this model, there was evidence of electrical remodelling with shortening of the atrial refractory period compared to control within 24 h of atrial fibrillation. In addition, there was a loss of rate adaptation of atrial refractoriness manifested by short atrial effective refractory periods (AERPs) even at slower heart rates. The decrease in atrial refractory periods resulted in an increase in the rate of atrial fibrillation, which therefore became more complex. Perpetuation of atrial fibrillation resulted in even shorter atrial fibrillatory intervals.

Role of Calcium Currents in Atrial Electrical Remodelling

The cellular electrophysiological changes typical of rapid atrial pacing and atrial fibrillation are a decrease in action potential duration and a depression of the action potential plateau [4, 5]. It has been reported that L-type calcium current decreases within 24 h, consistent with the timing of the electrical

[1]Division of Cardiology, Penn State University College of Medicine, Hershey, PA, USA;
[2]Maastricht University, Maastricht, The Netherlands

remodelling noted above. Lai et al. [6] reported that mRNA of the L-type calcium channel and of calcium-ATPase was significantly ($P < 0.05$) down-regulated in patients with atrial fibrillation of more than 3 months duration. It has also been documented that outward K_{ACh} currents increase.

Some of the biochemical mechanisms explaining tachycardia-induced changes on AERPs in humans have been described. Yu et al. [7] reported on 60 patients before and after induced atrial fibrillation. They documented that AERP was shortened by 30 ms after induced atrial fibrillation ($P < 0.0001$) and that shortening was attenuated by verapamil but unchanged by procainamide, propafenone, propranolol, sotalol, or amiodarone. In addition, verapamil shortened the time course of post-atrial-fibrillation AERP changes from 6.1 to 3.1 min ($P < 0.001$). Wijfells et al. [8] documented that electrical remodelling was not mediated by changes in autonomic tone ischaemic stretch or levels of atrial natriuretic factor. In a human study by Daoud et al. [9], verapamil attenuated shortening of atrial refractory periods after atrial fibrillation; procainamide was ineffective in preventing this remodelling. Thus, the above cascade of electrical remodelling starts with a decreased L-type calcium current and a decrease in action potential duration followed by a decrease in the atrial fibrillation cycle length, which decreases wave length and circuit size. Further evidence that verapamil reduces tachycardia-induced remodelling of the atrium was reported by Tieleman et al. [10]. They documented that electrical remodelling of the atrium during rapid atrial pacing was attenuated ($P < 0.01$) by verapamil with only a minimal decrease in the induction of atrial fibrillation by verapamil (34% vs control 39%; $P = 0.03$). These data suggest that electrical remodelling is at least partially triggered by high calcium influx during rapid atrial pacing rates.

Electrical remodelling has important clinical significance. In the short-term (hours–days), it appears to be completely reversible and to play a role in the immediate (IRAF) and early (ERAF) recurrence of atrial fibrillation. These changes also make atrial fibrillation more likely to be persistent and to reduce the likelihood that class III drugs will be effective. Several investigators have shown that calcium channel blockade may minimise electrical remodelling and ERAF [11, 12]. Also, beta-blockers prevent ERAF but only in hypertensive patients with persistent atrial fibrillation, not in those with isolated atrial fibrillation [13].

If atrial fibrillation begets atrial fibrillation, the opposite may be true. Several studies support the concept that sinus rhythm begets sinus rhythm. Dell'Orfano et al. [14] reported that spontaneous conversion was highest in patients with the shortest episodes of atrial fibrillation. Dietrich et al. [15] reported that the longer a patient remains in atrial fibrillation the harder it is to cardiovert and maintain sinus rhythm. Hobbs et al. [16] documented that the atrial fibrillation cycle length is shortest after prolonged atrial fibrillation and progressively prolongs after cardioversion, with prolonged periods of sinus rhythm. Rapid conversions of atrial fibrillation by internal atrial defibrillators prolong the time to its next occurrence.

Structural and Contractile Remodelling of the Atria

During atrial fibrillation remodelling, there are different time domains [1, 2, 17]. In the short term, within seconds to minutes, metabolic changes, including ion concentration, pump activity, and phosphorylation, take place. The next step is an intermediate phase, lasting hours to days, that is characterised by altered gene expression and calcium down-regulation. Longer term effects, lasting weeks to months, include cellular changes, such as dedifferentiation and myolysis. Finally, there is a very long-term phase, involving the persistence of atrial fibrillation from months to years. In this phase, there is irreversible tissue damage, with histological changes showing fibrosis, fatty degeneration, and cell death.

Structural changes from remodelling show left atrial appendage enlargement, reduced atrial contractility, decreasing cardiac output, and an increased propensity for clot formation. Whether histological changes occur due to cardiomyocyte degeneration depends on the duration of the remodelling. Using atrial pressure volume-loop studies, Schotten et al. [18] reported that there is atrial stunning and contractile remodelling even 48 h after atrial fibrillation. Although the refractory period is shortened during this phase, once conversion of atrial fibrillation occurs, not only do the atrial refractory periods return to normal but the atrial work index and contractile function also return. Thus, with dilatation of the atrium, sinus rhythm also reverts to atrial fibrillation, and once sinus rhythm returns the atrium shrinks back to a more normal size. This has been documented in multiple studies, while left atrial volume increases have been shown in echo studies [19]. In addition, the return to improved left atrial function after cardioversion of persistent atrial fibrillation has been documented in echo Doppler studies [20]. Left atrial emptying, after DC cardioversion of atrial fibrillation, takes up to 3 weeks to return to normal baseline due to atrial stunning. AVE0118 has been documented to enhance atrial contractility in the isolated right atrium in atrial fibrillation patients [21]. This positive chronotropic effect may be an added benefit of such drugs.

As noted above, heart failure provokes dilatation and left atrial volume increases over time. In turn, dilatation can provoke stretched-induced arrhythmias [22, 23]. Regional stretch for even 30 min can alter stretch-activated channels. This may also augment the synthesis of angiotensin II, which induces myocyte hypertrophy, increases L-type calcium current, and decreases I_{to}. In addition to increased atrial size, increases in atrial pressure load can alter the electrophysiologic properties of the atrium through stretch receptors purportedly located in the sarcolemmal membrane. Acute and chronic atrial dilatation diminishes resting-membrane potential and action-potential amplitude, thereby decreasing conduction velocity and increasing the heterogeneity of atrial repolarisation. Although atrial stretch may increase calcium influx through stretch-activated and L-type calcium channels in the short-term, long-standing atrial fibrillation leads to decreased inward L-type calcium currents by as much as 60–70%, accelerating repolarisation and thereby shortening the atrial action potential duration and effective refractory period. Atrial fibrillation can also stimulate transient calcium flux by substantial increases in the sodium–calcium exchanger, which is thought to be responsible for delayed after-depolarisations and triggered activity.

Several investigators [24–26] have documented histological remodelling of the atrium by 4 months of atrial fibrillation, as evidenced by myolysis, enlarged atrial cells, glycogen accumulation, and a reduction in connexin 40 expression. The development of small islands without connexin make atrial fibrillation more complex; and in the presence of fibrosis and conduction abnormalities atrial fibrillation can persist through micro-reentrant mechanisms. This structural remodelling appears to be a slow process, often taking as long as 2–3 months.

Does Blockade of the Angiotensin System Have Benefit?

Li et al. [27] have shown that fibrosis may be minimised by the addition of the ACE inhibitor enalapril. Other studies [28, 29] have demonstrated that ACE inhibitors and angiotensin receptor blockers can reverse some of the anatomic remodelling that occurs with atrial fibrillation. In addition, data from TRACE and SOLVD suggest that ACE inhibitors and angiotensin receptor blockers prevent atrial fibrillation [30, 31]. Madrid et al. [32] prospectively documented that patients with persistent atrial fibrillation treated with amiodarone plus irbesartan had a lower recurrence rate of atrial fibrillation post-conversion compared to patients receiving amiodarone alone. Murray et al. [33], based on an AFFIRM sub-study, documented that the benefits of ACE inhibition and angiotensin receptor blockers in preventing atrial fibrillation appear to be limited to patients with congestive heart failure and left ventricular dysfunction. Whether the benefit of angiotensin II blockade is secondary to decreasing atrial stretch, minimising and reversing atrial fibrosis, and other structural changes, or occurs through some direct antagonistic effect on the angiotensin system is not clear.

Can Atrial Selective Potassium Channel Blockade Attenuate Atrial Remodelling?

As noted above, classic class III agents that block the I_{Kr} channel seem to be ineffective once the atrium has remodelled. Newer drugs targeting the I_{Kur} and the I_{KACh} channel, which are not expressed in the ventricle, appear to have different results [34]. Thus, the efficacy of drugs like D-sotalol in blocking I_{Kr} decreased as a result of electrical remodelling during 48 h of atrial fibrillation, whereas newer antiarrhythmic drugs, such as AVE0118, which blocks I_{Kur}, I_{to}, and I_{KACh}, do not lose efficacy by electrical remodelling [35]. AVE0118 significantly increased AERP in the remodelled compared to the normal atrium [35]. Hopefully, this unique electrophysiological action will lead to better efficacy for termination and prevention of atrial remodelling in patients with persistent atrial fibrillation. These newer drugs, due to their relative atrial selectivity, may also minimise problems with ventricular proarrhythmias, such as torsades de pointes [34].

Can Catheter Ablation Reverse Atrial Remodelling?

Whether histological changes can be reversed in advance stages of atrial fibrillation is controversial. An encouraging report showed that following pulmonary vein isolation procedures in congestive heart failure, that left ventricular ejection fraction, fractional shortening improved, with a decrease in left ventricular dimensions in addition to an improvement in exercise capacity and quality of life [36].

Conclusions

The progression of atrial fibrillation may be explained by the above-described effects of atrial remodelling. Maintaining sinus rhythms in atrial fibrillation by whatever means may slow the progression of remodelling and give patients benefit until safer antiarrhythmic drugs and ablation procedures are developed.

References

1. Allessie MA, Ausma J, Schotten U (2002) Electrical, contractile and structural remodeling in atrial fibrillation. Cardiovasc Res 54:230–246
2. Schotten U, Duytschaever M, Ausma J et al (2003) Electrical and contractile remodeling during the first days of atrial fibrillation go hand in hand. Circulation 107:1433–1439

3. Wijffels MC, Kirchhof CJ, Dorland R et al (1995) Atrial fibrillation begets atrial fibrillation. A study in awake chronically instrumented goats. Circulation 92:1954–1968
4. Allessie MA, Konings KTS, Kirchhof CJHJ et al (1996) Electrophysiologic mechanisms of perpetuation of atrial fibrillation. Am J Cardiol 77:10A-23A
5. Goette A, Honeycutt C, Langberg JJ (1996) Electrical remodeling in atrial fibrillation. Time course and mechanisms. Circulation 94:2968–2974
6. Lai LP, Su MJ, Lin JL et al (1999) Down-regulation of L-type calcium channel land sarcoplasmic reticular Ca(2+)-ATPase mRNA in human atrial fibrillation without significant change in the mRNA of ryanodine receptor, calsequestrin and phospholamban: an insight into the mechanism of atrial electrical remodeling. J Am Coll Cardiol 33:1231–1237
7. Yu W-C, Chen S-A, Lee S-H et al (1998) Tachycardia-induced change of atrial refractory period in humans: rate dependency and effects of antiarrhythmic drugs. Circulation 97:2331–2337
8. Wijffels MC, Kirchhof CJ, Dorland R et al (1997) Electrical remodeling due to atrial fibrillation in chronically instrumented conscious goats: roles of neurohumoral changes, ischemia, atrial stretch, and high rate of electrical activation. Circulation 96:3710–3720
9. Daoud EG, Knight BP, Weiss R et al (1997) Effect of verpamil and procainamide on atrial fibrillation-induced electrical remodeling in humans. Circulation 95:1542–1550
10. Tieleman RG, Van Gelder IC, Crijns HJ et al (1998) Early recurrences of atrial fibrillation after electrical cardioversion: a result of fibrillation-induced electrical remodeling of the atria? J Am Coll Cardiol 31:167–173
11. Tieleman RG, De Langen C, Van Gelder IC et al (1997) Verapamil reduces tachycardia-induced electrical remodeling of the atria. Circulation 95:1945–1953
12. De Simone A, Stabile G, Vitale DF et al (1999) Pretreatment with verapamil in patients with persistent or chronic atrial fibrillation who underwent electrical cardioversion. J Am Coll Cardiol 34:810–814
13. Van Noord T, Tieleman RG, Bosker HA et al (2004) Beta-blockers prevent subacute recurrences of persistent atrial fibrillation only in patients with hypertension. Europace 6:343–350
14. Dell'Orfano JT, Patel H, Wolbrette DL et al (1999) Acute treatment of atrial fibrillation: Spontaneous conversion rates and cost of care. Am J Cardiol 83:788–790
15. Dittrich HC, Ericson JS, Schneiderman T et al (1989) Echocardiographic and clinical predictors for outcome of elective cardioversion of atrial fibrillation. Am J Cardiol 63:193–197
16. Hobbs WJ, Van Gelder IC, Fitzpatrick AP et al (1999) The role of atrial electrical remodeling in the progression of focal atrial ectopy to persistent atrial fibrillation. J Cardiovasc Electrophysiol 10:866–870
17. Allessie MA, Boyden PA, Camm AJ et al (2001) Pathophysiology and prevention of atrial fibrillation. Circulation 103:769–777
18. Schotten U, Ausma J, Stellbrink C et al (2001) Cellular mechanisms of depressed atrial contractility in patients with chronic atrial fibrillation. Circulation 103:691–698
19. San Fillippo AJ, Abascol VM, Sheehan M et al (1990) Atrial enlargement as a consequence of atrial fibrillation: A prospective echocardiographic study. Circulation 82:792–797
20. Manning WJ, Silverman DI, Katz SE et al (1994) Impaired left atrial mechanical

function after cardioversion: relationship to the duration of atrial fibrillation. J Am Coll Cardiol 23:1535–1540
21. De Haan S, Blaauw Y, Van Hunnik A et al (2005) The novel I_{to}/I_{Kur} blocker AVE0118, but not the IKr blocker dofetilide, restores atrial contractility after cardioversion of atrial fibrillation in the goat. Heart Rhythm 2:S181 (abs)
22. Allessie MA, Boyden PA, Camm AJ et al (2001) Pathophysiology and prevention of atrial fibrillation. Circulation 103:769–777
23. Solti F, Vecsey T, Kékesi V et al (1989) The effect of atrial dilatation on the genesis of atrial arrhythmias. Cardiovasc Res 23:882–886
24. Ausma J, Wijffels M, Thone F et al (1997) Structural changes of atrial myocardium due to sustained atrial fibrillation in the goat. Circulation 96(9):3157–3163
25. van der Velden HMW, van Kempen MJA, Wijffels MCEF et al (1998) Altered pattern of connexin-40 distribution in persistent atrial fibrillation in the goat. J Cardiovasc Electrophysiol 9:596–607
26. Kanagaratnam P, Cherian A, Stanbridge RDL et al (2004) Relationship between connexins and atrial activation during human atrial fibrillation. J Cardiovasc Electrophysiol 15:206–213
27. Li D, Fareh S, Leung TK et al (1999) Promotion of atrial fibrillation by heart failure in dogs: atrial remodeling of a different sort. Circulation 100(1):87–95
28. Nakashima H, Kumagai K, Urata H et al (2000) Angiotensin II antagonist prevents electrical remodeling in atrial fibrillation. Circulation 101(22):2612–2617
29. Kumagai K, Nakashima H, Urata H et al (2003) Effects of angiotensin II type 1 receptor antagonist on electrical and structural remodeling in atrial fibrillation. J Am Coll Cardiol 41(12):2197–2204
30. Pedersen OD, Bagger H, Kober L et al (1999) Trandolapril reduces the incidence of atrial fibrillation after acute myocardial infarction in patients with left ventricular dysfunction. Circulation 100(4):376–380
31. Vermes E, Tardif JC, Bourassa MG et al (2003) Enalapril decreases the incidence of atrial fibrillation in patients with left ventricular dysfunction: insight from the Studies Of Left Ventricular Dysfunction (SOLVD) trials. Circulation 107:2926–2931
32. Madrid AH, Bueno MG, Rebollo JM et al (2002) Use of irbesartan to maintain sinus rhythm in patients with long-lasting persistent atrial fibrillation: a prospective and randomized study. Circulation 106:331–336
33. Murray KT, Rottman JN, Arbogast PG et al for the AFFIRM Investigators (2004) Inhibition of angiotensin II signaling and recurrence of atrial fibrillation in AFFIRM. Heart Rhythm 1: 669–675
34. Ross HM, Kowey PR, Naccarelli GV (2005) New antiarrhythmic pharmacologic therapies and regulatory issues in antiarrhythmic drug development. In: Wang P (ed) New Arrhythmia technologies. Oxford, Blackwell Publishing (in press)
35. Blaauw Y, Gogelein H, Tieleman RG et al (2004) 'Early' class III drugs for the treatment of atrial fibrillation. Efficacy and atrial selectivity of AVE0118 in remodeled atria of the goat. Circulation 110:1717–1724
36. Hsu LF, Jaïs P, Sanders P et al (2004) Catheter ablation for atrial fibrillation in congestive heart failure. N Engl J Med 351:2373–2383

Atrial Fibrillation and Heart Failure: Does One Epidemic Feed the Other?

G. Boriani, M. Biffi, C. Martignani, C. Valzania, I. Diemberger, M. Ziacchi, D. Saporito, P. Artale, G. Domenichini, L. Frabetti, A. Branzi

The Epidemiology of Atrial Fibrillation and Heart Failure

Atrial fibrillation (AF) and chronic heart failure (HF) are two common cardiac diseases, affecting 1–2% of the population [1–3] with a prevalence that rises steeply with age. AF and HF are conditioned by common risk factors and frequently coexist [3].

AF is the most common sustained arrhythmia, and the need for treatment constitutes an important burden on health care systems. It is estimated that 2.3 million Americans and probably a similar number of Europeans are affected by AF. Projected data from the ATRIA study indicate that the number of people in the United States affected by AF will increase to more than 5.6 million in the coming decades, corresponding to a 2.5-fold increase [4]. HF is also a very frequent cardiovascular disorder, and it is estimated that it affects 15–20 million people worldwide. HF represents the most important risk factor for AF in developed countries where the prevalence of rheumatic heart disease has declined and a large amount of patients affected by various heart diseases survive to old age. Approximately two thirds of patients with HF are older than 65 years of age and thus have a high probability of AF presenting as a comorbidity [3]. In the Framingham study, HF was associated with a five- to six-fold increased risk of AF, which was higher than the risk related to valvular heart disease [5].

The most impressive data on the risk of developing AF or HF during life come from two studies from the Framingham cohort, where the cumulative, lifetime risk of developing AF [6] or HF [7] was evaluated in more than 8000

Institute of Cardiology, University of Bologna, Azienda Ospedaliera S.Orsola-Malpighi, Bologna, Italy

patients followed from 1968 through 1999. In these studies, the lifetime risk of developing AF and HF, for subjects aged 40 years or more, was 1 in 4 and 1 in 5, respectively.

The true epidemiological burden of AF–HF comorbidity in the 'real world' is only partially known and is surely underestimated by any analysis based on randomised clinical trials examining HF, where AF is often one of the exclusion criteria. Indeed, as shown in Fig. 1, the prevalence of AF is higher in hospitalised HF patients or in community HF patients than in HF patients participating in randomised clinical trials [8].

The Euro Heart Failure survey, conducted in 24 countries in Europe, showed that up to 45% patients with HF presented with AF, in the intermittent or chronic form. According to the Euro Heart Failure survey, the overall prevalence of new onset AF in patients with HF requiring hospitalisation was 13%, ranging from 8% to 36% [9]. The prevalence of AF was related to the severity of HF, varying between 10% and 20% in mild to moderate HF to 50% in patients with more advanced HF [3, 9–11].

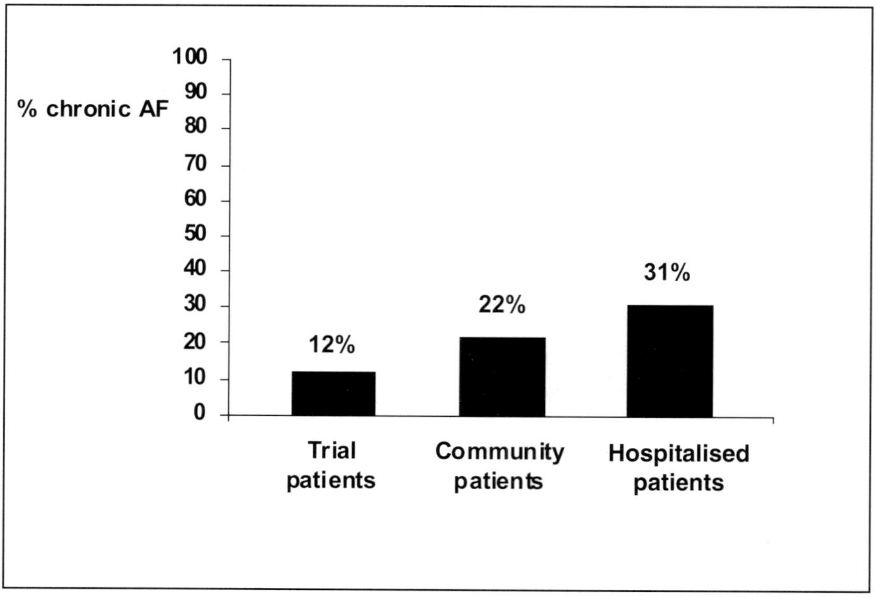

Fig. 1. Prevalence of chronic atrial fibrillation (AF) in various settings of heart-failure patients, according to the literature

The Interplay Between Atrial Fibrillation and Heart Failure

A temporal sequence of AF preceding HF gains further support from a prospective epidemiologic investigation. The Manitoba Follow-Up Study examined the relationship of AF to the development of HF in a cohort of men fit for pilot training in the Canadian Air Force [2]. Adjusting for other cardiovascular conditions and risk factors, the investigators found that subjects with AF had an independent 3-fold increase in the risk for developing congestive heart failure during follow-up. Since HF is a well known risk factor for AF, the extent to which AF causes HF, as opposed to HF causing AF, remains unclear. In many instances, the conditions are interdependent.

In clinical practice, the relationship between AF and HF, or left ventricular dysfunction, is intriguing. Indeed, AF may cause HF, particularly when there is a fast uncontrolled ventricular response. This form of HF may be reversible after rhythm or rate-control and is called tachycardiomiopathy [12–14]. At the initial patient observation, it may be quite difficult to distinguish it from the most common phenomenon of AF facilitated by the mechanical, electrophysiological, and neurohormonal derangements caused by HF in a background of primary ventricular dilation and ipokinaesia.

The haemodynamic consequences of AF are related to the loss of atrial contribution to cardiac output, to an increase in heart rate with shortening in the duration of diastole, and to irregularity in the diastolic intervals. The loss of atrial contribution to ventricular filling may be well-tolerated in a healthy heart but may have adverse consequences in the presence of left ventricular dysfunction. Loss of atrial transport is particularly significant if there is impairment in left ventricular filling due to reduced diastolic compliance or to mitral stenosis. In this kind of patient, a high heart rate or an irregular heart rate with frequent short diastolic intervals will be poorly tolerated. Over the long term, a sustained uncontrolled tachycardia with heart rate higher than 120 beats/min gives rise to an impairment of left ventricular function with various degrees of ventricular dysfunction. This may result in an important worsening of the patient's condition, unless heart rate can be controlled or sinus rhythm restored. This clinical condition is known as 'tachycardiomyopathy' or 'tachycardia-induced cardiomyopathy' [12–14].

The Relationship Between Atrial Fibrillation and Heart Failure: A Chicken–Egg Dilemma?

In clinical practice, the diagnosis of tachycardiomyopathy remains a difficult issue, since characterisation of patients with pure reversible tachycardia-induced cardiomyopathy and differentiation from other patients with dilated cardiomyopathy is very difficult 'a priori' and constitutes a 'chicken–egg type of dilemma' [12–16]. Tachycardiomyopathy may be suspected by the coexistence of chronic AF and of left ventricular dysfunction with improvement in cardiac performance following rate control or rhythm control. However, even the absence of improvement does not demonstrate that a tachycardiomyopathy component was not present, since it may reflect an advanced stage of irreversible tachycardia-related myocardial injury [12–16]. Indeed, the degree of regression of ventricular dysfunction with rate control depends on several factors and may be total, partial, or absent.

Apart from clear cases of tachycardiomyopathy secondary to AF, there is also the possibility that AF may have a subtle long term deleterious effect on left ventricular function [14]. Indeed, a subtle form of cardiomyopathy secondary to chronic AF may be related to a series of factors including: (1) controlled heart rate at rest but with disproportionately high rates (> 120 beats/min) during minor exercises and normal daily activity [16], (2) lack of physiological rate-response during daily activity, and (3) irregularity of the ventricular cycle during AF. Patients with already impaired left ventricular function and excessive sympathetic activation may be particularly prone to this possibility. The real prevalence of these forms of occult or latent tachycardiomyopathy among patients with chronic persistent AF is unknown, but a series of observations suggests its relevance [14–16].

Clinical Significance of Atrial Fibrillation in Heart Failure

In the Framingham Study, the development of AF in patients with HF was associated with a 2.7-fold increased risk of death in women and a 1.6-fold risk in men [17]. Middlekauff et al. analysed a series of 390 patients with advanced HF and found that AF was associated with a higher risk of all-cause and sudden death mortality compared with sinus rhythm [10]. In the SOLVD trials, a 1.3-fold greater risk of all-cause death related to AF was found [18]. This increase was probably linked to an increase risk of death from progressive pump failure. In the DIAMOND trial, the presence of AF in HF patients was associated with significantly lower survival compared with patients in sinus rhythm [19].

Costs of Atrial Fibrillation and Heart Failure

The cost of hospitalising patients with AF in the United States has been estimated to be approximately $1 billion annually. According to Medicare data, the relative hospital costs in 1991 of 12 625 elderly Medicare patients with recent-onset AF compared to matched patients without AF ranged from $1442 in 75- to 84-year-old women, to $3250 in 65- to 74-year-old women. In both men and women, and across the two decades of age studied, patients with AF had significantly higher annual hospital costs than subjects without AF [20]. Similarly, and even more impressively, the costs of HF are becoming a major threat to health care systems, especially in relationship with increasing costs for hospitalisation [21]. According to data reported by the American Heart Association, the treatment of HF in the United States in 2004 accounted for an overall cost of 26.8 billion dollars.

Therapeutic Implications of Atrial Fibrillation and Heart Failure Comorbidity

The multiple relationships between AF an HF make the therapeutic approach extremely complex and multifactorial. Indeed, for both AF and HF a wide variety of therapeutic endpoints can be considered, ranging from symptom relief to mortality prevention, and including the prevention of major events, an improvement in quality of life, and a reduction in hospitalisation. Even limiting this analysis of potential therapeutic endpoints to AF, a complex picture emerges, as shown in Table 1. The complexity of any therapeutic approach to AF–HF comorbidity is magnified by the wide range of potential treatment options for AF, including atrial cardioversion and rhythm control [3, 22, 23], pharmacological or non-pharmacological rate control [3, 15], ablation directed on the atrial substrate with the aim to suppress AF [25], and algorithms for atrial pacing combined with cardiac resynchronisation therapy [26]. With regard to the treatment of HF, a favourable effect on AF has been documented for a series of drugs used in HF treatment (angiotensin converting enzyme inhibitors and AT-1 receptor blockers) [11].

Conclusions

The interplay between AF and HF is complex, and the clinical implications of this relationship are currently enhanced by the epidemiological relevance of both HF and AF. Until more precise clinical data are available, from prospective controlled evaluations, rate control and rhythm control should be pursued in all patients with a clinical picture of unrecognised and unexplained HF/ventricular dysfunction coupled with AF at relatively fast ventricular response. This may allow interruption of the vicious cycle existing between AF and HF, in which each disease facilitates, promotes, and worsens the other. A wide range of pharmacological and non-pharmacological treat-

Table 1. Potential therapeutic endpoints in the treatment of atrial fibrillation (AF)

Symptoms
• Palpitations
• Dyspnoea
• Fatigue
• Dizziness/syncope
• Others
Clinical events
• Stroke/ thromboembolism
• Haemorrhagic complications
• Onset/ worsening of heart failure
• Death
• Others
Medical interventions
• Hospitalisation
• Hospitalisation for heart failure
• Electrical cardioversion
Rhythm endpoints
• Measures of rhythm control
• Measures of rate control
• Days spent in AF
• AF burden
• Others
Other clinical measures
• Functional capacity
• Quality of life
• Ventricular function
• Cognitive function
• Other
Economic endpoints
• Cost
• Cost-effectiveness

ments is currently available, and, in view of the variable clinical picture of the patients and the clinical priorities, tailoring of medical decisions appears to be mandatory.

References

1. Kannel WB, Abbott RD, Savage DD et al (1982) Epidemiologic features of chronic atrial fibrillation: the Framingham Study. N Engl J Med 306:1018–1022
2. Krahn AD, Manfreda J, Tate RB et al (1995) The natural history of atrial fibrillation: incidence, risk factors, and prognosis in the Manitoba Follow-Up Study. Am J Med 98:476–484
3. Khand AU, Rankin AC, Kaye GC et al (2000) Systematic review of the management of atrial fibrillation in patients with heart failure. Eur Heart J 21:614–632
4. Go AS, Hylek EM, Phillips KA et al (2001) Prevalence of diagnosed atrial fibrillation in adults: national implications for rhythm management and stroke prevention: the AnTicoagulation and Risk Factors in Atrial Fibrillation (ATRIA) Study. JAMA 285:2370–2375
5. Benjamin EJ, Levy D, Vaziri SM et al (1994) Independent risk factors for atrial fibrillation in a population-based cohort. The Framingham Heart Study. JAMA 16:840–844
6. Lloyd-Jones DM, Wang TJ, Leip EP et al (2004) Lifetime risk for development of atrial fibrillation: the Framingham Heart Study. Circulation 110:1042–1046
7. Lloyd-Jones DM, Larson MG, Leip EP et al (2002) Lifetime risk for developing congestive heart failure: the Framingham Heart Study. Circulation 106:3068–3072
8. Badano LP, Di Lenarda A, Bellotti P et al (2003) Patients with chronic heart failure encountered in daily clinical practice are different from the 'typical' patient enrolled in therapeutic trials. Ital Heart J 4:84–91
9. Cleland JG, Swedberg K, Follath F et al (2003) The EuroHeart Failure survey programme: a survey on the quality of care among patients with heart failure in Europe. Part 1: patient characteristics and diagnosis. Eur Heart J 24:442–463
10. Middlekauff HR, Stevenson WG, Stevenson LW (1991) Prognostic significance of atrial fibrillation in advanced heart failure. A study of 390 patients. Circulation 84:40–48
11. Savelieva I, Camm AJ (2004) Atrial fibrillation and heart failure: natural history and pharmacological treatment. Europace 5:S5-S19
12. Grogan M, Smith HC, Gersh BJ et al (1992) Left ventricular dysfunction due to atrial fibrillation in patients initially believed to have idiopathic dilated cardiomyopathy. Am J Cardiol 69:1570–1573
13. Shinbane JS, Wood MA, Jensen DN et al (1997) Tachycardia-induced cardiomyopathy: a review of animal models and clinical studies. J Am Coll Cardiol 29:709–715
14. Boriani G, Biffi M, Rapezzi C et al (2003) Late improvement in ventricular performance following internal cardioversion for persistent atrial fibrillation: an argument in support of concealed cardiomyopathy. Pacing Clin Electrophysiol 26:1218–1226
15. Boriani G, Biffi M, Diemberger I et al (2003) Rate control in atrial fibrillation: choice of treatment and assessment of efficacy. Drugs 63:1489–1509
16. Van Den Berg MP, Tuinenburg AE, Crijns HJGM et al (1997) Heart failure and atrial fibrillation: current concepts and controversies. Heart 77:309–313

17. Wang TJ, Larson MG, Levy D et al (2003) Temporal relations of atrial fibrillation and congestive heart failure and their joint influence on mortality: the Framingham Heart Study. Circulation 107:2920–2925
18. Dries DL, Exner DV, Gersh BJ et al (2001) Atrial fibrillation is associated with an increased risk for mortality and heart failure progression in patients with asymptomatic and symptomatic left ventricular systolic dysfunction: a retrospective analysis of the SOLVD trials. Studies of Left Ventricular Dysfunction. J Am Coll Cardiol 32:695–703
19. Pedersen OD, Bagger H, Keller N et al (2001) Efficacy of dofetilide in the treatment of atrial fibrillation-flutter in patients with reduced left ventricular function: a Danish investigations of arrhythmia and mortality on dofetilide (Diamond) substudy. Circulation 104:292–296
20. Wolff PA, Mitchell JB, Baker CS et al (1995) Mortality and hospital costs associated with atrial fibrillation. Circulation 92:I-140 (abs)
21. Berry C, Murdoch DR, McMurray JJ (2001) Economics of chronic heart failure. Eur J Heart Fail 3:283–291
22. Boriani G, Biffi M, Camanini C et al (2004) Efficacy of internal cardioversion for chronic atrial fibrillation in patients with and without left ventricular dysfunction. Int J Cardiol 95:43–47
23. Boriani G, Diemberger I, Biffi M et al (2004) Pharmacological cardioversion of atrial fibrillation: current management and treatment options. Drugs 64:2741–2762
24. Hsu LF, Jaïs P, Sanders P et al (2004) Catheter ablation for atrial fibrillation in congestive heart failure. N Engl J Med 351:2373–2383
25. Jessup M, Brozena S (2003) Heart failure. N Engl J Med 348:2007–2018
26. Boriani G, Biffi M, Martignani C et al (2004) Cardiac resynchronization by pacing: an electrical treatment of heart failure. Int J Cardiol 94:151–161

Atrial Fibrillation: What Is the Impact of the Different Therapies on Quality of Life?

B. LÜDERITZ

Atrial fibrillation (AF) is a frequent and costly health care problem. In patients with AF, the restoration and maintenance of sinus rhythm is the primary therapeutic goal. The most frequent strategy for maintaining sinus rhythm after restoration is the use of anti-arrhythmic drugs. The efficacy of therapy in AF has been predominantly measured using objective criteria such as mortality and morbidity. In recent years, the importance of quality of life as an outcome measure has been recognised. However, few published studies have examined quality of life in patients with AF using properly validated tools. In addition, the specific impact of anti-arrhythmic treatment on quality of life in patients with AF has not been assessed. These issues are now being addressed in several ongoing studies. This article attempts to define quality of life, makes recommendations on how it might be assessed, and reviews our current knowledge regarding quality of life in patients with AF.

AF is the most frequently experienced cardiac arrhythmia, affecting an estimated 2.2 million people in the United States, and approximately 6 million in Europe. Approximately 1.2 million patients are suffering from paroxysmal AF, and about 1 million from persistent AF. A rate of conversion from paroxysmal AF to persistent AF of 30% is anticipated [1]. The prevalence of AF increases with age [2], ranging from less than 1% at 50–59 years to nearly 9% at 80–89 years [3]. In addition to palpitations, patients with AF have an increased risk of stroke and can develop decreased exercise tolerance and left ventricular dysfunction [4]. All of these problems may be reversed with restoration and maintenance of sinus rhythm. Thus, treatment of AF is

Department of Medicine – Cardiology, University of Bonn, Germany

warranted in the hope of eliminating symptoms, preventing complications, and possibly decreasing the excess mortality associated with this arrhythmia [5]. The primary intervention for maintaining sinus rhythm after restoration is use of anti-arrhythmic drugs. However, many of the existing drugs have only limited efficacy and are associated with considerable undesirable adverse effects. Current treatment is therefore suboptimal [6].

In patients with AF, the restoration and maintenance of sinus rhythm is the primary therapeutic goal. Once sinus rhythm is maintained, physiological rate control is restored and left ventricular ejection fraction, cardiac output, and exercise capacity are increased. This improved cardiovascular performance enhances the patient's ability to perform the functions of normal daily life. Effective treatment of AF is based on these objective criteria, but subjective criteria such as quality of life are important. To address the quality-of-life issues, rigorous yet practical approaches are needed to enable a comprehensive understanding of quality of life in patients with AF [7]. Different instruments can be used to measure various parameters reflecting quality of life. The most important items to be considered for endpoints and outcome events for the assessment of therapy for AF, as agreed by the European Society of Cardiology Atrial Fibrillation Endpoints Working Group in June 2000, are listed in Table 1 [8–13].

Table 1. Meaningful endpoints for quality of life evaluation in AF patients

Frequency of episodes
Duration of episodes
Hospitalisations
Frequency of symptoms
Type of AF: 'Paroxysmal, Persistent, Permanent' or 'Initial, Recurrent, Established' respectively
AF and NYHA classification
General life satisfaction (general health and well being)
Cardiac symptom frequency / cardiac symptom severity (symptom burden)
SF-36 category
Mental health / social functioning (emotional/social functioning)
Physical role, vitality (physical functioning)
Somatisation
Gender men/women (SF-36)
Outcome scores (follow-up)
Silent AF vs symptomatic AF
Age < 50 years, > 50 years

continue →

Table 1, *continue*

Comparison to other settings (Post Myocardial Infarction, Implantable Cardioverter/ Defibrillator
Congestive Heart Failure
Therapeutic interventions: radiofrequency catheter and atrioventricular node ablation
Medical therapy vs ablation
AV junction ablation
Cardiac Output-change (rest, exercise) after cardioversion
Effects of Maze operation
New technology for therapy (new leads, new algorithms, ATP, stabilisation features)

Rhythm Control or Rate Control and Anticoagulation

The clinical categorisation relating to quality of life of patients who present with AF is a major determinant of the most appropriate strategy for rhythm management. For patients with recurrent AF that has not become permanent, the two available strategies are (1) rhythm control and anticoagulation and (2) rate control and anticoagulation. There is no clear evidence that one of these strategies is superior to the other [14]. Our knowledge about the efficacy and safety of various therapeutic strategies is insufficient, especially with respect to the direct comparison of re-establishment of sinus rhythm by drugs in comparison to rate control [14].

Ventricular Rate Control By AV Junction Ablation

Haemodynamic effects of complete atrioventricular (AV) junction ablation with subsequent regular ventricular pacing are exclusively due to rate control and regularisation of ventricular contraction rather than to atrial contractile function and previous AV synchrony. Several studies have been published that underline the beneficial effects of complete AV junction ablation in patients with AF, fast ventricular response, and depressed left ventricular function (Table 2) [9, 15–21].

RFC Ablation

The frequency of hospital admissions and emergency room visits and the number of anti-arrhythmic drugs taken decreased significantly after

Table 2. Impact of complete atrioventricular (AV) junction ablation and pacemaker implantation on left ventricular haemodynamics, exercise capacity, and quality of life

Author	No. of patients	Haemodynamics	Exercise capacity	Quality of life
Heinz et al. [15]	10 (10/0)	+	0	–
Twidale et al. [16]	14 (7/7)	+	+	–
Rodriguez et al. [17]	30 (3/2)	+	–	–
Brignole et al. [18]	23 (23/0)	+	+	+
Edner et al. [19]	29 (17/12)	+	+	–
Fitzpatrick et al. [20]	90 (54/46)	+	+	+
Natale et al. [21]	29 (17/12)	+	+	+
Schumacher and Lüderitz [9]	45 (27/18)	+	+	+

+ Significant improvement, *0* no significant improvement, – no data available

radiofrequency catheter (RFC) ablation and pacemaker implantation. Activity capacity improved significantly after ablation in patients with depressed left ventricular function. All improvements after ablation were maintained over 6 months follow-up. However, compared with patients without AF before ablation, patients who did have AF before ablation had less improvement in general quality of life, frequency of significant symptoms, and symptoms during attacks [22].

In summary, it has been shown that not only pharmaceutical but, even more, electrical treatment can enhance quality of life in patients with AF (Table 3) [23].

Table 3. Estimates by scorig points of health-related quality of life (SF-36 categories), medical therapy vs ablation therapy [16]. Higher score indicates higher quality of life

SF-36 category	Medical therapy			Ablation therapy		
	Baseline	Follow-up	*P* value	Baseline	Follow-up	*P* value
Physical function	71 ± 26	81 ± 24	< 0.05	70 ± 25	83 ± 27	< 0.005
Physical role	54 ± 41	65 ± 38	< 0.05	47 ± 38	81 ± 31	< 0.001
Bodily pain	67 ± 17	63 ± 245	ns	72 ± 15	81 ± 20	< 0.05
General health	68 ± 19	69 ± 21	ns	65 ± 21	79 ± 21	< 0.001
Vitality	50 ± 16	55 ± 21	ns	51 ± 22	66 ± 22	< 0.005
Social function	68 ± 24	78 ± 26	< 0.01	72 ± 26	83 ± 29	< 0.001
Emotional role	74 ± 40	78 ± 36	ns	79 ± 37	94 ± 17	< 0.05
Mental health	69 ± 15	73 ± 19	< 0.05	68 ± 19	77 ± 18	< 0.01

ns Not significant

References

1. Feinberg WM, Blackshear JL, Laupacis A et al (1995) Prevalence, age distribution, and gender of patients with atrial fibrillation: analysis and implications. Arch Intern Med 155:469–473
2. Benjamin EJ, Levy D, Vaziri SM et al (1994) Independent risk factors for atrial fibrillation in a population-based cohort: the Framingham Heart Study. JAMA 271:840–844
3. Kannel WB, Wolf PA, Benjamin EJ et al (1998) Prevalence, incidence, prognosis, and predisposing conditions for atrial fibrillation: population-based estimates. Am J Cardiol 82:2N-9N
4. Krahn AD, Manfreda J, Tate RB et al (1995) The natural history of atrial fibrillation: incidence, risk factors, and prognosis in the Manitoba Follow-Up Study. Am J Med 98:476–484
5. Benjamin EJ, Wolf PA, D'Agostino RB et al (1998) Impact of atrial fibrillation on the risk of death: the Framingham Heart Study. Circulation 98:946–952
6. Lüderitz B, Jung W (2000) Quality of life in patients with atrial fibrillation. Arch Intern Med 160:1749–1757
7. Jung W, Lüderitz B (1998) Quality of life in patients with atrial fibrillation. J Cardiovasc Electrophysiol 9(suppl 8):S177-S186
8. Crijns HJGM, Van Gelder IC, Tieleman RG et al (1997) Why is atrial fibrillation bad for you? In: Murgatroyd FD, Camm AJ (eds) Nonpharmacological management of atrial fibrillation. Futura, Armonk, NY, pp 3–13
9. Schumacher B, Lüderitz B (1998) Rate issues in atrial fibrillation: consequences of tachycardia and therapy for rate control. Am J Cardiol 82:29N-36N
10. Lönnerholm S, Blomström P, Nilsson L et al (2000) Effects of the maze operation on health-related quality of life in patients with atrial fibrillation. Circulation 101:2607–2611
11. Wellens JJW, Lau CP, Lüderitz B et al for the METRIX Investigators (1998) Atrioverter: an implantable device for the treatment of atrial fibrillation. Circulation 98:1651–1656
12. Lüderitz B, Jung W (2000) Quality of life in atrial fibrillation. J Intervent Card Electrophysiol 4:201–209
13. Savelieva I, Paquette M, Dorian P (2001) Quality of life in patients with silent atrial fibrillation. Heart 85:216–217
14. Wyse DG (2000) The AFFIRM trial: Main trial and substudies – what can we expect? J Interv Card Electrophysiol 4:171–176
15. Heinz G, Siostrzonek P, Kreiner G et al (1992) Improvement in left ventricular systolic function after successful radiofrequency His bundle ablation for drug refractory, chronic atrial fibrillation and recurrent atrial flutter. Am J Cardiol 69:489–492
16. Twidale N, Sutton K, Bartlett L et al (1993) Effects on cardiac performance of atrioventricular node catheter ablation using radiofrequency current for drug-refractory atrial arrhythmias. Pacing Clin Electrophysiol 16:1275–1284
17. Rodriguez LM, Smeets JL, Xie B et al (1993) Improvement in left ventricular function by ablation of atrioventricular nodal conduction in selected patients with lone atrial fibrillation. Am J Cardiol 72:1137–1141
18. Brignole M, Gionfranchi L, Menozzi C et al (1994) Influence of atrioventricular junction radiofrequency ablation patients with chronic atrial fibrillation and flutter on quality of life and cardiac performance. Am J Cardiol 74:242–246

19. Edner M, Caidahl K, Bergfeldt L et al (1995) Prospective study of left ventricular function after radiofrequency ablation of atrioventricular junction in patients with atrial fibrillation. Br Heart J 74:261–267
20. Fitzpatrick AP, Kourouyan HD, Siu A et al (1996) Quality of life and outcomes after radiofrequency His-bundle catheter ablation and permanent pacemaker implantation: impact of treatment in paroxysmal and established atrial fibrillation. Am Heart J 131:499–507
21. Natale A, Zimerman L, Tomassoni G et al (1996) Impact on ventricular function and quality of life of transcatheter ablation of the atrioventricular junction in chronic atrial fibrillation with a normal ventricular response. Am J Cardiol 78:1431–1433
22. Steinbeck G (1996) Drug therapy of atrial fibrillation: control of heart rate versus establishing sinus rhythm (in German). Z Kardiol 85(Suppl 6):69–74
23. Bathina MN, Mickelsen S, Brooks C et al (1998) Radiofrequency catheter ablation versus medical therapy for initial treatment of supraventricular tachycardia and its impact on quality of life and healthcare costs. Am J Cardiol 82:589–593

'Pill-In-The-Pocket' Approach for Outpatient Treatment of Recent Onset Atrial Fibrillation: The Obvious Solution?

P. Alboni

In the clinical setting, some patients with recurrent atrial fibrillation (AF) present with episodes that are not frequent (< 1 per month) and are haemodynamically well tolerated, but which are long enough to require emergency room (ER) intervention or hospitalisation. These patients need treatment, but long-term oral prophylaxis or catheter ablation may not be the most appropriate first-line therapy. Rather, a good method of treatment in this group of patients might be the 'pill-in-the-pocket' approach, consisting of single-dose oral ingestion at the time and place of palpitation onset. This type of treatment has already been investigated in studies carried out in hospital in patients with recent-onset AF. The oral drugs that have been used to convert recent-onset AF to sinus rhythm are class IA, class IC, and class III anti-arrhythmic agents [1–7]. The class IC agents flecainide and propafenone have the advantage of being conveniently administered in a single oral dose that acts rapidly and causes minimal side effects [1, 6, 8–16]. The efficacy of a single oral loading dose of flecainide and propafenone in converting recent-onset AF to sinus rhythm has been documented by several placebo-controlled trials [1, 6, 8, 9, 11, 13, 16]. Both drugs showed similar efficacy, and their success rate varied from 58% to 95% [1, 6, 8–13], depending on the duration of AF and the observation period after drug administration. In all controlled studies, a low incidence of adverse effects has been reported [1–6, 8–13, 15, 16]. The most serious side effect seems to be the appearance of a transient atrial flutter with high ventricular rate owing to 1:1 atrioventricular (AV) conduction (in about 1% of patients).

Very recently, out-of-hospital treatment with the 'pill-in-the-pocket'

Division of Cardiology and Arrhythmologic Centre, Ospedale Civile, Cento (Ferrara), Italy

approach has been investigated in an Italian multi-centre study [17]. Inclusion criteria were as follows:

- Age between 18 and 75 years with requirement for ER intervention for recent onset AF (< 48 h).
- History of palpitation with abrupt onset, haemodynamically well tolerated (absence of symptoms such as dyspnoea, pre-syncope, or syncope).
- Number of episodes in the last year < 1 per month.
- Absence of cardiological symptoms apart from the arrhythmic episodes.

Patients with contraindications to class IC agents were excluded. The patients could be treated either in the ER or in the cardiology ward. For AF conversion, oral propafenone and flecainide were administered in a single dose according to the weight of the patient: flecainide 300 mg if the patient weighed ≥ 70 kg, otherwise 200 mg; propafenone 600 mg if the patient weighed ≥ 70 kg, otherwise 450 mg. The drug treatment was considered 'successful' if the conversion time to sinus rhythm was within 6 h after drug administration, without severe side effects.

Two hundred and sixty-eight patients with recent-onset AF received an in-hospital oral loading dose of flecainide and propafenone. Of these, 58 were ruled out of the out-of-hospital treatment: in 3 (1%) exclusion criteria emerged during echocardiographic recording, in 41 (14%) the drug was not effective in restoring sinus rhythm within 6 h, and in 14 (6%) the drug induced side effects (transient hypotension in 4, atrial flutter in 7, one of whom had 1:1 AV conduction, and slightly symptomatic bradycardia in 3). The remaining 210 patients (age 59 ± 11 years) were discharged on flecainide or propafenone for 'pill-in-the-pocket' treatment of recurrent AF. One hundred and eighteen patients had no signs of heart disease and the remaining 92 (43%) had mild heart disease. The mean follow-up was 15 ± 5 months; 4 patients were lost just after enrolment. Of the remaining 206 patients, 41 (20%) did not experience any arrhythmic recurrences during the follow-up period and 165 reported 618 episodes of palpitation with abrupt onset, 569 of which were treated with flecainide (64 patients) or propafenone (101 patients). The drug was effective in 534 out of 569 arrhythmic episodes (94%).

Similar results on the efficacy of class IC drugs were recently reported by Capucci et al. [16], who investigated in hospital the reproducibility of efficacy of an oral loading dose of propafenone in restoring sinus rhythm in patients with recurrent AF. Efficacy was evaluated by electrocardiographic monitoring and was reproducible in 93% of the patients. In the Italian multicentre study, time to symptom resolution after drug ingestion was 113 ± 84 min (median 98 min). Sixteen arrhythmic episodes were interrupted after an interval of more than 6 h without the patients contacting the ER. Twenty-six episodes (5%) required ER intervention, and 10 of these (2%) also required hospitalisation of the patient. Out of the 618 episodes, 49 were not treated, mainly because of drug unavailability, and 5 (10%) of these required ER intervention. Thus, during the follow-up period, the number of ER contacts among the treated and untreated arrhythmic episodes was 31 (5%), and 10 of them also needed hospitalisation. Out of the 31 calls for ER intervention, 19 were due to AF lasting more than 6 h, 1 to acceleration of heart rate after drug ingestion (atrial flutter with 1:1 AV conduction), and 11 to anxiety (request for ER intervention although palpitation had ceased).

During follow-up, the number of calls for ER intervention per month was significantly lower than in the year before the target episode (4.9 versus 45.6, $P < 0.001$). The number of hospitalisations per month during the follow-up period was also significantly lower (1.6 versus 15.0 $P < 0.001$). Adverse effects during one or more arrhythmic episodes were reported in 12 out of the 165 patients (7%) who utilised the drug during the follow-up. One patient (0.7%) felt a marked acceleration of heart rate after drug ingestion and contacted the ER; electrocardiogram showed atrial flutter with 1:1 AV conduction. This means that successful in-hospital treatment does not completely prevent the appearance of atrial flutter at high rate during follow-up. The remaining 11 patients reported non-cardiac side effects such as nausea, asthenia, or vertigo.

These results show that out-of-hospital treatment of recurrent AF using the 'pill-in-the-pocket' approach is feasible and safe, in view of the high rate of patient compliance and the very low incidence of adverse effects. Data from the Italian study show that the 'pill-in-the-pocket' strategy with flecainide or propafenone is effective in over 90% of arrhythmic episodes after patient selection on clinical grounds and on the basis of the results of in-hospital treatment. Episodic treatment minimises the need for ER and hospital admission during the acute event. It is noteworthy that about one-third of ER contacts were due to anxiety. Therefore, psychological management of these patients (particularly reassurance) could further reduce calls for ER intervention. The marked reduction in ER and hospital admissions, besides avoiding prophylactic treatment, will help to reduce the economic impact of AF, although in only quite a small group of patients with this tachyarrhythmia. The safety of this approach without previous evaluation of in-hospital treatment remains to be investigated; therefore, at present, oral flecainide or propafenone must be tested once in hospital before prescription for out-of-hospital treatment.

Contraindications to this treatment, listed in Table 1, must always be considered. If the patient is undergoing chronic treatment with anti-arrhythmic drugs, the loading dose of flecainide or propafenone cannot be utilised, but if the patient appears suitable for the 'pill-in-the-pocket' treatment, the chronic therapy can be suspended and the loading dose given during the

Table 1. Contraindications to treatment using the 'pill-in-the-pocket' approach

Hyperthyroidism
Left bundle branch block or bifascicular block
Ischaemic heart disease
Dilated or hypertrophic cardiomyopathy
History of heart failure
Severe valvular heart disease
Chronic cor pulmonale
Left ventricular dysfunction (ejection fraction < 50%)
Long QT interval or Brugada syndrome
Bradycardia–tachycardia syndrome (resting sinus rate < 50 bpm)
Documentation of previous episodes of second- or third-degree AV block
Acute disease
Very severe chronic disease
Renal or hepatic insufficiency
Previous hypokalaemia (potassium level < 3 mmol/l)
Suspected or known pregnancy
Current prophylactic anti-arrhythmic treatment

next AF relapse. AV nodal blockers (β-blockers, verapamil, diltiazem) for treatment of hypertension or other diseases can be administered chronically.

Before discharge, patients should be given some recommendations:

- They should take the drug 5 min after any onset of typical palpitation
- After taking it, they should rest (sitting or lying down) until the palpitation has stopped or at least 4 h have passed
- They should contact the ER if palpitation has not ceased 8 h after they took the drug, or if they have symptoms that have not occurred during previous arrhythmic episodes (e.g. dyspnoea, pre-syncope, or syncope), or if they feel a marked increase in heart rate after taking the drug
- They must take no more than one oral dose during any 24-h period
- They must not take less than the prescribed dosage of the drug

The practical management of patients suitable for out-of-hospital treatment with the pill-in-the-pocket approach is summarised in Fig. 1.

Patients ≤ 75 years with mild heart disease or none, requiring ER intervention for an episode of recent-onset AF (< 48 h), with a history of palpitations of abrupt onset, not very frequent (≤1 per month), haemodynamically well tolerated but lasting long enough to require hospital intervention, with no contraindications to class IC drugs after clinical and electrocardiographic evaluation.

↓

In-hospital treatment (ER or ward) with a loading dose of flecainide (300 mg, or 200 mg if body weight < 70 kg) or propafenone (600 mg, or 450 mg if body weight < 70 kg).

↓

If treatment successful (AF interruption within 6 h, without severe side effects), an echocardiogram and some laboratory tests (thyroid hormones, creatinine, transaminases, kalaemia) must be requested.

↓

If contraindications do not emerge, the drug used in hospital can be prescribed at the same dose for out-of-hospital interruption of AF episodes.

Fig. 1. Practical management of patients suitable for the 'pill-in-the-pocket' approach

References

1. Villani GQ, Rosi A, Piepoli M et al (1990) The efficacy of oral treatment with flecainide for paroxysmal atrial fibrillation: correlation with plasma concentration. G Ital Cardiol 20:564–568
2. Capucci A, Lenzi T, Boriani G et al (1992) Effectiveness of loading oral flecainide for converting recent-onset atrial fibrillation to sinus rhythm in patients without organic heart disease or with only systemic hypertension. Am J Cardiol 70:69–72

3. Botto GL, Bonini W, Broffoni T et al (1994) Regular ventricular rhythms before conversion of recent onset atrial fibrillation to sinus rhythm. Pacing Clin Electrophysiol 17:2114–2117
4. Capucci A, Boriani G, Botto GL et al (1994) Conversion of recent onset atrial fibrillation by a single oral loading dose of propafenone or flecainide. Am J Cardiol 74:503–505
5. Capucci A, Boriani G, Rubino I et al (1994) A controlled study on oral propafenone versus digoxin plus quinidine in converting recent-onset atrial fibrillation to sinus rhythm. Int J Cardiol 43:305–313
6. Boriani G, Capucci A, Lenzi T et al (1995) Propafenone for conversion of recent-onset atrial fibrillation; a controlled comparison between oral loading dose and intravenous administration. Chest 108:355–358
7. Halinen MO, Huttunen M, Paakkinen S et al (1995) Comparison of sotalol with digoxin-quinidine for conversion of acute atrial fibrillation to sinus rhythm (the sotalol-digoxin-quinidine trial). Am J Cardiol 76:495–498
8. Botto GL, Bonini W, Broffoni T et al (1996) Conversion of recent onset atrial fibrillation with single oral dose of propafenone: is in-hospital admission absolutely necessary? Pacing Clin Electrophysiol 19:1939–1943
9. Azpitarte J, Alvarez M, Baun O et al (1997) Value of single oral loading dose of propafenone in converting recent onset atrial fibrillation: results of a randomized, double-blind, controlled study. Eur Heart J 18:1649–1654
10. Boriani G, Biffi M, Capucci A et al (1997) Oral propafenone to convert recent-onset atrial fibrillation in patients with and without underlying heart disease: a randomized, controlled trial. Ann Intern Med 126:621–625
11. Botto GL, Capucci A, Bonini W et al (1997) Conversion of recent onset atrial fibrillation to sinus rhythm using a single loading oral dose of propafenone: comparison of two regimens. Int J Cardiol 58:55–61
12. Botto GL, Bonini W, Broffoni T et al (1998) A randomized, crossover, controlled comparison of oral loading versus intravenous infusion of propafenone in recent-onset atrial fibrillation. Pacing Clin Electrophysiol 21:240–244
13. Blanc JJ, Voinov C, Maarek M for the PARSIFAL Study Group (1999) Comparison of oral loading dose of propafenone and amiodarone for converting recent-onset atrial fibrillation. Am J Cardiol 84:1029–1032
14. Kishikawa T, Maruyoma T, Kaji Y et al (1999) Effects of oral disopyramide on acute-onset atrial fibrillation with concurrent monitoring of serum drug concentration. Int J Cardiol 68:57–62
15. Khan IA (2001) Single oral loading dose of propafenone for pharmacological cardioversion of recent onset atrial fibrillation. J Am Coll Cardiol 37:542–547
16. Capucci A, Villani GQ, Piepoli MF (2003) Reproducible efficacy of loading oral propafenone in restoring sinus rhythm in patients with paroxysmal atrial fibrillation. Am J Cardiol 92:1345–1347
17. Alboni P, Botto GL, Baldi N et al (2004) Outpatient treatment of recent-onset atrial fibrillation with the 'pill-in-the-pocket' approach. N Engl J Med 351:2384–2391

Pharmacological Cardioversion of Atrial Fibrillation: Which Drugs Are Preferred, Class IC or Class III?

N. Baldi, V. A. Russo, L. Di Gregorio, V. Morrone, L. Liconso, G. Polimeni

Introduction

It is accepted that pharmacological treatment of recent-onset atrial fibrillation (AF) in order to reset sinus rhythm restoration, if effective and safe, is doubtless the favourite approach, since it is preferred by patients over electrical cardioversion. Nonetheless, it must be remembered that the placebo effect is very consistent (> 50% at 12–24 h) for AF duration of 48 h or less. Also, class I and class III antiarrhythmic drugs are not equivalent, and should be used according to their electrophysiological and pharmacokinetic properties and to their effect on cardiac inotropism, which must be strictly connected to the clinical condition of the patient. Pharmacological treatment can be carried out either intravenously or per os; and the availability of orally administered drugs has made it possible for some AF patients to treat themselves at home.

There are three main factors that must be taken into consideration in choosing the appropriate drug for AF cardioversion: the duration of the arrhythmia, the clinical context in which it takes place, and the ventricular function. AF duration is also the most important factor influencing the possibility of sinus rhythm restoration.

The present review discusses two types of AF: AF of less than 48-h duration and AF of more than 48-h duration. According to the guidelines of the American College of Chest Physicians, in AF of < 48-h duration, antithrombotic treatment can be avoided due to a low thromboembolic risk linked with cardioversion (< 1%) [1].

Dipartimento di Cardiologia, Ospedale SS. Annunziata, Taranto, Italy

Paroxysmal Atrial Fibrillation (Duration < 48 h)

In this condition, the clinical context and left ventricular function are the most important factors in choosing an antiarrhythmic drug. For lone AF or AF associated with mild hypertension, the class IC antiarrhythmic drugs propafenone and flecainide, administered intravenously, have a priority indication. In patients treated in this manner, the percentage of success is between 85% and 93% for flecainide [2–4] and between 57% and 87% for propafenone [4–6]. The use of these drugs depends not only on their effectiveness, but also on the time until sinus rhythm restoration occurs (generally within 1 h and often during the drug infusion). In our opinion, the above-mentioned drugs are preferred due to their quick action, which in most cases allows the patient to return home after only a short hospital stay. Also, in AF complicating Wolff-Parkinson-White (WPW) syndrome, propafenone and flecainide can be considered as the drugs of choice. Many studies have show that in such patients the two drugs prolong the anterograde and retrograde refractory periods of the accessory pathway – in patients with either a long or a short refractory period – as well as the complete block of conduction via the accessory pathway [7–16].

These drugs considerably slow down the ventricular response during AF with pre-excited ventricular response [7, 9, 12, 15, 16]. Thus, their effects are two-fold: restoration of sinus rhythm and prolongation of pre-excited beat intervals or block of conduction via the accessory pathway, with slowing down of the ventricular rate. It must be emphasised, however, that drugs such as amiodarone, a class III antiarrhythmic drug, are contraindicated because of their depressive actions on nodal conduction, which may speed up the ventricular response during AF and increase the risk of degeneration to ventricular fibrillation [17]. Instead, in recent years, a single oral loading dose of propafenone and flecainide has been proposed [18–20].

The efficacy of such a regimen is indisputable: a percent conversion of 52–82% and 45–63% has been obtained within 3 h after ingestion of flecainide and propafenone, respectively. The aim of this regimen is to allow the patient to continue treatment at home, if it proves to be efficacious and safe. After a pilot study [21], a clinical trial was recently published [22] in which the safety of home treatment was verified. The study also confirmed the efficacy of treatment (success rate 94%), a low incidence of side effects, and a significantly lower number of monthly visits to the emergency room or hospitalisation. Therefore, in a selected, risk-stratified population of patients with recurrent AF, a 'pill-in-the-pocket' approach is feasible and safe, is associated with a low rate of adverse events, mostly non-cardiac, and results in a marked reduction on emergency room visits and hospital admissions. In patients with bundle-branch block or multifascicular block, there is a potential risk of complete paroxysmal atrioventricular block due to drugs that considerably depress conduction through the His-Purkinje system. The H–V interval is actually prolonged by class IC drugs such as flecainide and propafenone [23, 24]. However, amiodarone does not substantially modify the H–V interval, and in some studies it has been proved to be safe for patients with bundle-branch block [25, 26] and efficacious (50–60%, with a mean time to efficacy of 12 h) [27]. Ibutilide, another class III antiarrhythmic drug, may also be used (mean efficacy rate of 30–40% within 90 min) [28, 29] because it does not modify the H–V interval. In the presence of left ventricular dysfunction, the drugs of choice are amiodarone, ibutilide, and dofetilide, since they have been shown to be effective in this clinical setting [29–32]. The most significant potential adverse effect of ibutilide and, with minor misuse, of dofetilide is polymorphic ventricular tachycardia in association with excess Q–T interval. Class I antiarrhythmic drugs are contraindicated due to their specific negative inotropic effect. Amiodarone is the drug of choice in patients with coronary heart disease and after coronary artery by-pass grafting.

Persistent Atrial Fibrillation (Duration > 48 h)

In these patients, the efficacy of antiarrhythmic drugs is progressively lower (not more 50%) with increasing duration of AF. The procedure of choice is external cardioversion with a biphasic waveform (rate of efficacy > 90%) preceded by transoesophageal echocardiography [33] to be sure there are no auricular thrombi. If pharmacological treatment is preferred, the drugs of choice are ibutilide (expected efficacy rate 30–40%, usually within 60 min in a patient population with long-lasting AF and underlying heart disease) [29] and dofetilide; however, these drug are not on the market in Italy. Also the expected efficacy of dofetilide in the treatment of, mainly, long-lasting AF is about 30% [31, 34, 35]. In this clinical context, intravenous amiodarone is probably less effective. However, if a cardioversion attempt has to be made, especially in patients with left ventricular dysfunction, amiodarone is likely to be the most suitable drug. A review of the literature [36–38] by the author revealed the following: of the patients tested, many of whom presented with underlying NYHA III–IV [38] heart disease of 3–75 months (on average) duration, sinus rhythm restoration occurred in 20% administered drug alone and in 51% administered drug and treated with direct current cardioversion, whereas other antiarrhythmic drugs had frequently failed. In spite of the uncertainty surrounding the real efficacy of amiodarone – since the studies were not controlled – it is clear that amiodarone at least does not reduce performance, in contrast to the majority of class I drugs. Also, dofetilide administered per os restores sinus rhythm in about one third of patients with AF > 48 h in a relatively short time (91% within 3 days) in a patient population in which myocardial infarction, congestive heart failure, ischaemic heart disease, valvular heart disease, and dilated and obstructive cardiomyopathy were present in > 50% of patients [39].

In conclusion knowledge of both the physiopathology of the different clinical conditions in which AF can occur, and the haemodynamic and electrophysiologic effects of the various antiarrhythmic drugs must be used in order to choose the most appropriate drug for restoring sinus rhythm.

References

1. Singer DE, Albers GW, Dalen JE et al (2004) Antithrombotic therapy in atrial fibrillation. The Seventh ACCP Conference on antithrombotic and thrombolytic therapy. Chest 126:429S–456S
2. Borgeat A, Goy JJ, Maendly R et al (1986) Flecainide versus quinidine for conversion of atrial fibrillation to sinus rhythm. Am J Cardiol 58:496–498
3. Suttorp MJ, Kingma JH, Lie-A-Hauel et al (1989) Intravenous flecainide versus verapamil for acute conversion of paroxysmal atrial fibrillation or flutter to sinus rhythm. Am J Cardiol 63:693–696
4. Suttorp MJ, Kingma JH, Jessuron EK et al (1990) The value of class IC antiarrhythmic drugs for acute conversion of paroxysmal atrial fibrillation or flutter to sinus rhythm. J Am Coll Cardiol 16:1722–1727
5. Bianconi L, Boccadamo R, Pappalardo A et al (1989) Effectiveness of intravenous propafenone for conversion of atrial fibrillation and flutter of recent onset. Am J Cardiol 64:335–338
6. Bertini G, Conti A, Fradella G et al (1990) Propafenone versus amiodarone in field treatment of primary atrial tachydysrhythmias. J Emerg Med 8:15–20
7. Neuss M, Buss J, Schlepper M et al (1983) Effects of flecainide on electrophysiological properties of accessory pathways in the Wolff-Parkinson-White syndrome. Eur Heart J 4:347–353
8. Hellenstrand KJ, Nathan AW, Bexton RS et al (1984) Electrophysiologic effects of flecainide acetate on sinus node function anomalous, atrioventricular connections and pacemaker threshold. Am J Cardiol 53(Suppl B):30–38
9. Breithardt G, Borggrefe M, Wiebringhaus E et al (1984) Effect of propafenone in the Wolff-Parkinson-White syndrome: electrophysiological findings and long-term follw-up. Am J Cardiol 54:29D–39D
10. Kim SS, Lae R, Ruffy R (1986) Treatment of paroxysmal supraventricular tachycardia with flecainide acetate. Am J Cardiol 58:80–85
11. Shen EN, Keung E, Huicke E et al (1986) Intravenous propafenone for termination of reentrant supraventricular tachycardia. A placebo-controlled, randomized, double-blind, cross-over study. Ann Intern Med 105:655–659
12. Hammil SC, Mc Laran CJ, Wood DL et al (1987) Double blind study of intravenous propafenone for paroxysmal supraventricular re-entrant tachycardia. J Am Coll Cardiol 9:1364–1368
13. Ludmer PL, Mc Cowan NE, Antman EM et al (1987) Efficacy of propafenone in Wolff-Parkinson-White syndrome: electrophysiologic findings and long-term fol-

low-up. J Am Coll Cardiol 9:1357–1363
14. Dubuc M, Kus T, Campa MA et al (1989) Electrophysiologic effects of intravenous propafenone in Wolff-Parkinson-White syndrome. Am Heart J 117:370–376
15. Kappenberger LJ, Fromer MA, Shenasa M et al (1985) Evaluation of flecainide acetate in rapid atrial fibrillation complicating Wolff-Parkinson-White syndrome. Clin Cardiol 8:321–326
16. Manolis AS, Salen DN, Estes NAM et al (1989) Electrophysiologic effects, efficacy and tolerance of class IC antiarrhythmic agent in Wolff-Parkinson-White syndrome. Am J Cardiol 63:746–750
17. Vitale P, Stefano R, Auricchio A (1986) Possibile pericolosità dell'amiodarone per via endovenosa rapida nel corso di tachicardia da rientro in soggetti con Wolff-Parkinson-White. G It Cardiol 16:969–974
18. Capucci A, Lenzi T, Boriani G et al (1992) Effectiveness of loading oral flecainide for converting recent-onset atrial fibrillation to sinus rhythm in patients without organic heart disease or with only systemic hypertension. Am J Cardiol 70:69–72
19. Capucci A, Boriani G, Rubino I et al (1994) A controlled study on oral propafenone versus digoxin plus quinidine in converting recent-onset atrial fibrillation to sinus rhythm. Int J Cardiol 43:305–313
20. Capucci A, Boriani G, Botto GL et al (1994) Conversion of recent-onset atrial fibrillation by a single oral loading dose of propafenone or flecainide. Am J Cardiol 74:503–505
21. Baldi N, Russo VA, Morrone V et al (1998) Home treatment of recent-onset atrial Fibrillation with a single oral dose of flecainide or propafenone: an efficacious, reproducible and safe procedure. G It Cardiol 29 (Suppl 5):380–383
22. Alboni P, Botto GL, Baldi N et al (2004) Out patients treatment of recent-onset atrial fibrillation with the 'pill in the pocket' approach. N Engl J Med 351:2384–2391
23. Hellenstrand KJ, Bexton RS, Nathan AW et al (1982) Acute electrophysiological effects of flecainide acetate on cardiac conduction and refractoriness in man. Br Heart J 48:140–148
24. Pristowsky EN, Heger JJ, Chilson DA et al (1984) Antiarrhythmic and electrophysiologic effect of oral propafenone. Am J Cardiol 54:26D–28D
25. Benaim R, Uzan C (1978) Les effects antiarythmiques de l'amiodarone injectable (à propos de 153 cas). Rev Med 19:1959–1963
26. Morady F, Scheinman MM, Shen E et al (1983) Intravenous amiodarone in the acute treatment of recurrent symptomatic ventricular tachycardia. Am J Cardiol 51:156–159
27. Galve E, Rius T, Ballester R et al (1996) Intravenous amiodarone in treatment of recent-onset atrial fibrillation:results of a randomized, controlled study. J Am Coll Cardiol 27:1079–1082
28. Vos MA, Golitsyn RS, Stangl K et al (1998) Superiority of ibutilide (a new class III agent) over DL-sotalol in converting atrial flutter and atrial fibrillation. The Ibutilide-Sotalol Comparator Study Group. Heart 79:568–575
29. Stambler BS, Wood MA, Ellenbogen KA et al (1996) Efficacy and safety of repeated doses of ibutilide for rapid conversion of atrial fibrillation and flutter. Ibutilide Repeat Dose Study Investigators. Circulation 94:1613–1621
30. Deedwania PC, Singh BN, Ellenbogen K et al (1998) Spontaneos conversion and maintenance of sinus rhythm by amiodarone in patients with heart failure and atrial fibrillation: observations from the veterans affairs congestive heart failure survival trial of antiarrhythmic therapy (CHF-STAT). Circulation 98:2574–2579
31. Falk RH, Pollak A, Singh SN et al (1997) Intravenous dofetilide, a class III

antiarrhythmic agent, for termination of sustained atrial fibrillation or flutter. J Am Coll Cardiol 29:385–390

32. Top-Pedersen, Moller M, Bloch-Thomsen PE et al (1999) Dofetilide in patients with congestive heart failure and left ventricular dysfunction. Danish Investigations of Arrhythmias and Mortality on Dofetilide Study Group. N Engl J Med 341:857–865
33. Klein AL, Grimm RA, Murray RD et al (2001) Use of trans-oesophageal echocardiography to guide cardioversion in patients with atrial fibrillation. N Engl J Med 344:1411–1420
34. Norgaard BL, Wachtell K, Christensen PD et al (1999) Efficacy and safety of intravenously administered dofetilide in acute termination of atrial fibrillation and flutter: a multicenter, randomized, double-blind, placebo-controlled trial. Danish Dofetilide in Atrial Fibrillation and Flutter Study Group. Am Heart J 137:1062–1069
35. Lindeboon JE, Kingma JH, Crjins HJ et al (2000) Efficacy and safety of intravenous dofetilide for rapid termination of atrial fibrillation and atial flutter. Am J Cardiol 85:1031–1033
36. Horowitz LN, Spielman SR, Greenspan AM et al (1985) Use of amiodarone in the treatment of persitent and paroxysmal atrial fibrillation resistant to quinidine therapy. J Am Coll Cardiol 6:1402–1407
37. Blevius RD, Kerin NZ, Benaderet D et al (1987) Amiodarone in the management of refractory atrial fibrillation. Arch Intern Med 147:1401–1404
38. Gosselink ATM, Crijns HJ, Van Gelder IC et al (1992) Low-dose amiodarone for maintenance of sinus rhythm after cadioversion of atrial fibrillation or flutter. JAMA 267:3289–3293
39. Singh S, Zoble RG, Yellen L et al (2000) Efficacy and safety of oral dofetilide in converting to and maintaining sinus rhythm in patients with chronic atrial fibrillation or atrial flutter: the Symptomatic Atrial Fibrillation Investigative Research on Dofetilide (SAFIRE-D) Study. Circulation 102:2385–2390

Early Recurrences of Atrial Fibrillation: How To Predict Them?

G.L. Botto, M. Luzi, F. Ruffa, M.G. Gorgoglione, G. Ferrari

Introduction

Atrial fibrillation (AF) is the most common sustained tachyarrhythmia encountered in clinical practice [1], causing the highest number of days of hospitalisation for arrhythmia admission in the United States [2]. It affects more than 2.2 million individuals in the USA: the overall prevalence in the adult population is 0.4%, and its incidence increases with age (up to 8–10% of persons older than 80 years) and with the presence of heart disease [3–5]. The AFFIRM study demonstrated equivalent survival between patients treated using rate control versus rhythm control strategy [6]; however, converting the rhythm electrically and preventing recurrences with drugs remains a standard approach to reducing symptoms [1]. With all of these options, embolic risk stratification and proper anticoagulation strategies are required for each patient [1, 6, 7].

Electrical cardioversion (ECV) is currently the most effective way to convert persistent AF to sinus rhythm (SR), with success rates of approximately 75–95% with the use respectively of monophasic or biphasic defibrillators [8–10]. Unfortunately, because of the high recurrence rate, no more than 40–50% of patients maintain SR for 6 months or more with anti-arrhythmic drug prophylaxis different from amiodarone [11]. Thus, the main limitation on cardioversion success is not 'technical failure' – impossibility of restoring SR – but recurrence of the arrhythmia, which may occur in different time frames following the procedure.

Department of Cardiology, Sant' Anna Hospital, Como, Italy

Time Course and Definition of Recurrence of AF

The aetiology of reinitiation of AF after external ECV is obscure and its incidence is unknown. It can occur in a significant proportion of patients following successful ECV using either internal [12, 13] or external methods [14]. It is a phenomenon that was only described in the late 1990s, in part because the increasing use of internal ECV [11], the catheters for which enable recording of atrial electrograms, and the employment of atrial defibrillator devices [12], which make possible the analysis of stored atriograms, provide the motive and the means for its study. The recurrence phenomena have acquired their own acronyms: recurrence may occur in a very early phase (minutes) after electrical shock, and this is now called IRAF (immediate recurrence of AF); it may occur in an early phase (first 24–48 h to 5–7 days; ERAF, or early recurrence of AF); or it may occur weeks to months after the successful procedure (LRAF, or late recurrence of AF).

In a retrospective study of 85 patients with AF, the functional and pharmacological variables which could possibly influence the long-term outcome after first ECV were analysed [15]. Multivariate analysis confirmed the duration of the treated episode and age below 75 years as prognostic factors that predict persistence of SR 100 days after successful ECV, whereas echocardiographic parameters and the presence of organic heart disease played no role. The phenomena of IRAF and ERAF are the most difficult to characterise because they would require continuous monitoring of an AF patient's cardiac rhythm, and few studies are available concerning this. However, understanding these phenomena and the potential factors affecting them may improve the efficacy of maintaining SR in the long run. For instance, IRAF can occur within seconds after ECV and may be difficult to distinguish from shock failure. In a small study, 27 patients who experienced unsuccessful ECV were treated with a 1-month load of amiodarone, after which ECV was repeated. Of the patients in whom the initial ECV failed due to technical failure, only 31% were in SR at 1 month, compared with 91% for those with initial failure due to IRAF [16].

Early Recurrences of AF

The phenomenon of ERAF following successful ECV is a clinical setting in which two important concepts are implicated and may strongly interact. The first is that an increasingly recognised and growing number of patients have AF initiated, and possibly maintained, by an ectopic focus of repetitive atrial activity [17]. The second is that AF itself causes changes in cellular electrophysiology that, at least in animal models, have the effect of further increasing the tendency to fibrillation [18], and there is a reversal of this electrophysiological remodelling after a certain period of SR [19]. The first of these two concepts relates to the triggers for initiation of the arrhythmia and the second to the myocardial substrate predisposing to and maintaining the arrhythmia. However, the extent to which ERAF is due either to enhanced frequency of atrial ectopic activity as potential triggers or to enhanced vulnerability of the remodelled, recently defibrillated atrium to the effects of the atrial ectopy remains uncertain.

Several authors have reported premature atrial beats causing ERAF. Premature atrial beats initiated ERAF in 91% of cases after internal ECV [20], and a short interval predicted an early relapse in patients with AF recurrences [21]. A recurrence rate of up to 27% within the first minute after external ECV has been reported. An high incidence of premature atrial beats, with particular specific sequences such as long–short, were responsible for 70% of cases of ERAF after external ECV [22].

It has been demonstrated that prolonged atrial pacing in goats at rates sufficiently rapid to produce AF causes reversible electrophysiological and structural changes in the atria. Whereas during the control condition no sustained AF could be induced, after several days to weeks of rapid pacing in these animals, AF had become sustained.

In the study of Wijffels et al. [18] the refractory period was measured at multiple sites by programmed electrical stimulation. AF was produced by burst pacing (1 s, 50 Hz). In the normal goat, electrically induced AF lasted only for a short time and terminated promptly within a few seconds. After the baseline study was completed, the animals were connected to an external automatic atrial fibrillator. The device detected spontaneous cardioversion of AF and delivered a burst of stimuli to promptly reinduce the arrhythmia. Within the first 24 h of AF, both the duration and the rate of the arrhythmia increased significantly and AF cycle length shortened progressively until after about 4–6 days a new steady state was reached. The most important atrial parameter of AF-induced electrical remodelling is the refractory period. During control, early premature beats did not induce any arrhythmia. After few hours of AF, the atrial refractory period was shortened and a premature stimulus was followed by a short run of rapid atrial responses. Twenty-four hours of AF further shortened the atrial refractory period and now early premature beats triggered paroxysms of AF. Moreover, during control, the refractory period showed a short-term rate adaptation to pacing intervals. After hours of AF, the relationship between refractory period and rate become reversed, so that instead of lengthening at slow rate, the refractory period actually shortens [18]. The loss of the physiological prolongation of the refractory period in response to a sudden decrease in rate has also been observed in other studies [23, 24].

In this condition, the physiological normalisation of atrial refractoriness after SR restoration was lost, and it was recovered only after several days of stable sinus rhythm [19]. Of note is the finding that the time course of electrical remodelling parallels the timing when likelihood of recurrence is highest [21].

Novel Techniques to Predict Recurrences of AF

Prediction of the outcome of electrical cardioversion is not perfect: clinical and laboratory variables have not always been predictive [15]. This constitutes the background of the need for new parameters that can identify patients who will have recurrence after successful ECV, and distinguish them from those that will not.

Changes in autonomic milieu probably play a role in the occurrence of relapse into AF. Lombardi et al. [25] demonstrated increased sympathetic tone and decreased vagal modulation of the sinus node in patients prone to ERAF. The authors analysed short-term heart rate variability in 93 patients with persistent AF and on chronic amiodarone treatment, after restoration of SR by ECV. Patients with ERAF (25/93, 27%) were characterised by a greater LF/HF ratio than those in SR. In univariate analysis no clinical parameters distinguished the two groups, and no correlation was observed between LF/HF ratio and late recurrences.

Bollmann et al. [26] analysed the meaning of AF frequency obtained from the surface ECG for prediction of early arrhythmia relapse in patients undergoing internal ECV of persistent AF. AF relapse occurred in 11 out of 19 (58%) patients, but in 7 out of 8 (88%) patients with a high fibrillatory frequency (≥ 7 Hz). A high fibrillatory frequency reflects a high AF complexity (that is, the number of simultaneous wandering wavelets) [27] and correlates inversely to the refractory period [28].

AF is an irregularly irregular (random) heart beat [29], and the randomness of ventricular rhythm is primarily a consequence of the inherent randomness of atrial activity. However, controversy exists as to whether the ventricular rhythm in AF is truly random, and some investigators using a variety of mathematical techniques have shown that a certain degree of clustering may be present [30]. Everett et al. [31] confirmed in a dog model that AF is characterised by varying degrees of organisation, and demonstrated that the efficacy of electrical shock in restoring SR is increased when shocks are delivered during periods of high AF organisation. Based on this premise, Van den Berg et al. [32] demonstrated in humans that ECV is more effective in restoring SR in AF patients with clustering than in patients in whom no clustering is apparent in plots obtained from Holter monitoring. In addition, the degree of clustering appears to be predictive of the overall outcome of ECV: the higher the degree of clustering, the higher the likelihood of SR at follow-up.

Conclusions

The heterogeneous nature of AF dictates that a variety of treatment modalities should be used to manage this disease. Recent studies have shown that strategy of rate control is not inferior to a strategy of rhythm control in terms of mortality [6]. However, in highly symptomatic patients restoration of SR is still desirable, and selection of patients with a high likelihood of clinically effective ECV remains critical.

The therapeutic efficacy of this treatment modality is likely to be affected by early recurrences of AF noted soon after cardioversion. The mechanism underlying early recurrence of AF is unclear for the majority of patients, but is probably multifactorial. Contributing factors may include complex electrophysiological remodelling which strongly interacts with triggering factors such as atrial ectopic beats, both probably modulated by the autonomic nervous system.

Several clinical factors and laboratory variables that are predictive of poor arrhythmia outcome after ECV have been identified, but their efficacy in the clinical setting is not completely satisfactory [15]. Novel and simple techniques are expected to permit identification of patients likely to experience a better outcome of ECV of AF.

Future larger studies are warranted to establish further the potential clinical role of these new techniques.

References

1. Anonymous (2001) ACC/AHA/ESC Guidelines for the management of patients with atrial fibrillation: executive summary. J Am Colls Cardiol 38:1231–1265
2. Bialy D, Lehmann MH, Schumacher DN et al (1992) Hospitalization for arrhythmias in the United States: importance of atrial fibrillation. J Am Coll Cardiol 19:41A (abs)
3. Kannel WB, Wolf PA (1992) Epidemiology of atrial fibrillation. In: Falk RH, Podrid PJ (eds) Atrial fibrillation: mechanisms and management. Raven, New York, pp 81–92
4. Brand FN, Abbot RD, Kannel WB et al (1985) Characteristics and prognosis of lone atrial fibrillation. J Am Med Assoc 254:3449–3516
5. Feinberg WM, Blackshear JL, Laupacis A et al (1995) Prevalence, age distribution, and gender of patients with atrial fibrillation. Arch Intern Med 155:469–473
6. The Atrial Fibrillation Follow-up Investigation in Rhythm Management (AFFIRM) Investigators (2002) A comparison of rate control and rhythm control in patients with atrial fibrillation. N Engl J Med 347:1825–1833

7. Laupacis A, Albers G, Dalen J et al (2004) Antithrombotic therapy in atrial fibrillation. Chest 126:429S-456S
8. Lown B, Perlroth MG, Bey SK et al (1963) Cardioversion of atrial fibrillation. A report on the treatment of 65 episodes in 59 patients. N Engl J Med 269:325–331
9. Botto GL, Politi A, Bonini W et al (1999) External cardioversion of atrial fibrillation: role of paddle position on technical efficacy and energy requirements. Heart 82:726–730
10. Mittal S, Ayati S, Stein KM et al (2000) Transthoracic cardioversion of atrial fibrillation. Comparison of rectilinear biphasic versus damped sine wave monophasic shocks. Circulation 101:1282–1287
11. Roy D, Talajic M, Dorian P et al (2000) Amiodarone to prevent recurrence of atrial fibrillation. Canadian Trial of Atrial Fibrillation Investigators. N Engl J Med 342:913–920
12. Timmermans C, Rodriguez LM, Smeets JLRM et al (1998) Immediate reinitiation of atrial fibrillation following internal defibrillation. J Cardiovasc Electrophysiol 9:122–128
13. Wellens HJJ, Lau CP, Luderiz B et al for the Metrix Investigators (1998) Atrioverter, an implantable device for the treatment of atrial fibrillation. Circulation 98:1651–1656
14. Bianconi L, Mennuni M, Lukic V et al (1996) Effects of oral propafenone administration before electrical cardioversion of chronic atrial fibrillation: a placebo-controlled study. J Am Coll Cardiol 28:700–706
15. Daytschaever M, Haerynck F, Tevernier R et al (1998) Factors influencing long-term persistence of sinus rhythm after first electrical cardioversion of atrial fibrillation. Pacing Clin Electrophysiol 21: 284–287
16. Van Noord T, Van Gelder IC, Schoonderwoerd BA et al (2000) Immediate reinitiation of atrial fibrillation after electrical cardioversion predicts subsequent pharmacologic and electrical conversion to sinus rhythm on amiodarone. Am J Cardiol 86:1384–1385
17. Jaïs P, Haïssaguerre M, Shah DC et al (1997) A focal source of atrial fibrillation treated by discrete radiofrequency ablation. Circulation 95:572–576
18. Wijffels MCEF, Kirchhof CJHJ, Dorland R et al (1995) Atrial fibrillation begets atrial fibrillation: a study in awake chronically instrumented goats. Circulation 92:1954–1968
19. Yu WC, Lee SH, Tai CT et al (1999) Reversal of atrial electrical remodeling following cardioversion of long standing atrial fibrillation in man. Cardiovasc Res 42:470–476
20. Tse HF, Lau CP, Ayers GM (1999) Incidence and mode of onset of early reinitiation of atrial fibrillation following internal cardioversion, and its prevention by intravenous sotalol. Heart 82:319–324
21. Tieleman RG, Van Gelder IC, Crijns HJGM et al (1998) Early recurrence of atrial fibrillation after electrical cardioversion: a result of fibrillation-induced electrical remodeling of the atria? J Am Coll Cardiol 31:167–173
22. Gorenek B, Kudaiberdieva G, Goktekin O et al (2003) Long-short sequences may predict immediate recurrence of atrial fibrillation after external cardioversion of atrial fibrillation. Europace 5:11–16
23. Goette A, Honeycutt C, Langberg JJ (1996) Electrical remodeling in atrial fibrillation. Time course and mechanism. Circulation 94:2968–2974
24. Tieleman RG, De Langen CDJ, Van Gelder IC et al (1997) Verapamil reduces tachycardia-induced electrical remodeling of the atria. Circulation 95:1945–1953

25. Lombardi F, Colombo A, Basilico B et al (2001) Heart rate variability and early recurrence of atrial fibrillation after electrical cardioversion. J Am Coll Cardiol 37:157–162
26. Bollmann A, Mende M, Neugebauer A et al (2002) Atrial fibrillatory frequency predicts atrial defibrillation threshold and early arrhythmia recurrence in patients undergoing internal cardioversion of persistent atrial fibrillation. Pacing Clin Electrophysiol 25:1179–1184
27. Konings KT, Kirchhof CJ, Smeets JR et al (1994) High-density mapping of electrically induced atrial fibrillation in humans. Circulation 89:1665–1680
28. Capucci A, Biffi M, Boriani G et al (1995) Dynamic electrophysiological behaviour of human atria during paroxysmal atrial fibrillation. Circulation 92:1193–1202
29. Hering HE (1903) Analyse des Pulsus irregularis perpetuus. Prager Med Wochenschr 28:377–381
30. Rawles JM, Rowland E (1986) Is the pulse in atrial fibrillation irregularly irregular? Br Heart J 56:4–11
31. Everett TH, Moorman JR, Kok LC et al (2001) Assessment of global atrial fibrillation organization to optimize timing of atrial fibrillation. Circulation 103:2857–2861
32. Van den Berg MP, Van Noord T, Brouwer J et al (2004) Clustering of RR intervals predicts effective electrical cardioversion for atrial fibrillation. J Cardiovasc Electrophysiol 15:1027–1033

Dronedarone for Prevention of Atrial Fibrillation: An Unfulfilled Promise?

A. Capucci, G.Q. Villani, D. Aschieri, M. Piepoli

The prophylactic treatment for many patients with atrial fibrillation (AF) remains unsatisfactory. The ideal anti-arrhythmic drug for the prevention of recurrences of both AF after cardioversion and paroxysmal AF is still a long way off. AF has an high propensity to recur, and only one-quarter of patients who undergo successful cardioversion remain in sinus rhythm at 1 year if no additional therapy is used [1].

Since the publication of studies documenting that certain class I drugs may increase mortality in high-risk post-infarction patients, basic science and clinical studies have focused on class III anti-arrhythmic drugs. Class III agents remain the focus of drug development efforts because they lack negative haemodynamic effects, affect both atrial and ventricular tissue, and can be administered as either parenteral or oral preparations. Amiodarone is one of the most effective, and is associated with a comparatively low risk of drug-induced pro-arrhythmia, probably due to its multiple pharmacological actions on cardiac ion channels and receptors. However, amiodarone is associated with significant extra-cardiac side effects, and this has driven development of amiodarone analogues [2].

Developers of newer anti-arrhythmic agents have focused on identifying anti-arrhythmic medications with the following characteristics: appropriate modification of the arrhythmia substrate, suppression of arrhythmia triggers, efficacy in pathological tissues and states, positive rate dependency, appropriate pharmacokinetics, equally effective oral and parenteral formulations of similar efficacy in arrhythmias and their surrogates, few side effects, positive frequency blocking actions, and cardiac-selective ion channel block-

Cardiology Department, Guglielmo da Saliceto Hospital, Piacenza, Italy

ade. New and investigational agents include azimilide, dofetilide, ersentilide, ibutilide, tedisamil, and trecetilide [3].

Dronedarone is one of a number of analogues that derive from the currently most successful class III anti-arrhythmic drug, amiodarone [4]. This review describes some new studies providing insight into the mechanism of its action and the latest developments in the clinical usage of this drug.

Electrophysiological Properties

Dronedarone is a non-iodinated amiodarone derivative that inhibits Na^+, K^+, and Ca^{2+} currents. It is a potent inhibitor of the acetylcholine-activated K^+ current from atrial and sinoatrial nodal tissue, and inhibits the rapid delayed rectifier more potently than slow and inward rectifier K^+ currents and inhibits the L-type calcium current. It is also an antagonist at α- and β-adrenoceptors and, unlike amiodarone, has little effect at thyroid receptors. It is more potent than amiodarone in inhibiting arrhythmias and death in animal models of ischaemia- and reperfusion-induced arrhythmias [4].

Gautier et al. [5] studied the electrophysiological properties of dronedarone on the action potential (AP) and contraction of papillary muscle and on membrane ionic currents, Ca^{2+} transient, and shortening of ventricular cells of the guinea pig heart. The effects of dronedarone on AP durations (APDs) at different percentages of repolarisation were not significantly changed, except for a slight decrease in APD_{30} and APD_{50} at the highest concentration. In isolated ventricular myocytes, dronedarone inhibited rapidly activating delayed rectifier K^+ current (I_{Kr}), slowly activating delayed-rectifier K^+ current (I_{Ks}), and voltage-dependent and time-, frequency-, or use-independent and inward rectifier potassium current (I_{K1}). Moreover, dronedarone blocked L-type Ca^{2+} current ($I_{Ca(L)}$) in a use- and frequency-dependent manner. Simultaneously with these electrophysiological effects, dronedarone reduced contraction amplitudes of papillary muscle and decreased Ca^{2+} transient and shortening of ventricular myocytes. The results show that dronedarone is a multi-channel blocker because it decreases dV/dt_{max} (I_{Na}), $I_{Ca(L)}$, I_{Kr}, I_{Ks}, and I_{K1} very similarly to amiodarone in cardiac ventricle, despite the absence of iodine in its molecular structure.

Sun et al. [6] compared the acute and chronic electrophysiological effects of dronedarone and amiodarone in isolated rabbit atrial muscle by microelectrode techniques. Four-week oral treatment with dronedarone or amiodarone increased the action potential duration (APD_{90}) and effective refractory period with an inverse rate dependency. In contrast to this, acute superfusion with 10 μM dronedarone or amiodarone decreased APD_{90}, the effective refractory period, and the maximum upstroke slope of the action potential.

However, dronedarone can not be considered a simple copy of amiodarone. Varro et al. [7] studied the electrophysiological effects of dronedarone after chronic and acute administration in dog Purkinje fibres, papillary muscle, and isolated ventricular myocytes, and compared them with those of amiodarone by applying conventional microelectrode and patch-clamp techniques. Chronic treatment with dronedarone, unlike chronic administration of amiodarone, did not significantly lengthen the QTc interval of the electrocardiogram or the APD in papillary muscle. After chronic oral treatment with dronedarone, a small but significant use-dependent V_{max} block was noticed, while after chronic amiodarone administration a strong use-dependent V_{max} depression was observed.

Acute superfusion of dronedarone, like that of amiodarone, moderately lengthened APD in papillary muscle but shortened it in Purkinje fibres. Both dronedarone and amiodarone superfusion reduced the incidence of early and delayed in Purkinje fibres. The authors showed that after acute administration dronedarone exhibits effects on cardiac electrical activity similar to those of amiodarone, but it lacks the 'amiodarone-like' chronic electrophysiological characteristics.

Pantos et al. [8] investigated the effects of dronedarone and amiodarone administered for 2 weeks in normal and thyroxine-treated animals on plasma thyroid hormones and the possible consequences on the response of the heart to ischaemia. Amiodarone resulted in increased T_4, T_4/T_3, and rT_3, whereas dronedarone did not alter the thyroid hormone profile in normal animals. In thyroxine-treated animals, amiodarone increased the T_4/T_3 ratio but T_4, T_3, and rT_3 levels were not altered. Baseline functional parameters and ischaemic contracture were not changed by amiodarone and/or dronedarone in either normal or thyroxine-treated hearts.

Clinical Studies

At present three clinical studies have demonstrated that the drug is safe and effective for the maintenance of normal sinus rhythm in patients with atrial fibrillation (AF) or atrial flutter (AFl).

In the Dronedarone Atrial Fibrillation Study After Electrical Cardioversion (DAFNE), a phase IIb clinical trial, a dose of 800 mg dronedarone per day was established as effective and safe for the prevention of AF relapses after cardioversion [9]. Patients with persistent AF were randomly allocated to receive a daily dose of 800 mg, 1200 mg, or 1600 mg dronedarone or placebo. The main analysis was conducted on 199 of 270 patients who entered the maintenance phase following pharmacological cardioversion or, if that was unsuccessful, DC cardioversion. Within a 6-month follow-up period, the time to AF relapse increased in the group receiving dronedarone 800 mg, with a median of 60 days compared to 5.3 days in the placebo group [relative risk reduction 55% (95% CI, 28 to 72%) $P = 0.001$]. No significant effect was seen at higher doses. Spontaneous conversion to sinus rhythm on dronedarone occurred in 6–15% of patients ($P = 0.026$). There were no proarrhythmic reactions. Drug-induced QT prolongation was only noticed in the 1600 mg group. Premature drug discontinuation affected 23% of subjects given 1600 mg dronedarone versus 4% on 800 mg and was mainly due to gastrointestinal side effects. No evidence of thyroid, ocular, or pulmonary toxicity was found.

Recently the results of two phase III trials were reported at the 2004 European Society of Cardiology Congress [10]. In the European Trial In Atrial Fibrillation or Flutter Patients Receiving Dronedarone for the Maintenance of Sinus Rhythm (EURIDIS) and the American–Australian Trial With Dronedarone in Atrial Fibrillation or Flutter Patients for the Maintenance of Sinus Rhythm (ADONIS), dronedarone administered at a dose of 400 mg twice daily was effective in preventing both symptomatic and asymptomatic recurrences of AF or AFl and had a safety profile similar to that of placebo. Patients enrolled in EURIDIS and ADONIS were men and women aged > 21 years who had been in sinus rhythm for ≥ 1 h at the time of randomisation and had experienced at least one electrocardiogram (ECG)-documented episode of AF/AFl during the previous 3 months. After a screening period (pre-trial day 6 to day 1), patients in both trials were randomised 2:1 (dronedarone:placebo) to receive either 400 mg twice daily of dronedarone or matching placebo twice daily for 12 months. A total of 1237 patients were enrolled in both trials, 828 randomised to dronedarone and 409 to placebo.

The primary endpoint of both trials – time from randomisation to first documented AF/AFl occurrence – was defined as an episode lasting ≥ / = 10 minutes as indicated by 2 consecutive 12-lead ECGs or trans-telephonic electrocardiographic monitoring (TTEM) tracings recorded approximately 10 min apart, with both showing AF/AFl.

Both trials showed a significant decrease in the risk of recurrence of AF/AFl (Table 1). In EURIDIS, the median time to first recurrence of AF/AFl was 2.3 times longer in the dronedarone group than in the placebo group, with a 22% lower risk of a recurrence during the study. In ADONIS, there was an almost three-fold increase in the median time to recurrence with dronedarone and a 28% reduction in the risk of AF/AFl recurrence. However, the arrhythmic recurrence was quite high (around 75% for placebo and 65% for dronedarone in EURIDIS), but it must be remembered that the trials enrolled patients with different types of symptoms; there might be differences according to duration of symptoms and also between patients with AF and AFl.

Table 1. Patients with adjudicated first recurrence of atrial fibrillation (AF)/flutter (AFl)

	Placebo	Dronedarone	RR	95% CI	*P* value*
EURIDIS					
Patients with AF/AFl	155	272	0.78	0.64–0.95	0.0318
Median time to relapse (days)	41	96			
ADONIS					
Patients with AF/AFl	146	246	0.72	0.59-0.89	0.0017
Median time to relapse (days)	58	158			

*Log-rank test

There were three subgroups of the primary endpoint prespecified for analysis, according to whether patients had cardioversion within 5 days of randomisation, prior amiodarone treatment, or structural heart disease. All three subanalyses showed the benefit of dronedarone over placebo in all groups. Furthermore, fewer patients had symptomatic recurrence of AF/AFl with dronedarone in EURIDIS ($P = 0.055$) and ADONIS ($P = 0.021$). The other secondary endpoint of both trials, mean ventricular rate during AF/AFl at first recorded recurrence (12-lead ECG or TTEM), was significantly reduced in both trials (Table 2).

Table 2. Ventricular rate (bpm) at first recurrence of atrial fibrillation

Ventricular rate (bpm)	Placebo	Dronedarone	*P* value
EURIDIS			
Mean	117.5	102.3	0.0001
SD	29.1	24.7	
Min–max	70–204	53–173	
ADONIS			
Mean	116.6	104.6	0.001
SD	31.9	27.1	
Min–max	56–226	57–173	

bpm beats per minute, *SD* standard deviation

The incidence of adverse events was similar in the dronedarone and placebo groups (Table 3). In addition, there was no evidence of pro-arrhythmia in the patients receiving dronedarone; in particular, no case of torsades de pointes was reported during the 12-month follow-up period. There was also no evidence of amiodarone-related toxicities (thyroid or pulmonary). However, few data are available on the side effects with longer follow-up. Some studies have suggested that dronedarone is an antagonist of the thyroid hormone receptor-α_1, and experimental data have indicated that it may be associated with more side effects on lung tissue than amiodarone. These may not be of clinical importance, but they should be investigated long term, along with any ophthalmological and liver-related side effects. Another question that remains unanswered is how safe dronedarone is in patients with depressed left ventricular ejection fraction. One trial in the phase III development program, the Anti-arrhythmic Trial with Dronedarone in Moderate-to-Severe Congestive Heart Failure Evaluating Morbidity Decrease (ANDROMEDA), carried out in Europe and evaluating high-risk patients, was stopped in January 2003 after an interim safety analysis identified a potential increased risk of heart failure death in the dronedarone group.

Table 3. EURIDIS and ADONIS pooled tolerability and safety data

Incidence of treatment-emergent adverse events (TEAEs)	Placebo ($n = 409$)	Dronedarone 800 mg ($n = 828$)
Any adverse events (%)	65.8	69.8
Any serious adverse events (%)	24.4	19.8
Deaths (%)	0.7	1.0
Permanent drug discontinuations following TEAE (%)	7.1	9.7

Future Perspectives

The results of another phase III trial with dronedarone, the Efficacy and Safety of Dronedarone for the Control of Ventricular Rate (ERATO), in patients with AF/AFl are expected to be reported in 2005. In addition, a phase II study in patients with AF is ongoing in Japan.

Results of a pilot study of dronedarone in patients with an implantable cardioverter defibrillator (ICD) and an indication for adjunctive antiarrhythmic therapy were reported at the 2004 annual meeting of the Heart

Rhythm Society. Dronedarone at doses below 2000 mg/day was found to be safe, did not cause deterioration in ICD function, and reduced the need for ICD therapy. However, further clinical studies are required before we have a definitive answer to whether dronedarone has real advantages over amiodarone and other amiodarone analogues in this clinical setting.

References

1. Coplen SE, Antman EM, Berlin JA et al (1990) Efficacy and safety of quinidine therapy for maintenance of sinus rhythm after cardioversion: a meta-analysis of randomized control trials. Circulation 82:1106–1116
2. Khan MH (2004) Oral class III antiarrhythmics: what is new? Curr Opin Cardiol Jan 19:47–51
3. Camm AJ (2000) Clinical differences between the newer antiarrhythmic agents. Europace 1:C16–C22
4. Doggrell SA, Hancox JC (2004) Dronedarone: an amiodarone analogue. Expert Opin Investig Drugs 13:415–426
5. Gautier P, Guillemare E, Marion A (2003) Electrophysiologic characterization of dronedarone in guinea pig ventricular cells. J Cardiovasc Pharmacol 41:191–202
6. Sun W, Sarma JS, Singh BN (2002) Chronic and acute effects of dronedarone on the action potential of rabbit atrial muscle preparations: comparison with amiodarone. J Cardiovasc Pharmacol 39:677–684
7. Varro A, Takacs J, Nemeth M et al (2001) Electrophysiological effects of dronedarone (SR 33589), a noniodinated amiodarone derivative in the canine heart: comparison with amiodarone. Br J Pharmacol 133:625–634
8. Pantos C, Mourouzis I, Delbruyere M et al (2002) Effects of dronedarone and amiodarone on plasma thyroid hormones and on the basal and postischemic performance of the isolated rat heart. Eur J Pharmacol 444:191–196
9. Touboul P, Brugada J, Capucci A et al (2003) Dronedarone for prevention of atrial fibrillation: a dose-ranging study. Eur Heart J 24:1481–1487
10. Hohnloser SH (2004) EURIDIS and ADONIS: maintenance of sinus rhythm with dronedarone in patients with atrial fibrillation or flutter. Hot Line II: Acute coronary syndromes /medical treatment II. Program and abstracts from the European Society of Cardiology Congress, 28 August–1 September, 2004, Munich, Germany

Prognosis and Management of Atrial Fibrillation in Patients Without Structural Heart Disease

M. Di Biase, R. Troccoli

Atrial fibrillation (AF), the most common sustained cardiac rhythm disturbance, is increasing in prevalence as the population ages. Although it is often associated with heart disease, AF occurs in many patients with no detectable disease.

AF may be related to acute, temporary causes, including alcohol intake ('holiday heart syndrome'), surgery, electrocution, myocardial infarction, pericarditis, myocarditis, pulmonary embolism or other pulmonary diseases, and hyperthyroidism or other metabolic disorders. In such cases, successful treatment of the underlying condition may eliminate AF. AF may be associated with another supraventricular tachycardia, the Wolff-Parkinson-White (WPW) syndrome, or atrioventricular (AV) nodal re-entrant tachycardias, and treatment of these primary arrhythmias reduces the incidence of recurrent AF. AF is a common early postoperative complication of cardiac or thoracic surgery. Specific cardiovascular conditions associated with AF include valvular heart disease (most often mitral valve disease), coronary artery disease, and hypertension, particularly when left ventricular hypertrophy is present. In addition, AF may be associated with hypertrophic or dilated cardiomyopathy or with congenital heart disease, especially atrial septal defect in adults. The list of aetiologies also includes restrictive cardiomyopathies (such as amyloidosis, haemochromatosis, and endomyocardial fibrosis), cardiac tumours, and constrictive pericarditis. Other heart diseases, such as mitral valve prolapse even without mitral regurgitation, calcification of the mitral annulus, cor pulmonale, and idiopathic dilation of the right atrium, have been associated with a high incidence of AF. AF is commonly encoun-

Institute of Cardiology, University of Foggia, Foggia, Italy

tered in patients with the sleep apnoea syndrome, but whether the arrhythmia is provoked by hypoxia or another biochemical abnormality or mediated by changes in pulmonary dynamics or right atrium factors has not been determined.

AF and Hyperthyroidism

AF occurs in 10–25% of patients with hyperthyroidism, more commonly in men and the elderly than in women or patients less than 75 years old [1, 2]. Treatment is primarily directed toward restoring a euthyroid state, which is usually associated with a spontaneous reversion to sinus rhythm. Antiarrhythmic drugs and electrical cardioversion are generally unsuccessful while the thyrotoxic condition persists [3, 4]. β-Blockers are somewhat effective in controlling the ventricular rate in this situation, and aggressive treatment with intravenous β-blockers is particularly important in cases of thyroid storm, for which high doses may be required. Calcium channel antagonists may also be useful [4]. Although specific evidence is lacking in AF caused by hyperthyroidism, oral anticoagulation is recommended to prevent systemic embolism [5].

AF and Pulmonary Diseases

Supraventricular arrhythmias, including AF, are common in patients with chronic obstructive lung disease [6, 7] and have adverse prognostic implications in patients with acute exacerbations of chronic obstructive pulmonary disease [8]. Treatment of the underlying lung disease and correction of hypoxia and acid–base imbalance are of primary importance.

AF and Wolff-Parkinson-White Syndrome

AF may induce ventricular fibrillation and sudden death in patients with the WPW syndrome when atrial impulses are conducted antegrade across a bypass tract. This complication is feared but infrequent. The incidence of sudden death ranges from 0 to 0.6% per year in patients with WPW syndrome.

Radiofrequency ablation of the accessory pathway is usually the preferred therapy for patients with pre-excitation syndromes and AF. Antiarrhythmic drugs may be useful in selected cases. Digoxin should be avoided because of the risk of paradoxical acceleration of the ventricular rate during AF. β-Blockers do not decrease conduction over accessory pathways during pre-excited periods of AF and could cause hypotension or other complications in patients with tenuous haemodynamics.

AF and Pregnancy

AF is rare during pregnancy [9] and is usually associated with another underlying cause, such as mitral stenosis [10], congenital heart disease [11], or hyperthyroidism [12]. A rapid ventricular response to AF can have serious haemodynamic consequences for both the mother and the fetus. In a pregnant woman who develops AF, diagnosis and treatment of the underlying condition causing the dysrhythmia is the first priority. The ventricular rate should be controlled with digoxin, a β-blocker, or a calcium channel antagonist [13–15].

References

1. Davidson E, Weinberger I, Rotenberg Z et al (1989) Atrial fibrillation: cause and time of onset. Arch Intern Med 149:457–459
2. Agner T, Almdal T, Thorsteinsson B et al (1984) A reevaluation of atrial fibrillation in thyrotoxicosis. Dan Med Bull 31:157–159
3. Nakazawa HK, Sakurai K, Hamada N et al (1982) Management of atrial fibrillation in the post-thyrotoxic state. Am J Med 72:903–906
4. Clozel JP, Danchin N, Genton P et al (1984) Effects of propranolol and of verapamil on heart rate and blood pressure in hyperthyroidism. Clin Pharmacol Ther 36:649
5. Hirsh J (1991) Oral anticoagulant drugs. N Engl J Med 324:1865–1875
6. Shih HT, Webb CR, Conway WA et al (1988) Frequency and significance of cardiac arrhythmias in chronic obstructive lung disease. Chest 94:44–48
7. Hudson LD, Kurt TL, Petty TL et al (1973) Arrhythmias associated with acute respiratory failure in patients with chronic airway obstruction. Chest 63:661–665
8. Fuso L, Incalzi RA, Pistelli R et al (1995) Predicting mortality of patients hospitalized for acutely exacerbated chronic obstructive pulmonary disease. Am J Med 98:272–277
9. Bhanderi AK, Isher N (1998) Cardiac arrhythmias and pregnancies. In: Gleicher N, Galbraith RM, Gall SA, Buttino L, Sibai BM (eds) Principles and practice of medical therapy in pregnancy. Appleton & Lange, Stanford, pp 975–987
10. Bryg RJ, Gordon PR, Kudesia VS et al (1989) Effect of pregnancy on pressure gradient in mitral stenosis. Am J Cardiol 63:384–386
11. Whittemore R, Hobbins JC, Engle MA (1982) Pregnancy and its outcome in women with and without surgical treatment of congenital heart disease. Am J Cardiol 50:641–651
12. Forfar JC, Miller HC, Toft AD (1979) Occult thyrotoxicosis: a correctable cause of 'idiopathic' atrial fibrillation. Am J Cardiol 44:9–12
13. Page RL (1995) Treatment of arrhythmias during pregnancy. Am Heart J 130:871–876
14. Cox JL, Gardner MJ (1998) Cardiovascular drugs in pregnancy and lactation. In:

Gleicher N, Galbraith RM, Gall SA, Buttino L, Sibai BM (eds) Principles and practice of medical therapy in pregnancy. Appleton & Lange, Stanford, pp 911–926
15. Chow T, Galvin J, McGovern B (1998) Antiarrhythmic drug therapy in pregnancy and lactation. Am J Cardiol 82:58I–62I

Primary Prevention of Atrial Fibrillation in Hypertensive Patients: What Is New from the LIFE Trial?

K. Wachtell[1,2], M.H. Olsen[1], B. Dahlöf[3], R.B. Devereux[2]

Introduction

Atrial fibrillation (AF) is associated with increased cardiovascular risk and the incidence of AF is increased in hypertensive patients [1–3]. Furthermore, patients with AF have a high prevalence of hypertension [4]. Although antihypertensive treatment reduces new-onset AF, it is unclear whether there is difference in the risk of new-onset AF with different antihypertensive drugs. Several studies suggest that renin-angiotensin-aldosterone system (RAAS) blockade, compared to placebo, reduces new-onset AF and helps maintain sinus rhythm [5–8]. Experimental studies have suggested that this benefit is due to the antiarrhythmic properties of RAAS-blocking drugs [9–12]. However, because of the placebo-controlled design of previous clinical studies, it is uncertain whether the reduction in new-onset AF was a result of blood pressure reduction per se or a direct effect of RAAS blockade. Furthermore, although AF is a frequent complication of hypertension, there is little evidence that choosing beta-blockade with combined antiarrhythmic and antihypertensive properties is better than other antihypertensive treatments in preventing AF [13]. A striking result of the Losartan Intervention For Endpoint reduction in hypertension (LIFE) study was a 25% reduction of fatal and non-fatal stroke by losartan-based treatment [14]. This result can in part be explained by a 45% lower rate of stroke (24.1 vs 46.5 strokes per 1000 patient-years of follow-up) in patients on losartan treatment who have a history of AF [15], but could also reflect benefits of reduced new-onset AF.

[1]Department of Medicine, Glostrup University Hospital, Glostrup, Denmark; [2]Division of Cardiology, Weill Medical College of Cornell University, New York, NY, USA; [3]Department of Medicine, Sahlgrenska University Hospital/Östra, Gothenburg, Sweden

The LIFE study was a prospective, randomised, double-masked, parallel group study ($n = 9193$) with double-dummy technique that evaluated the long-term effects of losartan-based vs atenolol-based antihypertensive therapy on cardiovascular morbidity and mortality in patients with hypertension and ECG left ventricular (LV) hypertrophy. The main outcome [14] as well as the complete study protocol with study design, organisation, clinical measures, exclusion criteria, basis for choice of comparative agents, statistical considerations, and baseline characteristics [16, 17] have been published. Sinus rhythm was documented by ECG in 8851 patients with no history of AF at baseline who were at risk of developing AF during the study. These patients are the focus of this article.

New-Onset Atrial Fibrillation

New-onset AF was identified from annual in-study ECGs that underwent Minnesota coding for AF at a single ECG Core Center [16]. Care of the patients with new-onset AF was left to the discretion of local investigators. New-onset AF occurred in 150 losartan-treated patients (6.8 per 1000 person-years of follow-up) and 221 atenolol-treated patients (10.1 per 1000 person-years of follow-up); HR = 0.67 [95% CI: 0.55–0.83], $P < 0.001$. Adjustment for differences in LV hypertrophy by Cornell voltage-duration and Sokolow-Lyon criteria as well as Framingham risk score had only minimal effect on the reduction of new-onset AF associated with losartan (Fig. 1). Furthermore, patients on losartan tended to stay in sinus rhythm longer from baseline (1809 ± 225 vs 1709 ± 254 days from baseline, $P = 0.057$) than those on atenolol.

New-Onset AF and Cardiovascular Outcome

Although patients with new-onset AF treated with losartan vs atenolol had similar baseline characteristics, losartan-treated patients with new-onset AF had a 40% lower rate of subsequent cardiovascular events (first occurrence of myocardial infarction, stroke, or cardiovascular death) than atenolol-treated patients ($n = 31$ vs 51, HR = 0.60 [95% CI: 0.38–0.94], $P = 0.03$). As shown in Fig. 2, there were substantially fewer subsequent strokes, a trend toward fewer myocardial infarctions, and no difference in cardiovascular mortality in losartan- compared to atenolol-treated patients with new-onset AF.

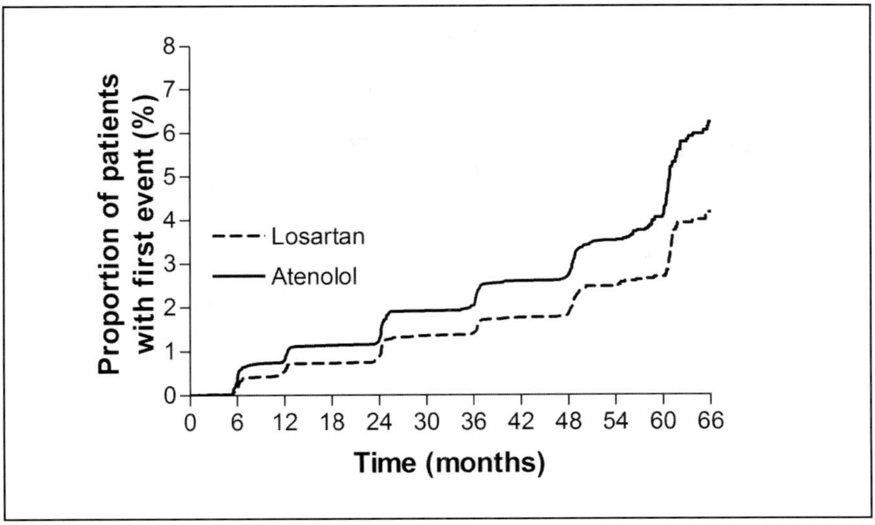

Fig. 1. Kaplan-Meier curves illustrating new-onset ECG-verified atrial fibrillation during follow-up. (From [8] with permission of the American College of Cardiology)

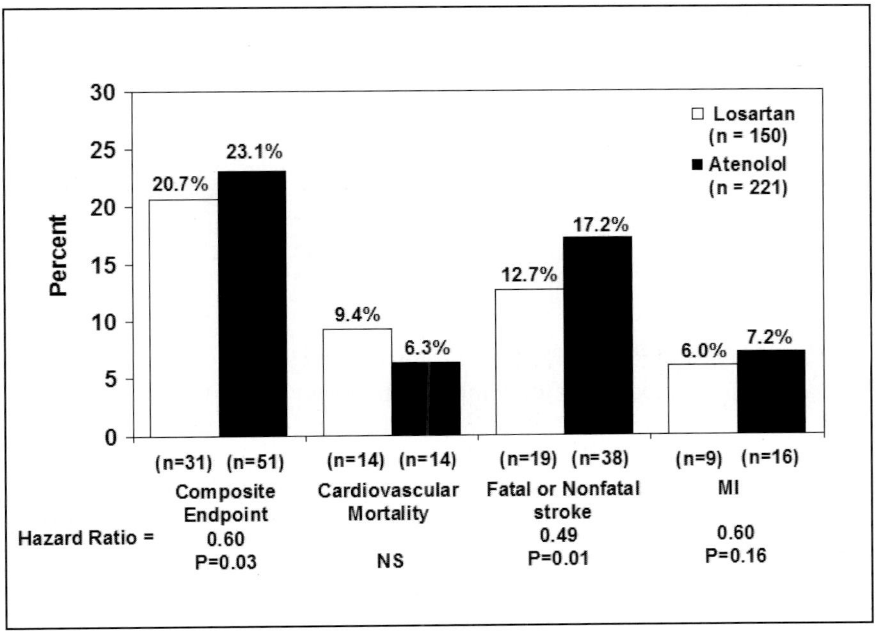

Fig. 2. Patients with new-onset AF on losartan have a lower risk of cardiovascular events

Prediction of New-Onset Atrial Fibrillation

To identify the most important factors associated with development of new-onset AF, we developed a multivariate prediction models (Table 1). In the model, age was by far the most important predictor of new-onset AF, with each year of age associated with a 9% higher rate of new-onset AF. Age was followed, in order, by male gender (56% increase in risk compared with women), systolic blood pressure (6% increase per 10 mmHg), and ECG LV hypertrophy by Cornell product (4% increase per 100 mV ms). Addition of study treatment to the model indicated that randomisation to losartan was associated with a 33% lower rate of new-onset AF, independent of other risk factors ($P < 0.001$).

Table 1. Multivariate predictors of new-onset atrial fibrillation (From [8] with permission of the American College of Cardiology)

Variable	χ^2	Hazard ratio (95% CI)	P
Age (year)	106.2	1.09 (1.07–1.11)	< 0.001
Male gender	17.7	1.56 (1.27–1.92)	< 0.001
Systolic blood pressure (10 mmHg)	5.2	1.09 (1.01–1.18)	0.023
Cornell voltage-duration (mV msec/100)	4.3	1.01 (1.001–1.02)	0.030
Randomisation to losartan	15.1	0.67 (0.54–0.82)	< 0.001

The 33% reduction in the rate of new-onset AF obtained with losartan-based therapy compared to atenolol-based therapy with similar blood pressure reduction suggests the need for a change of paradigm. Guidelines recommend beta-blockade, especially atenolol, as a first-line therapy to prevent AF as well as the preferred treatment for rate control in established AF [13]. In contrast to expectations from these recommendations, in the LIFE study, patients on losartan-based therapy tended to stay in sinus rhythm longer and had fewer cardiovascular events, especially fatal and non-fatal stroke, associated with new-onset AF. In addition, losartan-based therapy was equally effective in reducing the rate of cardiovascular events and stroke in hypertensive patients with pre-existing AF. The lower stroke rates associated with new-onset AF and in patients with pre-existing AF explained about half of the stroke reduction in the entire LIFE study [14], although a significant risk reduction was found in the remaining patients with neither pre-existing nor new-onset AF.

Finally, the magnitude of losartan's antiarrhythmic effect is substantial. The multivariate Cox regression model revealed that a reduction in systolic blood pressure by 30 mmHg would have similar effect as the benefit of losartan-based treatment compared with atenolol-based treatment. We speculate that the reduction in heart rate in patients without tachycardia might be 'a double-edged sword' because reducing heart rate increases LV stroke volume in order to maintain cardiac output, thereby increasing LV chamber volume and wall stress in both systole and diastole. These effects may, in turn, lead to less reduction in left atrial size, which has been shown to be associated with new-onset AF [18].

Conclusions

New-onset AF and associated stroke were significantly reduced by losartan-based compared with atenolol-based antihypertensive treatment, with similar blood pressure reduction, as shown in the LIFE study. The antiarrhythmic effect of losartan was, in multivariate analysis, similar to that of a 30 mmHg difference in systolic blood pressure.

References

1. Stewart S, Hart CL, Hole DJ et al (2002) A population-based study of the long-term risks associated with atrial fibrillation: 20-year follow-up of the Renfrew/Paisley study. Am J Med 113:359–364
2. Vidaillet H, Granada JF, Chyou PH et al (2002) A population-based study of mortality among patients with atrial fibrillation or flutter. Am J Med 113:365–370
3. Tsang TS, Petty GW, Barnes ME et al (2003) The prevalence of atrial fibrillation in incident stroke cases and matched population controls in Rochester, Minnesota: changes over three decades. J Am Coll Cardiol 42:93–100
4. Wyse DG, Waldo AL, DiMarco JP et al (2002) A comparison of rate control and rhythm control in patients with atrial fibrillation. N Engl J Med 347:1825–1833
5. Pedersen OD, Bagger H, Køber L et al (1999) Trandolapril reduces the incidence of atrial fibrillation after acute myocardial infarction in patients with left ventricular dysfunction. Circulation 100:376–380
6. Vermes E, Tardif JC, Bourassa MG et al (2003) Enalapril decrease the incidence of atrial fibrillation in patients with left ventricular dysfunction. Insight from the Studies Of Left Ventricular Dysfunction (SOLVD) Trials. Circulation 107:2926–2931
7. Madrid AH, Bueno MG, Rebollo JM et al (2002) Use of irbesartan to maintain sinus rhythm in patients with long-lasting persistent atrial fibrillation: a prospective and randomized study. Circulation 106:331–336
8. Wachtell K, Lehto M, Gerdts E et al (2005) Angiotensin II receptor blockade reduces new-onset atrial fibrillation and subsequent stroke compared to atenolol: The LIFE

study. J Am Coll Cardiol 45:712–719
9. Kumagai K, Nakashima H, Urata H et al (2003) Effects of angiotensin II type 1 receptor antagonist on electrical and structural remodeling in atrial fibrillation. J Am Coll Cardiol 41:2197–2204
10. Li D, Shinagawa K, Pang L et al (2001) Effects of angiotensin-converting enzyme inhibition on the development of the atrial fibrillation substrate in dogs with ventricular tachypacing-induced congestive heart failure. Circulation 104:2608–2614
11. Shi Y, Li D, Tardif JC et al (2002) Enalapril effects on atrial remodeling and atrial fibrillation in experimental congestive heart failure. Cardiovasc Res 54:456–461
12. Nakashima H, Kumagai K, Urata H et al (2000) Angiotensin II antagonist prevents electrical remodeling in atrial fibrillation. Circulation 101:2612–2617
13. Fuster V, Ryden LE, Asinger RW et al (2001) ACC/AHA/ESC guidelines for the management of patients with atrial fibrillation: executive summary. A Report of the American College of Cardiology/American Heart Association Task Force on Practice Guidelines and the European Society of Cardiology Committee for Practice Guidelines and Policy Conferences (Committee to Develop Guidelines for the Management of Patients With Atrial Fibrillation): developed in Collaboration With the North American Society of Pacing and Electrophysiology. J Am Coll Cardiol 38:1231–1266
14. Dahlöf B, Devereux RB, Kjeldsen SE et al (2002) Cardiovascular morbidity and mortality in the Losartan Intervention For Endpoint reduction in hypertension study (LIFE): a randomised trial against atenolol. Lancet 359:995–1003
15. Wachtell K, Hornestam B, Lehto M et al (2005) Cardiovascular morbidity and mortality in hypertensive patients with a history of atrial fibrillation: The LIFE study. J Am Coll Cardiol 45:705–711
16. Dahlöf B, Devereux RB, de Faire U et al (1997) The Losartan Intervention For Endpoint reduction (LIFE) in Hypertension Study. Am J Hypertens 10:705–713
17. Dahlöf B, Devereux RB, Julius S et al (1998) Characteristics of 9194 patients with left ventricular hypertrophy: The LIFE study. Hypertension 32:989–997
18. Wachtell K, Palmieri V, Gerdts E et al (2005) Left ventricular structural and functional response in hypertensive patients with new-onset atrial fibrillation and left ventricular hypertrophy: The LIFE Study. J Am Coll Cardiol 45:374A (abs)

Prognosis and Management of Atrial Fibrillation in Different Clinical Settings: Acute Myocardial Infarction

G. Zuin, M. Celestre, F. Di Pede

Introduction

Atrial fibrillation (AF) is a common arrhythmia in patients with acute myocardial infarction (AMI) found in around 10–20% of all such patients. AF is caused by ischemic myocardium (atrial and ventricular), pericarditis, and left ventricular dysfunction. In a large, community study [1] conducted in the pre-fibrinolytic era over the 10-year period from 1975 to 1986, the incidence of AF was 16.6%. Mortality was higher in the AF group than in the non-AF group both in-hospital (27.6% vs 16.6%) and after a 5-year follow-up period. Congestive heart failure, cardiogenic shock, and other signs of left ventricular dysfunction were frequently found in patients with AF. However, a multivariate analysis showed that both in-hospital and long-term prognosis were not affected by AF (OR 1.18, 95% CI 0.90–1.52), suggesting that the prognostic impact of AF may be mediated by left ventricular dysfunction.

In a large study conducted in the fibrinolytic era (GUSTO-I trial) [2], AF was present on admission in 2.5 % of patients and developed during hospitalisation in an additional 7.9% of cases. Patients with AF were more often affected by three-vessels disease and in-hospital stroke , and the adjusted 30-day mortality rate was significantly higher (OR 1.3, 95% CI 1.3–1.5).

Data derived from the GISSI-3 trial [3], which included 17.944 patients receiving fibrinolytic therapy, within the first 24 h after AMI, showed an incidence of in-hospital AF of 7.8%. AF correlated with advanced age, female sex, higher Killip class, previous myocardial infarction, hypertension, diabetes, and heart failure. After adjustment for other prognostic factors, AF remained an independent predictor of increased in-hospital (RR 1.98, 95%

Division of Cardiology, Cardiovascular Department, Umberto I Hospital, Mestre-Venice, Italy

CI 1.67 to 2.34) and long-term (RR 1.78, 95% CI 1.60 to 1.99) mortality. Similar results were found in other studies [4–6]. In the GRACE registry [4], 5.0% of the patients with AMI had previous AF and 7.7% had a new onset of AF. Patients with AF were older, more likely to be women, with previous MI, stroke, or congestive heart failure, and previous revascularisation, and had an in-hospital complicated course. However, only new-onset AF was an independent predictor of all adverse in-hospital outcomes.

In the GUSTO 3 trial [7] 3906 patients (6.5%) out of 13 858 with AMI treated with fibrinolytic therapy who were in sinus rhythm at the time of enrolment developed AF. Worsening heart failure, hypotension, third-degree heart block, and ventricular fibrillation were independent predictors of new-onset AF. Patients with AF had an increased 30-day and 1-year mortality rate even after adjustment for baseline factors and pre-AF complications. These data suggest that AF is often a consequence of post-AMI complications, but is itself an independent predictor of a worse outcome.

The effects of fibrinolysis on AF were analysed by the authors of the SPRINT registry [8], who compared the incidence of AF in patients with AMI treated in the prefibrinolytic era vs those treated in the fibrinolytic era. They reported an overall incidence of AF of 9.9% and 8.9%, respectively, and a similar 30-day (27.6% vs 25.1%) and 1-year (42.5 % vs 38.4%) mortality. However, AF in the fibrinolytic era occurred in older and sicker patients. Therefore, the mortality rate, after adjustment for confounding factors during these two periods was significantly reduced (more than 30%) in mortality treated with fibrinolysis.

The effects of primary percutaneous coronary intervention (PCI) on AF have been rarely evaluated. In patients treated with primary PCI [9], 4.3% had AF on admission and 7.7% developed AF during hospitalisation. AF correlated with age, Killip class, previous infarction and stroke, shock, multivessel disease, and poor reperfusion of the infarct-related artery. AF was not an independent predictor of in-hospital mortality but was an independent predictor of 1-year mortality (OR 1.64, 95% CI 1.05–2.55).

Pharmacological treatment with drugs aimed to reduce the size of the infarct and ventricular remodelling has also been beneficial in reducing the incidence of AF. In the GISSI-3 [3], patients treated with nitrates and ACE inhibitors showed a trend towards a reduced incidence of AF, suggesting that haemodynamic impairment was the most likely mechanism underline this arrhythmia. In the TRACE study [5], patients with AMI between day 2 and day 6 after the onset of symptoms were included and randomised to ACE-inhibitor treatment or placebo. The risk of new, in-hospital AF was reduced by 45% with trandolapril treatment. Beta-blockers such as carvedilol seem to reduce atrial arrhythmias. In the CAPRICORN study [10], patients with left ventricular dysfunction were treated with carvedilol added to an ACE inhibitor 3–21 days after AMI. The incidence of AF was 5.4% in the placebo group and 2.3 % in the carvedilol group, with a carvedilol/placebo hazard ratio (HR) of 0.41 (95% CI 0.25–0.68 , $P = 0.0003$).

The occurrence of AF increases the risk of ischaemic stroke. Data obtained from patients enrolled in the GRACE registry [11] showed a 1.3% incidence of in-hospital stroke in patients with AMI. AF was one of the strongest risk factors for in-hospital non-haemorrhagic stroke, together with in-hospital CABG, previous stroke, and advanced age. These data are consistent with the findings of the GUSTO-I study [2].

Management

The management of AF includes antiarrhythmic therapy or electrical cardioversion. Recent ACC/AHA practice guidelines [12] for the management of patients with ST-elevation myocardial infarction, give the following suggestions:

1. Patients with a sustained AF and haemodynamic compromise should be treated with direct cardioversion, preceded by brief general anaesthesia. For episodes of AF that do not respond to electrical cardioversion or recur after a brief period of sinus rhythm, antiarrhythmic drugs are recommended, with the aim of slowing the ventricular response. The agents that we use are: i.v. amiodarone or i.v. digoxin.
2. Patients with sustained AF and ongoing ischaemia but without haemodynamic compromise should be treated with one or more of the following : beta-blocker and/or i.v. diltiazem or verapamil and/or direct cardioversion.
3. In patients with sustained AF without haemodynamic compromise or ischaemia, rate control is indicated.

In addition, patients with sustained AF should be treated with anticoagulants.

Conclusions

Atrial fibrillation in AMI is often secondary to other post-AMI complications, but is itself an independent predictor of a worse outcome. AF can be prevented by optimising the treatment of AMI with reperfusion therapy, beta-blockers, and ACE inhibitors. When AF occurs, it should be treated with DC shock as soon as possible and/or drugs with little haemodynamic impact according to the clinical status.

References

1. Goldberg RJ, Seeley D, Becker RC et al (1990) Impact of atrial fibrillation on the in-hospital and long term survival of patients with acute myocardioal infarction: A community-wide perspective. Am Heart J 119:996–1001
2. Crenshaw BS, Ward SR, Granger CB et al for the GUSTO-I Trial Investigators (1997) Atrial fibrillation in the setting of acute myocardial infarction: the GUSTO-I experience. J Am Coll Cardiol 30:406–413
3. Pizzetti F, Turazza FM, Franzosi MG et al GISSI-3 Investigators (2001) Incidence and prognostic significance of atrial fibrillation in acute myocardial infarction: the GISSI-3 data. Heart 86:527–532
4. Mehta RH, Dabbous OH, Granger CB et al for the GRACE Investigators (2003) Comparison of outcomes of patients with acute coronary syndromes with and without atrial fibrillation. Am J Cardiol 92:1031–1036
5. Pedersen OD, Bagger H, Kober L et al on behalf of the TRACE Study Group (1999) The occurence and prognostic significance of atrial fibrillation/flutter following acute myocardial infarction. Eur Heart J 20:748–754
6. Lehto M, Snapinn S, Dickstein K et al behalf of the OPTIMAAL Investigators (2005) Prognostic risk of atrial fibrillation in acute myocardial infarction complicated by left ventricular dysfunction: the OPTIMAAL experience. Eur Heart J 26:350–356
7. Wong CK, White HD, Wilcox RG et al for the GUSTO III Investigators (2000) New atrial fibrillation after acute myocardial infarction indipendently predicts death: the GUSTO III experience. Am Heart J 140:878–885
8. Eldar M, Canetti M, Rotstein Z et al for the SPRINT and Thrombolytic Survey Group (1998) Significance of paroxysmal atrial fibrillation complicating acute myocardial infarction in the thrombolytic era. Circulation 97:965–970
9. Kinjo K, Sato H, Ohnishi Y et al for Osaka Acute Coronary Insufficiency Study (OACIS) Group (2003) Prognostic significance of atrial fibrillation/atrial flutter in patientas with acute myocardial infarction treated with percutaneous coronary intervention. Am J Cardiol 92:1150–1154
10. McMurray J, Kober L, Robertson M et al (2005) Antiarrhytmic effect of carvedilol after acute myocardial infarction. Results of Carvedilol Post Infarct Survival Control in Left Ventricular Dysfunction (CAPRICORN) Trial. J Am Coll Cardiol 45:525–530
11. Budaj A, Flasinka K, Gore JM et al for the GRACE Investigators (2005) Magnitude of and risk factors for in hospital and postdischarge stroke in patients with acute coronary syndromes. Findings from a Global Registry of Acute Coronary Events. Circulation 111:3242–3247
12. Antman EM, Anbe DT, Armstrong PW et al (2004) AHA Guedelines for the management of patients with ST-elevation myocardial infarction. Executive summary: a report of the American College of Cardiology/American Heart Association Task Force on practice guidelines. Circulation 110:588–636

Post-CABG Atrial Fibrillation: What Are the Incidence, Predictors, Treatment, and Long-Term Outcome?

C. Blomström Lundqvist

Post operative atrial fibrillation (AF) is a common complication of coronary artery bypass surgery (CABG), occurring in 5–40% of patients during the first postoperative week, depending on definitions and methods of detection. A meta-analysis of controlled randomised trials confirmed that in trials using 24-h Holter ECG monitoring, the incidence of supraventricular arrhythmias was higher with Holter recordings (41.3 %) than in trials without (19.9 %) [1]. Despite recent improvements in surgical techniques and postoperative patient care, the incidence of postoperative AF seems to increase, most likely related to the existence of an increasing number of elderly patients with co-morbidities. In the majority of cases postoperative AF is transient and not life-threatening, although it may cause marked subjective symptoms, congestive heart failure, hypotension, and ischaemia, requiring pharmacological treatment or electrical cardioversion, resulting in prolonged hospital stay and additional costs in medical care [2].

Stroke is a major adverse event, complicating the immediate outcome of CABG in about 2% of cases. AF was reported to be a major determinant of stroke after CABG, preceding the occurrence of neurological complications in approximately 37% of the patients [3]. Apart from a higher risk of stroke (odds ratio, OR 2.02), postoperative AF was associated with greater in-hospital mortality (OR 1.7) and worse survival (74% versus 87%) at long-term follow-up (4–5 years) [2]. In a multivariate analysis it was an independent predictor of long-term mortality [2]. The complexity of distinguishing the intrinsic hazards due to postoperative AF from the risks related to its aetiological factors and treatment should, however, be recognised in this retrospective cohort study.

Department of Cardiology, University Hospital in Uppsala, Uppsala, Sweden

The mechanisms responsible for postoperative AF are still unclear and are probably multifactorial. Since risk stratification strategies for patients undergoing CABG could lead to more targeted preventive or therapeutic interventions, large number of trials have aimed at identifying risk factors for the development of postoperative AF. Risk factors associated with AF include advanced age (OR for 10-year increase, 1.75); history of AF (OR 2.11) or chronic obstructive lung disease (OR 1.43); valve surgery (OR 1.74); peripheral vascular disease (OR 1.54); and postoperative withdrawal of β-blockers (OR 1.91) or angiotensin-converting enzyme inhibitors (OR 1.69) [2, 4].

Among preoperative risk factors, advancing age has a significant association with the incidence of AF, a relationship that is particularly important as the number of elderly patients considered for CABG steadily increases. Advanced age was associated with increased levels of circulating norepinephrine, which could be related to imbalance in the autonomic nervous system, previously reported in some but not other studies as an independent risk factor for postoperative AF. Thoracic epidural anaesthesia, aimed at blocking excessive sympathetic activity, was, however, not effective in preventing postoperative AF [5].

There is still no consensus as to whether operative clinical and/or electrocardiographic characteristics further distinguish patients who would develop postoperative AF. Prolonged P-wave duration consistent with intra-atrial conduction delay, the presence of preoperative supraventricular arrhythmias, and fluctuations in autonomic balance as measured by heart rate variability were identified in some but not other studies as independent risk factors for postoperative AF [6].

Postoperative AF is probably the most important potentially reversible health care expenditure related to CABG. The recognition of the potential benefits of preventing AF after CABG is reflected by the large number of prophylactic strategies reported in the literature. In a meta-analysis including 42 randomised controlled trials, β-blocking agents, sotalol, and amiodarone significantly reduced the incidence of postoperative AF compared with placebo, and with no marked difference between them [7]. The three drugs each prevented AF with the following odds ratios: β-blockers 0.39, sotalol 0.35, and amiodarone 0.48 [7]. From the analysis of 10 pacing trials, atrial pacing was shown to be effective, with an odds ratio of 0.46 for biatrial pacing [7]. Biatrial pacing significantly reduced length of hospital stay by 1.5 days, but there was no evidence that the stroke rate was lowered. In another meta-analysis of prophylactic anti-arrhythmic therapy (amiodarone, sotalol, procainamide, pacing) for the prevention of postoperative AF, the incidence of AF varied from 8% to 37% in the treatment groups and from 29% to 53% in the control groups, with a combined overall significant decrease of 0.52 (OR) in the treatment groups [8]. When the studies were combined there was

1.0 ± 0.2 day overall decrease in length of hospital stay, but no significant effect on the incidence of stroke or mortality. Data on costs, available for five of the six studies that used amiodarone and one of the studies that used pacing, showed a combined insignificant decrease in cost [8].

In a randomised study, amiodarone plus pacing significantly decreased the frequency of AF after open heart surgery, compared with amiodarone alone, pacing alone, and placebo [9]. In the cost-effectiveness analysis, when compared with placebo, the probability of lower cost but higher effect (superiority) was 67% for amiodarone, 15% for pacing, and 97% for amiodarone plus pacing [9]. In the multivariate analysis, preoperative β-blockers and amiodarone were negatively associated with hospital costs ($P < 0.05$). Data suggest that both amiodarone alone and the combination of amiodarone plus pacing are cost-effective compared with placebo.

A meta-analysis of 8 prophylactic pacing trials, with 776 patients enrolled, demonstrated a significant anti-arrhythmic effect of biatrial overdrive and fixed high-rate pacing and overdrive right atrial pacing, with a relative risk reduction of approximately 2.5-fold for new-onset AF at open heart surgery [10]. Another, larger meta-analysis of 58 studies (8565 patients) demonstrated that prophylactic therapies (amiodarone, β-blockers, sotalol, and pacing) favoured treatment for postoperative AF with an odds ratio of 0.43 [11]. A positive result for cost of hospitalisation in favour of treatment was achieved, but the statistic was not significant due to low power and large standard deviations. β-Blockers had the greatest magnitude of effect across 28 trials (4074 patients), with an odds ratio of 0.35. The data for stroke favoured treatment by a non-significant effect size of 0.81. Similarly, a positive indication for length of stay was derived, but it too was not significant, with a weighted mean difference of –0.66.

Hypomagnesaemia is frequently observed after cardiac surgery and is related to the extracorporeal circulation and the use of diuretics In a meta-analysis of 17 trials with 2069 patients, magnesium supplementation reduced the risk of supraventricular arrhythmias (relative risk 0.77) but had no effect on the length of the hospital stay or mortality [12]. Administration of prophylactic magnesium reduced the risk of postoperative AF by 29%, although the homogeneity among trials may limit the formulation of definitive conclusions.

The effect of cardiopulmonary bypass on the incidence of AF after CABG has been addressed in several trials. A meta-analysis of all observational studies comparing cardiac pulmonary bypass (2253 patients) and off-pump techniques (764 patients) in elderly patients demonstrated a significantly lower incidence of postoperative AF (odds ratio 0.70) after off-pump surgery [13]. The results were confirmed in another meta-analysis of 37 randomised trials (3369 patients), in which off-pump CABG significantly decreased AF

(OR, 0.58) and hospital stay (weighted mean difference, –1.0 days) but without affecting 30-day mortality or stroke rate (OR, 0.68) [14]. It should be emphasised, though, that the lower risk profile of patients undergoing off-pump CABG could contribute to a lower AF risk.

Radiofrequency ablation of pulmonary vein triggers has had a remarkable high success rate for non-postoperative AF. Our own data showed that onset of AF after CABG was triggered by premature beats in 72% of patients with postoperative AF, which implies that atrial triggers may be important in the postoperative setting. It is, however, as yet unclear whether a surgical epicardial approach would be effective and safe if implemented during routine CABG procedures.

The importance of the parasympathetic nervous system for the initiation of AF is still incompletely understood, although it is thought to play a role in the subsets of patients with paroxysmal non-postoperative AF. Vagal postganglionic neurons are located in well-defined anatomic fat pads situated in two posterior epicardial regions around the heart and adjacent structures. Transvenous radiofrequency (RF) ablation at such sites has resulted in vagal denervation and improved outcome in patients with non-postoperative AF subjected to circumferential pulmonary vein ablation [15]. In animal studies the destruction of an anterior fat pad shown to contain vagal neurons resulted in decreased susceptibility to AF. The anterior fat pad, located in the aortopulmonary window, was therefore studied in humans with respect to its role in postoperative AF [16]. The authors' question was whether its removal, as routinely done during the process of placing the aortic cross-clamp, would decrease subsequent AF [16]. By stimulating the anterior fat pad in patients undergoing CABG, the sinus rate was slowed with no change in PR interval, consistent with innervation of the sinus node but not the atrioventricular node [16]. Since enhanced vagal tone is pro-fibrillatory in the atria by shortening refractoriness, the underlying theory was that removal of tissue responsible for vagal atrial influences would improve AF outcome. In the randomised study, paradoxically, 37% of patients in whom the interior fat pad was dissected developed postoperative AF compared with 7% in whom the fat pad was preserved [16]. Supportive of these findings is the reported lower incidence of AF after off-pump CABG, during which the anterior fat pad is often preserved [13]. Animal experiments support vagal denervation as an effective anti-arrhythmic strategy, which is consistent with the finding of a lower incidence of AF following vagal denervation during catheter ablation procedures. The importance of vagal influences and the role of the cardiac fat pads for developing postoperative AF demand further clinical research to determine the optimal surgical technique.

The class I recommendations for prevention and management of postoperative AF are: (1) an oral β-blocker for prevention, and (2) atrioventricular nodal blocking agents for rate control [17]. Class IIa recommendations are: (1) prophylactic sotalol or amiodarone for patients at increased risk of developing postoperative AF; (2) electrical or pharmacological cardioversion to restore sinus rhythm, as recommended for non-surgical patients; (3) attempt at maintenance of sinus rhythm by administration of anti-arrhythmic medications if there is recurrent or refractory postoperative AF, as recommended for patients with coronary artery disease who develop AF; and (4) anti-thrombotic medication, as recommended for non-surgical patients.

References

1. Andrews T, Reimold S, Berlin J et al (1991) Prevention of supraventricular arrhythmias after coronary artery bypass surgery. A meta-analysis of randomized control trials. Circulation 84(5 Suppl):III236–III244
2. Villareal R, Hariharan R, Liu B et al (2004) Postoperative atrial fibrillation and mortality after coronary artery bypass surgery. J Am Coll Cardiol 43:742–748
3. Lahtinen J, Biancari F, Salmela E et al (2004) Postoperative atrial fibrillation is a major cause of stroke after on-pump coronary artery bypass surgery. Ann Thorac Surg 77:1241
4. Mathew JP, Fontes ML, Tudor IC et al (2004) A multicenter risk index for atrial fibrillation after cardiac surgery. JAMA 291:1720–1729
5. Jidéus L, Joachimsson P-O, Stridsberg M et al (2001) Thoracic epidural anaesthesia does not influence the occurrence of postoperative sustained atrial fibrillation. Ann Thorac Surg 72:65–71
6. Jidéus L, Blomström P, Nilsson L et al (2000) Tachyarrhythmias and triggering factors for atrial fibrillation after coronary artery bypass operations. Ann Thorac Surg 69:1064–1069
7. Crystal E, Connolly SJ, Sleik K et al (2002) Interventions on prevention of postoperative atrial fibrillation in patients undergoing heart surgery a meta-analysis. Circulation 106:75–80
8. Zimmer J, Pezzullo J, Choucair W et al (2003) Meta-analysis of antiarrhythmic therapy in the prevention of postoperative atrial fibrillation and the effect on hospital length of stay, costs, cerebrovascular accidents, and mortality in patients undergoing cardiac surgery. Am J Cardiol 91:1137–1140
9. Reddy P, Kalus J, Caron M et al (2004) Economic analysis of intravenous plus oral amiodarone, atrial septal pacing, and both strategies to prevent atrial fibrillation after open heart surgery. Pharmacotherapy 24:1013–1019
10. Daoud EG, Snow R, Hummel JD et al (2003) Temporary atrial epicardial pacing as prophylaxis against atrial fibrillation after heart surgery: a meta-analysis. J Cardiovasc Electrophysiol 14:127–132
11. Crystal E, Garfinkle MS, Connolly SS et al (2004) Interventions for preventing postoperative atrial fibrillation in patients undergoing heart surgery. Cochrane Database Syst Rev CD003611
12. Shiga T, Wajima Z, Inoue T et al (2004) Magnesium prophylaxis for arrhythmias after cardiac surgery: a meta-analysis of randomized controlled trials. Am J Med 117:325–333
13. Athanasiou T, Aziz O, Mangoush O et al (2004) Do off-pump techniques reduce the

incidence of postoperative atrial fibrillation in elderly patients undergoing coronary artery bypass grafting? Ann Thorac Surg 77:1567–1574
14. Cheng D, Bainbridge D, Martin J et al (2005) Does off-pump coronary artery bypass reduce mortality, morbidity, and resource utilization when compared with conventional coronary artery bypass? A meta-analysis of randomized trials. Anesthesiology 102:188–203
15. Pappone C, Santinelli V, Manguso F et al (2004) Pulmonary vein denervation enhances long-term benefit after circumferential ablation for paroxysmal atrial fibrillation. Circulation 109:327–334
16. Cumming J, Gill I, Akhrass R et al (2004) Preservation of the anterior fat pad paradoxically decreases the incidence of postoperative atrial fibrillation in humans. J Am Coll Cardiol 43:994–1000
17. Fuster V, Ryden LE, Asinger RW et al (2001) ACC/AHA/ESC guidelines for the management of patients with atrial fibrillation. A report of the American College of Cardiology/American Heart Association Task Force on Practice Guidelines and the European Society of Cardiology Committee for Practice Guidelines and Policy Conferences (committee to develop guidelines for the management of patients with atrial fibrillation) developed in collaboration with the North American Society of Pacing and Electrophysiology. Eur Heart J 22:1852–1923

Post-PCI Atrial Fibrillation: Possible Clinical and Prognostic Significance

B. Gorenek

Atrial fibrillation (AF) is a major arrhythmia that has a high prevalence among the population. It is clinically important because affected patients have a higher risk of mortality; a deterioration in haemodynamics due to increased heart rate, loss of atrioventricular synchrony, and progressive dysfunction of the left atrium and left ventricle; and stroke and other embolic events resulting from atrial thrombi [1, 2]. In addition, AF may cause significant symptoms and impair both functional status and the quality of life.

Percutaneous coronary interventions (PCI) have been the fastest growing major invasive procedure in the past decade. Accompanying the obvious benefit, there are certain risks, including cardiac arrhythmias. Several kind of arrhythmias, especially ventricular arrhythmias and conduction disturbances, can occur during PCI. These arrhythmias may result from excess catheter manipulation, intracoronary dye injection, new ischaemic events, or reperfusion injury. Lethal ventricular arrhythmias, including serious ventricular tachycardia and ventricular fibrillation, have been reported to occur in 1.5–4.4% of patients undergoing coronary angioplasty. The frequency of these arrhythmias after primary PCI was analyzed in a study of 3065 patients participating in the PAMI trials [3]. Ventricular arrhythmias occurred in 133 patients (4.3%). Smoking, lack of preprocedural beta-blockers, shorter time from symptom onset to emergency room arrival, initial TIMI flow grade 0, and infarct of the right coronary artery were variables independently associated with a risk of serious ventricular arrhythmias. Those patients also had higher rates of complications, including cardiopulmonary resuscitation and intubation, in the catheterisation laboratory but had similar frequencies of major adverse cardiac events in-hospital and at 1 year.

Osmangazi University, Cardiology Department, Eskisehir, Turkey

Supraventricular arrhythmias, including atrial flutter and atrial AF, may also occur during or after PCI, as a complication or a sequel of the revascularisation procedure. However, these are not as frequent as ventricular arrhythmias. In general, AF has prognostic significance in patients treated with PCI, as it can be induced by cardiac catheterisation, especially in response to catheter placement into or out of the right atrium. Atrial dysfunction (due to atrial ischaemia or atrial stretching in heart failure), sinoatrial and AV nodal ischaemia, congestive heart failure, sympathetic stimulation, and iatrogenic factors are the possible causes of AF in patients undergoing primary PCI for acute myocardial infarction (MI). AF, by contrast, can cause clinical sequelae in the setting of a rapid ventricular response or if the loss of atrial systole results in hypotension, as in a patient with mitral stenosis or diastolic ventricular dysfunction.

Importance of Clinical Features

The clinical characteristics of patients play important roles in the occurrence of AF in PCI. Kinjo et al. assessed the prognostic significant of AF and atrial flutter in patients with acute MI that had been treated with PCI [4]. In their study, patients with AF were older, were in higher Killip classes, had higher rates of previous MI and previous cerebrovascular accident, had systolic blood pressures of < 100 mmHg and heart rates ≥ 100 beats/min, were less likely to smoke, and had higher prevalence of multivessel disease and poorer reperfusion of infarct-related artery than those without AF. AF was a common complication in patients with MI who were treated with PCI and independently influenced 1-year mortality. Cardiogenic shock, congestive heart failure, cardiac rupture, ventricular tachycardia and/or ventricular fibrillation, and stroke occurred more often in patients with AF than in those without AF. No significant difference was observed in the rates of recurrent infarction or recurrent ischaemia. The unadjusted in-hospital mortality rate was significantly higher in patients with AF than in those without AF. But, after adjustment for demographic characteristics and clinical factors, AF was not associated with in-hospital mortality. Furthermore, when stratified by the timing of AF, both AF at admission and AF that developed during hospitalisation were not independent predictors for in-hospital mortality. Therefore, AF was not significantly associated with in-hospital mortality in patients with MI who underwent PCI. One-year mortality was higher in patients with AF than in those without AF. Most deaths were due to cardiovascular causes. Patients with AF had a greater incidence of death due to pump failure than those without AF. After adjustment for demographic characteristics and clinical factors, patients with AF remained at significantly greater risk for mortality at 1 year. Furthermore, when stratified by the timing of AF, AF during hospitalisation was independently associated with 1-year mortality but AF at admission was not. The 1-year mortality of patients discharged alive was higher in those with AF than in those without AF. After adjustment for demographic characteristics, clinical factors, and antiarrhythmic drug use at discharge, patients with AF remained at significantly greater risk for mortality at 1 year [4].

Importance of Electrophysiological Predictors

Inhomogeneous prolongation of sinus impulses may predict the recurrence of AF [5, 6]. The heterogeneity of the structural and electrophysiological properties of the atrium prone to fibrillate results in an inhomogeneous and discontinuous prolongation of sinus impulses [7]. Electrophysiological studies have demonstrated that individuals with a clinical history of AF have a significantly longer intra-atrial and inter-atrial conduction time of sinus impulses [8–10]. This has been confirmed by the finding of P-wave prolongation on 12-lead surface ECG and signal-averaged ECG recordings [11–13]. The importance of P-wave dispersion in predicting recurrence of AF in patients with paroxysmal AF has also been elucidated [5, 14]. Thus, P-wave signal-averaged ECG could be useful to identify patients at risk for recurrence of AF after internal cardioversion [15].

Ozmen et al. investigated the effects of angioplasty induced-ischaemia on atrial conduction abnormalities as estimated by P-wave maximum and P-wave dispersion [16]. Both were significantly higher during balloon occlusion compared with the baseline condition in coronary dilatation procedures. However, the P-wave minimum was not found to differ between baseline and during balloon occlusion. These data demonstrate that prolongation of P-wave dispersion might be a simple and useful additional marker of myocardial ischaemia during PCI.

Budeus et al. examined the incidence of atrial late potentials in patients with a proximal stenosis of the right coronary artery and new onset of AF [17]. They also investigated the anti-ischaemic effect of a successful percutaneous transluminal coronary angioplasty (PTCA) of the right coronary artery. After successful PTCA only three out of 15 patients were affected after 1 day, as well as after 1 month. None of the patients with a history of AF suffered from an arrhythmic recurrence within the following 6 months after successful PTCA. In that study, stenosis of the right coronary artery was associated with atrial late potentials. The authors concluded that a successful PTCA of the right coronary artery eliminates pre-existent atrial late potentials and may reduce the risk of AF.

Atrial Fibrillation in Acute MI. Thrombolytic Therapy vs Primary PCI

Given the primary role of thrombus in the genesis of acute coronary occlusion, the introduction of thrombolytic therapy was a major advance in the treatment of acute ST-elevation MI. But, compared to thrombolysis, primary PCI achieves a higher rate of TIMI 3 flow, does not carry the risk of intracranial haemorrhage, and is associated with improved outcomes. The ACC/AHA task force gave a class I recommendation to the use of primary PCI for any patient with an acute MI who presents within 12 h of symptom onset and who can undergo the procedure within 90 min of presentation by persons skilled in the procedure [18]. The task force also identified specific considerations for choosing primary PCI, including the experience of the person performing the procedure, the timing of the procedure, and the specific clinical setting.

Several studies in the thrombolytic era showed that the prognostic significance of AF on mortality was attenuated by improved treatment [19, 20]. Randomised studies performed in the past few years have demonstrated that PCI is a more effective reperfusion strategy than intravenous thrombolysis [21, 22]. Therefore, the incidence of AF may have decreased and the prognostic significance of AF may have been attenuated in patients with AMI who underwent PCI. However, little is known concerning the incidence of AF and its effects on the prognosis of patients with AMI who are treated with PCI.

A study was conducted to compare the effects of reperfusion either by thrombolytic therapy or primary PTCA on P-wave duration and dispersion in patients with acute anterior-wall MI. The authors evaluated 72 consecutive patients retrospectively experiencing acute anterior-wall MI for the first time. Patients were grouped according to the reperfusion therapy, PTCA versus thrombolytic therapy. There were no significant differences between the groups regarding age, gender, left ventricular ejection fraction (LVEF), left atrial diameter and volume, cardiovascular risk factors, and duration from symptom onset to treatment. P-wave dispersions and P-wave durations were significantly decreased after PTCA. In that study, primary PTCA reduced the incidence of AF by decreasing the P-wave maximum and P-wave dispersion [23].

We investigated the coronary angiographic findings of patients who developed AF during acute MI, and the effects of primary PCI and thrombolytic therapy for restoration of sinus rhythm [24]. The study consisted of 52 patients with acute MI who underwent primary PCI or had thrombolytic therapy and developed AF during the first 12 h of hospitalisation. On admission, and 1 month later, coronary angiography was performed in all patients. In 26 of the 52 patients primary PCI was performed and in the other 26 patients thrombolytic therapy was applied (streptokinase or r-TPA) following angiography. Right coronary artery occlusions were the most frequent causes of AF (73%). In repeated coronary angiography, the coronary artery affected by the infarct was still totally occluded in five patients in the primary PCI group and eight patients in the thrombolytic therapy group ($P < 0.01$). At least TIMI-3 flow was observed in rest of the patients. Twenty-one patients in PCI group, and 16 patients in thrombolytic therapy group were in sinus rhythm (SR) at the time of second coronary angiography, although there was no difference between the LVEFs of the groups, as determined by echocardiography at the time of the first coronary angiography. However, the LVEF of patients in the PCI group was higher at the time of second angiography. Our data showed that, because the patency of the infarct-related artery is better with primary PCI, this mode of treatment is superior to thrombolytic therapy in restoring sinus in acute MI patients.

Recommendations for Management

Post-PCI AF tends to revert spontaneously over a period of minutes to hours, and thus usually does not usually require immediate treatment unless it produces ischaemia or haemodynamic instability. Specific recommendations for therapy in those patients are preliminary and based on consensus since no adequate trials have tested alternate strategies.

Electrical cardioversion is very rarely required. But, when haemodynamic decompensation is prominent, electrical cardioversion is indicated, beginning with 50–100 joules with gradual increase if the initial shock is not successful. When necessary, a beta-blocker can be used for rate control because of the combined effects of ischaemia and sympathetic tone which usually present in patients with AF. If an intravenous beta-blocker is preferred but it is uncertain whether such therapy will be tolerated by the patient, esmolol may be cautiously administrated since its very short half-life permits a therapeutic trial to be performed at reduced risk. If esmolol is tolerated, then a moderate or long-acting beta-blocker can be given. These drugs can be administered in combination as indicated. Intravenous doses of verapamil or diltiazem are attractive alternatives because of their ability to slow the ventricular rate promptly, but they should be used with caution if at all in patients with pulmonary congestion. Due to the increased risk of embolism, intravenous anticoagulation with heparin should be instituted in the absence of any contraindications and if it is still present while the patient is in the coronary care unit or in his or her room. Amidorone and dofetelide are also effective for acute control of the ventricular response, but generally are not recommended as the drug of choice for rate control. Digoxin is one of the drugs of choice and can be used especially in patients with congestive heart failure. Atrial flutter is generally well tolerated and also tends to revert spontaneously; when necessary, it can be treated with either burst atrial pacing or electrical or pharmacologic cardioversion.

Conclusions

Atrial flutter may occur as a complication of PCI, but most of the time the patients' characteristics play important roles in the occurrence of this type of arrhythmia. For instance, ongoing acute MI can be the real reason for AF. Generally, AF tends to revert spontaneously, but when necessary treatment must be given promptly. If the patient is compromised by ventricular rate or by the loss of atrial contribution to cardiac output, synchronised DC cardioversion should be performed without delay. Intravenous beta-blockade can be effective for acute rate control. Calcium-channel blockers can be administered to promptly control ventricular rate. Digoxin, amiodarone and dofetilide are the drugs of choice for treating patients with acute MI with heart failure.

References

1. Benjamin EJ, Wolf PA, D'Agostino RB et al (1998) Impact of atrial fibrillation on the risk of death: the Framingham Heart Study. Circulation 98:946–952
2. Chugh SS, Blackshear JL, Shen WK et al (2001) Epidemiology and natural history of atrial fibrillation: clinical implications. J Am Coll Cardiol 37:371–378
3. Mehta RH, Harjai KJ, Grines L et al (2004) Sustained ventricular tachycardia or fibrillation in the cardiac catheterization laboratory among patients receiving primary percutaneous coronary intervention: incidence, predictors, and outcomes. J Am Coll Cardiol 43:1765–1772
4. Kinjo K, Sato H, Sato H et al (2003) Prognostic significance of atrial fibrillation/atrial flutter in patients with acute myocardial infarction treated with percutaneous coronary intervention. Am J Cardiol 92:1150–1154
5. Dilaveris PE, Gialafos EJ, Sideris SK et al (1998) Simple electrocardiographic markers for the prediction of paroxysmal idiopathic atrial fibrillation. Am Heart J 135:733–738
6. Gorenek B, Kudaiberdieva G, Cavusoglu Y (2002) Immediate recurrence of atrial fibrillation after internal cardioversion: importance of right atrial conduction variations. J Electrocardiol 35:313–320
7. Gialafos JE (1999) P-wave dispersion. Eur Heart J 20:317
8. Tanigawa M, Fukatani M, Konoe A et al (1991) Prolonged and fractionated right atrial electrograms during sinus rhythm in patients with paroxysmal atrial fibrillation and sinus sick node syndrome. J Am Coll Cardiol 17:403–408
9. Centurion OA, Isomoto S, Fukatani M et al (2002) Relationship between atrial conduction defects and fractioned atrial endocardial electrocardiograms in patients with sick sinus syndrome. PACE 16:2022–2023
10. Papageoriou P, Monahan K, Boyle NG et al (1996) Site dependent intra-atrial con-

duction delay: Relationship to initiation of atrial fibrillation. Circulation 94:348–349
11. Steinberg JS, Zelenkofske S, Wong SC et al (1993) Value of P-wave signal-averaged ECG for predicting atrial fibrillation after cardiac surgery. Circulation 88:2618–2622
12. Vilani GQ, Piepoli M, Cripps T et al (1994) Atrial late potentials in patients with paroxysmal atrial fibrillation detected using a high gain, signal-averaged esophageal lead. PACE 17:1118–1123
13. Klein M, Evans SJL, Cataldo L et al (1995) Use of P-wave-triggered, P-wave signal-averaged electrocardiogram to predict atrial fibrillation after coronary artery bypass surgery. Am Heart J 129:895–901
14. Yamada T, Fukunami M, Shimonagata T et al (1999) Dispersion of signal-averaged P wave duration on precordial body surface in patients with paroxysmal atrial fibrillation. Eur Heart J 20:211–220
15. Aytemir K, Aksoyek S, Yildirir A et al (1999) Prediction of atrial fibrillation recurrence after cardioversion by P wave signal-averaged electrocardiography. Int J Cardiol 70:15–21
16. Ozmen F, Atalar E, Aytemir K, Ozer N, et al (2001) Effect of balloon-induced acute ischemia on P wave dispersion during percutaneous transluminal coronary angioplasty. Europace 3:299–303
17. Budeus M, Hennersdorf M, Dierkes S et al (2003) Effects of right coronary artery PTCA on variables of P-wave signal averaged electrocardiogram. Ann Noninvasive Electrocardiol 8:150–156
18. Antman EM, Anbe DT, Armstrong PW et al (2004) ACC/AHA guidelines for the management of patients with ST-elevation myocardial infarction-executive summary: a report of the American College of Cardiology/American Heart Association Task Force on Practice Guidelines (Writing Committee to Revise the 1999 Guidelines for the Management of Patients With Acute Myocardial Infarction). Circulation 110:588
19. Eldar M, Canetti M, Rotstein Z, Boyko V et al (1998) Significance of paroxysmal atrial fibrillation complicating acute myocardial infarction in the thrombolytic era. SPRINT and Thrombolytic Survey Groups. Circulation 97:965–970
20. Goldberg RJ, Yarzebski J, Lessard D et al (2002) Recent trends in the incidence rates of and death rates from atrial fibrillation complicating initial acute myocardial infarction: a community-wide perspective. Am Heart J 143:519–527
21. Grines CL, Browne KF, Marco J et al (1993) A comparison of immediate angioplasty with thrombolytic therapy for acute myocardial infarction. The Primary Angioplasty in Myocardial Infarction Study Group. N Engl J Med 328:673–679
22. Zijlstra F, de Boer MJ, Hoorntje JC et al (1993) A comparison of immediate coronary angioplasty with intravenous streptokinase in acute myocardial infarction. N Engl J Med 328:680–684
23. Akdemir R, Ozhan H, Gunduz H et al (2005) Effect of reperfusion on P-wave duration and P-wave dispersion in acute myocardial infarction: primary angioplasty versus thrombolytic therapy. Ann Noninvasive Electrocardiol 10:35–40
24. Gorenek B, Birdane A, Unalir A et al (2000) Restoring sinus rhythm in patients with atrial fibrillation complicating acute myocardial infarction: comparison of outcomes of primary angioplasty and thrombolytic therapy. Eur J Heart Fail, Suppl 1:32 (abs)

Perioperative Interruption of Warfarin: How Effective and Safe Is Bridging Therapy with Low-Molecular-Weight Heparin?

F. Di Pede, P. Buja

Nowadays many patients are treated with warfarin for a variety of reasons, and the question of how to manage these patients when they are undergoing surgery or other procedures is of great clinical relevance. In the majority of cases warfarin is given to prevent thromboembolic events in patients with supraventricular arrhythmias, mechanical heart valves, and other disorders that carry a high risk of thromboembolism [1]: stroke represents a frequent devastating consequence of thromboembolism, resulting in major neurological deficit or death in more than half of patients [2]. Atrial fibrillation (AF) is the most common cardiac abnormality requiring warfarin therapy. Its prevalence increases with age and it affects approximately 6% of people over 65 years of age [3].

Warfarin has been shown to reduce the risk of stroke associated with AF, while the risk of haemorrhage remains small [4]. By contrast, excessive bleedings occur when patients undergo several invasive and surgical procedures while continuing warfarin therapy [5].

The optimal management of patients receiving long-term warfarin treatment when they are to undergo surgical or invasive procedures is still debated. Three aspects need to be discussed [6]: first, the risk of thromboembolism due to warfarin interruption, and to the procedure itself as well as to the postoperative risk related to the procedure. Secondly, the risk of bleeding if anti-coagulation treatment is continued during the procedure. And, finally, the effectiveness and safety of various bridging strategies: several reports suggest a substitute therapy with a short-acting anti-coagulant to prevent the risk of thromboembolism when the oral anti-coagulation treatment is

Division of Cardiology, Cardiovascular Department, Umberto I Hospital, Mestre-Venice, Italy

interrupted, especially in high-risk patients [1, 5, 7, 8]. Low-molecular weight heparin (LMWH) is playing an emerging role as a perioperative substitute of unfractionated heparin (UFH) in such cases.

Thromboembolic Risk Related to Warfarin Interruption for Surgical/Invasive Procedures

The risk of thromboembolism during warfarin discontinuation depends on four major variables: (1) the duration of warfarin interruption, (2) the indication for anti-coagulation, (3) the perioperative risk related to the procedure, and (4) the bridging therapy during anti-coagulant interruption. If warfarin is stopped 4 days before the procedure and restarted as soon as possible after the intervention, patients should have a sub-therapeutic INR for approximately 2 days before and 2 days after the procedure [8]. However, the INR should be raised to some extent during this period, and consequently patients should be at least partially protected against thromboembolic events. Finally, because the coagulation state needs to be normal or nearly normal during the perioperative period, an increased risk of thromboembolism cannot be completely avoided.

The risk of thromboembolism due to warfarin interruption can be stratified as low, intermediate, or high according to the underlying disease [5]. Briefly, patients at low risk of thromboembolism (< 4% per year) are those with atrial fibrillation without a history of stroke or other risk factors. Patients at intermediate risk (4–7% per year) are those with a mechanical aortic valve. Patients at high risk (> 7% per year) are those with a mechanical mitral valve or atrial fibrillation with a history of thromboembolic stroke or with heart valvular disease.

The perioperative thromboembolic risk is also related to other factors such as the rebound of hypercoagulability due to warfarin interruption [9] and the pro-thrombotic state following from the intervention itself [10].

Risk of Bleeding

The assessment of bleeding risk, is very important to estimate the risk/benefit ratio of bridging therapy. Bleeding rates for invasive and surgical procedures are often not analysed separately, the definitions of minor and major bleeding are often different, and treatment strategies are various. However, on the basis of available data, the increase in major bleeding over 2 days in the postoperative period is approximately 2–4% for major surgery and 0–2% for invasive procedures [5].

Low-Molecular-Weight Heparin Versus Unfractionated Heparin

The advantages of LMWH over UFH can be summed up in four main characteristics:

1. LMWH may reduce the incidence of major bleedings [11, 12].
2. LMWH can be given in a subcutaneous fixed weight-based dose without laboratory monitoring [13].
3. Patients can easily self-inject LMWH at home, shortening hospital stays and reducing costs [14–17].
4. LMWH carries a risk of heparin-induced thrombocytopenia lower than that associated with UFH [18].

On the other hand, no antidote exists to neutralise LMWH, although protamine can partially reverse it [19], and no laboratory test is easily available for monitoring the amount of anti-coagulation effect at the time of the procedure.

Several studies relating to different clinical settings and indications analysed LMWH and compared it to UFH, but no randomised trial exists that addresses this issue. Furthermore, published data are often small, underpowered, and associated with statistical bias [12, 13, 16, 20–29]. Although a firm conclusion is difficult to draw in terms of superiority of LMWH over UFH, LMWH therapy appears to be a safe and effective alternative in this setting. In fact, the American College of Cardiology/American Heart Association [1] and the American College of Chest Physicians (ACCP) [7] do not indicate significant differences between LMWH and UFH as bridging therapies in the context of perioperative warfarin discontinuation.

Recommendations

The decision of how to manage patients receiving long-term warfarin treatment who need an invasive procedure is based on the estimation of the risks associated with stopping or continuing anti-coagulation and the cost/risk ratio of alternative anti-coagulant therapy. No large randomised trial exists to support our decision. On the basis of data available in 2004, the seventh ACCP conference on anti-thrombotic and thrombolytic therapy gave the following recommendations [7]:

- For patients with a low risk of thromboembolism, stop warfarin approximately 4 days before surgery; briefly use postoperative prophylaxis if the intervention increases the risk of thrombosis with a low dose of UFH (5000 U s.c.) or a prophylactic dose of LMWH and simultaneously begin warfarin therapy. Alternatively, a low dose of UFH or a prophylactic dose of LMWH can be used preoperatively (grade 2C).

- For patients with an intermediate risk of thromboembolism, stop warfarin 4 days before surgery; cover the patient 2 days before with a low dose of UFH (5000 U SC) or a prophylactic dose of LMWH, and than commence with low-dose UFH or LMWH and warfarin postoperatively, (grade 2C).
- For patients with a high risk of thromboembolism, stop warfarin 4 days before surgery and begin full-dose UFH or full-dose LMWH as the INR falls. Intravenous UFH can be stopped approximately 5 h before surgery. If LMWH is used, it should be stopped 12–24 h before surgery. Then full-dose UFH (or LMWH) and warfarin is given after surgery (grade 2C). In selected cases (for example in major surgery) several authors suggest restarting anti-coagulation the day after surgery, or when adequate haemostasis is obtained.
- Patients at low risk of bleeding will continue warfarin therapy at a lower dose that allows an INR of 1.3–1.5 at the time of surgery. Then warfarin can be restarted postoperatively (grade 2C).

Minor surgeries do not require anti-coagulation interruption, but the INR should be within the therapeutic range at the time of the intervention. Among these are dental extractions, joint and soft tissue injections, arthrocentesis, cataract surgery, upper gastrointestinal endoscopy of or colonoscopy with biopsy [5].

In conclusion, on the basis of current available data, LMWH seems a good alternative to UFH as bridging therapy in patients requiring warfarin interruption.

References

1. Hirsh J, Fuster V, Ansell J et al (2003) AHA/ACC Foundation Guide to Warfarin Therapy. J Am Coll Cardiol 41:1633–1652
2. Longstreth WT Jr, Bernick C, Fitzpatrick A et al (2001) Frequency and predictors of stroke death in 5888 participants in the Cardiovascular Health Study. Neurology 56:368–375
3. Feinberg WM, Blackshear JL, Laupacis A et al (1995) Prevalence, age distribution and gender of patients with atrial fibrillation. Analysis and implications. Arch Intern Med 155:469–473
4. Go AS, Hylek EM, Chang Y et al (2005) Anticoagulation therapy for stroke prevention in atrial fibrillation. How well do randomized trials translate into clinical practice? JAMA 290:2685–2692
5. Dunn AS, Turpie AGG (2003) Perioperative management of patients receiving oral anticoagulants. Arch Intern Med 163:901–908
6. Ansell JE (2003) The perioperative management of warfarin therapy. Arch Intern Med 163:881–883
7. Ansell J, Hirsh J, Poller L et al (2004) The pharmacology and management of the vitamin K antagonists. The Seventh ACCP Conference on Antithrombotic and Thrombolytic Therapy. Chest 126:204–233

8. Kearon C, Hirsh J (1997) Management of anticoagulation before and after elective surgery. N Engl J Med 336:1506–1511
9. Gould MK, Dembitzer AD, Doyle RL et al (1999) Low-molecular-weight heparins compared with unfractioned heparin for treatment of acute deep venous thrombosis: a meta-analysis of randomized, controlled trials. Ann Intern Med 130:800–809
10. Poller L, Thomson J (1964) Evidence for 'rebound' hypercoagulability after stopping anticoagulants. Lancet 2:62–64
11. Lopez Y, Paramo JA, Valenti JR et al (1997) Hemostatic markers in surgery: a different fibrinolytic activity may be of pathophysiological significance in orthopedic versus abdominal surgery. Int J Clin Lab Res 27:233–237
12. Van Den Belt AGM, Prins MH, Lensing AWA et al (2000) Fixed dose subcutaneous low-molecular-weight heparins versus adjusted dose unfractioned heparin for venous thromboembolism. Cochrane Database Syst Rev 2:CD001100
13. Hirsh J, Warkentin TE, Shaughnessy SG et al (2001) Heparin and low-molecular-weight heparin: mechanism of action, pharmacokinetics, dosing, monitoring, efficacy and safety. Chest 119:S64–S94
14. Goldstein JL, Larson LR, Yamashita BD et al (2001) Low molecular weight heparin versus unfractionated heparin in the colonoscopy periprocedure period: a cost modeling study. Am J Gastroenterol 96:2360–2366
15. Groce JB (1998) Patient outcomes and cost analysis associated with an outpatient deep venous thrombosis treatment program. Pharmacotherapy 18:S175–S180
16. Tsilimingras K, Grasso-Correnti N, Fanikos J et al (2002) Initiation of anticoagulation after cardiac surgery: a prospective cohort study of efficacy, safety, and cost with low-molecular-weight heparin bridging in lieu of continuous intravenous unfractionated heparin. J Am Coll Cardiol 39(Suppl):836–837
17. Spyropoulos AC, Frost FJ, Hurley JS et al (2004) Costs and clinical outcomes associated with low-molecular-weight heparin vs unfractionated heparin for perioperative bridging in patients receiving long-term oral anticoagulant therapy. Chest 125:1642–1650
18. Warkentin TE, Levine MN, Hirsh J et al (1995) Heparin-induced thrombocytopenia in patients treated with low-molecular-weight heparin or unfractionated heparin. N Engl J Med 332:1330–1335
19. Holst J, Lindblad B, Berqvist D et al (1994) Protamine neutralization of intravenous and subcutaneous low-molecular weight heparin (tinzaparin, Logiparin): an experimental investigation in healthy volunteers. Blood Coagul Fibrinolysis 5:783–795
20. Douketis JD, Johnson JA, Turpie AG (2004) Low-molecular-weight heparin as bridging anticoagulation during interruption of warfarin: assessment of a standardized periprocedural anticoagulation regimen. Arch Intern Med 164:1319–1326
21. Akopov SE, Suzuki S, Fredieu A et al (2004) Withdrawal of warfarin prior to a surgical procedure: time to follow the guidelines? Cerebrovasc Dis 19:337–342
22. Kalafut MA, Gandhi R, Kidwell CS et al (2000) Safety and cost of low-molecular-weight heparin as bridging anticoagulant therapy in subacute cerebral ischemia. Stroke 31:2563–2568
23. Ferreira IJ, Dos L, Tornos MP et al (2000) Is low molecular weight heparin a safe alternative to unfractionated heparin in patients with prosthetic mechanical heart valves who must interrupt antithrombotic therapy? Eur Heart J 21(Suppl):301
24. Stellbrink C, Nixdorff U, Hofmann T et al (2004) Safety and efficacy of enoxaparin compared with unfractionated heparin and oral anticoagulants for prevention of thromboembolic complications in cardioversion of nonvalvular atrial fibrillation. The Anticoagulation in Cardioversion using Enoxaparin (ACE) Trial. Circulation

109:997–1003

25. Cohen M, Demers C, Gurfinkel EP et al (1997) A comparison of low-molecular-weight-heparin with UFH for unstable coronary artery disease: Efficacy and Safety of Subcutaneous Enoxaparin in Non-Q-Wave Coronary Events Study Group. N Engl J Med 337:447–452
26. Spandorfer JM, Lynch S, Weitz HH et al (1999) Use of enoxaparin for the chronically anticoagulated patient before and after procedures. Am J Cardiol 84:478–480
27. Johnson J, Turpie AGG (1999) Temporary discontinuation of oral anticoagulants: role of low-molecular-weight heparin (dalteparin). Thromb Haemost 82(Suppl):62–63
28. Tinmouth AH, Morrow BH, Cruickshank MK et al (2001) Dalteparin as periprocedure anticoagulation for patients on warfarin and at high risk of thrombosis. Ann Pharmacother 35:669–674
29. Montalescot G, Polle V, Collet JP et al (2000) Low molecular weight heparin after mechanical heart valve replacement. Circulation 101:1083–1086

How Safe Is Anticoagulant Therapy in Older Patients and What Should Be the INR Target?

G. Di Pasquale, M. di Niro, G. Casella, P.C. Pavesi, A. Rubboli, C. Greco, V. Carinci

Epidemiology

Atrial fibrillation (AF) is the most common arrhythmia in clinical practice, and its prevalence increases substantially with age. In the ATRIA study, AF occurred in 4% of people aged 60 years and older and in 9% of people aged 80 years and older [1]. The authors estimated that approximately 2.3 million US adults currently have AF, projecting that this figure will increase to more than 5.6 million by the year 2050, with more than 50% of affected individuals aged 80 years or older. The estimate of AF in Italy is about 500 000 subjects with an incidence of 60 000 new cases per year.

Thromboembolic Risk

In the absence of any antithrombotic therapy, the annual risk of stroke and systemic thromboembolism is 4.5% and rises to 8% in subjects older than 75 years of age. Taking into account also the risk of transient ischaemic attack (TIA) and silent cerebral infarction, the risk of cerebral embolism exceeds 7% per year [2, 3]. Clinical features independently associated with a high risk of stroke in AF patients have been defined and integrated into several risk stratification schemes. High-risk factors include age > 75 years, prior stroke/TIA or systemic embolism, history of hypertension, congestive heart failure or poor left ventricular systolic function, diabetes mellitus, rheumatic mitral valve disease, and prosthetic heart valves.

Moderate risk factors include age 65–75 years, and coronary artery dis-

Unità Operativa di Cardiologia, Ospedale Maggiore, Bologna, Italy

ease with preserved left ventricular function.

It is evident from thromboembolic risk stratification that older age (> 75 years) per se is a high-risk factor for thromboembolism and all patients older than 75 years should receive oral anticoagulant treatment (OAT) for effective prophylaxis. This represents a therapeutic dilemma because of the higher risk of life-threatening haemorrhages, in particular cerebral haemorrhage, in these patients during OAT.

Indications for Oral Anticoagulant Therapy

The effectiveness of OAT for the prevention of thromboembolism and stroke has been assessed by a number of randomised clinical trials [4, 5]. Six trials (AFASAK, SPAF, BAATAF, CAFA, SPINAF, and EAFT) compared the therapeutic effects of adjusted-dose warfarin with placebo. Overall adjusted-dose warfarin reduced stroke by 62% (95% CI, 48–72%); absolute risk reductions were 2.7% per year for primary prevention [number needed to treat (NNT) for 1 year to prevent one stroke = 37] and 8.4% per year (NNT = 12) for secondary prevention.

The efficacy of aspirin for stroke prevention in AF patients is unclear and more controversial [4, 5]. Six trials (AFASAK, SPAF I, EAFT, ESPS II, LASAF, and UK TIA) compared the therapeutic effects of antiplatelet therapy with placebo. Meta-analysis of all six trials showed that aspirin reduced the incidence of stroke by 22% (CI, 2–38%). On the basis of these six trials, the absolute risk reduction was 1.5% per year (NNT = 67) for primary prevention and 2.5% per year (NNT = 40) for secondary prevention. Although all six trials showed trends toward reduced stroke with aspirin, this result was statistically significant only in the SPAF I study.

Recommendations for treatment, based on the evidence from clinical trials and thromboembolic risk stratification, were reconfirmed in the 2001 ACC/AHA/ESC guidelines for the management of patients with AF [5] and in the Seventh 2004 Consensus Conference on antithrombotic therapy of the American College of Chest Physicians [6]. OAT is mandatory in AF high-risk patients (those with any high-risk factor or with more than one moderate-risk factor), provided that high-quality monitoring of OAT is possible and no risk factors for bleeding are present. These two last requirements are particularly important when deciding on OAT in patients older than 75 years.

Aspirin is a possible and acceptable alternative to OAT in moderate-risk patients (those without high-risk factors and with only one moderate-risk factor). In this group of patients, the choice between aspirin and OAT is based on the assessment of the risk/benefit ratio of OAT and also on the patient's preference [7].

Finally, aspirin is the treatment of choice in low-risk patients (those without high-risk or moderate-risk factors). This group is represented by patients with no clinical or echocardiographic evidence of cardiovascular disease.

Despite the strong evidence for the efficacy of OAT, the use of warfarin for stroke prevention in patients with AF is still low in general clinical practice [8–10]. Underutilisation of OAT is especially evident among elderly people with AF, in whom, paradoxically, the thromboembolic risk is higher. In fact, anticoagulation treatment decreases with age (44% of eligible patients age 65–75 years are treated with anticoagulants as opposed to less than 20% after 80 years) and it is estimated that less than 40% of eligible patients receive OAT.

A recent study has shown that, despite the known increased risk for stroke with advancing age in AF patients, there is a 14% reduction in warfarin use with each advancing decade of life [11].

Major reasons for the underuse of OAT are the difficulty of high-quality monitoring of OAT, especially in older patients, and the fear of bleeding. Therefore new, safer and effective thromboprophylactic strategies for AF are warranted, particularly for older patients, who represent a substantial proportion of the AF population.

Bleeding Risk of Oral Anticoagulant Therapy

Bleeding is the most important complication of OAT, even if the risk of bleeding in patients receiving OAT in randomised clinical studies was quite low. The annual frequency of major bleeding events was 1.3% in warfarin-treated patients (vs 1.0% in patients receiving placebo or controls, and 1.0% in aspirin-treated patients). However the bleeding risk is likely higher in patients treated in general clinical practice. Patients included in the clinical trials were carefully selected (representing only 7–39% of the screened patients) and followed up carefully according to strict protocols. This can explain the low bleeding risk during warfarin therapy. Moreover, the safety and tolerability of long-term anticoagulation at conventional levels has not been completely defined among patients older than 75 years. In the AFASAK study [12], which involved AF patients older than those enrolled in every other trial (mean age of 75 years), the withdrawal rate from warfarin was 38% after 1 year. In the SPAF II study [13] (INR 2.0–4.5, mean 2.7), the risk of major haemorrhage, mainly cerebral, was substantially higher among AF patients older than 75 years.

In the the real world, bleeding is often a major concern regarding anticoagulation of elderly patients for stroke prevention. In particular, conventional intensities of anticoagulation increase the risk of intracranial haemorrhage 7- to 10-fold, and the risk of cerebral bleeding is significantly higher in the elderly. The key issue in using warfarin to prevent stroke and systemic embolism in AF patients is whether the benefit of therapy outweighs the risk of bleeding in an individual patient.

Risk factors for bleeding during OAT include advanced age, intensity of anticoagulation, recent initiation of warfarin therapy, and comorbid conditions.

Patients with advanced age are more prone to complications of OAT than younger patients [14, 15]. Only a few studies have shown that advanced age by itself does not increase the complication rate of OAT. In a large prospective Italian collaborative study (ISCOAT), the frequency of bleeding complications was studied in outpatients treated routinely in anticoagulation clinics [16]. The rate of fatal, major and minor bleeding events was quite low, 1.1 and 6.2 per patient-years of follow-up, respectively. The rate was higher in older patients and during the first 90 days of treatment. The risk of bleeding was related to the intensity of anticoagulation, even if a fifth of the bleeding events occurs at INR < 2.0.

A subsequent analysis of patients age > 75 years who were included in ISCOAT showed a nonsignificant trend toward a higher rate of both bleeding and thrombotic complications in elderly versus matched younger patients [17]. In addition, intracranial bleedings and fatal thrombotic events were more frequent in the elderly. The results of this analysis also indicated that INRs < 2.0 do not preclude bleeding in the elderly nor offer adequate protection from thrombotic events. In the subset of patients with AF, major bleeding occurred more frequently in patients over 75 years of age (5.1% per year) than in younger patients (1.0% per year) [18]. Univariate analysis revealed a higher frequency of major bleeding in females, in diabetics, and in those who had suffered a previous thromboembolic event.

A clear correlation was reported between intensity of anticoagulation and risk of bleeding. In ISCOAT, the risk of bleeding in patients aged > 75 years markedly increased with INR values of 3.0–4.4, and became disproportionately high for INR values > 4.5 [17]. However, a substantial number of events (10%) occurred in association with very low INR values (< 2.0), confirming previous reports that bleeding during OAT is not always related to the intensity of OAT but that OAT can unmask a local bleeding source.

A higher frequency of bleeding early in the course of OAT was reported in a number of studies [16, 17, 19]. Several factors may contribute to the increased risk of bleeding within the first months of each course of OAT. First, OAT can unmask a cryptic, often neoplastic, lesion. Second, dose adjustment may be less well-controlled at the start of treatment.

Furthermore, multiple drug therapies are quite common in elderly patients and this increases the risk of adverse drug interaction with OAT. In a recent large study [20] in patients treated with OAT, subjects receiving more than three drugs had a six-fold higher risk of bleeding or embolic complications than patients receiving less than three drugs (24.4%/100 patient-years versus 4.3%; $P = 0.01$). Since the complication rate did not differ between patients taking drugs known to interact with OAT and those who did not take interacting drugs, it may be inferred that the increased complication rate of patients with multiple medications was a consequence of comorbidity rather than of drug interaction.

The quality of anticoagulation laboratory control is also affected by the mental status of the patient. Palareti et al. [21] found a previously unsuspected reduction of mental status or attention level in a number of elderly patients receiving OAT; these patients had been exposed to longer periods of either under- or over-anticoagulation and therefore to a higher risk of thrombotic or bleeding complications.

A recent combined retrospective and prospective study [22] comprising a large group of older patients evaluated the importance of OAT education. This study showed that the rate of bleeding complications, especially major bleeding, is low in well-informed elderly patients.

Recommendations

The management of OAT in older subjects needs regular monitoring of INR, which should be kept in the narrow therapeutic range of 2.0–3.0 most of the time, with adjustments of the dose as required [23]. Moreover, elderly patients should be administered a low dose of warfarin during the induction phase, because of their increased sensitivity to the drug [24].

In older patients, a risk/benefit assessment is warranted before initiating OAT. Major considerations should include:

1. Decision for AF electrical cardioversion which, at least in some cases, could obviate the need of long-term OAT
2. Thromboembolic risk stratification in the individual patient; the prevalence of additional risk factors for thromboembolism beside advanced age (i.e. hypertension, prior stroke or TIA, heart failure or left ventricular dysfunction, or diabetes mellitus, should reinforce the decision for OAT
3. Ability to provide high-quality monitoring of OAT through coordinated medical care (e.g. anticoagulation clinics)
4. Patient's inherent risk of bleeding with OAT
5. Evaluation of risk factors for OAT-related bleeding complications.

When deciding whether to initiate OAT in older patients, patient education and optimal OAT monitoring are key issues for minimising the risk of bleeding. An Italian study has shown that, in a group of elderly patients followed by their general practitioner with the support of a specialised cardiologic unit, OAT was well-tolerated and associated with a significant decrease in mortality and hospitalisation, in the absence of an increase of major bleeding [25].

High-quality monitoring of OAT is of utmost importance. A systematic approach to anticoagulation management, as offered by anticoagulation clinics, can improve the safety and effectiveness of warfarin therapy by reducing related and unrelated complications. This coordinated care can be contrasted with that provided by a patient's own physician, without systematic coordination (routine medical care). Available data indicate that coordinated care, compared with routine medical care, reduces the incidence of adverse outcomes and also the cost of OAT [26–28].

References

1. Go AS, Hyiek EM, Phillips KA et al (2001) Prevalence of diagnosed atrial fibrillation in adults. National implications for rhythm management and stroke prevention: the Anticoagulation and Risk Factors In Atrial Fibrillation (ATRIA) Study. JAMA 285:2370–2375
2. Atrial Fibrillation Investigators (1994) Risk factors for stroke and efficacy of antithrombotic therapy in atrial fibrillation: analysis of pooled data from five randomized controlled trials. Arch Intern Med 154:1449–1457
3. Hart RG, Pearce LA, Me Bride R et al, on behalf of the Stroke Prevention in Atrial Fibrillation (SPAF) Investigators (1999) Factors associated with ischemic stroke during aspirin therapy in atrial fibrillation. Analysis of 2012 participants in the SPAF I-III clinical trials. Stroke 30:1223–1229
4. Hart RG, Benavente 0, McBride R, Pearce LA (1999) Antithrombotic therapy to prevent stroke in patients with atrial fibrillation: a meta-analysis. Ann Intern Med 131:492–501
5. Fuster V, Ryden L et al (2001) ACC/AHA/ESC guidelines for the management of patients with atrial fibrillation: executive summary. Am J Cardiol 38:1231–1265
6. Singer DE, Albers GW, Dalen JE et al (2004) Antithrombotic therapy in atrial fibrillation. The seventh ACCP conference antithrombotic and thrombolytic therapy. Chest 126:429S-256S
7. Di Pasquale G, Cere E, Biancoli S et al (2002) Antiplatelet agents for prevention of thromboembolism in atrial fibrillation : when, why, and which one? In: Raviele A (ed) Cardiac Arrhythmias 2001, Springer Verlag Italia, Milan, pp 422–435
8. Bungard TJ, Ghali WA, Teo KK et al (2000) Why do patient with atrial fibrillation not receive warfarin? Arch Intern Med 160:41–46
9. Cohen N, Sarafian DA, Alon I et al (2000) Warfarin for stroke prevention still underused in atrial fibrillation. Stroke 31:1217–1222
10. Frykman V, Beermann B, Ryden L, Rosenqvist M (2001) Management of atrial fibrillation: discrepancy between guideline recommendations and actual practice exposes patients to risk for complications. Eur Heart J 22:1954–1959
11. Brophy MT, Snyder KE, Gaehde S et al (2004) Anticoagulant use for atrial fibrillation in the Elderly. J Am Geriatr Soc 52:1151–1156

12. Petersen P, Boysen G, Godtfredsen J et al (1989) Placebo-controlled, randomised trial of warfarin and aspirin for prevention of thromboembolic complications in chronic atrial fibrillation. The Copenhagen AFASAK Study. Lancet 1:175–179
13. Stroke Prevention in Atrial Fibrillation Investigators (1994) Warfarin versus aspirin for prevention of thromboembolism in atrial fibrillation: Stroke Prevention in Atrial Fibrillation II Study. Lancet 343:687–691
14. Sebastian J, Tresch DD (2000) Use of oral anticoagulants in older patients. Drugs Aging 16:409–435
15. Beyth RJ, Landefeld S (1995) Anticoagulants in older patients: a safety perspective. Drugs Aging 6:45–54
16. Palareti G, Leali N, Coccheri S et al on behalf of the Italian Study on Complications of Oral Anticoagulant Therapy (1996) Bleeding complications of oral anticoagulant treatment: an inception-cohort, prospective collaborative study (ISCOAT). Lancet 348:423–428
17. Palareti G, Hirsh J, Legnani C et al (2000) Oral anticoagulation treatment in the elderly: a nested prospective, case-control study. Arch Intern Med 160:470–478
18. Pengo V, Legnani C, Noventa F, Palareti G, on behalf of the ISCOAT Study Group (2001) Oral anticoagulant therapy in patients with nonrheumatic atrial fibrillation and risk of bleeding. Thromb Haemost 85:418–422
19. Landefeld CS, Goldman L (1989) Major bleeding in outpatients treated with warfarin. Incidence and prediction by factors known at the start of outpatient therapy. Am J Med 87:144–152
20. Wehinger C, Stollberger C, Langer T et al (2001) Evaluation of risk factors for stroke/embolism and of complications due to anticoagulant therapy in atrial fibrillation. Stroke 32:2246–2252
21. Palareti G, Poggi M, Guazzaloca G et al (1997) Assessment of mental ability in elderly anticoagulated patients: its reduction is associated with a less satisfactory quality of treatment. Blood Coagul Fibrinolysis 8:411–417
22. Kagansky N, Knobler H, Rimon E et al (2004) Safety of anticoagulation therapy in well-informed older patients. Arch Intern Med 164:2044–2050
23. American Geriatrics Society (2002) The use of oral anticoagulants (warfarin) in older people. J Am Geriatr Soc 50:1439–1532
24. Siguret V, Gouin I, Debray et al (2005) Initiation of warfain therapy in elderly medical patients: a safe accurate regimen. Am J Med 118(2):137–140
25. Bordin P, Mazzone C, Pandullo C et al (2003) Morbidity and mortality in 229 elderly patients with nonrheumatic atrial fibrillation. A five-year follow-up. Ital Heart J 4(8):537–543
26. Ansell JE, Hirsh J, Dalen J et al (2001) Managing oral anticoagulant therapy. Chest 119: 22S-38S
27. Chiquette E, Amato MG, Bussey HI (1998) Comparison of an anticoagulation clinic with usual medical care: anticoagulation control, patient outcomes, and health care costs. Arch Intern Med 158:1641–1647
28. Fitmaurice DA, Hobbs FD, Delaney BC et al (1998) Review of computerized decision support system for oral anticoagulation management. Br J Hematol 102:907–909

Oral Antithrombin Agents: Will They Replace Warfarin?

G. Grönefeld, D. Pajitnev, F. Wegener, J.R. Ehrlich, S.H. Hohnloser

Introduction

Three cornerstones constitute the current treatment of atrial fibrillation: rhythm control, rate control, and antithrombotic therapy for the prevention of systemic thromboembolic events. The loss of mechanical atrial contraction leads to altered blood flow characteristics that can result in clot formation; particularly, the left atrial appendage is the most important area of clot formation within the fibrillating atria. Left atrial thrombi can subsequently embolise to the brain, coronary arteries, peripheral limb arteries, or other end organs, resulting in irreversible and in many patients functionally devastating sequelae. The risk of systemic thromboembolism in patients with atrial fibrillation (AF) is well-established [1, 2]. Five randomised controlled trials have convincingly demonstrated that the risk of AF-associated thrombembolic events (predominantly strokes) can be reduced by 65% by therapy with vitamin K antagonists [2]. Accordingly, current guidelines strongly recommend preventive oral anticoagulation in the presence of valvular heart disease, for patients with non-valvular AF who are age 65 years or older, or in the presence of additional risk factors (Table 1) [3–6]. The results from the AFFIRM [7] and other prospective trials comparing rhythm versus rate control have additionally shown that, even when the strategy of rhythm control is effectively pursued, effective oral anticoagulation should be maintained in high-risk patients [8]. Despite this overwhelming body of evidence, however, there is a considerable underutilisation of vitamin K antagonists (Table 2) due to patients' or doctors' concerns as well as to an unwillingness to comply with the necessary modes of monitoring and dosage adjustments during

Division of Cardiology, Department of Medicine, J.W.Goethe-University, Frankfurt am Main, Germany

Table 1. Recommendations for antithrombotic therapy in patients with AF

Annual stroke risk (%)	Risk stratification	Recommendations	NNT (95% CI)
Low (1%)	Age < 65 years without additional risk factors (such as: previous stroke, TIA, or systemic embolism hypertension, heart failure, or LVEF < 50%)	ASA	227 (135–2500)
Low-moderate (1.5%)	Age 65–74 years without additional risk factors	ASA	152 (88–1667)
Moderate (2.5%)	Age 65–74 years without additional risk factors but comorbidity of diabetes or coronary artery disease	Warfarin	32 (28–42)
High (6%) (such as: hypertension, heart failure, or LVEF or: age ≥ 75 years without any risk factor < 50%)	Age < 75 years with additional risk factors	Warfarin	14 (12–17)
Very high (10%)	Age ≥ 75 years with additional risk factors (such as: hypertension, heart failure, or LVEF or: any age with previous history of stroke, TIA or systemic embolism < 50%)	Warfarin	8 (7–10)

NNT Number needed to treat, *ASA* Acetyl salicylic acid, *TIA* transient ischaemic attack, *LVEF* left ventricular ejection fraction

Table 2. The real world: prescription of oral anticoagulants as reported in studies after 1992

Study	Number of patients population	Patient prescription (%)	OAC
Albers et al. 1997	171 mean age of 75 years	AF and stroke,	19.8
Antani et al. 1996	98	AF, mean age of 76 years	36.7
Bath et al. 1993	95	AF, age 32–100 years	29.3
Beyth et al. 1996	189	NVAF	24.0
Brass et al. 1997	488 were age 65–74 years with additional risk factor	AF, age 65 years; 54%	38.4
Gottlieb et al. 1994	238	AF, mean age of 69 years	78.8
Gurwitz et al. 1997	413	AF, 66% age 85 years	31.5
Hendry et al. 1994	131	NVAF, age 53–95 years	15,2
Lip et al. 1997	111	AF, age 50–105 years	22.3
Lip et al. 1994	170	AF, aged 38–95 years	36.0
Munschauer et al. 1997	651	Chronic AF	38.1
O´Connell and Gray, 1996	91	AF, mean age of 77 years	24.1
Sudlow et al. 1998	207	AF, age 65 years	23.0
CQIN Investigators, 1998	3575	AF, aged 19–104 years	23.8
Whittle et al. 1997	172	AF, mean age of 80 years	44.1

NVAF non valvular atrial fibrillation, *OAC* oral anticoagulation

long-term treatment [9]. Hence, more convenient and equally effective treatment alternatives to warfarin are currently under evaluation for the purpose of thromboembolic prophylaxis in patients with AF. The present short review provides an overview of the current state of development of an alternative to vitamin K antagonists for the prevention of AF-associated stroke.

Underuse of Vitamin K Antagonists

The use of oral vitamin K antagonist in patients with AF has stagnated during more than 15 years that have passed since the publication of the large anticoagulation trials [10]. At present, only 30–50% of high-risk AF patients without contraindications for oral anticoagulation receive this treatment [11]. The major reasons for this underutilisation include the reluctance of physicians and patients to follow the somewhat complicated and time-consuming procedures of monitoring and patient counseling (Table 3). A frequent concern is the narrow therapeutic window of warfarin which may result in an increased bleeding risk, particularly in patients above the age of 80 years [11]. In addition, in many regions of the world, the health care system may be unable to provide the necessary resources.

Table 3. Main reasons for the underutilisation of warfarin

Patient-related reasons
- Advanced age
- Suspected or given lack of compliance
- Inconvenience of monitoring
- Impaired quality of life
Physician-related reasons
- Failure to detect atrial fibrillation (i.e. in pacemaker patients)
- Estimation of individual risk for embolism too low
- Estimation of individual risk for bleeding too high
- Results of randomised controlled trials (RCTs) not known or not accepted
- INR-target range not achievable or not maintainable
- Guidelines not applicable for own patients
Health-care-system-related reasons
- Limited coverage of frequent INR checks
- Lack of specialised anticoagulation-clinics

Moreover, even when warfarin is appropriately prescribed, international normalized ratio (INR) values vary considerably due to individual metabolism and food or drug interactions, resulting in over- or undercoagulation. Even in patients enrolled in prospective trials, the quality of anticoagulation therapy offers room for improvement. For instance, in the Stroke Prevention Using Oral Thrombin Inhibitor in Atrial Fibrillation (SPORTIF III) trial [12], patients kept on open-label warfarin showed an INR within the target range of 2.0–3.0 only during 66% of the monitored intervals. After including a range of borderline effectiveness (INR 1.8–3.2), still 19% of the checked intervals were outside that target range. Accordingly, despite frequent clinical visits and well-supervised treatment, consistent levels of anticoagulation during vitamin K antagonist treatment are difficult to achieve.

Alternative Pharmacological Treatment Options

For many years, acetyl salicylic acid (ASA) has been used as an alternative for treating AF patients with contraindications to warfarin treatment. However, ASA has limited effectiveness for stroke prevention compared to warfarin [13]. There is ample evidence from experimental and clinical studies that a combination of different antiplatelet agents may increase antithrombotic efficacy compared to monotherapy. A currently ongoing prospective trial investigates the hypothesis that the addition of clopidogrel improves the effectiveness of ASA for the prevention of stroke. The Atrial Fibrillation Clopidogrel Trial with Irbesartan for prevention of Vascular Events (ACTIVE) represents the largest prospective study ever performed in patients with AF and additional risk factors for stroke [14]. In this trial program, the combination of Clopidogrel and ASA compared to warfarin in patients without contraindications and compared to ASA alone in patients with contraindications for oral anticoagulation will be assessed in more than 14 000 patients [14].

Heparin and the low-molecular-weight heparins have gained wide spread acceptance during short-term therapy, i.e. for bridging warfarin treatment pauses due to concomitant interventions. In a prospective multicentre trial, the use of enoxiparin was compared against unfractionated heparin followed by phenprocoumon in patients scheduled for cardioversion of persistent AF (duration > 48 h, < 1 year). Enoxaparin was noninferior to the standard regimen with regard to the incidence of embolic events, all-cause death, and major bleeding complications on per-protocol analysis (7 of 216 patients vs 12 of 212 patients, respectively; P for noninferiority = 0.016) and in an intention-to-treat analysis (7 of 248 patients vs 12 of 248 patients, P = 0.013), respectively [15]. There are, however, only limited data from prospective studies addressing the benefits of long-term heparin therapy in patients with AF. Ultimately, cost and compliance issues may be seen as a limitation for further research along this avenue.

Thrombin plays a major role in thrombus formation through activation of platelets and conversion of fibrinogen to fibrin. Accordingly, a novel class of effective anticoagulants has been derived from hirudin, the first known direct thrombin inhibitor. More recently, the oral formulation of a direct thrombin inhibitor, ximelagatran, was developed. Hepatic transformation after oral administration leads to the active drug melagatran, which has been shown to be a potent, rapidly binding, competitive inhibitor of human alpha-thrombin that inhibits both, thrombin activity and generation. Melagatran also effectively inhibits both, free and clot-bound thrombin. This drug has a wide therapeutic interval that enables it to be administered safely across a wide range of doses with no increased risk of bleeding [16]. Recently, two prospective studies (SPORTIF III and V) demonstrated the effectiveness of this new compound in AF patients.

Ximelagatran for Stroke Prevention in Atrial Fibrillation

In clinical trials for the prevention and treatment of venous thrombosis, administration of ximelagatran in a fixed dose was comparable with conventional therapy (warfarin and/or low-molecular-weight heparin) [17, 18]. Similarly, a prospective study program with this drug for prevention of systemic thrombembolism in patients with non-valvular AF was performed. The SPORTIF trials comprised the SPORTIF II study, a dose-finding trial that was continued during open-label long-term follow up as the SPORTIF IV study. SPORTIF III [12] was an open-label trial and SPORTIF V [19] was a double-blind trial comparing ximelagatran (fixed dose of 36 mg bid) to warfarin with an meticulously monitored treatment to keep the INR between 2.0 and 3.0.

In SPORTIF III, 3410 patients were prospectively randomised to warfarin or ximelagatran [12]. The primary endpoint was the occurrence of stroke (ischaemic and haemorrhagic) or peripheral arterial embolism. After a mean follow-up period of 17.4 months, this endpoint was observed in 56 patients on warfarin (2.3% per year) compared to 40 patients on ximelagatran (1.6% per year). The sample size of this study was based on a non-inferiority hypothesis which was confirmed by the results. Total mortality did not differ between treatment groups (79 patients on warfarin vs 78 patients on ximelagatran). Major bleedings were observed in 41 patients on warfarin (1.8%) compared to 29 patients on ximelagatran (1.3%). Combined analysis of major and minor bleeding resulted in a significantly lower event rate for patients on ximelagatran (478 patients = 25.8%) than for those on warfarin (547 patients = 29.8%; $P = 0.007$). The overall incidence of side effects was similar between treatment groups. Abnormal liver function, (elevation of alanine transferase), however, occurred significantly more often in patients on ximelagatran (6% vs 1%, $P < 0{,}0001$). Forty-nine of the affected patients discontinued treatment and liver enzymes returned to normal in 42 of them; while in 55 out of 59 patients, laboratory values returned to normal during continued therapy.

The second pivotal study (SPORTIF V) enrolled 3922 patients with non-valvular AF who were assigned in a double-blind fashion to treatment with either ximelagatran (36 mg bid) or warfarin. During a mean follow-up period of 20 months, a primary endpoint event was observed in 37 patients randomised to warfarin compared to 51 patients randomised to receive ximelagatran ($P = 0.13$) (Table 4). There was a reduced incidence of major and minor bleedings in ximelagatran-treated patients. However, similar to SPORTIF III, a significant elevation of the L-alanine aminotransferase (ALAT) of more than three times the upper normal limit was observed in 6% of patients receiving ximelagatran. In a pooled analysis of both studies, ximelagatran was found to significantly reduce the combined endpoint of major bleeding or death (Table 4).

Table 4. Results from the SPORTIF V trial and combined endpoint analysis from SPORTIF III and V trials

Endpoint	Ximelagatran *n* (% per year)	Warfarin *n* (% per year)	*P* value
Stroke or embolism	51 (1.6)	37 (1.2)	0.13
Intracranial haemorrhage	(0.06)	(0.06)	1
Major bleeding	(2.4)	(3.2)	0.16
Major and minor bleeding	37	47	< 0.001
ALAT > 3 upper limit	(6.0)	(0.8)	< 0.001
Combined SPORTIF III+V			
Major bleeding and death	(5.2)	(6.2)	0.038

ALAT L-Alanine aminotransferase

Conclusions

The benefits of oral anticoagulation have been consistently proven in many prospective studies. Hence, all patients at risk for thromboembolism due to AF and without contraindications for oral anticoagulants should receive appropriate treatment. According to more recent findings, thrombembolic prophylaxis should be continued even with the strategy of rhythm control since many paroxysmal episodes of AF may be asymptomatic and will go unrecognised by patients and doctors. The availability of oral direct thrombin inhibitors may become a preferable alternative to warfarin. Ximelagatran has shown equal effectiveness compared to warfarin and has a lower risk of bleeding complications. Currently, the occurrence of liver toxicity has jeopardised approval of this drug for wider applications in Europe and the USA. Other substances from the same class are currently under investigation in clinical phase I and phase II trials, but it may take more than 5 years until a protocol comparable to that of the SPORTIF trials and using any of these new compounds has been evaluated.

References

1. Albers GW, Dalen JE, Laupacis A et al (2001) Antithrombotic therapy in atrial fibrillation. Chest 119:S194-S206
2. Anonymous (1994) Risk factors for stroke and efficacy of antithrombotic therapy in atrial fibrillation. Analysis of pooled data from five randomized controlled trials. Arch Intern Med 154:1449–1457
3. Anonymous (1998) ASHP therapeutic position statement on antithrombotic therapy in chronic atrial fibrillation. American Society of Health-System Pharmacists. Am J Health Syst Pharm 55:376–381
4. Fuster V, Ryden LE, Asinger RW et al (2001) ACC/AHA/ESC guidelines for the management of patients with atrial fibrillation. A report of the American College of Cardiology/American Heart Association Task Force on Practice Guidelines and the European Society of Cardiology Committee for Practice Guidelines and Policy Conferences (Committee to develop guidelines for the management of patients with atrial fibrillation) developed in collaboration with the North American Society of Pacing and Electrophysiology. Eur Heart J 22:1852–1923
5. Singer DE, Albers GW, Dalen JE et al (2004) Antithrombotic therapy in atrial fibrillation: the Seventh ACCP Conference on Antithrombotic and Thrombolytic Therapy. Chest 126:S429–S456
6. Fuster V, Ryden LE, Asinger RW et al (2001) ACC/AHA/ESC Guidelines for the Management of Patients With Atrial Fibrillation: Executive Summary A Report of the American College of Cardiology/American Heart Association Task Force on Practice Guidelines and the European Society of Cardiology Committee for Practice Guidelines and Policy Conferences (Committee to Develop Guidelines for the Management of Patients With Atrial Fibrillation) Developed in Collaboration With the North American Society of Pacing and Electrophysiology. Circulation 104:2118–2150
7. Wyse DG, Waldo AL, DiMarco JP et al (2002) A comparison of rate control and rhythm control in patients with atrial fibrillation. N Engl J Med 347:1825–1833
8. Gronefeld G, Hohnloser SH (2003) Rhythm or rate control in atrial fibrillation: insights from the randomized controlled trials. J Cardiovasc Pharmacol Ther 8(suppl 1):S39–S44
9. Buckingham TA, Hatala R (2002) Anticoagulants for atrial fibrillation: why is the treatment rate so low? Clin Cardiol 25:447–454

10. Portnoi VA (1999) The underuse of warfarin treatment in the elderly. Arch Intern Med 159:1374–1375
11. Flaker GC, Schutz J (2004) Why is warfarin underutilized in patients with atrial fibrillation? J Interv Card Electrophysiol 10(suppl 1):21–25
12. Olsson SB (2003) Stroke prevention with the oral direct thrombin inhibitor ximelagatran compared with warfarin in patients with non-valvular atrial fibrillation (SPORTIF III): randomised controlled trial. Lancet 362:1691–1698
13. Taylor FC, Cohen H, Ebrahim S (2001) Systematic review of long term anticoagulation or antiplatelet treatment in patients with non-rheumatic atrial fibrillation. BMJ 322:321–326
14. Hohnloser SH, Connolly SJ (2003) Combined antiplatelet therapy in atrial fibrillation: review of the literature and future avenues. J Cardiovasc Electrophysiol 14:S60-S63
15. Stellbrink C, Nixdorff U, Hofmann T et al (2004) Safety and efficacy of enoxaparin compared with unfractionated heparin and oral anticoagulants for prevention of thromboembolic complications in cardioversion of nonvalvular atrial fibrillation: the Anticoagulation in Cardioversion using Enoxaparin (ACE) trial. Circulation 109:997–1003
16. Gustafsson D, Elg M (2003) The pharmacodynamics and pharmacokinetics of the oral direct thrombin inhibitor ximelagatran and its active metabolite melagatran: a mini-review. Thromb Res 109:S9–S15
17. Fiessinger JN, Huisman MV, Davidson BL et al (2005) Ximelagatran vs low-molecular-weight heparin and warfarin for the treatment of deep vein thrombosis: a randomized trial. JAMA 293:681–689
18. Francis CW, Berkowitz SD, Comp PC et al (2003) Comparison of ximelagatran with warfarin for the prevention of venous thromboembolism after total knee replacement. N Engl J Med 349:1703–1712
19. Albers GW, Diener HC, Frison L et al (2005) Ximelagatran vs warfarin for stroke prevention in patients with nonvalvular atrial fibrillation: a randomized trial. JAMA. 293:690–698

Guidelines for Anticoagulation of Atrial Fibrillation: Is It Time for an Update?

A.L. Waldo

Introduction

Atrial fibrillation is the most common arrhythmia in the Western world. In the United States, it currently affects about 2.4 million people, and by the year 2050 the number will be about 5.6 million [1]. Two principal clinical problems are associated with atrial fibrillation [2]. One is that if the ventricular response rate is not adequately controlled, patients may develop a tachycardia-mediated cardiomyopathy. The other problem is the risk of stroke. Patients with atrial fibrillation have a five-fold increased risk of stroke compared to those in sinus rhythm [3]. And, as patients get older, the prevalence of atrial fibrillation increases, roughly doubling with each decade beginning with the seventh; so that 2–3% of people in their 60s, 5–6% of people in their 70s, and 8–10% of people in their 80s have atrial fibrillation [1, 3, 4]. Moreover, the population-attributable risk also increases with age, as almost one-third of patients in their 80s who present with a stroke have atrial fibrillation [3]. There is also a 14.7–58% incidence of so-called silent strokes, i.e., strokes in which there are no manifestations of motor or sensory deficit, in patients with atrial fibrillation who are at risk for stroke but untreated with warfarin [5–8]. Such strokes are associated with senile dementia or Alzheimer's disease. Clearly, prevention of stroke in patients with atrial fibrillation is a key management goal.

Currently, the principal method of preventing strokes in patients with atrial fibrillation at risk of stroke is the use of oral anticoagulants, i.e., vitamin K antagonists. Over the years, guidelines have been proposed to guide physicians in the use of oral anticoagulants for the treatment of atrial fibril-

Case Western Reserve University/University Hospitals of Cleveland, Cleveland, OH, USA

lation. This chapter will deal with the recommendations of the two main sets of guidelines for the use of oral anticoagulation to prevent stroke in patients with atrial fibrillation, and will offer suggestions regarding some of the guidelines' recommendations which need updating. The two main sets of guidelines are those of the American College of Chest Physicians (ACCP), published in October of 2004 [9]; and the American College of Cardiology (ACC), the American Heart Association (AHA), and the European Society of Cardiology (ESC) guidelines, published in September of 2001 [10] and currently undergoing revision. These guidelines are generally quite compatible with each other, but there are some significant differences. Moreover, there are some sections of the guidelines which should be considered for an update.

Comparisons of the ACCP And ACC/AHA/ESC Guidelines

Both sets of guidelines generally indicate that if patients have risk factors for stroke [9, 10] (prior ischaemic stroke, transient ischaemic attack, or systemic embolism; age above 75 years; moderately or severely impaired left ventricular systolic function and/or congestive heart failure; history of hypertension; or diabetes mellitus), anticoagulation with an oral vitamin K antagonist, such as warfarin, is recommended. There is virtually universal acceptance of such recommendations. However, the ACC/AHA/ESC guidelines differ from the ACCP guidelines in several respects. First, the ACC/AHA/ESC guidelines use the age of 60 years as a cut-off for some considerations, whereas the ACCP uses the age of 65 years as a cut-off. If one is under the age of 60 years and has no heart disease, the ACC/AHA/ESC guidelines recommend aspirin (325 mg/day) or no therapy, and if one is under age 60 years of age with heart disease but no risk factors for stroke, they recommend aspirin (325 mg/day). The ACCP uses the same recommendation, but for age less than 65 years. It is not clear why the ACC/AHA/ESC guidelines chose age 60 as the cut-off, as the data regarding age per se as a risk factor for stroke start at age 65 [11].

Then, from age 60 to 75 years and with no risk factors, the ACC/AHA/ESC recommend aspirin (325 mg/day), but for the same age group when diabetes or coronary artery disease is present they recommend warfarin (International Normalised Ratio [INR] 2–3) with additional aspirin (81–162 mg) optional . It is clear that age is one of the risk factors for stroke. The new ACCP guidelines state that in patients with persistent atrial fibrillation or paroxysmal atrial fibrillation, aged 65–75 years, and with no other risk factors, they recommend anti-thrombotic therapy with either an oral vitamin K antagonist or aspirin (325 mg/day) in this group of patients who are at intermediate risk of stroke. We suggest that because the data indicate that beginning at age 65 there is 1.4 relative risk for stroke, and that this increases by 1.4 per decade, aspirin only may not be an appropriate recommendation for patients between 65–74 years of age without other risk factors for stroke. Over age 75, both guidelines agree that age per se is enough reason to recommend a vitamin K antagonist.

Is Aspirin Ever Sufficiently Effective as Prophylaxis Against Stroke in the Presence of Any Risk Factors?

This gets us to the question of whether aspirin is really ever sufficiently efficacious to use it in patients who are at any significant risk of stroke. As indicated in the most recent ACCP report [10], the evidence supporting the efficacy of aspirin is substantially weaker than the evidence supporting the efficacy of warfarin. Among the several studies that have compared aspirin with warfarin, it is clear that warfarin is far superior to aspirin in diminishing the risk of stroke [10, 12]. Moreover, of the several studies that have compared aspirin with placebo, only the Stroke Prevention in Atrial Fibrillation (SPAF) I trial demonstrated a relative risk reduction in stroke with aspirin [13]. Not only is that study an outlier, driving the meta-analysis of the several trials comparing aspirin with placebo, but also the data from the SPAF I trial demonstrate an internal inconsistency between patients in group I (patients eligible for warfarin) and patients in group II (patients with a relative or absolute contraindication to warfarin), both of which compared aspirin with placebo (Fig. 1). The analysis of these data throws yet more doubt on the efficacy of aspirin as an effective treatment for prevention of stroke in patients with atrial fibrillation [14]. For the most part, this is reflected in the guidelines regarding the type of anticoagulation therapy that is recommended for patients with atrial fibrillation who are at risk of stroke. Additionally, not only do we know that aspirin is a poor second best to warfarin in preventing stroke in patients with atrial fibrillation at risk of stroke, but also, should a stroke occur on aspirin, it is usually more severe, and is associated with significantly higher in-hospital mortality and 30-day mortality compared with warfarin therapy that maintains an INR in the therapeutic range [15]. In short, the data clearly indicate that aspirin not only is insufficiently effective in preventing stroke compared with warfarin, but also, should a stroke occur, the consequences are likely to be far more severe. Thus, the recommendations for the use of aspirin really need to be reconsidered or at least more seriously tested. A reasonable interpretation of the aspirin data is that they are consistent with the notion that, if one needs protection against stroke in the presence of atrial fibrillation, one needs a vitamin K antagonist.

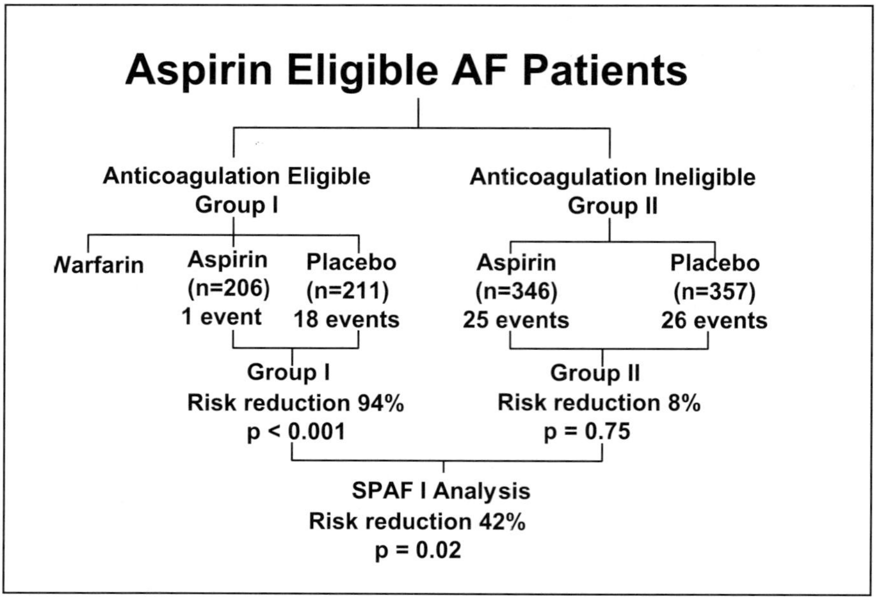

Fig. 1. Aspirin-eligible patients with atrial fibrillation: outcome of patients randomised to receive aspirin vs placebo in group I of the SPAF I trial. In group I, there was only one event (stroke) in patients receiving aspirin vs 18 events in the placebo group. This was a statistically highly significant difference. However, in group II, there were 25 events in patients receiving aspirin vs 26 events in patients receiving placebo. This difference was not statistically significant. Thus, there was internal inconsistency. When the data from both groups were combined, the data were significant, but this was driven by what appears to be the outlier data from group I. See text for discussion (modified from [14])

The question of whether a combination of aspirin and clopidogrel – two antiplatelet agents – will be effective as prophylaxis against stroke in patients with atrial fibrillation remains to be demonstrated. We await the results of the ACTIVE trials to give us clinical trial data in this regard.

Concerns About Intracerebral Bleeding Risk in Patients Taking Vitamin K Antagonists

The appropriate level of warfarin anticoagulation in elderly patients with atrial fibrillation has been debated because of an age-associated increase in intracerebral haemorrhage. The ACC/AHA/ESC guidelines, but not the ACCP guidelines, have suggested that if one is concerned about the risk of bleeding in patients over the age of 75 who have had no prior stroke, one can lower the target INR to 2.0 with a 'therapeutic range' of 1.6–2.5. It is unclear on what data that recommendation is based. It seems to have been based on a concern that there is an increased risk for intracranial haemorrhage in the elderly.

Although the relative risk of ischaemic stroke increases by 1.4 per decade beginning at the age of 65 years, so does the relative risk of intracranial bleeding while taking warfarin [16]. This seems to have led to the above recommendation for the primary prevention of ischaemic stroke and systemic embolism in patients older than 75 years who are considered at increased risk of bleeding complications, but have no frank contraindications to oral anticoagulant therapy (a class II recommendation). However, it is important to emphasise that because the base rate of ischaemic stroke is considerably greater than the risk of intracranial bleeding, the risk of ischaemic stroke in the absence of warfarin therapy is considerably greater that the risk of intracranial bleeding while receiving warfarin [16]. An additional perspective is that, although there is no increased therapeutic benefit associated with an INR greater than 3, an increased risk of bleeding does not occur until the INR reaches 3.9–4.0 [15, 16]. The most recent study [17] demonstrated that although intracerebral haemorrhage was associated with increasing age (especially > 85 years) and increasing INR (especially > 3.5), the incidence of intracerebral haemorrhage was not statistically different in patients with INRs below 2 and those with INRs between 2 and 3. This was true even among those older than 75 years of age. Thus, the risk of intracerebral haemorrhage is not diminished in elderly patients with atrial fibrillation when anticoagulation is maintained with an INR below 2.0. Therefore, there really seems no basis to support the idea that a target of 2.0 with a range of 1.6–2.5 of the INR is desirable in this patient age group.

Optimal Management of Interruption of Oral Anticoagulation

At present, there is a consensus that one can interrupt oral anticoagulation for 5–7 days if need be (e.g., for major or minor surgery) in patients with atrial fibrillation at risk of stroke. It is recognised that there is a small risk, but since the risk of stroke has been calculated on a yearly basis, it is thought that the risk of stroke with cessation of oral anticoagulation for 1 week is acceptable. But one wonders, particularly in the era of the ready accessibility and effectiveness of low-molecular-weight heparins, whether one should simply terminate warfarin treatment without providing a bridge during cessation of warfarin therapy to cessation by giving low-molecular-weight heparin until all anticoagulation must stop (e.g., for surgery), and a bridge to reinitiation of warfarin therapy by giving low-molecular-weight heparins after the need to withhold warfarin therapy is past.

Cessation of Oral Anticoagulation After Apparent Complete Suppression of Atrial Fibrillation with Drug Therapy or Cure with Radiofrequency Ablation or a Maze Surgical Procedure

One of the putative advantages of pursuing a rhythm control strategy (i.e., attempting to maintain sinus rhythm) in patients with atrial fibrillation at risk of stroke is that, with the absence of atrial fibrillation, the cause of clot formation in the left atrium is eliminated. For this reason, it has been a clinical assumption that there is no longer any need for oral anticoagulation with warfarin. Several factors have clearly affected this assumption. First are the data from the Atrial Fibrillation Follow-up Investigation of Rhythm Management (AFFIRM) trial examining the relationship of ischaemic stroke to INR and the presence of atrial fibrillation [18]. It is noteworthy that there was no significant difference in the incidence of stroke in the rate control versus the rhythm control arms. However, of the strokes that occurred in the rhythm control arm, 57% occurred in patients not taking warfarin, and 22% occurred in patients whose INR was less than 2. It is probable that these data are in part explained by a significant incidence of so-called silent or asymptomatic atrial fibrillation [19–22]. There is now a large body of evidence indicating a significant incidence of asymptomatic atrial fibrillation in patients with a history of atrial fibrillation who were thought to be in sinus rhythm. For instance, in a recent study in patients with a history of atrial fibrillation in whom atrial fibrillation recurred, in more than one-third (38%) the atrial fibrillation was both asymptomatic and of greater than 48 h duration [22]. Moreover, 16% of the patients developed asymptomatic atrial fibrillation of greater than 48 h duration, even after documented freedom from atrial fibrillation for 3 months. Data such as those from the AFFIRM trial and from the several trials demonstrating asymptomatic atrial fibrillation have led to the widely accepted conclusion that patients with atrial fibrillation and risk factors for stroke should receive anticoagulation indefinitely, even when sinus rhythm appears to be restored and maintained [18]. The point is that success rates of maintaining continuous sinus rhythm in patients with a history of atrial fibrillation are often grossly overestimated, with potentially serious consequences for the patient.

So the question then extends to patients who are ostensibly cured of atrial fibrillation with radiofrequency catheter ablation or a surgical maze procedure. Can we ever stop anticoagulation in those patients? At present, the patient follow-up is probably not long enough to make definitive declarations about the incidence of late recurrence of atrial fibrillation in these patients. The survey data recently published [23] indicate a late recurrence rate in patients months after undergoing radiofrequency catheter ablation. It is not clear whether those data are applicable to results from using current ablation techniques. Nor is the incidence of recurrence clear. However, a community standard seems to be developing in which many patients who are thought to be cured of atrial fibrillation are being advised to terminate oral anticoagulation therapy 3–6 months following apparent successful cure. Whether this turns out to be good medicine or not is yet to be determined. There are no good data relating to surgical ablation of which we are aware. A consensus regarding these issues ought to be updated in the guidelines. The most conservative approach for now would seem to be that there are no data yet available to support the safe cessation of oral anticoagulation in these patients.

Conclusions

Several areas regarding use of oral anticoagulation have been identified which are in need of updating or reconsideration. Recommendations are always best when data-driven. For some of these areas, the data are lacking, weak, or controversial. For others, the data seem clear. Because these several areas are important, we hope they will gain the attention they deserve from the ACC/AHA/ESC and ACCP guideline committees.

References

1. Go AS, Hylek EM, Phillips KA et al for the AnTicoagulation and Risk factors In Atrial Fibrillation (ATRIA) Study (2001) Prevalence of diagnosed atrial fibrillation in adults: national implications for rhythm management and stroke prevention. JAMA 285:2370–2375
2. Waldo AL (2003) Stroke prevention in atrial fibrillation. JAMA 209:1093–1095
3. Wolf PA, Abbott RD, Kannel WB (1987) Atrial fibrillation: a major contributor to stroke in the elderly. The Framingham Study. Arch Intern Med 147:1561–1564
4. Feinberg WM, Blackshear JL, Laupacis A et al (1995) Prevalence, age distribution, and gender of patients with atrial fibrillation: analysis and implications. Arch Intern Med 155:469–473
5. Petersen P, Madsen EB, Brun B et al (1987) Silent cerebral infarction in chronic atrial fibrillation. Stroke 18:1098–1100 (abs)
6. Guidotti M, Tadeo G, Zanasi S et al (1990) Silent cerebral ischemia in patients with chronic atrial fibrillation: a case-control study. Irish J Med Sci 159:96–97
7. Feinberg WM, Seeger JF, Carmody RF et al (1990) Epidemiologic features of asymptomatic cerebral infarction in patients with nonvalvular atrial fibrillation. Arch Intern Med 150:2340–2344 (abs)
8. Ezekowitz MD, James KE, Nazarian SM et al for the Veterans Affairs Stroke Prevention in Nonrheumatic Atrial Fibrillation Investigators (1995) Silent cerebral infarction in patients with nonrheumatic atrial fibrillation. Circulation 92:2178–2182
9. Singer DE, Albers GW, Dalen JE et al (2004) Antithrombotic therapy in atrial fibril-

lation: the Seventh ACCP Conference on Antithrombotic and Thrombolytic Therapy. Chest 126:429S–456S
10. Fuster V, Ryden LE, Asinger RW et al (2002) ACC/AHA/ESC guidelines for the management of patients with atrial fibrillation: executive summary: A report of the American College of Cardiology/American Heart Association Task Force on Practice Guidelines and the European Society of Cardiology Committee for Practice Guidelines and Policy Conferences (Committee to Develop Guidelines for the Management of Patients with Atrial Fibrillation): developed in collaboration with the North American Society of Pacing and Electrophysiology. J Am Coll Cardiol 38:1231–1266
11. Ezekowitz MD, Levine JA (1999) Preventing stroke in patients with atrial fibrillation. JAMA 281:1830–1835
12. van Walraven C, Hart RG, Singer DE et al (2002) Oral anticoagulants vs aspirin in nonvalvular atrial fibrillation: an individual patient meta-analysis. JAMA 288:2441–2448
13. Hart RG, Benavente O, McBride R, Pearce LA (1999) Antithrombotic therapy to prevent stroke in patients with atrial fibrillation: a meta-analysis. Ann Intern Med 131:492–501
14. Anonymous (1993) A differential effect of aspirin in prevention of stroke on atrial fibrillation. Stroke Prevention in Atrial Fibrillation Investigators. J Stroke Cerebrovasc Dis 3:181–188
15. Hylek EM, Go AS, Chang Y et al (2003) Effect of intensity of oral anticoagulation on stroke severity and mortality in atrial fibrillation. N Engl J Med 349:1019–1026
16. Hylek EM, Singer DE (1994) Risk factors for intracranial hemorrhage in outpatients taking warfarin. Ann Intern Med 120:897–902
17. Fang MC, Chang Y, Hylek EM et al (2004) Advanced age, anticoagulation intensity, and risk for intracranial hemorrhage among patients taking warfarin for atrial fibrillation. Ann Intern Med 141:745–752
18. Wyse DG, Waldo AL, DiMarco JP et al (2002) A comparison of rate control and rhythm control in patients with recurrent persistent atrial fibrillation. N Engl J Med 34:1825–1833
19. Bhandari AK, Anderson JL, Gilbert M et al; Flecainide Supraventricular Tachycardia Study Group (1992) Correlation of symptoms with occurrence of paroxysmal supraventricular tachycardia or atrial fibrillation: a transtelephonic monitoring study. Am Heart J 124:381–386
20. Page RL, Wilkerson WE, Clark WK et al (1994) Asymptomatic arrhythmias in patients with symptomatic paroxysmal atrial fibrillation and paroxysmal supraventricular tachycardia. Circulation 89:224–227
21. Savelieva I, Camm AJ (2000) Clinical relevance of silent atrial fibrillation: prevalence, prognosis, quality of life, and management. J Intervent Cardiac Electrophysiol 4:369–382
22. Israel C, Ehrlich JR, Gronefeld G et al (2004) Long-term risk of recurrent atrial fibrillation as documented by an implantable monitoring device: implications for optional patient care. J Am Coll Cardiol 43:47–52
23. Cappato R, Calkins H, Chen SA et al (2005) Worldwide survey on the methods, efficacy and safety of catheter ablation for human atrial fibrillation. Circulation 111:1100–1105

ATRIAL FIBRILLATION: CATHETER ABLATION AND OTHER NON-PHARMACOLOGICAL THERAPIES

Anatomy of the Left Atrium and Pulmonary Veins: What Have We Learned in Recent Years?

J. Kautzner, H. Mlcochova, P. Peichl

Introduction

Although atrial fibrillation (AF) can be adequately controlled by drugs in the majority of patients, medicaments may fail in certain proportion of cases. In recent years, substantial progress has been made in both the elucidation of AF mechanisms and non-pharmacological treatment of this arrhythmia. Catheter ablation is now considered to be a highly effective treatment option for the cure of symptomatic, drug-resistant AF [1–5]. Since 1998, when catheter ablation of focal sources of AF was first reported by Haïssaguerre et al. [1], several ablation techniques have been developed. Despite the diversity of individual ablation strategies, all of them have something in common: the ablation is performed either within or around the ostia of the pulmonary veins (PVs). Contrary to initial belief, pulmonary venous anatomy has been shown to be highly variable, and this increases the importance of imaging before or during the procedure. The aim of this review is to discuss what have we learned in recent years about the anatomy of the left atrium and PVs, and to illustrate the impact of this on the practice of catheter ablation.

Anatomical Studies

Probably the first mention of myocardial sleeves around pulmonary and caval veins originates from one of the Purkinje's pupils, Ferdinandus Raeuschel, and dates back to 1836 [6]. In his medical dissertation, Raeuschel described muscular fibres on the surface of both caval veins and PVs up to

Department of Cardiology, Institute for Clinical and Experimental Medicine, Prague, Czech Republic

their branching to secondary vessels. Muscular sleeves around the PVs were later rediscovered in 1907 by Keith and Flack [7]. A detailed morphological description was published in the late 1960s [8]. However, the importance of PV anatomy went unrecognised until the era of catheter ablation for AF.

Reflecting the need of electrophysiologists for detailed knowledge of the pulmonary venous anatomy, Ho et al. carried out a thorough investigation of the arrangement and dimensions of the PVs in postmortem hearts [9]. Although some changes in the macroscopic anatomy and diameters were possible owing to fixation of the specimens, four distinct PV ostia were reported in 77% of cases and the rest presented with variant anatomy. In the second study by these authors [10], a common vestibule of the left PVs was described in three cases and a common orifice of the right PVs was found in a further two subjects (accounted for 25% incidence of variant PV anatomy). Discounting the common ostia, the diameter of the PV ostia ranged from 8 mm to 21 mm (mean 12.5 mm). An identical proportion of common ostia of PVs (25%), usually on the left side of the left atrium, was reported in the study by Moubarak et al. [11]. Thus, the concept of four PVs with distinct ostia originating from the left atrium was debated for the first time in these early anatomical studies.

Pulmonary Venous Angiography

Pulmonary venous angiography was often used during the early period of our experience with catheter ablation for AF. The main purpose was to determine the position and size of the PV ostia and, additionally, to detect possible stenosis of the veins after the procedure. Some of the studies revealed that patients with AF have larger PV diameters in proportion to the enlarged left atrium [12]. The average diameter, of superior PV ostia were 10.9–11.0 mm in controls, and 13.1–13.6 mm in patients with AF. The corresponding diameters of the inferior PVs were 7.5 mm and 8.3 mm, respectively. In the light of contemporary experience, the above data suggest that the PV diameters were measured within the tube-like portions of PVs and not at the level of the actual PV–atrial junction. More realistic values of PV ostial diameters (ranging between 16.9 and 19.4 mm) were reported by Vasamreddy et al. [13], who defined the PV ostium angiographically as the junction of the PV with the left atrium and measured from both projections with correction for a degree of magnification. The study revealed excellent correlation between the angiographic measurements and MR angiographic (MRA) measurements as analysed from 2D maximum intensity projections and multiplanar reformations. Surprisingly, ostial diameters were found to be similar in the two perpendicular planes, implying that the PV ostia are circular in shape.

Wittkampf et al. [14] demonstrated for the first time how contrast angiography can be misleading in its representation of PVs. Comparing this method with 3D reconstruction of MRA images, they showed that the majority of the PV ostia are oval in shape, being longer in the superoinferior dimension than in the anteroposterior dimension. The mean ratios between maximum and minimum dimensions were 1.5 for left veins and 1.2 for right veins, which corresponds with a more circular shape of the right PVs. Maximum diameters of PVs ranged between 15.9 and 18.7 mm, and left common PV ostium measured 27.3 mm on average.

The above experience suggests that neither PV angiography nor 2D viewing format of MRA data provides an exact description of the true PV ostial shape. Despite this, many electrophysiologists still rely solely on PV angiography to guide catheter ablation of AF.

3D Imaging Techniques

The advent of modern 3D imaging techniques such as MRA and/or multidetector CT angiography enabled detailed anatomical studies of PV anatomy and non-invasive assessment of PV stenosis after catheter ablation [15–19]. The PV ostia were found to be oval in shape with the anteroposterior dimension less than the superoinferior dimension. Subjects with AF also presented with complex branching patterns, especially in the inferior PVs [16]. However, individual authors identified variant PV ostial anatomy in a variable proportion of subjects. For instance, the occurrence of a common left vestibule of PVs ranged from 3% to 32%. Even the largest study, by Mansour et al. [19], suggested that only 17% of cases presented with a common left trunk and 29% with additional right-sided PVs. Our experience suggests that the above inconsistency may arise from the fact that the majority of the studies used 2D formatting of data instead of true 3D reconstructions. Using special software for digital subtraction of arterial and venous phase and subsequent 3D reconstruction of the data (Fig. 1), we have demonstrated that the majority of patients (i.e. 75%) present with a common left vestibule [20]. Such a high occurrence of a common left vestibule suggests that this pattern should be defined as the 'normal' PV arrangement. In addition, comparing 2D and 3D formats we have shown that the true PV arrangement is often underestimated from 2D maximum intensity projections. Thus, only 3D reconstructions of the segmented MRA data can reveal the true anatomy of the left atrium, appendage, and PVs from different views.

A similar observation was made by Schwartzman et al. [21] using 3D reconstructions of CT images, which they then correlated with those obtained from intracardiac echocardiography. They revealed sligtly more frequent occurrence of common vestibules on the left side and confirmed by

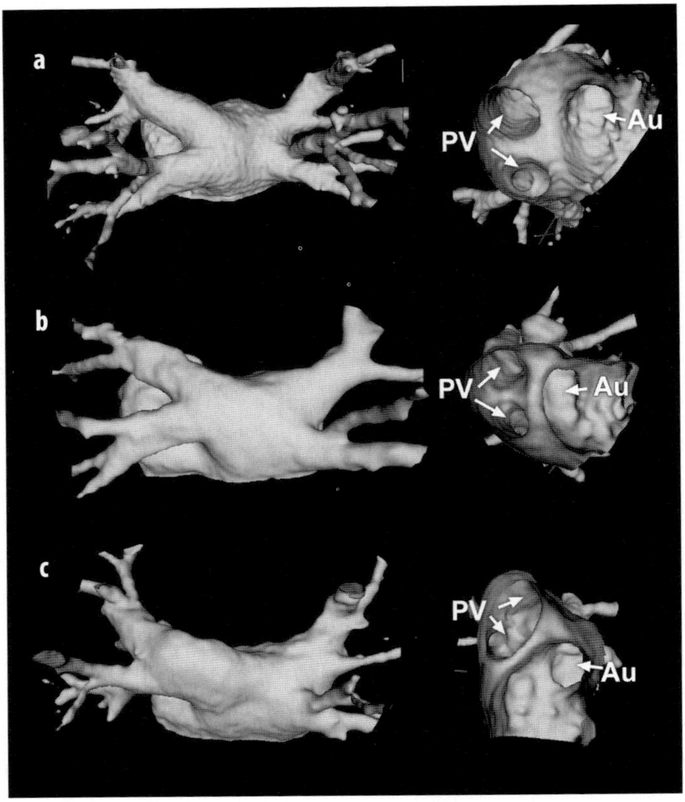

Fig. 1a–c. Different types of pulmonary vein branching patterns as assessed by 3D reconstructions of MRA imaging including virtual endoscopic images of the left pulmonary veins: **a** less common pattern of four separate ostia and early branching of the right superior vein, **b** prevailing pattern of short common vestibule or antrum of left-sided pulmonary veins, **c** long common left trunk and early branching of both right pulmonary veins. *Au* auricle, *PV* pulmonary veins

analysis of local electrograms the presence of typical fractionated or bifid potentials at these sites. Left atrial and PV dimensions were significantly greater in the AF group. However, after correcting for left atrial volume, all PV diameters were similar.

Thus, the use of 3D imaging techniques has changed our understanding of PV ostial anatomy significantly and has helped to identify PV vestibules that make up real PV–left atrial junctions. Their shape is predominantly oval and they tend to extend to various degrees into the posterior wall of the left atrium, especially on the left side. As a result, in many patients both left and right-sided vestibules are close to each other on the posterior wall. This may have important implications for the strategy of catheter ablation.

Intracardiac Echocardiography

Recently, studies have been published on the use of intracardiac echocardiography (ICE) during catheter ablation [22–26]. The most widely used imaging modalities are either a mechanical system with rotating transducer obtaining images in 360° radial fashion (Boston Scientific, Natick, Mass., USA) or a phased-array system (Acuson, Mountain View, Calif., USA) with steerable 90° longitudinal imaging. The latter system offers a greater depth of penetration and the possibility of Doppler imaging including colour coding. It has been reported that ICE can facilitate catheter ablation of AF by increasing efficacy and reducing complications [22]. The main advantages ICE offers are: (1) real-time delineation of cardiac anatomy, especially of PV ostia; (2) positioning of the catheter tip and assessment of its contact with the atrial wall; (3) visualisation of microbubble formation as a sign of tissue overheating; (4) assessment of PV flow and recognition of PV stenosis; and (5) early detection of thrombus and/or char formation. An ICE catheter positioned in the middle of the right atrium provides clear images of the fossa ovalis and allows safe trans-septal puncture even in anticoagulated patients. Given the high variability in PV arrangement, ICE provides very accurate information about the position of the catheter tip around the PV ostia, allowing precise positioning of the circular mapping catheter (Lasso, Biosense Webster, Diamond Bar, Calif., USA) at the exact level of the ostium. It has been shown to visualise PV ostia better than angiography (Fig. 2), and

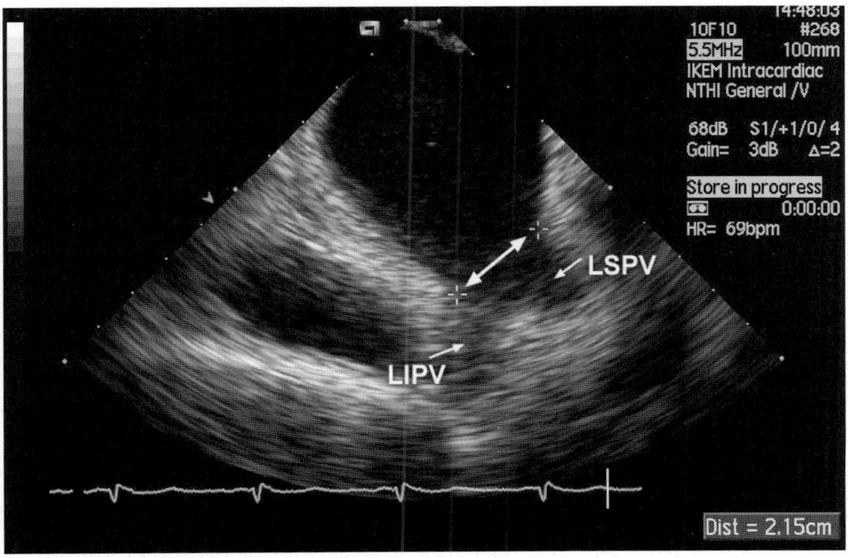

Fig. 2. Common vestibule of the left-sided pulmonary veins (*doubleheaded arrows*) as depicted by intracardiac ultrasound (ACUSON, Siemens, Mountain View, Calif., USA). *LIPV* left inferior pulmonary vein, *LSPV* left superior pulmonary vein

to ensure proper electrode alignment and contact [23]. Monitoring of microbubble formation can reveal tissue overheating [24–25] and thus minimise the risk of thrombus formation and other complications such as atrio-oesophageal fistula. At the same time, ICE navigation minimises the risk of PV stenosis [26]. For attempts to use novel devices such as a balloon catheter for circumferential ultrasound ablation and/or a focused ultrasound balloon, ICE may provide an excellent tool for navigation within the PV ostia. On the basis of previous experience, ostial anatomy and resulting misalignment of the catheter were identified as the main reason for ineffective energy delivery and failure of catheter ablation [27].

Implications for Catheter Ablation

All the above data suggest that the arrangement of the PV ostia is highly variable, and even results obtained by the same imaging technique may vary significantly. Pre-procedural 3D imaging appears to be the best tool to provide an understanding of the anatomy and provides a basis for subsequent assessment of PV stenosis. True 3D reconstructions of images allow not only visualisation of supernumerary PVs but, especially, an appreciation of the morphology and size of PV ostia. This morphological knowledge may the modify strategy of catheter ablation in a given case. Repeat studies during follow-up can reveal PV stenosis. However, apart from PV angiography and/or fluoroscopy guidance around the circular mapping catheter in the PV, no on-line imaging was available until recently. Many electrophysiologists turned to an electroanatomical mapping system (CARTO, Biosense-Webster, Diamond Bar, Calif., USA) to reconstruct a virtual 3D anatomy of the left atrium and tag the position of the PV ostia as identified from PV angiography and/or from evaluation of catheter tip impedance during mapping. The advent of ICE provides real on-line control of the position of the catheter with respect to the PV ostia, and thus an additional potential benefit in catheter ablation of AF. There is mounting evidence that on-line imaging by means of ICE increases the success rate and minimises all potential complications of the procedure. Besides the imaging itself, ICE allows titration of power delivery through monitoring for microbubbles as a sign of tissue overheating. It may also enable proper placement of novel devices such as the focused ultrasound catheter into the PV ostia.

Reflecting the need for intra-procedural navigation, various techniques of image integration are being developed. One of them that is ready for clinical use (CARTO Merge, Biosense-Webster, Diamond Bar, Calif., USA) integrates pre-procedural 3D images (either 3D CT angiography or MRA) with the virtual electroanatomical CARTO map constructed during the procedure. After the initial process of registration, the imported 3D anatomical map of the left atrium and PVs could be used for catheter navigation. ICE guidance could be used in order to improve the registration process (Fig. 3). According to our early experience with this software, reliable correlation between anatomical reconstructions and real-time CARTO maps of the left atrium and PVs can be obtained in a good proportion of patients. Image integration with other mapping modalities such as NAVx (St. Jude Medical, Minneapolis–St Paul, Minn., USA) is under development.

Conclusions

Lessons learned from sophisticated imaging techniques such as MRA or CT angiography suggest that the anatomy of the left atrium and PVs is very complex and highly variable. The most important discovery appears to be the fact that in a large proportion of patients left-sided PVs merge into a common vestibule or antrum. Recent evidence suggests that ablation at the level of this common antrum, if present, may have better efficacy and carry less risk of PV stenosis. This increases the need for either pre-procedural 3D imaging (and image integration) or intra-procedural imaging using ICE. The latter technology, especially, may become a universal guiding tool that allows precise catheter positioning, monitoring of energy delivery, and/or reduction of complications during these complex procedures.

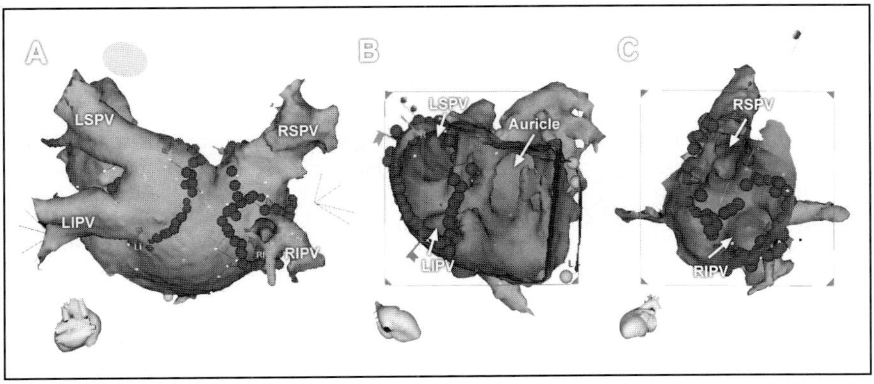

Fig. 3. Computer tomography angiographic 3D image integrated with electroanatomical mapping system (CARTO Merge, Biosense-Webster). After initial registration under intracardiac echocardiographic guidance, the anatomical image was fitted to an electroanatomical map and subsequently used to deploy ablation lines around pulmonary veins (*black dots*). *A* shows the left atrium in posterior view; *B* and *C* show virtual endoscopic images of the left- and right-sided pulmonary veins, respectively. *LIPV* left inferior pulmonary vein, *LSPV* left superior pulmonary vein, *RIPV* right inferior pulmonary vein, *RSPV* right superior pulmonary vein

References

1. Haïssaguerre M, Jais P, Shah DC et al (1998) Spontaneous initiation of atrial fibrillation by ectopic beats originating in the pulmonary veins. N Engl J Med 98:1769–1775
2. Haïssaguerre M, Shah DC, Jais P et al (2000) Mapping-guided ablation of pulmonary veins to cure atrial fibrillation. Am J Cardiol 86(Suppl 1):K9-K19
3. Pappone C, Rosanio S, Oreto G et al (2000) Circumferential radiofrequency ablation of pulmonary vein ostia: a new anatomic approach for curing atrial fibrillation. Circulation 102:2619–2628
4. Pappone C, Oreto G, Rosanio S et al (2001) Atrial electroanatomic remodeling after circumferential radiofrequency pulmonary vein ablation: efficacy of an anatomical approach in a large cohort of patients with atrial fibrillation. Circulation 104:2539–2544
5. Nademanee K, McKenzie J, Kosar E et al (2004) A new approach for catheter ablation of atrial fibrillation: mapping of the electrophysiologic substrate. J Am Coll Cardiol 43:2044–2053
6. Raeuschel F. De arteriarum et venarum structura. Dissertatio inauguralis anatomico-physiologica, Universitate Viadrina, Vratislaviae, 29 October 1836
7. Keith A, Flack M (1907) The form and the nature of muscular connections between the primary divisions of the vertebrate heart. J Anat Physiol 41:172 -189
8. Nathan H, Eliakin M (1966) The junction between the left atrium and the pulmonary veins. Circulation 34:412–422
9. Ho SY, Sanchez-Quintana D, Cabrera JA et al (1999) Anatomy of the left atrium: implications for radiofrequency ablation of atrial fibrillation. J Cardiovasc Electrophysiol 10:1525–1533
10. Ho SY, Cabrera JA, Tran VH et al (2001) Architecture of the pulmonary veins: relevance to radiofrequency ablation. Heart 86:265–270
11. Moubarak JB, Rozwadowski JV, Strzalka CT et al (2000) Pulmonary veins – left atrial junction: anatomic and histological study. Pacing Clin Electrophysiol 23:1836–1838
12. Lin WS, Prakash VS, Tai CT et al (2000) Pulmonary vein morphology in patients with paroxysmal atrial fibrillation initiated by ectopic beats originating from the pulmonary veins: implications for catheter ablation. Circulation 101:1274–1281
13. Vasamreddy CR, Jayam V, Lickfett L et al (2004) Technique and results of pulmonary vein angiography in patients undergoing catheter ablation of atrial fibrillation. J Cardiovasc Electrophysiol 15:21–26
14. Wittkampf FHM, Vonken EJ, Derksen R et al (2003) Pulmonary vein ostium geometry: analysis by magnetic resonance angiography. Circulation 107:21–23
15. Dill T, Neumann T, Ekinci O et al (2003) Pulmonary vein diameter reduction after radiofrequency catheter ablation for paroxysmal atrial fibrillation evaluated by contrast-enhanced three-dimensional magnetic resonance imaging. Circulation 107:845–850
16. Kato R, Lickfett L, Meininger G et al (2003) Pulmonary vein anatomy in patients undergoing catheter ablation of atrial fibrillation: lessons learned by use of magnetic resonance imaging. Circulation 107:2004–2010
17. Takase B, Nagata M, Matsui T et al (2004) Pulmonary vein dimensions and variation of branching pattern in patients with paroxysmal atrial fibrillation using magnetic resonance angiography. Jpn Heart J 45:81–92
18. Scharf C, Sneider M, Case I et al (2003) Anatomy of the pulmonary veins in

patients with atrial fibrillation and effects of segmental ostial ablation analyzed by computed tomography. J Cardiovasc Electrophysiol 14:150–155
19. Mansour M, Holmvang G, Sosnovik D et al (2004) Assessment of pulmonary vein anatomic variability by magnetic resonance imaging: implications for catheter ablation techniques for atrial fibrillation. J Cardiovasc Electrophysiol 15:387–393
20. Mlcochova H, Cihak R, Tintera J et al (2004) Variability of pulmonary veins in patients undergoing ablation of AF. Europace 6(1):80
21. Schwartzman D, Lacomis J, Wigginton WG (2003) Characterisation of left atrium and distal pulmonary vein morphology using multidimensional computed tomography. J Am Coll Cardiol 16:1349–1357
22. Cooper JM, Epstein LM (2001) Use of intracardiac echocardiography to guide ablation of atrial fibrillation. Circulation 104:3010–3013
23. Kalman JM, Fitzpatrick AP, Olgin JE et al (1997) Biophysical characteristics of radiofrequency lesion formation in vivo: dynamics of catheter tip-tissue contact evaluated by intracardiac echocardiography. Am Heart J 133:8–18
24. Marrouche N, Martin D, Wazni O et al (2003) Phased-array intracardiac echocardiography monitoring during pulmonary vein isolation in patients with atrial fibrillation: impact on outcome and complications. Circulation 107:2710–2716
25. Wood MA, Shaffer KM, Ellenbogen AL et al (2005) Microbubbles during radiofrequency ablation: composition and formation. Heart Rhythm 2:397–403
26. Saad EB, Rosillo A, Saad CP et al (2003) Pulmonary vein stenosis after radiofrequency ablation of atrial fibrillation: functional characterisation, evolution, and influence of the ablation strategy. Circulation 108:3102–3107
27. Saliba W, Wilber D, Packer D et al (2002) Circumferential ultrasound ablation for pulmonary vein isolation: analysis of acute and chronic failures. J Cardiovasc Electrophysiol 13:957–961

Imaging in Arrhythmic Syndromes: What Is the Role of Cardiac Radiology?

R.D. White

Introduction

The field of cardiac radiology is now primarily concerned with applications of tomographic imaging modalities, especially magnetic resonance imaging (MRI) [1] and multi-detector computed tomography (MDCT) [2], to the diagnostic evaluation of acquired and congenital cardiovascular diseases. The value of MRI and MDCT in assessing conditions predisposing to the development of atrial or ventricular arrhythmias, in addressing their complications, and/or in guiding and monitoring treatments of such arrhythmias, has grown rapidly in recent years.

Atrial Arrhythmias

Atrial fibrillation is the most common form of atrial arrhythmia. While the atrial myocardial histopathology leading to atrial fibrillation cannot be readily detected by MRI or MDCT, signs of cardiac disease (e.g. coronary artery disease, mitral valve disease) leading to the development of atrial fibrillation, as well as the resulting gross morphological abnormalities in the atria (e.g. left atrial body and appendage dilatation) are easily assessed. In addition, thrombus within the distended appendage can be identified using either imaging modality; however, distinguishing it from stagnating flow is not always possible [3].

In patients undergoing evaluation for pulmonary vein isolation for treatment of atrial fibrillation, MRI and MDCT are also capable of delineating

Center for Integrated Non-Invasive Cardiovascular Imaging, Cleveland Clinic Foundation, Cleveland, OH, USA

patterns of pulmonary venous drainage which may influence the planning of pulmonary vein ostial ablation [4–11]. Such 'roadmaps' of left atrial and pulmonary vein anatomy can be co-registered with electrical-wavefront maps for image-directed intervention [8, 12]. Following pulmonary vein isolation, pulmonary vein luminal stenosis can be detected using MRI [13–16]. However, MDCT is especially well suited to the detection of changes in the pulmonary vein wall (e.g. thickening from oedema), as well as the commonly associated mediastinal (e.g. enlarged nodes), hilar (e.g. increased lymphoid tissue), pericardial (e.g. effusion) or lung parenchymal abnormalities (e.g. infarct) which may result from the pulmonary vein isolation procedure (Fig. 1) [17–20].

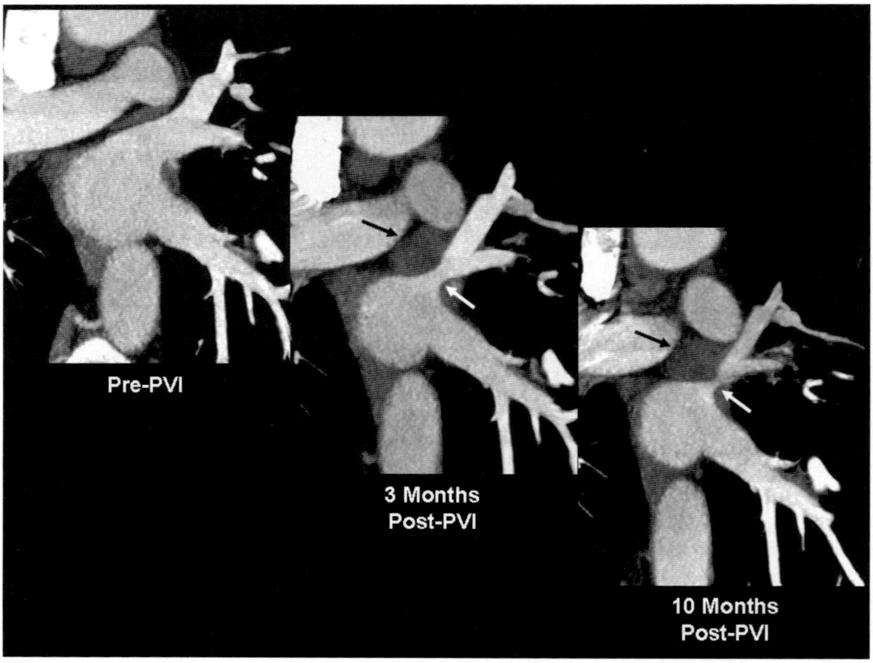

Fig. 1. Pulmonary venous stenosis after pulmonary vein isolation for treatment of atrial fibrillation (MDCT). Despite successful radiofrequency ablation of the ostium of the left superior pulmonary vein for pulmonary vein isolation (*PVI*), there was subsequent development by 3 months and progression to 10 months of luminal stenosis (*white arrows*) with adjacent soft tissue or fluid (*black arrows*)

Ventricular Arrhythmias

Left Ventricular Arrhythmias

Ventricular arrhythmias originating from the left ventricle often result from a wide range of ischaemic or non-ischaemic myocardial insults which lead to characteristic patterns detectable by tomographic imaging. MRI, in particular, is uniquely capable of identifying gross morphological changes in the cardiac chambers, intra-cardiac haemodynamic abnormalities, and myocardial histopathology associated with the various diseases predisposing to left ventricular arrhythmia [1, 21].

Dynamic MRI techniques (e.g. cine and cine-tagging) can be used to detect global dysfunction in which the systolic component predominates over the diastolic component (e.g. dilated cardiomyopathy) or vice versa (e.g. restrictive cardiomyopathy) [1]. Regional dysfunction can also be evaluated using the same dynamic techniques, with patterns of systolic mechanics of myocardium particularly useful for differentiating between thick-wall conditions (e.g. concentrically hyper-contracting in physiological left ventricular hypertrophy due to systemic arterial hypertension vs asymmetrically depressed contraction of the interventricular septum in hypertrophic obstructive cardiomyopathy vs concentric hypo-contracting in infiltrative myocardial conditions such as amyloid heart disease). While these approaches provide indirect functional indicators of myocardial disease, direct indications of myocardial histopathology are provided by tissue-characterising techniques (e.g. delayed-enhancement and T2-weighted fast spin-echo). Patterns of myocardial necrosis which indicate the presence of ischaemic damage (predominantly subendocardially distributed) from non-ischaemic damage (patchy and/or non-subendocardial in myocarditis and non-ischaemic cardiomyopathies) can be appreciated (Fig. 2) [22]. In patients with coronary artery disease, myocardial infarct surface area and mass on MRI have been shown to be better identifiers of a substrate for inducible monomorphic ventricular tachycardia than reduction in left ventricular ejection fraction [23]. In addition, acute and/or inflammatory stages can be distinguished from chronic and/or fibrotic stages [24].

In the presence of contraindications to the performance of MRI (e.g. permanent pacemakers and implanted defibrillators), MDCT can be employed to provide valuable gross morphological and functional information. MDCT can also provide important additional insights into the condition of the heart (e.g. coronary artery atherosclerosis) which can help to identify the underlying cause of myocardial disease [2, 21]. Last, MDCT may be used in the planning of therapy for ventricular arrhythmias (e.g. delineation of coronary venous anatomy for deciding pacemaker/defibrillator lead placement).

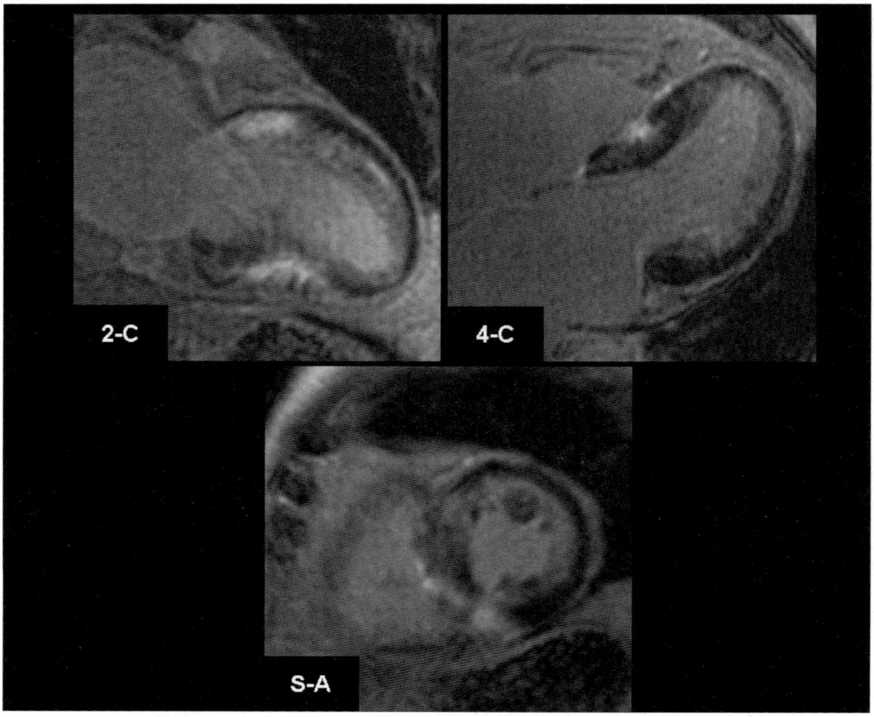

Fig. 2. Myocardial scarring in hypertrophic obstructive cardiomyopathy (MRI). Two-chamber (*2-C*), four-chamber (*4-C*), and mid short-axis (*S-A*) delayed enhancement images demonstrate patchy myocardial scarring (bright) intermixed with more normal-appearing myocardium (dark). The non-subendocardial distribution of the scarring within the hypertrophic left ventricle with asymmetric septal prominence is characteristic of non-ischaemic myocardial disease

Right Ventricular Arrhythmias

Right ventricular cardiomyopathy, especially arrhythmogenic right ventricular dysplasia, is a major cause of ventricular arrhythmia of right ventricular origin. MRI has been widely used for many years to evaluate arrhythmogenic right ventricular dysplasia due to its ability to reveal overall right ventricular dilation, aneurysmal outpouchings, global or regional systolic dysfunction, and fibrofatty myocardial replacement, which characterise this condition and are related to inducible ventricular tachycardia [25–31] (Fig. 3). In addition, in the setting of idiopathic right ventricular outflow tract tachycardia [32, 33] and Brugada syndrome [34], MRI has demonstrated milder morphological and functional abnormalities associated with the site of origin of ectopy. More recently, MDCT has been shown to have comparable capabilities and can be effectively used when there are contraindications to MRI (e.g. implanted defibrillator) [35, 36] (Fig. 4).

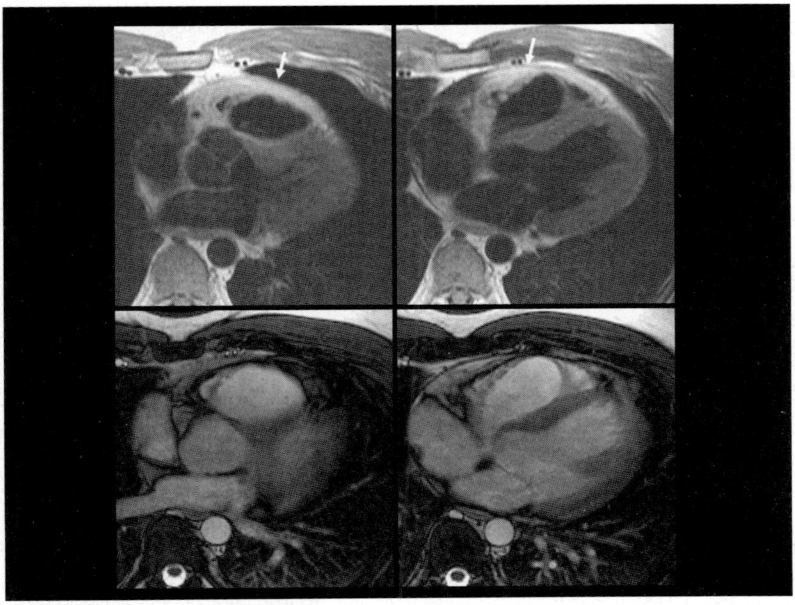

Fig. 3. Arrhythmogenic right ventricular dysplasia (MRI). Adjacent oblique-transaxial 'dark blood' images (*upper images*) and corresponding images from cine 'bright blood' image loops (*lower images*) are shown. The former reveal bright fatty tissue replacing the musculature of the anterior surface of the lower outflow tract and upper body of the right ventricle; the latter demonstrate systolic dysfunction in the same areas

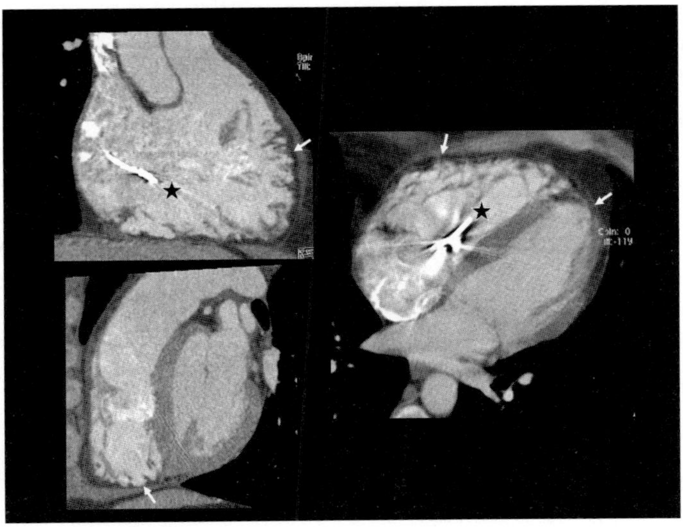

Fig. 4. Arrhythmogenic right ventricular dysplasia (MDCT). Oblique multiplanar reconstructions demonstrate diffuse dark fatty replacement (*arrows*) of both the right ventricular myocardial wall, which also shows prominent irregularity and multiple small outpouchings, and the apical portion of the left ventricular wall. Owing to the presence of an implanted defibrillator (*stars*), MRI could not be performed

Conclusions

MRI and MDCT can play important roles in understanding the underlying causes of atrial and ventricular arrhythmias. In addition, they are becoming more and more often incorporated into the development of new interventional therapies for these clinical conditions.

References

1. Schvartzman PR, White RD (2002) Magnetic resonance imaging. In: Topol EJ (ed) Textbook of cardiovascular medicine, 2nd edn. Lippincott Williams & Wilkins, Philadelphia, pp 1214–1256
2. Halliburton SS, Stillman AE, White RD (2005) Multi-slice computed tomography. In: Bergmann SR (ed) Cardiac imaging: The clinical guide. Humana Press, Inc, Potowa, NJ (in press)
3. Jaber WA, White RD, Kuzmiak SA et al (2004) Comparison of ability to identify left atrial thrombus by three-dimensional tomography versus transesophageal echocardiography in patients with atrial fibrillation. Am J Cardiol 93:486–489
4. Wittkampf FHM, Vonken E-J, Derksen R et al (2003) Pulmonary vein ostium geometry: Analysis by magnetic resonance angiography. Circulation 107:21–23
5. Cirillo S, Bonamini R, Gaita F et al (2004) Magnetic resonance angiography virtual endoscopy in the assessment of pulmonary veins before radiofrequency ablation procedure for atrial fibrillation. Eur Radiol 14:2053–2060
6. Mansour M, Holmvang G, Sosnovik D et al (2004) Assessment of pulmonary vein anatomic variability by magnetic resonance imaging: Implications for catheter ablation techniques for atrial fibrillation. J Cardiovasc Electrophysiol 15:387–393
7. Wood MA, Wittkamp M, Henry D et al (2004) A comparison of pulmonary vein ostial anatomy by computerized tomography, electrocardiography, and venography in patients with atrial fibrillation having radiofrequency catheter ablation. Am J Cardiol 93:49–53
8. Cronin P, Sneider MB, Kazerooni EA et al (2004) MDCT of the left atrium and pulmonary veins in planning radiofrequency ablation for atrial fibrillation: A how-to guide. AJR Am J Roentgenol 183:767–778
9. Lacomis JM, Wigginton W, Fuhrman C et al (2003) Multi-detector row CT of the left atrium and pulmonary veins before radio-frequency catheter ablation for atrial fibrillation. Radiographics 23:S35-S50
10. Jongbloed MR, Dirksen MS, Bax JJ et al (2005) Atrial fibrillation: Multi-detector row CT of pulmonary vein anatomy prior to radiofrequency catheter ablation – initial experience. Radiology 234:702–709
11. Schwartzman D, Lacomis J, Wigginton WG (2003) Characterization of left atrium and distal pulmonary vein morphology using multidimensional computed tomography. J Am Coll Cardiol 41:1349–1357
12. Sra J, Krum D, Hare J et al (2005) Feasibility and validation of registration of three-dimensional left atrial models derived from computed tomography with a noncontact cardiac mapping system. Heart Rhythm 2:55–63
13. Kluge A, Dill T, Ekinci O et al (2004) Decreased pulmonary perfusion in pulmonary vein stenosis after radiofrequency ablation: Assessment with dynamic magnetic resonance perfusion imaging. Chest 126:428–437

14. Tsao HM, Wu MH, Huang BH et al (2005) Morphologic remodeling of pulmonary veins and left atrium after catheter ablation of atrial fibrillation: Insight from long-term follow-up of three-dimensional magnetic resonance imaging. J Cardiovasc Electrophysiol 16:7–12
15. Kato R, Lickfett L, Meininger G et al (2003) Pulmonary vein anatomy in patients undergoing catheter ablation of atrial fibrillation: Lessons learned by use of magnetic resonance imaging. Circulation 107:2004–2010
16. Dill T, Neumann T, Ekinci O et al (2003) Pulmonary vein diameter reduction after radiofrequency catheter ablation for paroxysmal atrial fibrillation evaluated by contrast-enhanced three-dimensional magnetic resonance imaging. Circulation 107:845–850
17. Tse H-F, Reek S, Timmermans C et al (2003) Pulmonary vein isolation using transvenous catheter cryoablation for treatment of atrial fibrillation without risk of pulmonary stenosis. J Am Coll Cardiol 42:752–758
18. Saad E, Rossillo A, Saad CP et al (2003) Pulmonary vein stenosis after radiofrequency ablation of atrial fibrillation: Functional characterization, evolution, and influence of the ablation strategy. Circulation 108:3102–3107
19. Ghaye B, Szapiro D, Dacher J-N et al (2003) Percutaneous ablation for atrial fibrillation: The role of cross-sectional imaging. Radiographics 23:S19-S33
20. Qureshi AM, Prieto LR, Latson LA et al (2003) Transcatheter angioplasty for acquired pulmonary vein stenosis after radiofrequency ablation. Circulation 108:1336–1342
21. White RD (2004) MR and CT assessment for ischemic cardiac disease. J Magn Reson Imaging 19:659–675
22. McCrohon JA, Moon JCC, Prasad SK et al (2003) Differentiation of heart failure related to dilated cardiomyopathy and coronary artery disease using gadolinium-enhanced cardiovascular magnetic resonance. Circulation 108:54–59
23. Bello D, Fieno DS, Kim RJ et al (2005) Infarct morphology identifies patients with substrate for sustained ventricular tachycardia. J Am Coll Cardiol 45:1104–1108
24. Abdel-Aty H, Zagrosek A, Schulz-Menger J et al (2004) Delayed enhancement and T2-weighted cardiovascular magnetic resonance imaging differentiate acute from chronic myocardial infarction. Circulation 109:2411–2416
25. Fattori R, Tricoci P, Russo V et al (2005) Quantification of fatty tissue mass by magnetic resonance imaging in arrhythmogenic right ventricular dysplasia. J Cardiovasc Electrophysiol 16:256–261
26. Tandri H, Saranathan M, Rodriguez ER et al (2005) Noninvasive detection of myocardial fibrosis in arrhythmogenic right ventricular cardiomyopathy using delayed-enhancement magnetic resonance imaging. J Am Coll Cardiol 45:98–103
27. Abbara S, Migrino RQ, Sosnovik DE et al (2004) Value of fat suppression in the MRI evaluation of suspected arrhythmogenic right ventricular dysplasia. AJR Am J Roentgenol 182:587–591
28. Castillo E, Tandri H, Rodriguez ER et al (2004) Arrhythmogenic right ventricular dysplasia: Ex vivo and in vivo fat detection with black-blood MR imaging. Radiology 232:38–48
29. Bluemke DA, Krupinski EA, Ovitt T et al (2003) MR imaging of arrhythmogenic right ventricular cardiomyopathy: Morphologic findings and interobserver reliability. Cardiology 99:153–162
30. Tandri H, Calkins H, Nasir K et al (2003) Magnetic resonance imaging findings in patients meeting task force criteria for arrhythmogenic right ventricular dysplasia. J Cardiovasc Electrophysiol 14:476–482

31. Kayser HWM, van der Wall EE, Sivananthan MU et al (2002) Diagnosis of arrhythmogenic right ventricular dysplasia: A review. Radiographics 22:639–650
32. Globits S, Kreiner G, Frank H et al (1997) Significance of morphological abnormalities detected by MRI in patients undergoing successful ablation of right ventricular outflow tract tachycardia. Circulation 96:2633–2640
33. White RD, Trohman RG, Flamm SD et al (1998) Right ventricular arrhythmia in the absence of arrhythmogenic dysplasia: MR imaging of myocardial abnormalities. Radiology 207:743–751
34. Papavassiliu T, Wolpert C, Fluchter S et al (2004) Magnetic resonance imaging findings in patients with Brugada syndrome. J Cardiovasc Electrophysiol 15:1139–1140
35. Kimura F, Sakai F, Sakomura Y et al (2002) Helical CT features of arrhythmogenic right ventricular cardiomyopathy. Radiographics 22:1111–1124
36. Tandri H, Bomma C, Calkins H et al (2004) Magnetic resonance and computed tomography imaging of arrhythmogenic right ventricular dysplasia. J Magn Reson Imaging 19:848–858

Value of Transoesophageal Echocardiography for the Ablation of Atrial Fibrillation

B. De Piccoli, A. Rossillo

Introduction

The ablation of atrial fibrillation by pulmonary vein antrum isolation (PVAI) through radiofrequency is an effective treatment of symptomatic, drug refractory arrhythmia. In this regard, transoesophageal echocardiography (TEE) is a useful tool to identify those patients eligible for the procedure [1] and to monitor its possible consequences.

Transoesophageal Echocardiography Before Ablation

Before the procedure, TEE examination of the patients mainly focuses on the interatrial septum (IAS), left atrial (LA) cavity, LA appendage and pulmonary veins (PVs). In people affected by atrial fibrillation, the IAS often exhibits minor abnormalities, such as a floating movement, an aneurism, a patent fossa ovalis or increased thickening [2]. These abnormalities, especially aneurism, can enhance thrombus deposition on the IAS surface; which constitutes a risk factor for embolic complications when the IAS is punctured by catheters aimed at the ostium of the PV. Conversely, a patent fossa ovalis can facilitate crossing of the IAS by the catheter; in this case, TEE can be used to determine the optimal approach to the PV.

The LA appendage is the structure most frequently involved [3] in cardiac thrombus formation; thus, it must be excluded before carrying out PVAI in order to avoid embolic complications. Spontaneous echo contrast (SEC) is also considered an embolic risk factor [4] and its presence and intensity are

Division of Cardiology, Cardiovascular Department, Umberto I Hospital, Mestre-Venice, Italy

strictly correlated with dilation of the LA appendage and reduction of its outward and inward flow velocities. Furthermore, Goldman et al. [5] used multivariate analysis to determine that an outward flow velocity < 20 cm/s correlated with the presence of thrombus, intense SEC and embolic events. If such information can be obtained for each patient, an optimal anticoagulant therapy before and during PVAI can be prescribed.

While LA morphology and contractility is adequately investigated by transthoracic echocardiography, TEE exhibits a higher sensitivity and specificity in thrombus detection [6] and can thus be used before PVAI to prevent subsequent embolic events.

The PV–LA junction and the antrum around the vein are the critical zones involved in the application of radiofrequency (RF) for PVAI. It is therefore important to determine the number of PVs, their dimensions, anatomical variants and the velocities of their flow in order to tailor the procedure to the individual patient. The most frequent variants are additional veins; these involve the right PV in near 30% of cases [7], and the common ostium, which involves the left PV in 10.5–32% of cases [1, 7, 8]. RF must be titrated only on the common ostium, not on the mouth of the single vein, in order to avoid future stenosis. Additional veins must also be treated since they can be the sites of foci triggering atrial fibrillation. Furthermore, the dimensions of the PV must also be determined before carrying out PVAI as it will facilitate choice of the best size Lasso catheter for use during the procedure.

Finally, by measuring the velocities (v) of pulmonary vein flow (pvf), we can calculate possible pressure gradients (gradient = 4v2) along the vein; that is, we can demonstrate PV stenosis, which is not a not rare occurrence in patients previously submitted to other ablation procedures, especially those done under the guidance of angiography or CARTO [9]. In this event, RF must be cautiously titrated so as not to worsen the anatomical features of the vein.

Transoesophageal Echocardiography During Ablation

The use of TEE in the cardiac electrophysiology lab during ablation has been reported in previous studies on RF treatment of supraventricular arrhythmias [10]. The method was shown to cause the prolonged discomfort of patients and was thus neglected after the introduction of intracardiac echocardiography.

Transoesophageal Echocardiography After Ablation

Early reports on the use of RF for PVAI in patients with atrial fibrillation [11] reported PV stenosis in subjects submitted to the procedure. Since then, follow-up studies of the treated patients have been carried out using multidimensional computed tomography (CT) [12], nuclear magnetic resonance [13] and TEE [13]. Each of these approaches can document the variations in the dimensions of the PV over time. Nevertheless, the documented calibre of the PV depends on the section of vein explored by the imaging technique and therefore may not reflect the real narrowing of the vein, owing to its elliptical shape [8]. However, TEE can also be used to calculate pvf velocities, whose variation better reflects the functional impact of the stenosis.

Personal Experience

We have recently conducted a follow-up study of 79 patients (65 males, 14 females, mean age 57 ± 9.9 years) who underwent ablation for the treatment of atrial fibrillation. In this series, 34% were affected by paroxysmal, 40% by persistent, and 17% by permanent atrial fibrillation. Many of the patients (35%) were free from cardiac diseases, while hypertensive cardiopathy was the prevailing (27%) pathology.

At the beginning of the study, PVAI was guided by angiography or CARTO, and later by intracardiac echocardiography. Each patient was examined by TEE both before and 48 h (first control), 3 months (second control) and 12 months (third control) after ablation.

A spiral CT was performed in each patient at the third month after the procedure, and was repeated at 6 and 12 months later in patients with suspected or certain PV stenosis.

In each study patient, the presence of IAS abnormalities such as floating movement, aneurism or shunt was searched for. In addition, the left atrium and LA appendage (LAa) were examined for the presence of thrombus, SEC, and we focused on the presence of a pericardial effusion. The dimension of each PV at the junction with the left atrium and the velocities of pvf by pulse wave were measured by Doppler. The peak (peak vel) and middle (mid vel) velocities and their ratio (mid vel/peak vel) were calculated.

Results

Qualitative Aspects

A floating IAS was documented in 33% and an aneurism in 4% of the study population. A patent fossa ovalis was observed in 10% of the patients at basal TEE. The incidence increased to 86% at the first control, but returned to the basal level of 10% at follow up. In 9% of the subjects, SEC with an intensity ≥ 2+/4+ was observed in the left atrium and LAa. The incidence increased to

19% at the first control but decreased subsequently. Thrombi were not detected at basal TEE or during the follow up. A pericardial effusion < 150 cc was observed in 26% of patients before ablation, and in 64%, with a maximal amount of 500 cc, at the first control; however, at the time of follow-up, the incidence had decreased to the basal level.

Quantitative Features of the Pulmonary Vein

Three months after ablation (second control), the average size of the PV in the study population had decreased (Table 1) by 7.8% ($P = 0.03$ compared to the basal values). The peak vel increased by 34.4% ($P = 0.0001$), the mid vel by 47.27% ($P = 0.0001$), and the mid vel/peak vel by 8% ($P = 0.002$). At the last control, there was a further but not significant narrowing of the PV and an increase in the parameters measuring velocity.

Spiral CT, 3 months after ablation, showed a < 50% narrowing of the PV in 75 patients, whereas in three patients there was 50–70% narrowing of the PV. In one patient narrowing was > 70%.

Table 1. Variation of the parameters 3 months after ablation

Parameters (average values of the 4 pulmonary veins)	Basal	3 months	Variation (%)	*P*
Dimension (mm)	13.7 ± 1.9	12.9 ± 1.8	≠ 7.8	0.03
Peak velocity (cm/s)	56 ± 6.5	75 ± 24.4	≠ 34.4	0.0001
Mid velocity (cm/s)	25.5 ± 8.4	37.8 ± 14.9	≠ 47.27	0.0001
Mid velocity/peak velocity	0.45 ± 0.05	0.49 ± 0.06	≠ 8	0.002

In the first group of 75 patients, the peak vel was 73.6 ± 21.1 cm/s, mid vel 36.9 ± 13 cm/s, and mid vel/peak vel 0.49 ± 0.06. In the four patients with a PV narrowing > 50%, peak vel was 107.7 ± 57.5 cm/s ($P = 0.009$), mid vel was 58.3 ± 33.6 cm/s ($P = 0.05$), and mid vel/peak vel 0.54 ± 0.05 ($P = 0.05$). In each PV with a stenosis > 50%, peak vel was > 139 cm/s, mid vel was > 92 cm/s and mid vel/peak vel was > 0.66, with a more than 100% increase compared to pre-ablation values.

Discussion

In present study, we observed a rather high prevalence of minor IAS abnormalities that could facilitate supraventricular arrhythmias, above all atrial fibrillation. This hypothesis is in agreement with the results of other authors [2], who observed a higher prevalence of atrial fibrillation in the presence of pathological IAS.

We did not detect a thrombus in the left atrium or LAa of any subject of the study population; in contrast with previous reports [14]. Nevertheless, we must emphasise that a high percentage of our patients was affected by paroxysmal or persistent atrial fibrillation, while previous reports mainly relate to permanent atrial fibrillation. Furthermore, our patients had been previously anticoagulated and thus were in an optimal therapeutic range for at least 4 weeks before ablation.

One day after ablation, there was a high prevalence of pericardial effusion. Affected patients were completely asymptomatic and pericardiocenthesis was not necessary. Moreover the effusion had been reabsorbed by the end of the study. It is likely that the effusion originated from an inflammation of the pericardium following the delivery of RF to the thin posterior wall of the left atrium during PVAI.

PV stenosis after RF of PVAI has been reported in previous studies, in which imaging studies were carried out [1, 8, 13]. The features of PV narrowing may not always provide information about the physiological significance of the stenosis; in fact, symptoms can be absent despite a visible reduction of PV calibre (Fig. 1). By calculating pvf velocities, we were able to document variations with respect to the basal value obtained before ablation and thus better able to quantify the haemodynamic consequences of RF to the ostium of the PV.

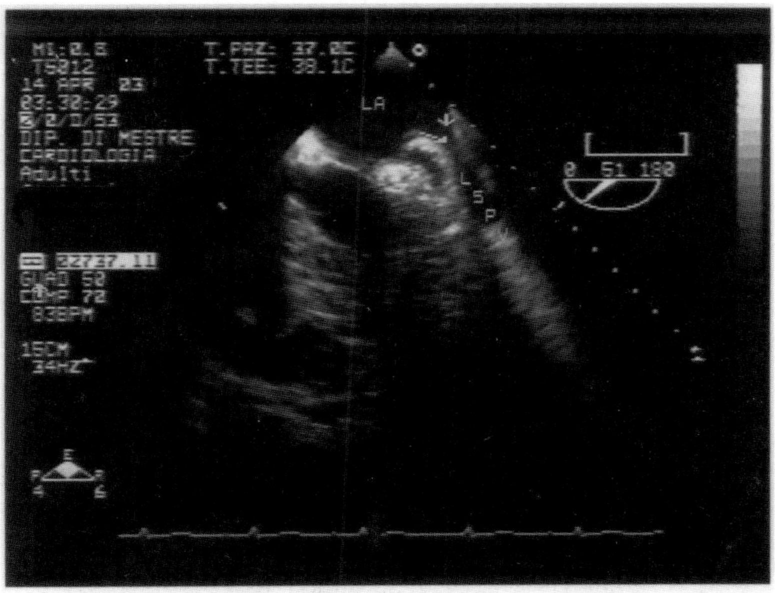

Fig. 1. Transoesophageal echocardiography (TEE) image of a pulmonary vein stenosis. The *arrows* point out the site of the stenosis. *LA* Left atrium, *LSPV* left superior pulmonary vein

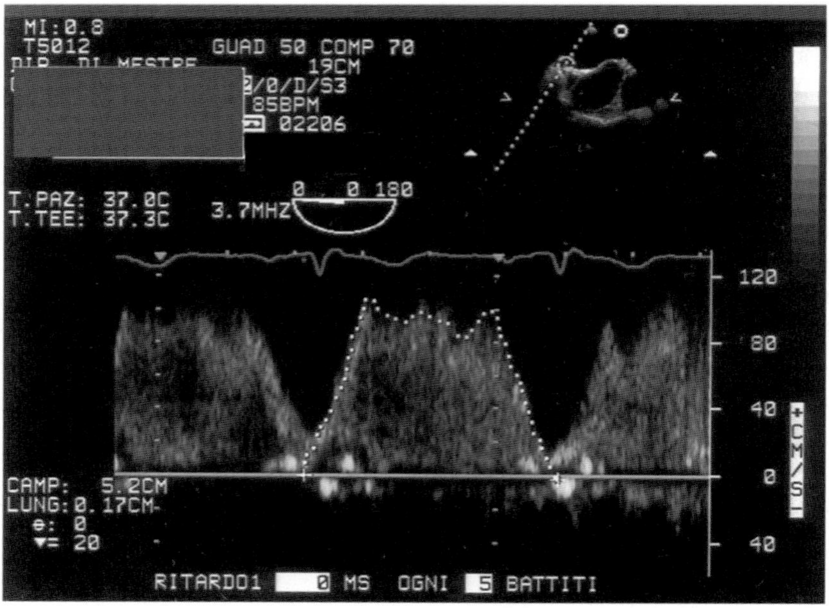

Fig. 2. Doppler flow of a critically stenosed pulmonary vein. The spectrum shows a 'plateau' configuration

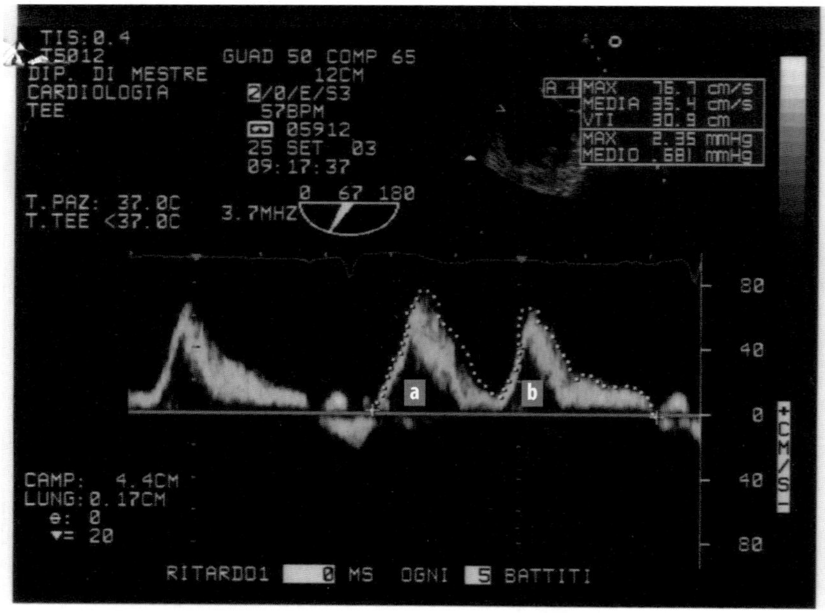

Fig. 3a, b. Normal pulmonary vein flow. **a** systolic wave, **b** diastolic wave

Our study also showed that, on average, pvf velocities increased, implying a slight narrowing of the PV. Three months after ablation there was a further but not significant increase in pvf. Only an increase over the basal value of more than 100% identified a > 50% stenosis of the PV at spiral CT. Moreover, the spectrum of the pulse-wave Doppler of the pvf of these patients was significantly altered owing to the large increase in the middle velocity. Figure 2 shows the Doppler flow spectrum of a patient with a PV stenosis > 70%. The peak vel was 210 cm/s, mid vel 120 cm/s and mid vel/peak vel 0.75. The normal systolic and diastolic waves (Fig. 3) are not distinguishable and the entire flow exhibits a 'plateau' configuration. The subject was symptomatic for dispnoea and haemoptysis and his stenosed left inferior PV was successfully treated by angioplasty and stent insertion.

Conclusions

TEE is a useful tool to investigate patients undergoing ablation therapy of atrial fibrillation. The technique provides important information about the presence of thrombus and SEC in the left atrium and LAa, and about minor IAS abnormalities, which seem to occur more frequently than in the normal population. Such information is necessary for planning the approach to the PV by catheters that must cross the septum and the atrial cavity.

After ablation, TEE can be used to monitor possible minor complications, such as a residual IAS shunt or pericardial effusion. It also allows the detection of PV stenosis, a rare but dreaded complication of PVAI. A control TEE examination 3 months after the ablation procedure is probably adequate for this purpose.

References

1. Marrouche NF, Martin DO, Wazni O et al (2003) Phased-array intracardiac echocardiography monitoring during pulmonary vein isolation in patients with atrial fibrillation. Impact on outcome and complications. Circulation 107:2710–2716
2. Lopez-Candales A, Grewal H, Katz W (2005) The importance of increased interatrial septal thickness in patients with atrial fibrillation: a transesophageal echocardiographic study. Echocardiography 22(5):408–414
3. Jordan RA, Scheifley CH, Edwards JE (1951) Mural thrombosis and arterial embolism in mitral stenosis: a clinical pathologic study of fifty-one cases. Circulation 3:363–367
4. Leung DYC, Black IW, Cranney GB et al (1994) Prognostic implications of left atrial spontaneous echocontrast in nonvalvular atrial fibrillation. J Am Coll Cardiol 24:755–762

5. Goldman ME, Pearce LA, Hart RG et al (1999) Pathophysiologic correlates of thromboembolism in nonvalvular atrial fibrillation: reduced flow velocity in the left atrial appendage (The Stroke Prevention in Atrial Fibrillation [SPAF-III] study). J Am Soc Echocardiogr 12(12):1080–1087
6. Kronzon I, Tunick PA, Glassman E et al (1990) Transesophageal echocardiography to detect atrial clots in candidates for percutaneous transseptal mitral balloon valvuloplasty. J Am Coll Cardiol 16:1320–1322
7. Piovesana P, Toffanin G, De Piccoli B et al (2005) Studio di confronto fra eco transesofageo e risonanza magnetica nucleare nella valutazione delle varianti anatomiche delle vene polmonari nei pazienti sottoposti ad ablazione della fibrillazione atriale. Ital Heat J 6:S28 (abs)
8. Kato R, Lickfett L, Meininger G et al (2003) Pulmonary vein anatomy in patients undergoing catheter ablation of atrial fibrillation: lessons learned by use of magnetic resonance imaging. Circulation 107(15):2004–2010
9. Saad EB, Rossillo A, Saad CP et al (2003) Pulmonary vein stenosis after radiofrequency ablation of atrial fibrillation: functional characterization, evolution, and influence of the ablation strategy. Circulation 108(25):3102–3107
10. Tucker KJ, Curtis AB, Murphy J et al (1996) Transesophageal echocardiographic guidance of transseptal left heart catheterisation during radiofrequency ablation of left-sided accessory pathways in humans. Pacing Clin Electrophysiol 19:272–281
11. Haïssaguerre M, Jaïs P, Shan DC et al (2000) Electrophysiological end point for catheter ablation of atrial fibrillation initiated from multiple pulmonary venous foci. Circulation 101:1409–1417
12. Schwartzman D, Lacomis J, Wigginton WG (2003) Characterization of left atrium and distal pulmonary vein morphology using multidimensional computed tomography. J Am Coll Cardiol 41:1349–1357
13. Yu W, Hsu T, Tai C et al (2001) Acquired pulmonary vein stenosis after radiofrequency catheter ablation of paroxysmal atrial fibrillation. J Cardiovasc Electrophysiol 12:887–892
14. Stoddart MF, Dawkins PR, Prince CR, Longaker RA (1995) Transesophageal echocardiographic guidance of cardioversion in patients with atrial fibrillation. Am Heart J 129:1204–1215

Value of the LocaLisa Non-fluoroscopic Mapping System in the Ablation of Atrial Fibrillation

P. SANDERS[1, 2], P. JAÏS[1], M. HOCINI[1], L.-F. HSU[1], G.D. YOUNG[2], C. SCAVÉE[1], P. KUKLIK[2], M. ROTTER[1], Y. TAKAHASHI[1], T. ROSTOCK[1], F. SACHER[1], B. JOHN[1], M. STILES[2], M. HAÏSSAGUERRE[1]

Background

Achieving and maintaining sinus rhythm in patients with atrial fibrillation (AF) is the optimal therapeutic outcome. While antiarrhythmic therapy to maintain sinus rhythm has been demonstrated to be of limited efficacy [1–3], preliminary evidence suggests a beneficial effect of catheter ablation strategies to achieve and maintain sinus rhythm [4, 5]. The importance of the interaction between the triggers and substrate in the development of AF is well-recognised. Catheter ablation strategies are centred on pulmonary vein (PV) ablation. However, it is becoming evident that most patients with permanent or persistent AF and 30–40% of those with paroxysmal AF will require additional substrate modification to improve the outcomes of AF ablation [6]. Several modalities of substrate modification have been proposed and include linear atrial ablation [7–9], ablation of fractionated electrograms [10], ablation at sites of high-frequency activity [11], and attempts at vagal denervation [12]. However, these procedures are technically challenging and associated with prolonged procedural and fluoroscopic durations.

Recently, several localising and three-dimensional mapping tools have emerged to facilitate and reduce the fluoroscopic exposure associated with AF ablation. This review will focus on the use of the LocaLisa (Medtronic) non-fluoroscopic mapping system for anatomical guidance during the ablation of AF.

[1]Hôpital Cardiologique du Haut-Lévêque, and Université Victor Segalen Bordeaux II, Bordeaux, France; [2]Department of Cardiology, Royal Adelaide Hospital, and Department of Medicine, University of Adelaide, Adelaide, Australia

The LocaLisa Mapping System

The LocaLisa mapping system has been developed to allow three-dimensional catheter localisation. This is based on externally applied electrical fields and works on the principle that a voltage drop occurs as the current passes through the various body structures. Three orthogonally placed pairs of skin electrodes are used to send small, 1-mA currents between each pair of skin electrodes (each at a slightly different frequency: 30.27 kHz, 30.70 kHz, and 31.15 kHz). Standard intra-cardiac catheters are used as sensors to detect these thoracic electrical fields. By digitally separating the three frequencies, the three-dimensional position (X, Y, and Z directions, respectively) of the catheter can be determined. Each electrode on the system can be used as a sensor and displayed in terms of its relative position. The location accuracy of the system has been demonstrated to be better than 2 mm, with a strong linear correlation with fluoroscopically determined catheter locations (correlation coefficient 0.996–0.999) [13].

Pulmonary Vein Isolation

While a number of sites within the atria have been reported to initiate AF, the PVs are recognised as the dominant source of triggers initiating AF in many clinical situations [14]. Spontaneous activity arising from the PVs can manifest in a spectrum of atrial arrhythmias, isolated extrasystoles, slow atrial rhythms, and atrial tachycardia [14]. Rapid sustained focal discharges (sometimes for hours, days, or longer) may drive sustained AF (true 'focal' AF), but more commonly short bursts initiate AF in patients with the appropriate atrial substrate [14]. More recently, it has been suggested that the PVs also have a role in the maintenance of a significant proportion of cases of paroxysmal AF [15, 16].

Circumferential mapping catheters have enabled evaluation of the perimetric distribution and activation sequence of PV activity to allow their effective isolation. Ablation of the PVs guided by circumferential mapping is performed 1 cm from the ostium of both right-PVs as well as for the posterior and superior aspects of the left-PVs, to minimise the risk of PV stenosis. However, when ablation is required at the anterior portions of the left-PVs, energy is delivered within the first millimetres of the PV (rather than the posterior wall of the appendage) to achieve effective disconnection. Radiofrequency (RF) energy is delivered for 30 s at each point and this application is prolonged for 1–2 min when a change occurs in the morphology or sequence of the PV potentials, as determined by circumferential mapping. The procedural endpoint is the total disconnection or dissociation of the PV. An immediate procedural success of 94–100% has been reported for this type of circumferential mapping. The long-term success rates for PV electrical isolation have been approximately 70% without antiarrhythmics.

Several mapping tools have been used for anatomical localisation during PV ablation, including for real-time demonstration of catheters and structures, tagging of ablation sites, and mapping of gaps in the ablation lines. Macle and colleagues prospectively randomised 52 patients undergoing PV ablation for paroxysmal AF to ablation using the LocaLisa mapping system or to fluoroscopy alone [17]. The LocaLisa system was used to visualise in real-time the circumferential mapping catheter positioned at the ostia of each PV and the ablation catheter location relative to this catheter, and to annotate ablated sites. While the total duration of RF energy delivered did not differ significantly between the groups, there was a significant decrease in the fluoroscopic duration (8.4 ± 4.3 min vs 23.7 ± 9.7 min, respectively; $P < 0.0001$) and time to achieve isolation of all four PVs (46.5 ± 12.0 min vs 66.3 ± 18.9 min, respectively; $P < 0.0001$). These results have recently been confirmed by Rotter et al. using a more advanced mapping system (NavX, Endocardial Solution) based on the same principles [18]. In this prospective randomised study evaluating the role of NavX in 72 patients with paroxysmal AF, a significant reduction in fluoroscopic duration (15.4 ± 3.4 min vs 21.3 ± 6.4 min, respectively; $P < 0.001$) and time to isolate all PVs (52 ± 12 min vs 61 ± 17 min; $P = 0.02$) was observed. Both these studies demonstrated the benefit of continuous real-time visualisation of catheters at the time of ablation to reduce the fluoroscopic exposure and procedural duration for the patient and the physician. While, theoretically, continuous monitoring of the ablation catheter may decrease the delivery of energy within the PV and therefore PV stenosis, neither of these studies were powered to establish this benefit.

Ablation of the Substrate for AF

Surgically created linear compartmentalisation of the atria (the MAZE operation) is associated with long-term suppression of AF. A number of groups have attempted to perform linear ablation to modify the atrial substrate. These studies have indicated that the most effective linear ablation for the prevention of AF needs to involve the left atrium or both atria [7–9, 19–22]. These procedures to achieve complete linear conduction block have been technically challenging, with incomplete linear lesions being associated with the frequent development of left atrial macroreentry and recurrence of arrhythmia; they were also associated with increased procedural risk and prolonged procedural and fluoroscopic durations.

Recently, ablation of the mitral isthmus (left inferior PV to the lateral mitral annulus) and the roofline (joining the two superior PVs) has become an increasingly popular approach. Mitral isthmus ablation is particularly attractive as target for substrate modification as it is short in length and its proximity to the coronary sinus allows optimal positioning of catheters to confirm linear conduction block. This short line, when combined with PV ablation results in a contiguous line of conduction block that transects the posterior lateral LA (analogous to the conduction block created by cavotricuspid isthmus ablation being extended by the crista terminalis). Conduction block at the mitral isthmus can be achieved in 92% of patients with paroxysmal AF and was associated with 88% of patients being arrhythmia-free without the use of anti-arrhythmic agents at 10 ± 5 months of follow-up [9]. Importantly, there was no change in atrial activation as a result of mitral isthmus ablation during sinus rhythm. Preliminary data concerning the use of this procedure in patients with chronic AF suggests that at a follow-up of 6 ± 5 months, 75% of patients remained in sinus rhythm. Scavee and colleagues presented data evaluating the role of LocaLisa navigation compared to fluoroscopy alone to undertake mitral isthmus ablation [23]. This group randomised 60 patients undergoing ablation of paroxysmal AF after PV isolation and found a significant reduction in the fluoroscopic duration (8 ± 4 min vs 20 ± 11 min, respectively; $P < 0.001$), procedural time (38 ± 18 min vs 62±38 min, respectively; $P = 0.004$), and the duration of RF energy to achieve bidirectional conduction block (1166 ± 652 s vs 1811 ± 922 s, respectively; $P = 0.04$). Similar results have been presented with the use of NavX mapping [24]. While the reduction in fluoroscopic and procedural duration is consistent with that observed with PV ablation and reflects the benefit of continuous online visualisation of the catheters, the reduction in the RF duration suggests a benefit in terms of tagging of previously ablated regions (Fig. 1).

Similarly, Rotter et al. evaluated the use of NavX navigation in performing roofline ablation and found a consistent reduction in the fluoroscopic (5.6 ± 2.2 min vs 9.9 ± 4.8 min, respectively; $P = 0.003$) and procedural durations (14.7 ± 5.5 min vs 26.6 ± 16.9 min; $P = 0.007$). While these results have not yet been confirmed using the LocaLisa mapping system, given the similarities of these systems it is anticipated that the benefit would extend to this system as well (Fig. 2).

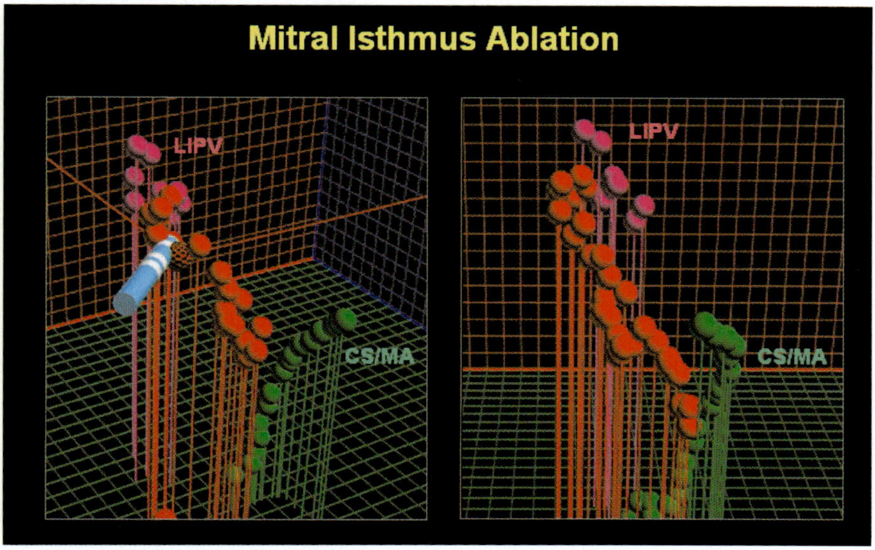

Fig. 1. Mitral isthmus ablation using the LocaLisa navigation system. *Left* right anterior oblique (*RAO*), *right* anterior posterior (*AP*). The left inferior PV (*LIPV*) is marked in purple and the mitral annulus (*MA*) marked through the coronary sinus (*CS*). The red tags demonstrate the linear ablation line

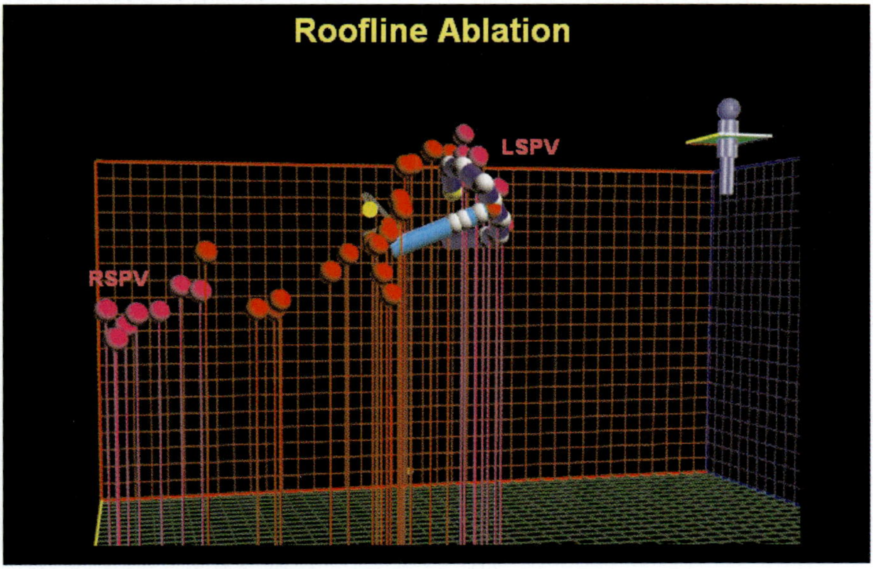

Fig. 2. Roofline ablation using the LocaLisa navigation system. The two superior PVs are marked in purple. The red tags demonstrate the ablation sequence joining the two superior PVs

Conclusions

The LocaLisa mapping system provides an economical means of continuous online monitoring of multiple catheters, the annotation of anatomic structures, and the tagging of previously ablated regions. These features significantly reduce the fluoroscopic exposure and procedural duration associated with PV isolation and linear substrate modification for AF.

Acknowledgments
Dr. Sanders is supported by the Neil Hamilton Fairley Fellowship from the National Health and Medical Research Council of Australia and the Ralph Reader Fellowship from the National Heart Foundation of Australia. Dr. Rotter is supported by the Swiss National Foundation for Scientific Research, Bern, Switzerland. Dr. Rostock is supported by the German Cardiac Society. Dr. Stiles is supported by an Overseas Research Fellowship from the National Heart Foundation of New Zealand.

References

1. Hohnloser SH, Kuck KH, Lilienthal J, for the PIAF investigators (2000) Rhythm or rate control in atrial fibrillation – pharmacological intervention in atrial fibrillation (PIAF): a randomised trial. Lancet 356:1789–1794
2. Anonymous (2002) A comparison of rate control and rhythm control in patients with atrial fibrillation. The atrial fibrillation follow-up investigation of rhythm management (AFFIRM) investigators. N Engl J Med 347:1825–1833
3. Van Gelder IC, Hagens VE, Bosker HA et al; Rate Control versus Electrical Cardioversion for Persistent Atrial Fibrillation Study Group (2002) A comparison of rate control and rhythm control in patients with recurrent persistent atrial fibrillation. N Engl J Med 347:1834–1840
4. Hsu LF, Jaïs P, Sanders P et al (2004) Catheter ablation of atrial fibrillation in congestive heart failure. N Engl J Med 351:2373–2383
5. Pappone C, Rosanio S, Augello G et al (2003) Mortality, morbidity, and quality of life after circumferential pulmonary vein ablation for atrial fibrillation: Outcomes from a controlled nonrandomized long-term study. J Am Coll Cardiol 42:185–197
6. Oral H, Knight BP, Tada H et al (2002) Pulmonary vein isolation for paroxysmal and persistent atrial fibrillation. Circulation 105:1077–1081
7. Haïssaguerre M, Jaïs P, Shah DC et al (1996) Right and left atrial radiofrequency catheter therapy of paroxysmal atrial fibrillation. J Cardiovasc Electrophysiol 7:1132–1144
8. Sanders P, Jaïs P, Hocini M et al (2004) Electrophysiologic and clinical consequence of linear catheter ablation to transect the anterior left atrium in patients with atrial fibrillation. Heart Rhythm 1:176–184
9. Jaïs P, Hocini M, Hsu LF et al (2004) Technique and results of linear ablation at the mitral isthmus. Circulation 110:2996–3002
10. Nademanee K, McKenzie J, Kosar E et al (2004) A new approach for catheter ablation of atrial fibrillation: mapping of the electrophysiological substrate. J Am Coll Cardiol 43:2044–2053

11. Sanders P, Berenfeld O, Hocini M et al (2005) Spectral analysis identifies sites of high frequency activity maintaining atrial fibrillation in humans. Circulation 112:789-797
12. Pappone C, Santinelli V, Manguso F et al (2004) Pulmonary vein denervation enhances long-term benefit after circumferential ablation for paroxysmal atrial fibrillation. Circulation 109:327–334
13. Wittkampf FHM, Wever EFD, Derksen R et al (1999) LocaLisa: new technique for real-time 3-dimensional localization of regular intracardiac electrodes. Circulation 99:1312–1317
14. Haïssaguerre M, Jaïs P, Shah DC et al (1998) Spontaneous initiation of atrial fibrillation by ectopic beats originating in the pulmonary veins. N Engl J Med 339:659–666
15. Haïssaguerre M, Sanders P, Hocini M et al (2004) Changes in atrial fibrillation cycle length and inducibility during catheter ablation and their relation to outcome. Circulation 109:3007–3013
16. Haïssaguerre M, Sanders P, Hocini M et al (2004) Pulmonary veins in the substrate for atrial fibrillation: the 'venous wave' hypothesis. J Am Coll Cardiol 43:2290–2292
17. Macle L, Jaïs P, Scavee C et al (2003) Pulmonary vein disconnection using the LocaLisa three-dimensional nonfluoroscopic catheter imaging system. J Cardiovasc Electrophysiol 14:693–697
18. Rotter M, Takahashi Y, Sanders P et al (2005) Reduction of fluoroscopy exposure and procedure duration during ablation of atrial fibrillation using a novel anatomical navigation system. Eur Heart J 26:1415-1421
19. Jaïs P, Shah DC, Takahashi A et al (1998) Long-term follow-up after right atrial radiofrequency catheter treatment of paroxysmal atrial fibrillation. Pacing Clin Electrophysiol 21:2533–2538
20. Ernst S, Ouyang F, Lober F et al (2003) Catheter-induced linear lesions in the left atrium in patients with atrial fibrillation: An electroanatomic study. J Am Coll Cardiol 42:1271–1282
21. Jaïs P, Shah DC, Haïssaguerre M et al (1999) Efficacy and safety of septal and left-atrial linear ablation for atrial fibrillation. Am J Cardiol 84:139R–146R
22. Packer DL (2002) Linear ablation for atrial fibrillation: the pendulum swings back. In: Zipes DP, Haïssaguerre M (eds) Catheter ablation of atrial arrhythmias. Futura Publishing, Armonk, pp 107–128
23. Scavee C, Jaïs P, Hsu LF et al (2003) Linear left atrial ablation of atrial fibrillation using a three-dimensional non-fluoroscopic mapping system. Eur Heart J 24:S–597
24. Takahashi Y, Rotter M, Sanders P et al (2005) Left atrial linear ablation to modify the substrate of atrial fibrillation using a new nonfluoroscopic imaging system. Pacing Clin Electrophysiol 28:S90–S93

Linear Atrial Lesions Should Always Be Performed in Addition to Circumferential Pulmonary Vein Isolation

D. Shah, H. Burri, H. Sunthorn, P. Gentil-Baron

Linear lesions are the equivalent of surgical atriotomies created by percutaneous catheter ablation, but in electrophysiological terms should be considered complete only if they create complete conduction block across two fixed or anatomic obstacles. Linear lesions increase the activation time of the atrium by enforcing a detour depending upon the site of impulse origin. By changing the sequence of activation of the atria they may alter electromechanical feedback. Depending upon the type and number of lesion(s) deployed, linear lesions can also debulk the atria. Theoretically, complete linear lesions should be the least pro-arrhythmic means of achieving debulking. They may also eliminate areas of slow conduction and affect the substrate of atrial fibrillation by modifying pivot points. If the linear lesions are incomplete, they may produce conduction delay and contribute to arrhythmogenicity.

Pulmonary vein isolation or encircling has been shown to be effective in eliminating atrial fibrillation in many patients. However, success rates for the elimination of persistent or permanent atrial fibrillation are consistently lower. In particular, circular mapping-guided percutaneous pulmonary vein isolation with radiofrequency (RF) energy and surgical open heart cryoablation have both led to disappointing initial results and high recurrence rates. Adjunctive linear left atrial lesions may improve results of curative ablation of persistent and permanent atrial fibrillation (AF).

In order to evaluate the mechanism of linear lesions and their effectiveness, we prospectively studied consecutive patients undergoing catheter ablation for drug-resistant and symptomatic atrial fibrillation. In view of the

Hôpital Cantonal Universitaire de Genève, Geneva, Switzerland

effectiveness of pulmonary vein isolation alone in patients with paroxysmal atrial fibrillation, adjunctive linear lesions were delivered only in patients with persistent or permanent atrial fibrillation.

Methods

Circular mapping-guided pulmonary vein (PV) isolation was performed followed when necessary by one or two linear lesions in the left atrium (LA) with irrigated-tip RF ablation (35–40 W max. for PVs, 45 W max. for linear lesions). Linear lesions were deployed from the left PV ostia to the posterolateral mitral annulus, and from the left to the right PV ostia guided by electroanatomic mapping. Their electrophysiology (EP) was assessed after ablation by complete electroanatomic mapping of the LA during distal coronary sinus pacing and correlated with rhythm outcome.

Results

Thirty-nine patients with persistent or permanent atrial fibrillation (5 with structural heart disease; 4 female patients; age 57 ± 10 years) underwent isolation of all PVs ($n = 155$). Cavotricuspid isthmus ablation was performed in 7 and linear LA ablation in 28 patients. The lesion from the left PV to the mitral annulus (27 ± 8 mm length, 14 ± 7 min RF) was incomplete in 14/28, with marked slow conduction in 5. The lesion from the left PV to the right PV (34 ± 10 mm, 11 ± 5 min RF) was incomplete in 9/23, with marked slow conduction in 3. Seventeen patients underwent reablation for recurrent atrial fibrillation ($n = 10$) or new-onset atrial flutter ($n = 10$). PV conduction recovery was observed in 12, while narrow channels near PV ostia acted as critical isthmuses of LA flutter in 8 (including 3 with complete linear lesions) and were successfully ablated. After a follow-up of 18 ± 8 months (range 6–37), 30/39 (77%) maintained stable sinus rhythm without anti-arrhythmic treatment. Nine of 12 with PV isolation alone, 9/10 patients with both linear lesions complete, and 12/17 patients with one or both linear lesions incomplete were in stable sinus rhythm.

Conclusions

1. Subsets of patients with persistent AF can be cured with PV isolation alone while others with persistent or permanent AF derive similar benefit from linear lesions. The challenge facing us is to identify those subsets of patients who benefit from supplementary linear lesions – such as those

with extensive LA scarring.

2. Complete conduction block across LA linear lesions does not eliminate the risk of subsequent LA macroreentry since slowly conducting channels adjacent to linear lesions or PV ostia can result in LA flutter in spite of complete conduction block across the linear lesions.

Suggested Readings

Shah DC, Haïssaguerre M, Jaïs P (2001) Towards a mechanism based on understanding of atrial fibrillation. J Cardiovasc Electrophysiol 12:600-601

Shah DC, Haïssaguerre M, Jaïs P, Hocini M (2003) Nonpulmonary vein foci: do they exist? Pacing Clin Electrophysiol 26:1631–1635

Shah D (2003) Curative ablation for atrial fibrillation: what clinical trials do we need to establish efficacy. J Cardiovasc Electrophysiol 14(suppl 9):S48-S51

Systematic Electrical Disconnection of Superior Vena Cava in Addition to Pulmonary Vein Ablation: Is It Worthwhile?

A. Bonso, S. Themistoclakis, A. Rossillo, M. Bevilacqua, A. Corrado, A. Raviele

Introduction

Many reports have focused attention on the pulmonary veins and posterior wall of the left atrium to explain the physiopathological mechanism of atrial fibrillation [1–3].

Anatomical observations have shown that sleeves of atrial myocardial tissue extend inside the pulmonary veins even for several centimetres [4] and they have peculiar electrophysiological properties that can be stimulated under pathological situations, such as wall stretching, or under neurovegetative stimulation [5]. In particular, the cells located inside the pulmonary veins, because of altered automatism or triggered activity [6], can provoke numerous supraventricular ectopic beats or even bursts of atrial tachycardia that are able to start paroxysmal atrial fibrillation episodes. Suppression of these ectopic foci inside the pulmonary veins by means of transcatheter ablation has provided effective treatment in about 70% of such patients [7]. The ablative techniques used to improve efficacy and safety, and to reduce the procedure time have simplified the ablative approach. Today, the electrical disconnection of pulmonary veins is carried out by a segmental or circumferential approach at the AV-junction or with antrum extension. These techniques have increased the success rate to 80–90% [8–10]. The evolution of ablative techniques and the extension of treatment to patients with persistent or permanent atrial fibrillation therefore allowed us to analyse the mechanisms of onset and maintenance of atrial fibrillation. It was observed that the AV-junction is another important factor in the physiopathology of atrial fibrillation [11]. Moreover, the electrical isolation of pulmonary veins

Division of Cardiology, Cardiovascular Department, Umberto I Hospital, Mestre-Venice, Italy

alone loses efficacy progressively when patients with persistent or permanent atrial fibrillation are treated; in these patients, both the substrate and electrical remodelling probably play important roles [12, 13].

Notwithstanding the different ablative techniques and the growing number of procedures, therapeutic success without antiarrhythmic treatment is rarely above 80%.

This is due to several fundamental reasons:

1. Electrical disconnection of the pulmonary veins is often incomplete, or, after a disconnection, some veins regain electrical conduction over time [14, 15].
2. It is possible that evolution of substrate and consequently of electrogenic disease is responsible for new recurrences.
3. The presence of different arrhythmogenic areas not included in the previous ablation can be responsible for recurrences of atrial fibrillation [16].

It has been pointed out that the triggers of atrial fibrillation can arise also from other structures of the atria, such as superior vena cava [17], Marshall vein [18, 19], coronary sinus [20], christa terminalis, as well as the free walls of the atria [16]. The superior vena cava has anatomical and electrical characteristics similar to those of the pulmonary veins [21–23] and its involvement in the genesis of episodes of atrial fibrillation can explain some of the failures after disconnection of the pulmonary veins alone [24]. It has been shown that ablation of other, non-pulmonary-vein foci that initiate paroxysmal atrial fibrillation episodes is efficient only in 60% of patients [16]. In addition, it seems that about 6% of cases of paroxysmal atrial fibrillation develop from ectopic beats starting from the superior vena cava [16, 24]. Disconnection of the superior vena cava proved successful in treating patients who had episodes of atrial fibrillation from foci arising from the superior vena cava [24, 25]. Moreover, recent findings in animals have demonstrated that the isolation of all thoracic veins can prevent episodes of permanent atrial fibrillation, when effective [26]. In this study, the importance of systematic electrical disconnection of the superior vena cava together with the disconnection of pulmonary veins was evaluated, and initial results of this approach vs disconnection of only the pulmonary veins are presented.

Study Conditions

From December 2004 to June 2005, 64 consecutive patients (45 males, mean age 58 ± 12) were treated with atrial fibrillation ablation. The patients were symptomatic for paroxysmal (28), persistent (20), permanent (16) atrial fibrillation and refractory to antiarrhythmic drug therapy. Structural heart disease was diagnosed in 61% (39/64) patients; 17 were hypertensive, 17 had mitral valvular prolapse, four had ischaemic heart disease, and 1 dilated cardiomyopathy). LVEF in this group of patients was 54 ± 10 , LAD 44 ± 6 mm. Patients were randomised in two groups: group I (30 patients) underwent circumferential electrical disconnection of the pulmonary veins and of the superior vena cava using a technique guided by intracardiac echocardiogram phased array. Group II (34 patients) underwent only circumferential electrical disconnection of the pulmonary veins. The procedure was carried out with two transeptal punctures. Mapping was done with a Lasso decapolar 2-cm-diameter catheter, while ablation was done using the large-curve 8-mm catheter (Byosence Webster). Energy was delivered at the AV-junction of the pulmonary veins with antrum extension according to titration and a flow-chart guided by microbubbles production, as described by Marrouche et al. [10]. The superior vena cava was disconnected at the junction of the vena cava and right atrium after positioning the mapping Lasso decapolar catheter, and guided by intracardiac echo. Before each radiofrequency delivery the ablation area was stimulated to reveal possible involvement of the right phrenic nerve, in which case no ablation was performed. In case of sudden sinus tachycardia during erogation in the juxta-sinus-node area, erogation was immediately interrupted and the ablating catheter moved to a more proximal position. In these cases, a partial disconnection of the superior vena cava was accepted as end-point. Energy was supplied at 50 Watts and the temperature was 50°C.

The end-point of the procedure was reached with complete disappearance of all sharp potentials at the AV-junction of the pulmonary veins and superior vena cava, and at the antrum of the pulmonary veins. All patients were in wash-out of antiarrhythmic drugs before the procedure and had undergone anticoagulant therapy for at least 1 month, Transoesophageal echo was done immediately before the procedure.

Follow-Up

Patients were discharged without antiarrhythmic therapy but they were provided with anticoagulant therapy for at least 3 months after the procedure. Antiarrhythmic therapy was administered only to those patients with many recurrences and, when necessary, within 2 months after ablation. Therapy was withdrawn after 2 months if effective. All patients received Holter monitoring before discharge for a week, had a routine follow-up visit and underwent further Holter monitoring at 1, 3, 6 and every 6 months. ECG and Holter monitoring were carried out at any other time if symptoms recurred. CT scan was performed at 3 months. Success was defined as total absence of recurrences of atrial fibrillation or atrial tachycardia/flutter.

Preliminary Results

All pulmonary veins were disconnected in the two study groups. The superior vena cava was not completely disconnected in 40% (12/30) of patients because of phrenic nerve stimulation. The mean time of the procedure for disconnecting the pulmonary veins in the two groups was 4. 05 ± 0.31 h. The mean procedure time for the vena cava disconnection was 25 ± 10 min. No lesions of the phrenic nerve were detected during the procedure and no other complications were found.

Follow-Up

The mean follow-up thus far is 3 ± 3 months. .At this writing, follow-up is incomplete and the patients are not evenly distributed between the two groups; nonetheless, early recurrence has been observed in the two groups: 30% (10/30) in group I and 38% (13/34) in group II. If we consider only the few patients with complete disconnection of the superior vena cava the rate of early recurrence is 22% (4/18) and 50% (6/12), respectively.

Conclusions

Although final results are not yet available, it is interesting to note that patients who had complete disconnection of the superior vena cava have had a good initial follow-up. However, these preliminary results must be confirmed by studies that include a larger number of patients and a longer follow-up time.

References

1. Jalife J, Berenfeld O, Mansour M (2002) Mother rotors and fibrillatory conduction: a mechanism of atrial fibrillation. Cardiovasc Res 54:204–216
2. Haïssaguerre M, Jaïs P, Shah DC et al (1998) Spontaneous initiation of atrial fibrillation by ectopic beats originating in the pulmonary veins. N Engl J Med 339:659–666
3. Chen SA, Hsieh MH, Tai CT et al (1999) Initiation of atrial fibrillation by ectopic beats originating from the pulmonary veins: electrophysiological characteristics, pharmacological responses, and effects of radiofrequency ablation. Circulation 100:1879–1886
4. Saito T, Waki K, Becker AE (2000) Left atrial extension onto pulmonary veins in humans: anatomic observations relevant for atrial arrhythmias. J Cardiovasc Electrophysiol 11:888–894
5. Pappone C, Santinelli V, Manguso F et al (2004) Pulmonary vein denervation

enhances long-term benefit after circumferential ablation for paroxysmal atrial fibrillation. Circulation 109:327–334
6. Wu TJ, Ong JJ, Chang CM et al (2001) Pulmonary veins and ligament of Marshall as sources of rapid activation in a canine model of sustained atrial fibrillation. Circulation 103:1157–1163
7. Haïssaguerre M, Jaïs P, Shah DC et al (2000) Electrophysiological end point for catheter ablation of atrial fibrillation initiated from multiple pulmonary venous foci. Circulation 101:1409–1417
8. Shah DC, Haïssaguerre M, Jaïs P et al (2001) Curative catheter ablation of paroxysmal atrial fibrillation in 200 patients: strategy for presentations from sustained atrial fibrillation to no arrhythmias. PACE 24:1541–1558
9. Pappone C, Oreto G, Rosanio S et al (2001) Atrial remodeling after circumferential radiofrequency pulmonary vein ablation. Efficacy of an anatomic approach in a large cohort of patients with atrial fibrillation.Circulation 104:2539–2544
10. Marrouche NF, Martin DO, Wazni O et al (2003) Phased-array intracardiac echocardiography monitoring during pulmonary vein isolation in patients with atrial fibrillation. Impact on outcome and complications. Circulation 107:2710–2716
11. Hocini M, Ho SY, Kawara T et al (2002) Electrical conduction in canine pulmonary veins: electrophysiological and anatomic correlation. Circulation 105:2442–2448
12. Ernst S, Ouyang F, Lober F et al (2003) Catheter-induced linear lesions in the left atrium in patients with atrial fibrillation: an electroanatomic study. J Am Coll Cardiol 42:1271–1282
13. Nademanee K, McKenzie J, Kosar E et al (2004) A new approach for catheter ablation of atrial fibrillation: Mapping of the electrophysiologic substrate. JACC 43:2044–2053
14. Cappato R, Negroni S, Pecora D et al (2003) Prospective assessment of late conduction recurrence across radiofrequency lesions producing electrical disconnection at the pulmonary vein ostium in patients with atrial fibrillation. Circulation 108:1599–1604
15. Nanthakumar K, Plumb VJ, Epstein AE et al (2004) Resumption of electrical conduction in previously isolated veins. Rationale for a different strategy? Circulation 109:1226–1229
16. Lin WS, Tai CT, Hsieh MH et al (2003) Catheter ablation of paroxysmal atrial fibrillation initiated by non-pulmonary vein ectopy. Circulation 107:3176–3183
17. Tsai CF, Tai CT, Hsiung MH et al (2000) Initiation of atrial fibrillation by ectopic beats originating from the superior vena cava. Circulation 102:67–74
18. Hwang C, Wu TJ, Doshi RN et al (2000) Vein of Marshall cannulation for the analysis of electrical activity in patients with focal atrial fibrillation. Circulation 101:1503–1505
19. Hsu LF, Jaïs P, Keane D et al (2004) Atrial fibrillation originating from persistent left superior vena cava. Circulation 109:828–832
20. Sanders P, Jaïs P, Hocini M et al (2004) Electrical disconnection of the coronary sinus by radiofrequency catheter ablation to isolate a trigger of atrial fibrillation. J Cardiovasc Electrophysiol 15:364–368
21. Yeh HI, Lai YJ, Lee SH et al (2001) Heterogeneity of myocardial sleeve morphology and gap junctions in canine superior vena cava. Circulation 104:3152–3157
22. Ooie T, Tsuchiya T, Ashikaga K et al (2002) Electrical connection between the right atrium and the superior vena cava, and the extent of myocardial sleeve in a patient with atrial fibrillation originating from the superior vena cava. J Cardiovasc Electrophysiol 13:482–485

23. Shah DC, Haïssaguerre M, Jaïs P et al (2002) High-resolution mapping of tachycardia originating from the superior vena cava. J Cardiovasc Electrophysiol 13:388–392
24. Goya M, Ouyang F, Ernst S et al (2002) Electroanatomic mapping and catheter ablation of breakthroughs from the right atrium to the superior vena cava in patients with atrial fibrillation. Circulation 106:1317–1320
25. Yamane T, Miyanaga S, Inada K et al (2004) A focal source of atrial fibrillation in the superior vena cava: isolation and elimination by radiofrequency ablation with the guide of basket catheter mapping. J Interv Card Electrophysiol 11:131–134
26. Park A, Chou CC, Drury PC et al (2004) Thoracic vein ablation terminates chronic atrial fibrillation in dogs. Am J Physiol Heart Circ Physiol 286:H2072–H2077

What Is the Outcome of Atrial Fibrillation Ablation in Patients with Left Ventricular Dysfunction?

L.-F. Hsu[1], P. Sanders[2], M. Hocini[2], F. Sacher[2], M. Rotter[2], Y. Takahashi[2], T. Rostock[2], C. Scavée[2], M. Haïssaguerre[2], P. Jaïs[2]

Introduction

Atrial fibrillation (AF) and congestive heart failure (CHF) are closely related conditions. While CHF promotes the development of AF, the presence of AF may exacerbate or, in some cases, cause left ventricular (LV) dysfunction, with symptoms of CHF as a consequence [1, 2]. In addition, each disease adversely affects the prognosis of the other [3, 4].

Cardiomyopathy due to rapid uncontrolled ventricular response has been implicated as the main mechanism by which AF results in LV dysfunction [5]. However, in the absence of a rapid ventricular rate during AF, LV dysfunction can still occur as a result of impaired atrial contractile function, loss of atrioventricular synchrony, or an irregular ventricular rhythm [58].

Rhythm vs Rate Control for AF in Heart Failure

The most effective strategy to prevent or reverse LV dysfunction associated with AF is the restoration and maintenance of sinus rhythm. However, to achieve this with the use of antiarrhythmic drugs is extremely challenging, owing to the limited efficacy and potentially deleterious effects of these drugs [9]. This has led to renewed interest in rate control, stimulated by reports from large randomised studies, especially the Atrial Fibrillation Follow-up Investigation of Rhythm Management (AFFIRM) and Rate Control versus Electrical Cardioversion (RACE) trials, suggesting a comparable outcome for strategies involving pharmacological rhythm or rate control

[1]National Heart Centre, Singapore; [2]Hôpital Cardiologique du Haut-Lévêque, Bordeaux-Pessac, France

[10-12]. However, recent evidence from these two studies not only confirmed the adverse prognostic effects of CHF, but also highlighted the potential benefits of sinus rhythm. In a recently reported substudy of the AFFIRM trial, restoration and maintenance of sinus rhythm was associated with a 47% reduction in mortality risk, while the use of antiarrhythmic drugs and the presence of CHF significantly increased the risk of death by 49% and 57%, respectively [13]. In a separate substudy, the RACE investigators also demonstrated that, although pharmacological rate control could prevent deterioration of LV function, restoration and maintenance of sinus rhythm were associated with improvement of LV function [14].

In patients with LV dysfunction, modest improvements in LV ejection fraction (LVEF) and fractional shortening can be achieved nonpharmacologically using the clinically proven and effective 'ablate and pace' strategy [15 17]. However, while it provides effective ventricular rate control and rhythm regularisation, it does not restore atrial contraction or atrioventricular or interventricular synchrony. In addition, the benefit of rhythm regularisation can be negated by the adverse haemodynamic effects of right ventricular (RV) pacing, which is commonly used in such patients. The use of LV or biventricular pacing, associated with a more favourable haemodynamic profile, may avoid this problem, although present evidence is inconclusive [18, 19]. Finally, long-term pacemaker dependence is also an important consideration for this strategy.

Catheter Ablation of AF in Heart Failure

The advent of catheter ablation as an effective therapy for AF resistant to pharmacologic rhythm or rate control has provided a viable strategy to restore and maintain sinus rhythm without the use of antiarrhythmic drugs. With current techniques and technology, long-term sinus rhythm can be restored in up to 90% of patients with paroxysmal AF, usually without the need for antiarrhythmic drugs [20]; however, ablation of permanent AF remains more difficult, often requiring extensive atrial ablation and multiple procedures.

Maintenance of Sinus Rhythm

Currently available results of patients with CHF who have undergone catheter ablation for AF are summarised in Table 1. A large proportion of these patients have permanent AF of significant duration (average of approximately 7 years) and other structural heart disease. In the two published studies, a significant number required multiple ablation procedures (27% and 50%, respectively) [21, 22]. Nonetheless, catheter ablation has been demonstrated to be feasible in these patients and is associated with a good success rate for sinus rhythm maintenance, ranging from 68% to 96%, mostly without use of antiarrhythmic drugs [21–25].

Table 1. Summary of results of atrial fibrillation (AF) ablation in patients with congestive heart failure (CHF)

	Patients (n)	Permanent AF	Duration of AF (years)	Repeat ablation	Sinus rhythm	Pre-ablation LVEF (%)	Post-ablation LVEF (%)
Chen/Natale (Cleveland Clinic) [21]	94	55 (56%)	6 ± 2	21 (22%)	90 (96%)	36 ± 7	41 ± 6
Hsu/Jaïs/Haïssaguere (Bordeaux) [22]	58	53 (91%)	7 ± 4	29 (50%)	45 (78%)	35 ± 7	56 ± 13
Pappone et al. (Milan) [23]	95	NA	6 ± 3	NA	77 (81%)	31 ± 9	44 ± 6
Cha/Packer (Mayo Clinic) [24]	19	7 (37%)	7 ± 5	NA	13 (68%)	34 ± 6	51 ± 7
Gentlesk /Marchlinski (Pennsylvania) [25]	53	17 (32%)	NA	NA	48 (90%)	42 ± 8	57 ± 8

LVEF Left ventricular ejection fraction, *NA* data not available

These results have also been achieved with an acceptable safety profile. In the two published studies, significant pulmonary vein (PV) stenosis was limited to < 1%, cardiac tamponade ~2%, and stroke ~2% [21, 22], results comparable to patients without CHF or structural heart disease [20]. An additional complication in CHF was the development of pulmonary oedema during the procedure, observed in one patient in the study by Chen et al. [21], and in two of our patients. These patients were treated for their acute decompensation, and AF was successfully ablated in a subsequent procedure.

Symptoms and Quality of Life

In patients without CHF, catheter ablation of AF has been demonstrated to improve symptoms and quality of life [26]. Similarly, these findings have been observed in CHF patients. CHF symptoms improved by approximately one NYHA class after ablation (Hsu et al. [22], from 2.3 to 1.5; Pappone et al. [23], from 2.8 to 1.6; and Cha et al. [24], from 2.3 to 1.5), while arrhythmia-related symptoms, as assessed by the Symptom Checklist-Frequency and Severity scores, also improved significantly [22]. Overall quality of life, assessed with the 36-item Short Form General Health Survey (SF-36) questionnaire, also improved significantly in all scales [21-23]. Among our patients, the summary scores for the physical and mental components increased by an average of 24 and 21 points, respectively [22].

Left Ventricular Function

An improvement in LV function after ablation has been demonstrated in all five studies currently available (Table 1), with mean improvements in LVEF ranging from 5% to 21% [21-25]. Importantly, Gentlesk et al. demonstrated a 'normalisation of LVEF' to > 55% in 87% of patients in their series [25], while 72% of our patients demonstrated a 'marked improvement of LVEF,' defined as an increase of ≥ 20% or to ≥ 55% [22].

Concurrently, LV dilatation was reduced significantly. Among our patients, LV end-systolic diameter was reduced by 6 ± 6 mm while end-systolic diameter was reduced by 8 ± 7 mm. Not surprisingly, recurrence of arrhythmia despite the use of antiarrhythmic drugs negatively affected the recovery of LVEF. However, LV function was still significantly improved in four of 12 patients with recurrent AF, as ablation had converted permanent AF to paroxysmal AF [22]. In addition, two of our three patients being considered for heart transplant improved sufficiently after ablation to merit removal from the active transplant list.

Effect of Coexisting Heart Disease

The presence of concurrent structural heart disease (ischaemic, valvular, hypertensive, or hypertrophic cardiomyopathy) did not significantly affect the outcome of ablation. Among our patients, sinus rhythm was maintained in 73% of patients with structural heart disease (66% without antiarrhythmic therapy) compared to 81% (73% without drugs) in patients without coexisting heart disease. Similarly, LVEF improved significantly in these patients by 16 ± 14% [22]. These findings were also observed in the series by Chen et al. [21].

Effect of Ventricular Rate Control

Effective ventricular rate control in AF using pharmacological measures or the 'ablate and pace' strategy have been demonstrated to improve LV dysfunction [5]. However, even in patients with adequate ventricular rate control, restoration and maintenance of sinus rhythm after catheter ablation resulted in further improvement of LVEF. Among our patients, LVEF increased by 17 ± 15% in those with good pre-ablation rate control (defined as mean ventricular rate < 80 beats/min at rest) [22]. Similarly, among 17 patients with persistent/permanent AF in Gentlesk's series, 10 had rate control < 90 beats/min at rest [25], while most of the patients with persistent/permanent AF in Chen's series were already well rate-controlled before ablation [21].

This finding could indicate that the degree of rate control was overestimated or, more likely, that the irregularity of the rhythm as well as the loss of atrial contractility and atrioventricular synchrony contributed to the LV dysfunction. Thus, restoration of sinus rhythm should be expected to confer additional haemodynamic benefits compared with pharmacological rate control.

Implications

Though the individual studies are small, their results have been remarkably consistent and challenge the notion that rate control is as good as rhythm control, especially in patients with CHF. A recent study evaluating an aggressive pharmacological rhythm-control strategy, utilising external or internal cardioversion and treatment with amiodarone, demonstrated long-term benefits in patients with advanced CHF [27]. Among 74 patients in this study, sinus rhythm was maintained in 70% and 55% at 1 and 3 years, respectively. LVEF was significantly improved, from 28 ± 7% at baseline to 38 ± 11% and 35 ± 12% at 1 and 3 years, while NYHA class significantly improved from 2.7 to 2.1 and 2.0, respectively. In addition, three patients were removed from the active heart transplant list due to marked clinical improvement.

While these observations are striking, it should be noted that sinus rhythm was maintained with high-dose amiodarone. A further issue not addressed in present drug or catheter ablation studies is the mortality benefit of restoring and maintaining sinus rhythm in patients with CHF, although several randomised trials have alluded to improved survival among patients with CHF and AF who reverted to sinus rhythm [13]. Presently a large multicentre study, the Atrial Fibrillation and Congestive Heart Failure (AF-CHF) trial, is being conducted to evaluate whether the benefits of sinus rhythm in CHF patients are sufficiently great to offset the risks of antiarrhythmic drug therapy.

Conclusions

Present evidence indicates that patients with CHF and AF may benefit from restoration and maintenance of sinus rhythm, if it can be achieved without the adverse effects of treatment. Further improvements are needed to make catheter ablation of AF easier and safer, in order to increase its availability outside experienced centres [28]. Nonetheless, curative ablation offers the unique opportunity to maintain sinus rhythm without the use of potentially harmful antiarrhythmic drugs, resulting in significant improvements in cardiac function, symptoms and quality of life.

References

1. Stevenson WG, Stevenson LW (1999) Atrial fibrillation in heart failure. N Engl J Med 341:910–911
2. Ehrlich JR, Nattel S, Hohnloser SH (2002) Atrial fibrillation and congestive heart failure: specific considerations at the intersection of two common and important cardiac disease sets. J Cardiovasc Electrophysiol 13:399–405
3. Middlekauff HR, Stevenson WG, Stevenson LW (1991) Prognostic significance of atrial fibrillation in advanced heart failure: a study of 390 patients. Circulation 84:40–48
4. Wang TJ, Larson MG, Levy D et al (2003) Temporal relations of atrial fibrillation and congestive heart failure and their joint influence on mortality: the Framingham Heart Study. Circulation 107:2920–2925
5. Shinbane JS, Wood MA, Jensen DN et al (1997) Tachycardia-induced cardiomyopathy: a review of animal models and clinical studies. J Am Coll Cardiol 29:709–715

6. Natale A, Zimerman L, Tomassoni G et al (1996) Impact on ventricular function and quality of life of transcatheter ablation of the atrioventricular junction in chronic atrial fibrillation with a normal ventricular response. Am J Cardiol 78:1431–1433
7. Clark DM, Plumb VJ, Epstein AE et al (1997) Hemodynamic effects of an irregular sequence of ventricular cycle lengths during atrial fibrillation. J Am Coll Cardiol 30:1039–1045
8. Daoud EG, Weiss R, Bahu M et al (1996) Effect of an irregular ventricular rhythm on cardiac output. Am J Cardiol 78:1433–1436
9. Falk RH (2001) Atrial fibrillation. N Engl J Med 344:1067–1078
10. The Atrial Fibrillation Follow-up Investigation of Rhythm Management (AFFIRM) Investigators (2002) A comparison of rate control and rhythm control in patients with atrial fibrillation. N Engl J Med 347:1825–1833
11. Van Gelder IC, Hagens VE, Bosker HA et al (2002) A comparison of rate control and rhythm control in patients with recurrent persistent atrial fibrillation. N Engl J Med 347:1834–1840
12. Hohnloser SH, Kuck KH et al (2000) Rhythm or rate control in atrial fibrillation—Pharmacological Intervention in Atrial Fibrillation (PIAF): a randomized trial. Lancet 356:1789–1794
13. Corley SD, Epstein AE, DiMarco JP et al (2004) Relationships between sinus rhythm, treatment, and survival in the Atrial Fibrillation Follow-up Investigation of Rhythm Management (AFFIRM) Study. Circulation109:1509–1513
14. Hagens VE, Van Veldhuisen DJ, Kamp O et al (2005) Effect of rate and rhythm control on left ventricular function and cardiac dimensions in patients with persistent atrial fibrillation: results from the Rate Control versus Electrical Cardioversion for persistent atrial fibrillation (RACE) study. Heart Rhythm 2:19–24
15. Wood MA, Brown-Mahoney C, Kay GN et al (2000) Clinical outcomes after ablation and pacing therapy for atrial fibrillation: a meta-analysis. Circulation 101:1138–1144
16. Brignole M, Menozzi C, Gianfranchi L et al (1998) Assessment of atrioventricular junction ablation and VVIR pacemaker versus pharmacological treatment in patients with heart failure and chronic atrial fibrillation: a randomized controlled study. Circulation 98:953–960
17. Ozcan C, Jahangir A, Friedman PA et al (2003) Significant effects of atrioventricular node ablation and pacemaker implantation on left ventricular function and long-term survival in patients with atrial fibrillation and left ventricular dysfunction. Am J Cardiol 92:33–37
18. Doshi R, Daoud E, Fellows C et al (2004) PAVE: the first prospective randomized study evaluating biventricular pacing after ablate and pace therapy. Presented at the American College of Cardiology Annual Scientific Session 2004, March 7–10, New Orleans, LA
19. Brignole M, Gammage M, Puggioni E et al on behalf of the Optimal Pacing Site (Opsite) Study Investigators (2005) Comparative assessment of right, left and biventricular pacing in patients with permanent atrial fibrillation. Eur Heart J:26:712–722
20. Cappato R, Calkins H, Chen SA et al (2005) Worldwide survey on the methods, efficacy and safety of catheter ablation for human atrial fibrillation. Circulation 111:1100–1115
21. Chen MS, Marrouche NF, Khaykin Y et al (2004) Pulmonary vein isolation for the treatment of atrial fibrillation in patients with impaired systolic function. J Am

Coll Cardiol 43:1004–1009

22. Hsu LF, Jaïs P, Sanders P et al (2004) Catheter ablation for atrial fibrillation in congestive heart failure. N Engl J Med 351:2373–2383
23. Pappone C, Augello G, Vicedomini G et al (2003) Circumferential pulmonary vein ablation in patients with atrial fibrillation and associated systolic or diastolic heart failure. Eur Heart J 24:494 (abs)
24. Cha YM, Asirvatham SJ, Friedman PA et al (2004) Improvement in left ventricular function following radiofrequency catheter ablation of atrial fibrillation in patients with congestive heart failure. Heart Rhythm 1:S139 (abs)
25. Gentlesk P, Sauer WH, Zado ES et al (2004) Ablation of atrial fibrillation in patients with decreased ejection fraction: outcome and evidence for reversible cardiomyopathy. Heart Rhythm 1:S171-S172 (abs)
26. Pappone C, Rosanio S, Augello G et al (2003) Mortality, morbidity and quality of life after circumferential pulmonary vein ablation for atrial fibrillation: outcomes from a controlled, nonrandomized long-term study. J Am Coll Cardiol 42:185–197
27. De Ferrari GM, Petracci B, Frattini F et al (2005) Long-term effects of an aggressive rhythm control strategy in patients with permanent atrial fibrillation and advanced heart failure. Heart Rhythm 2:S116 (abs)
28. Stevenson WG, Stevenson LW (2004) Atrial fibrillation and heart failure – five more years. N Engl J Med 351:2437–2440

Complications of Atrial Fibrillation Ablation: How to Prevent and Manage Cerebrovascular Accidents

A. Rossillo, A. Bonso, S. Themistoclakis, A. Corrado, B. De Piccoli, A. Raviele

Introduction

Atrial fibrillation is a common arrhythmia associated with significant morbidity and mortality. This arrhythmia increases the risk of ischaemic stroke, probably due to an atrioembolic mechanism. Without anti-thrombotic therapy, the incidence of this complication varies from fewer than 2 to more than 10 strokes per 100 patient-years [1, 2].

Warfarin substantially decreases the risk of stroke in patients with non-valvular atrial fibrillation (AF) by about 60% but increases the risk of major bleeding to about 1% per year [3–8]. Recently, many authors have had a high success rate in treating AF by means of radiofrequency catheter ablation and electrical isolation of the pulmonary veins [9–11]. However, the role of anticoagulation therapy in preventing atrioembolic stroke after such a procedure is still unclear. Thus, quantifying the efficacy of AF ablation in preventing cerebrovascular accident is crucial to determining whether oral anticoagulation therapy may be safely stopped or not after radiofrequency catheter ablation of AF, and perhaps which patients should continue it.

In the present study we evaluate the incidence of ischaemic stroke after the interruption of oral anticoagulation therapy after 3 months in patients in whom an intracardiac echocardiography-guided pulmonary vein antrum isolation procedure had been performed.

Division of Cardiology, Cardiovascular Department, Umberto I Hospital, Mestre-Venice, Italy

Methods

Patients

Between September 2002 and May 2004, 109 consecutive patients were referred to our institution for ablation of symptomatic drug-refractory AF. All patients gave their written informed consent for the procedure. Patients' characteristics are shown in Table 1. Amiodarone treatment was discontinued at least 3 months before the procedure. The other anti-arrhythmic drugs were discontinued at least five half-lives before ablation.

Table 1. Demographic characteristics of study population

	All patients (n = 109)
Age, years (mean ± SD)	58.0 ± 10.0
Male sex, n (%)	84 (77)
AF duration, years (mean, range)	8, 1–24
Left atrial size, cm (mean ± SD)	4.4 ± 0.6
Left ventricular ejection fraction (%)	58 ± 6
Structural heart disease, n (%)	73 (67)
Paroxysmal AF, n (%)	40 (36.7)
Persistent AF, n (%)	48 (44.0)
Permanent AF, n (%)	21 (19.3)

Oral anticoagulation therapy was started 1 month before the procedure in all patients.

Paroxysmal AF was defined as self-terminating episodes lasting less than 7 days. Persistent AF was defined as when AF episodes lasted longer than 7 days and when pharmacological or electrical cardioversion were necessary to restore sinus rhythm. AF episodes failing to respond to cardioversion or for which no cardioversion attempt was made were classified as permanent AF.

Procedure Description

Patients came to the electrophysiology laboratory fasting. Immediately prior to the procedure, trans-oesophageal echocardiography was performed in all cases to exclude the presence of left atrial thrombi. A 20-polar catheter (St. Jude Medical DAIG Division, Minnetonka, Minn., USA) was inserted into the coronary sinus from the right internal jugular vein. The proximal electrodes were positioned between the superior vena cava and the high crista terminalis, while the distal electrodes were placed laterally in the coronary sinus. A trans-oesophageal recording lead was used to record activation of the left atrial posterior wall and to define the position of the oesophagus. A 10-Fr phase array intracardiac echocardiography (ICE) catheter (Acunav Division, Acuson Inc., USA) was introduced into the right atrium from the left femoral vein.

Mapping of the left atrium and pulmonary veins was carried out after approaching the left atrium via the trans-septal puncture. The trans-septal sheaths were connected to continuous infusion of heparinised solution throughout the procedure.

Isolation of the pulmonary veins was performed using ICE to define the pulmonary vein ostium and to titrate the power. A decapolar circular catheter (Lasso-Biosense Webster, Diamond Bar, Calif., USA) was placed at the pulmonary vein–left atrium antrum as determined by ICE, where ablation was performed with an 8-mm tip catheter (Biosense-Webster, Diamond Bar) with power titration guided by the formation of microbubbles. According to Marrouche et al. [11], the delivery of radiofrequency energy is controlled by progressively increasing the power (watts) until scattered microbubbles are observed by ICE. When type I bubbles were seen, energy was immediately titrated downward by 5- W decrements until the microbubbles subsided. Energy delivery was also discontinued if microbubble generation did not settle, as this was considered to be an early manifestation of tissue overheating. Energy delivery was immediately interrupted if a brisk shower of microbubbles was observed in the left atrium cavity, although an effort was made to avoid this phenomenon. The decapolar circular catheter was placed at the superior vena cava–right atrium junction as defined by ICE, and ablation was performed in a temperature-controlled mode.

Anticoagulation Protocols

Anticoagulation therapy with intravenous heparin infusion was restarted after the first trans-septal puncture with a 10 000 IU intravenous bolus plus continuous infusion at a rate of 1000 IU/h. A second bolus of 5000 IU was repeated after the second puncture.

Activated clotting time was maintained at about 350–400 s throughout the entire procedure.

Follow-Up

At the end of the procedure a single dose of aspirin 325 mg was administered orally. All patients were discharged on oral anticoagulation therapy with warfarin, with the dose adjusted to reach a INR value between 2 and 3. Follow-up and Holter monitoring was scheduled at 1, 3, 6, and 12 months after ablation.

A trans-oesophageal echocardiographic evaluation was performed in all patients at 3 months' follow-up. A spiral computed tomogram (CT) of the pulmonary veins was obtained within 3 months after the procedure. If any pulmonary vein narrowing was detected at the first examination, CT was repeated at 6 and 12 months to evaluate progression of the lesion. CT was also performed as a diagnostic test whenever symptoms compatible with pulmonary vein stenosis developed. Pulmonary vein stenosis was defined as mild if less than 50% luminal narrowing was evident, moderate if it was between 50% and 69%, and severe if it was 70% or more. Patients with severe stenosis were referred for pulmonary vein angiography and angioplasty.

After 3 months, anticoagulation treatment was stopped in all patients except in cases where one of the following conditions was observed: (1) patients experienced recurrence of AF between 6 and 12 weeks after the procedure; (2) more than 60% narrowing of the treated pulmonary vein was demonstrated by spiral CT performed 3 months after ablation; (3) non-optimal atrial contractility was shown by echocardiography, or (4) other indications for oral anticoagulation therapy were present. In the case of recurrence of symptoms, event recorder monitoring was performed. The occurrence of AF during the first 6 weeks after ablation was not considered predictive of late recurrence and did not necessarily indicate continuation of oral anticoagulation therapy after 3 months follow-up.

Control Group

As control, we evaluated all the published data on patients with AF treated with oral anticoagulation therapy to prevent cerebrovascular accidents.

Statistical Analysis

Continuous variables were expressed as mean ± SD. Continuous variables were compared by Student's *t* test. Differences among groups of continuous variables were determined by analysis of variance (ANOVA). Categorical variables were compared by χ^2 analysis or using Fisher's exact test. A *P* value below < 0.05 was taken to indicate statistical significance.

Results

All four pulmonary veins were disconnected in all patients. In addition, complete electrical isolation of the superior vena cava was achieved in 95 patients (87%). In the other 14 patients this was not possible because of stimulation of the phrenic nerve or the presence of the sinus node on the ablation site. During the procedure a stroke occurred in a 74-year-old woman with a history of transient ischaemic attack and permanent AF after electrical cardioversion at the end of the ablation (0.9%).

After 15 ± 7 months' follow-up, 90 of 109 patients (82.5%) were in stable sinus rhythm. A previously ineffective anti-arrhythmic drug was necessary to maintain sinus rhythm in 16 of 109 patients (14.5%). Trans-oesophageal echocardiography showed good atrial contractility in all patients with stable sinus rhythm.

During the follow-up period, no pulmonary vein narrowing greater than 60% was detected by CT, and in only two patients was a pulmonary vein stenosis between 50% and 60% present(1.8%). No perfusion defects were documented by quantitative pulmonary V/Q scans. All patients with mild or moderate pulmonary vein stenosis were asymptomatic.

An iatrogenic post-AF-ablation left atrial flutter/tachycardia was documented in 7 patients (6.4%).

The risk factors for stroke are shown in Table 2. Oral anticoagulation therapy was stopped after 3 months in 73 patients (68%) and no cerebrovascular accidents occurred during the remaining follow up.

Table 2. Stroke risk factors

	All patients (n = 109)	
	n	%
Low risk (age < 65 years old, no hypertension, no diabetes, no CHF or previous cerebrovascular accidents)	41	37.6
Medium risk (age > 65 years old, no hypertension, no diabetes, no CHF or previous cerebrovascular accidents)	13	11.9
High risk (age > 65 years old, hypertension, diabetes, CHF or previous cerebrovascular accidents)	55	50.5

CHF congestive heart failure

Discussion

The main finding of the present study is that ICE-guided pulmonary vein antrum isolation seems to prevent cerebrovascular accidents in patients with symptomatic drug-refractory AF who are not receiving anticoagulation therapy.

Anticoagulant Prophylaxis Against Stroke After Pulmonary Vein Antrum Isolation

In the published literature the rate of cerebrovascular accident in patients with AF who are on warfarin therapy ranges between 1.6% and 4.8% [12]. The consumption of warfarin is associated with an increased risk of major bleeding, especially in subjects older than 85 years old [13, 14]. In the last 10 years various authors have tried to identify the clinical characteristics of patients who derive greater benefit from anticoagulant therapy [15–20]. Age greater than 65 years old and/or a history of hypertension, diabetes, congestive heart failure, or previous cerebrovascular event have been identified as increasing the risk of transient ischaemic attack or stroke in patients with AF.

Our data show a very low incidence of cerebrovascular accident in the medium-term follow-up after pulmonary vein antrum isolation. The cerebrovascular accident risk in our study population, according to the Stroke Prevention in Atrial Fibrillation (SPAF) trial criteria was high in 31 of 73 (43%), medium in 10 of 73 (13%), and low 32 of 73 (44%) of cases. These data are slightly different from the thromboembolic risk pattern shown in the SPAF trial. Our patients were younger and had a lower incidence of previous thromboembolic events. However, this was compensated by a higher percentage of permanent AF and a longer duration of the arrhythmia in our patients.

The lower risk profile of our patient population is clearly due to the policy on indication policy for pulmonary vein antrum isolation in our electrophysiology laboratory. We try to perform ablation in very high risk patients only if they are highly symptomatic. Moreover, it is well known that these classification schemes are variably effective in predicting stroke risk [21].

Even if we consider only the published data on patients with low risk of cerebrovascular accident, our data showed a reduction of stroke incidence (0% vs 1.1–2%) [17].

It is well known that restoring sinus rhythm with electrical cardioversion causes stunning of the left atrial appendage, and some authors have identified left atrial appendage stunning as a marker of future embolic events. As previously reported, we consider the presence of a higher peak velocity and prolonged duration of early diastolic ($E+E_1$) and end-diastolic ($A+A_1$) left appendage flow at trans-oesophageal echocardiography as a sign of better contractility and a mark of lower risk of stroke during the follow-up [22]. On the basis of these parameters we interrupted anticoagulation therapy at 3 months' follow-up in all patients in sinus rhythm with good contractility and no severe stenosis detected by spiral CT.

We also observed in our series a significant reduction of acute major bleeding and the absence of haematoma, pericardial effusion, or the need for transfusion during follow-up. It is known that in clinical trials warfarin increased the risk of major bleeding, and outside the trial this risk was greater depending on how the warfarin therapy was monitored and on the risk of haemorrhage [23].

Pulmonary Vein Antrum Isolation Results

Another important finding of our study is that ICE-guided pulmonary vein antrum isolation is a safe and effective treatment for AF. Our success rate was high (82.5%) and our complication rate was low in terms of the data previously reported by Marrouche et al. [11]. In our series we did not observe any severe pulmonary vein stenosis.

We had only one case of an embolic complication which occurred at the end of the ablation procedure in a 74-year-old woman with a history of transient ischaemic attack after electrical cardioversion. We hypothesised that this complication was due to the use of a larger trans-septal sheath (8.5 Fr). After this event we changed to 8-Fr trans-septal sheaths and saw no further embolic complications.

In 7 patients an iatrogenic post-AF-ablation atrial tachycardia/flutter was documented. This is similar to the data previously published by other groups.

Study Limitation

This is a retrospective analysis of consecutive patients. The lack of a matched control group may have affected the results. However, we consider our study to be a pilot and its aim was to evaluate two different therapeutic approaches. Of course, further randomised studies are needed to establish the safety of interrupting oral anticoagulation therapy after radiofrequency catheter ablation of AF in all patients.

Conclusions

ICE-guided pulmonary vein antrum isolation seems to prevent cerebrovascular accidents in patients with symptomatic drug-refractory AF who are not receiving anticoagulation therapy. ICE-guided pulmonary vein antrum isolation is an effective and safe treatment for AF.

References

1. Wolf PA, Dawber TR, Thomas HE et al (1978) Epidemiologic assessment of chronic atrial fibrillation and risk of stroke: the Framingham study. Neurology 28:973–977
2. Flegel KM, Shipley MJ, Rose G (1987) Risk of stroke in non rheumatic atrial fibrillation. Lancet 1:526–529
3. Man-Son-Hing M, Laupacis A, O'Connor AM et al (1999) A patient decision aid regarding antithrombotic therapy for stroke prevention in atrial fibrillation: a randomized controlled trial. JAMA 282:737–743
4. Petersen P, Boysen G, Godtfredsen J et al (1989) Placebo-controlled, randomised trial of warfarin and aspirin for prevention of thromboembolic complications in chronic atrial fibrillation. The Copenhagen AFASAK study. Lancet 1:175–179
5. Anonymous (1994) Risk factors for stroke and efficacy of antithrombotic therapy in atrial fibrillation. Analysis of pooled data from five randomized controlled trials. Arch Intern Med 154:1449–1457
6. Anonymous (1990) The effect of low-dose warfarin on the risk of stroke in patients with nonrheumatic atrial fibrillation. The Boston Area Anticoagulation Trial for Atrial Fibrillation Investigators. N Engl J Med 323:1505–1511
7. Anonymous (1991) Stroke Prevention in Atrial Fibrillation Study. Final results. Circulation 84:527–539
8. Anonymous (1994) Warfarin versus aspirin for prevention of thromboembolism in atrial fibrillation: Stroke Prevention in Atrial Fibrillation II Study. Lancet 343:687–691
9. Haïssaguerre M, Jaïs P, Shah DC et al (1998) Spontaneous initiation of atrial fibrillation by ectopic beats originating in the pulmonary veins. N Engl J Med 339:659–666
10. Chen SA, Hsieh MH, Tai CT et al (1999) Initiation of atrial fibrillation by ectopic beats originating from the pulmonary veins: electrophysiological characteristics, pharmacological responses, and effects of radiofrequency ablation. Circulation 100:1879–1886
11. Marrouche NF, Martin DO, Wazni O et al (2003) Phased array intracardiac echocardiography monitoring during pulmonary vein isolation in patients with atrial fibrillation: impact on outcome and complications. Circulation 107:2710–2716
12. Evans A, Perez I, Yu G et al (2000) Secondary stroke prevention in atrial fibrillation. Stroke 32:2106–2111
13. Evans A, Perez I, Yu G et al (2001) Should stroke subtype influence anticoagulation decision to prevent recurrence in stroke patients with atrial fibrillation? Stroke 32:2828–2832
14. Lightowlers S, McGuire A (1998) Cost-effectiveness of anticoagulation in non rheumatic atrial fibrillation in the primary prevention of ischemic stroke. Stroke 29:1827–1832
15. Connolly SJ, Laupacis A, Gent M et al (1991) Canadian Atrial Fibrillation Anticoagulation (CAFA) Study. J Am Coll Cardiol 18:349–355
16. Ezekowitz MD, Bridgers SL, James KE et al (1992) Warfarin in the prevention of stroke associated with nonrheumatic atrial fibrillation. Veterans Affairs Stroke Prevention in Nonrheumatic Atrial Fibrillation Investigators. N Engl J Med 327:1406–1412
17. Hart RG, Benavente O, McBride R (1999) Antithrombotic therapy to prevent stroke in patients with atrial fibrillation: a meta-analysis. Ann Intern Med 131:492–501
18. Hart RG, Pearce LA, McBride R et al (1999) Factors associated with ischemic stroke

during aspirin therapy in atrial fibrillation: analysis of 2012 participants in the SPAF I-III clinical trials. The Stroke Prevention in Atrial Fibrillation (SPAF) Investigators. Stroke 30:1223–1229
19. Hart RG, Halperin JL, Pearce LA et al (2003) Stroke Prevention in Atrial Fibrillation Investigators. Lessons from the Stroke Prevention in Atrial Fibrillation trials. Ann Intern Med 138:831–838
20. Sherman DG, Kim SG, Boop BS et al; National Heart, Lung, and Blood Institute AFFIRM Investigators (2005) Occurrence and characteristics of stroke events in the Atrial Fibrillation Follow-up Investigation of Sinus Rhythm Management (AFFIRM) study. Arch Intern Med 165:1185–1191
21. Go AS, Hylek EM, Philipps KA et al (2000) Implication of stroke risk criteria on the anticoagulation decision in non valvular atrial fibrillation. The anticoagulation and risk factors in atrial fibrillation (ATRIA study). Circulation 102:11–13
22. De Piccoli B, Rigo F, Ragazzo M et al (2001) Transthoracic and transesophageal echocardiographic indices predictive of sinus rhythm maintenance after cardioversion of atrial fibrillation. Echocardiography 18:545–552
23. Gage BF, van Walraven C, Pearce L et al (2004) Selecting patients with atrial fibrillation for anticoagulation: stroke risk stratification in patients taking aspirin. Circulation 110:2287–2292

Pulmonary Vein Stenosis After Catheter Ablation of Atrial Fibrillation

E.B. SAAD

Introduction

Catheter ablation around the pulmonary veins (PVs) has become the treatment of choice for symptomatic patients with atrial fibrillation (AF) who do not respond to pharmacological therapy [1–6]. Over the past few years, a variety of strategies have been developed to achieve cure of AF [7–16]. PV stenosis is a known potential complication of radiofrequency ablation (RF) around the PVs [17–24] and its recognition is important to avoid unnecessary workup and to initiate appropriate treatment.

Incidence and Clinical Manifestations

The incidence of PV stenosis following AF ablation has been variably reported, ranging from 0% to 42% depending on the ablative technique used and the method of assessment [7, 10, 20, 25, 26]. The latter number probably represents and overestimation since transoesophageal echocardiography (TEE) instead of an anatomical imaging modality was used to establish the diagnosis.

Several factors contribute to an increased risk of developing PV stenosis, such as RF delivery inside the PVs, increasing power and temperature settings, and a 'learning curve' effect [24, 27]. Recent reports have shown a trend towards a decreasing incidence of PV stenosis mainly due to limiting RF delivery at or outside the orifice of the veins, power titration based on monitoring of tissue effects of RF (as with microbubble formation on intrac-

Section of Cardiac Arrhythmias and Pacing, Center for Atrial Fibrillation, Hospital Pró-Cardíaco, Botafogo, Rio de Janeiro, Brazil

ardiac echocardiography) and increasing operator experience [10, 27]. In centres with a high volume of AF procedures, PV stenosis is becoming a 'disease in extinction.' However, with the widespread application of AF ablation in the electrophysiologic community more procedures are being performed by less experienced operators, increasing the chances that the incidence of PV stenosis will actually increase. In fact, a recently presented review of the European experience with AF ablation detected up to 20% of patients developing PV stenosis in centres performing less than 50 procedures.

Physicians in general should thus be ready to work up patients with symptoms developing after an ablation procedure. However, PV stenosis after RF ablation is frequently asymptomatic, especially when a mild or moderate degree of stenosis is present or a single vein is involved [21, 22]. Most important is the fact that, when present, symptoms appear to be largely respiratory in origin [23], usually developing between the first and fourth month after the index procedure. The spectrum of symptoms range from persistent cough and pleuritic chest pain to more dramatic presentations, such as haemoptysis and severe exertional dyspnoea (Table 1). The severity of symptoms may be related not only to the degree of stenosis but also to the number of PVs with stenosis, with almost all patients with ≥ 2 PVs with severe stenosis being symptomatic (Fig. 1). However, given the non-specific nature of these symptoms and the frequent association with radiological evidence of lung consolidation, it is not surprising that many patients are initially treated for other common conditions, such as pneumonia (Fig. 2) and

Table 1. Clinical presentation and CT findings in patients with severe pulmonary vein (PV) stenosis

Patients (n = 21)	n (%)
Clinical presentation	
Cough	8 (38.1)
Dyspnoea	11 (52.4)
Pleuritic chest pain	6 (28.6)
Haemoptysis	5 (23.8)
Asymptomatic	8 (38.1)
Spiral CT: > 70% PV stenosis (n = occluded PVs)	
LSPV	14 (6)
LIPV	15 (7)
RSPV	4 (1)
RIPV	3 (1)

LSPV Left superior PV, *LIPV* left inferior PV, *RSPV* right superior PV, *RIPV* right inferior PV

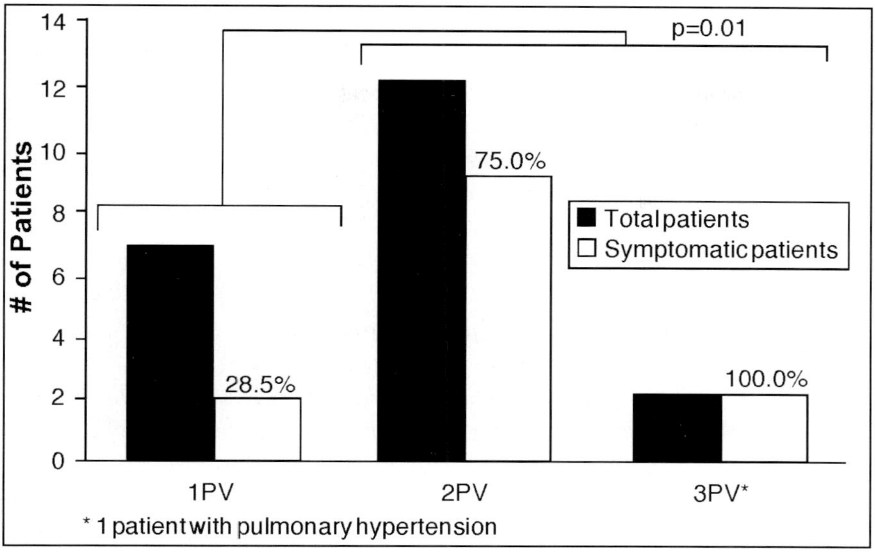

Fig. 1. Correlation between the presence of respiratory symptoms and number of pulmonary veins (PVs) with severe stenosis. While less than 1/3 of patients with single-vessel stenosis have symptoms, the majority of patients with more than one PV involved are symptomatic. Pulmonary arterial hypertension is rare and can be documented only in patients with multi-vessel involvement

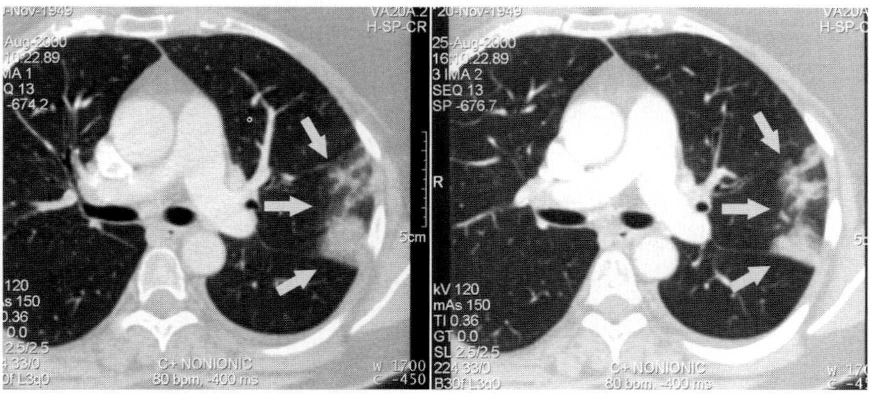

Fig. 2. CT scan of a patient with pulmonary consolidation initially attributed to pneumonia. There is a clear lung infiltrate in the periphery of the left lung (*arrows*). The patient did not respond to several antimicrobial regimens and was subsequently diagnosed with PV stenosis

pulmonary embolism, before the correct diagnosis is made [21, 23, 28]. Indeed, we published a series of 18 patients developing severe PV stenosis after AF ablation who were followed by their primary-care physicians, and in all patients PV stenosis was not considered in the differential diagnosis [21]. Misdiagnoses lead to improper diagnostic and therapeutic procedures, such as prolonged antibiotic treatment (5 patients), treatment for possible asthmatic syndrome and bronchitis (3 patients), placement of a vena cava filter (1 patient), and lung resection surgery (1 patient). Therefore, if a high degree of alertness and awareness is not present, this diagnosis can remain unknown.

Diagnostic Methods and Therapeutic Interventions

Strong suspicion is required to promptly diagnose PV stenosis, not only because it can mimic more prevalent respiratory and cardiovascular syndromes but also because diagnostic tests can be misleading, as we and others previously described [21–23, 28]. A number of imaging modalities have been used in the evaluation of PV stenosis. CT scanning is probably the most helpful since it can reliably identify the location and extension of the lesions (Fig. 3), while providing assessment of concomitant lung (e.g. consolidation or haemorrhage), mediastinal, and hilar (e.g. enlarged nodes) abnormalities

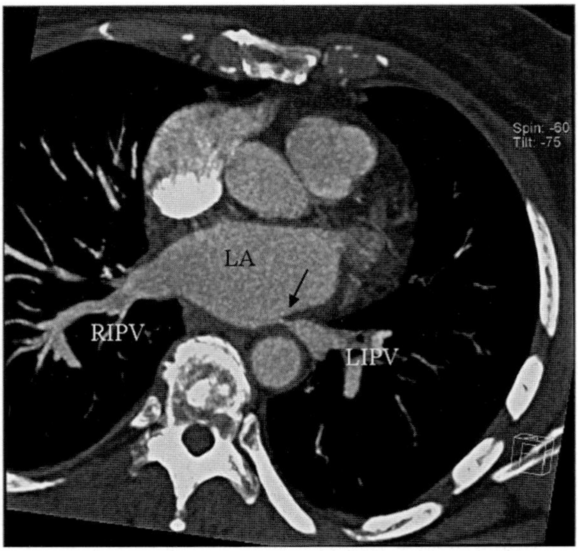

Fig. 3. Spiral CT scan at the level of the inferior PVs demonstrating a severe narrowing (*arrow*) of the proximal portion of the left inferior PV (*LIPV*). This location probably indicates that radiofrequency (RF) lesions were in fact placed inside the vein. *RIPV* Right inferior PV, *LA* left atrium

(Fig. 2). The only caveat is that some vessels that appear totally occluded on CT scanning are in fact patent when evaluated by PV angiography [29], the gold-standard diagnostic modality. Magnetic resonance angiography can also be performed with comparable results and has the advantage of avoiding iodine contrast injection [30–33].

Echocardiography has also been used to detect and predict the development of PV stenosis. TEE can provide accurate views of the superior PVs, and increased flow velocity on Doppler has been used as a surrogate for decreased luminal diameter. However, experience with intracardiac echocardiography (ICE) has demonstrated that even vessels with markedly increased flow velocities may not show significant stenosis when evaluated by CT or angiography [34]. As such, we believe that significant overestimation of the degree of stenosis may occur with an echo-based assessment.

Ventilation/perfusion (V/Q) scanning is a simple and accurate method to detect and evaluate the haemodynamic consequences of PV stenosis, the most common finding being a segmental perfusion abnormality in the presence of normal ventilation (similar to findings seen in pulmonary arterial embolism). In our experience, perfusion defects occur mainly when the degree of PV luminal narrowing is ≥ 70% [22], indicating that mild and moderate degrees of narrowing have minimal, if any, consequence on the physiology of the pulmonary circulation. Severe PV stenosis, in contrast, is associated with significant reduction in the pulmonary flow, which is only partially reversible even after successful treatment with PV dilatation. In our series evaluating 18 patients with severe PV stenosis, average pulmonary flow to the left lung increased from 11.7 ± 10.2% to 22.3 ± 10.8% after PV intervention [21].

Percutaneous PV dilatation is currently the treatment of choice for patients with symptoms attributable to severe PV stenosis, and it is associated with significant improvement in pressure gradients, venous diameter, lung perfusion, and symptoms [23, 29]. In a recent study involving 19 patients undergoing interventional procedures in 30 PVs, functional classification improved dramatically from a mean NYHA score of 3.1 to 1.7, with most patients able to perform their usual activities with no or only minimal limitation [29]. Unfortunately, the short-term results are not maintained, with approximately 50% of patients developing restenosis and necessitating repeat interventions [23, 29]. PV stenting does not appear to provide better results than simple balloon dilatation, at least when bare-metal stents are used. Currently, there is no published experience regarding the use of drug-coated stents, but better results are expected based on their successful use in the coronary arteries and in saphenous vein grafts.

Prognosis and Importance of Preventive Strategies

Progression of PV stenosis beyond the third month after ablation is rare but can occur in up to 10% of patients [22], indicating the need to repeat imaging evaluation every 3–6 months or if symptoms develop or worsen. More commonly, the degree of narrowing remains stable or improves (up to 30% of patients), probably reflecting the inflammatory nature of PV pathology. Based on these data, we recommend routine imaging evaluation with either CT or MRI 3 months after the procedure, irrespective of the presence of symptoms. If no stenosis is detected, no further evaluation is needed unless compatible symptoms develop. In the presence of luminal narrowing, repeat evaluation is undertaken at 6 and 12 months.

Development of pulmonary arterial hypertension appears to be extremely rare and occurs only in the presence of severe stenosis of several PVs (Fig. 1). Importantly, it is almost always associated with severe symptoms and appears to be reversible when PV dilatation is performed.

Risk factors for the development of PV stenosis, although yet to be completely defined, include energy delivery inside the veins [18, 24, 32], vein size, and use of excessive power during RF applications [22, 24]. As such, reliable and precise delineation of the PV–left atrium (LA) junction appears to be important. Our initial experience with ostial isolation based on electroanatomical mapping to delineate the PVs proved to be disappointing, with isolation observed in only 31% of treated veins and with severe stenosis developing in 15.5% of patients, comparable to the 20% severe stenosis rate obtained when we performed distal PV isolation based on a circular catheter in a selected group of patients.

Once it became clear that we had to avoid lesions inside the veins, selective PV angiography was utilised to determine the ostia. This approach decreased the incidence of severe stenosis to about 3%. However, in our experience the use of ICE was associated with the most considerable decrease in the occurrence of stenosis. When used to guide ostial positioning of the circular catheter (Fig. 4), it reduced severe stenosis to 1.4%. It is likely that angiography in not always reliable for adequate ostial visualisation because of the streaming effect of the contrast in the vein and the frequent gradual funnelling of the PV junction into the left atrial cavity.

Traditional methods for titration of energy delivery, such as tip temperature and impedance measures, may not be accurate [35]. This is especially true for left-side procedures, during which the use of excessive power may result in thromboembolic complications. Thus, the development of a reliable method to achieve more accurate energy delivery is needed and visualisation of microbubbles by ICE is a suitable option, being associated with a significantly reduced incidence of severe PV stenosis. Indeed, it is remarkable that

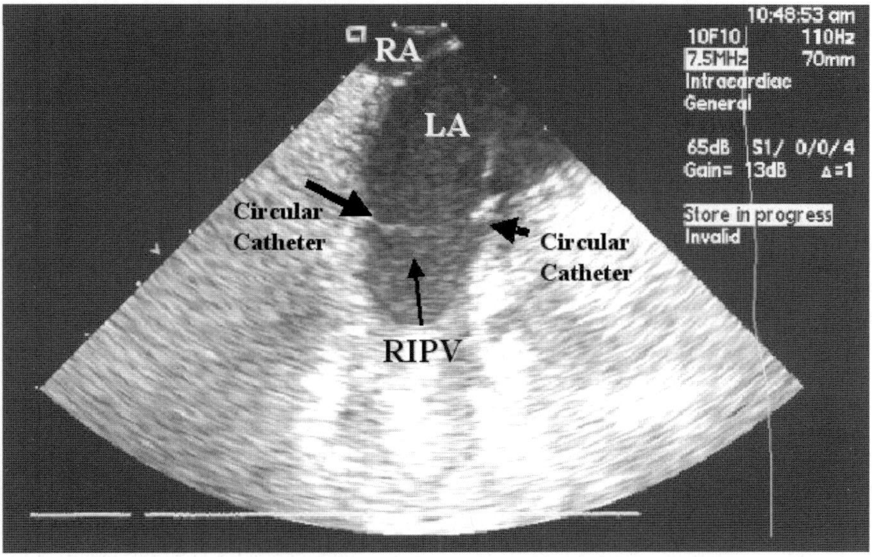

Fig. 4. Example of the use of intracardiac echocardiography (ICE) to guide ostial positioning of a circular mapping catheter in the right inferior PV (*RIPV*). The circular catheter is placed on the atrial side of the PV–LA junction, allowing real-time monitoring and avoiding the need for PV angiography. *LA* Left atrium, *RA* right atrium

none of our patients have developed severe stenosis since this strategy was introduced.

The rationale for microbubble-guided power titration lies in the premise that adequate tissue heating cannot be predicted simply by monitoring impedance and temperature. Instead, the formation of scattered microbubbles is believed to reflect significant tissue overheating [10, 36–38]. When this occurs, energy deliver has to be interrupted. However, if this phenomenon cannot be controlled, tissue desiccation will result, creating the milieu for coagulum formation and PV stenosis.

Other experienced groups also reported avoidance of PV stenosis just by performing circumferential ablation well outside the PVs [7, 12, 15, 39], usually up to 1 cm away from the PV–LA junction, a strategy that does not necessarily aim for PV isolation [39, 40].

Conclusions

Albeit almost an extinct complication in high-volume and experienced centres, PV stenosis most likely will continue to be a feared complication of AF ablative procedures, as they are more often performed in community settings by less-experienced operators. Severe PV stenosis is associated with a variety of respiratory symptoms that frequently mimic more common heart and lung diseases. A high degree of suspicion is necessary to avoid misleading diagnostic procedures and allow proper and prompt management of these patients.

PV dilatation is the treatment of choice for symptomatic patients but is still associated with a frequent need for repeat interventions due to restenosis. It remains to be seen whether the use of drug-coated stents will provide long-lasting results. Emphasis should be placed on prevention and imaging modalities that help to accurately delineate the PV–LA junction and guide power titration, both of which appear to provide the best means to avoid PV injury by RF energy.

References

1. Haïssaguerre M, Jaïs P, Shah DC et al (1998) Spontaneous initiation of atrial fibrillation by ectopic beats originating in the pulmonary veins. N Engl J Med 339:659–666
2. Marrouche NF, Dresing T, Cole C et al (2002) Circular mapping and ablation of the pulmonary vein for treatment of atrial fibrillation: impact of different catheter technologies. J Am Coll Cardiol 40:464–474
3. Pappone C, Oreto G, Rosanio S et al (2001) Atrial electroanatomic remodeling after circumferential radiofrequency pulmonary vein ablation: efficacy of an anatomic approach in a large cohort of patients with atrial fibrillation. Circulation 104:2539–2544
4. Chen SA, Tai CT, Tsai CF et al (2000) Radiofrequency catheter ablation of atrial fibrillation initiated by pulmonary vein ectopic beats. J Cardiovasc Electrophysiol 11:218–227
5. Oral H, Knight BP, Tada H et al (2002) Pulmonary vein isolation for paroxysmal and persistent atrial fibrillation. Circulation 105:1077–1081
6. Gerstenfeld EP, Guerra P, Sparks PB et al (2001) Clinical outcome after radiofrequency catheter ablation of focal atrial fibrillation triggers. J Cardiovasc Electrophysiol 12:900–908
7. Pappone C, Rosanio S, Oreto G et al (2000) Circumferential radiofrequency ablation of pulmonary vein ostia: A new anatomic approach for curing atrial fibrillation. Circulation 102:2619–2628
8. Natale A, Pisano E, Shewchik J et al (2000) First human experience with pulmonary vein isolation using a through-the-balloon circumferential ultrasound ablation system for recurrent atrial fibrillation. Circulation 102:1879–1882
9. Jaïs P, Hocini M, Macle L et al (2002) Distinctive electrophysiological properties of pulmonary veins in patients with atrial fibrillation. Circulation 106:2479–2485
10. Marrouche NF, Martin DO, Wazni O et al (2003) Phased-array intracardiac echocardiography monitoring during pulmonary vein isolation in patients with atrial fibrillation: impact on outcome and complications. Circulation 107(21):2710–2716
11. Kanagaratnam L, Tomassoni G, Schweikert R et al (2001) Empirical pulmonary vein isolation in patients with chronic atrial fibrillation using a three-dimensional

nonfluoroscopic mapping system: long-term follow-up. Pacing Clin Electrophysiol 24:1774–1779
12. Oral H, Scharf C, Chugh A et al (2003) Catheter ablation for paroxysmal atrial fibrillation: segmental pulmonary vein ostial ablation versus left atrial ablation. Circulation 108:2355–2360
13. Nademanee K, McKenzie J, Kosar E et al (2004) A new approach for catheter ablation of atrial fibrillation: mapping of the electrophysiologic substrate. J Am Coll Cardiol 43:2044–2053
14. Pappone C, Santinelli V, Manguso F et al (2004) Pulmonary vein denervation enhances long-term benefit after circumferential ablation for paroxysmal atrial fibrillation. Circulation 109:327–334
15. Ouyang F, Bansch D, Ernst S et al (2004) Complete isolation of left atrium surrounding the pulmonary veins: new insights from the double-Lasso technique in paroxysmal atrial fibrillation. Circulation 110:2090–2096
16. Cappato R, Calkins H, Chen SA et al (2005) Worldwide survey on the methods, efficacy, and safety of catheter ablation for human atrial fibrillation. Circulation 111:1100–1105
17. Scanavacca MI, Kajita LJ, Vieira M et al (2000) Pulmonary vein stenosis complicating catheter ablation of focal atrial fibrillation. J Cardiovasc Electrophysiol 11:677–681
18. Yu WC, Hsu TL, Tai CT et al (2001) Acquired pulmonary vein stenosis after radiofrequency catheter ablation of paroxysmal atrial fibrillation. J Cardiovasc Electrophysiol 12:887–892
19. Robbins IM, Colvin EV, Doyle TP et al (1998) Pulmonary vein stenosis after catheter ablation of atrial fibrillation. Circulation 98:1769–1775
20. Arentz T, Jander N, von Rosenthal J et al (2003) Incidence of pulmonary vein stenosis 2 years after radiofrequency catheter ablation of refractory atrial fibrillation. Eur Heart J 24:963–969
21. Saad EB, Marrouche NF, Saad CP et al (2003) Pulmonary vein stenosis after catheter ablation of atrial fibrillation: emergence of a new clinical syndrome. Ann Intern Med 138:634–638
22. Saad EB, Rossillo A, Saad CP et al (2003) Pulmonary vein stenosis after radiofrequency ablation of atrial fibrillation: functional characterization, evolution, and influence of the ablation strategy. Circulation 108:3102–3107
23. Packer DL, Keelan P, Munger TM et al (2005) Clinical presentation, investigation, and management of pulmonary vein stenosis complicating ablation for atrial fibrillation. Circulation 111:546–554
24. Purerfellner H, Cihal R, Aichinger J et al (2003) Pulmonary vein stenosis by ostial irrigated-tip ablation: incidence, time course, and prediction. J Cardiovasc Electrophysiol 14:158–164
25. Chen SA, Hsieh MH, Tai CT et al (1999) Initiation of atrial fibrillation by ectopic beats originating from the pulmonary veins: electrophysiological characteristics, pharmacological responses, and effects of radiofrequency ablation. Circulation 100:1879–1886
26. Haïssaguerre M, Jaïs P, Shah DC et al (2000) Electrophysiological end point for catheter ablation of atrial fibrillation initiated from multiple pulmonary venous foci. Circulation 101:1409–1417
27. Knight BP, Oral H, Chugh A et al (2003) Effects of operator experience on the outcome and duration of pulmonary vein isolation procedures for atrial fibrillation. Am J Cardiol 91:673–677

28. Ernst S, Ouyang F, Goya M et al (2003) Total pulmonary vein occlusion as a consequence of catheter ablation for atrial fibrillation mimicking primary lung disease. J Cardiovasc Electrophysiol 14:366–370
29. Qureshi AM, Prieto LR, Latson LA et al (2003) Transcatheter angioplasty for acquired pulmonary vein stenosis after radiofrequency ablation. Circulation 108:1336–1342
30. Carriero A, Marano R, Fossaceca R et al (1998) Pulmonary veins: magnetic resonance angiography anatomy. Magma 6:2–6
31. Yang M, Akbari H, Reddy GP et al (2001) Identification of pulmonary vein stenosis after radiofrequency ablation for atrial fibrillation using MRI. J Comput Assist Tomogr 25:34–35
32. Kato R, Lickfett L, Meininger G et al (2003) Pulmonary vein anatomy in patients undergoing catheter ablation of atrial fibrillation: lessons learned by use of magnetic resonance imaging. Circulation 107:2004–2010
33. Dill T, Neumann T, Ekinci O et al (2003) Pulmonary vein diameter reduction after radiofrequency catheter ablation for paroxysmal atrial fibrillation evaluated by contrast-enhanced three-dimensional magnetic resonance imaging. Circulation 107:845–850
34. Saad EB, Cole CR, Marrouche NF et al (2002) Use of intracardiac echocardiography for prediction of chronic pulmonary vein stenosis after ablation of atrial fibrillation. J Cardiovasc Electrophysiol 13:986–989
35. Farah A, Khan F, Machado C (2000) Thrombus formation at the site of radiofrequency catheter ablation. Pacing Clin Electrophysiol 23:538–540
36. Kalman JM, Fitzpatrick AP, Olgin JE et al (1997) Biophysical characteristics of radiofrequency lesion formation in vivo: dynamics of catheter tip-tissue contact evaluated by intracardiac echocardiography. Am Heart J 133:8–18
37. Bunch TJ, Bruce GK, Johnson SB et al (2004) Analysis of catheter-tip (8-mm) and actual tissue temperatures achieved during radiofrequency ablation at the orifice of the pulmonary vein. Circulation 110:2988–2995
38. Wood MA, Shaffer KM, Ellenbogen AL et al (2005) Microbubbles during radiofrequency catheter ablation: Composition and formation. Heart Rhythm 2:397–403
39. Cappato R, Negroni S, Pecora D et al (2003) Prospective assessment of late conduction recurrence across radiofrequency lesions producing electrical disconnection at the pulmonary vein ostium in patients with atrial fibrillation. Circulation 108:1599–1604
40. Hocini M, Sanders P, Jaïs P et al (2005) Prevalence of pulmonary vein disconnection after anatomical ablation for atrial fibrillation: consequences of wide atrial encircling of the pulmonary veins. Eur Heart J 26:696–704

Atrial Fibrillation Should Be Considered a First-Line Therapy – Or Not?

A. Pacifico, P.D. Henry

Introduction

In evidence-based medicine, the efficacy and toxicity of therapeutic options for a specific disease are assessed by carrying out comparative therapeutic trials. Only randomised placebo-controlled trials (RCT) can provide valid information on the merits of specific therapeutic manoeuvres in order to rank them as first-line, second-line, or third-line therapies. To the extent that valid RCT comparing ablation for atrial fibrillation (AF) with other AF treatments have never been published, the question whether ablation should be a first-line therapy appears premature and cannot be answered on the basis of available scientific information.

Our views on ablation for AF have not changed since our recent editorial on the subject [1]. Here, we will briefly enumerate arguments that cast doubts on recommending ablation for AF as a routine therapeutic procedure and certainly as a first choice or first-line treatment. This should not be misinterpreted to mean that clinical research in this field is not desirable.

Lack of Considering Extensive Epidemiologic Information

Extensive epidemiologic data indicate that AF in Western societies is a disease of old age [2, 3]. Consecutive enrolments of AF patients are unlikely to yield cohorts with mean ages of 60 years or below. Studies claiming consecutive enrolments yet exhibiting young cohorts are puzzling from an epidemiologic viewpoint and raise questions about the nature of the enrolment procedures [1, 4].

Texas Arrhythmia Institute and Baylor College of Medicine, Houston, TX, USA

In studies of AF, cardiovascular risk factors well known to represent AF risk factors, such as hypertension and diabetes [2], should be precisely defined and controlled. The recent demonstration that treatment with ACE inhibitors and/or statins may decrease AF risk appears to support the importance of controlling risk factors [5, 6]. Unfortunately, most AF ablation studies provide little information on risk factors and their control. Because AF relapse may occur as a nocturnal phenomenon [7], it would be important to monitor nocturnal blood pressure to determine whether lack of physiological nocturnal hypotensive dips in hypertensive patients can be correlated with the risk of AF relapse.

Lack of Considering Previous Trials and Previous Meta-Analyses

Placebo control groups in drug treatment trials of AF have exhibited extremely variable AF recurrence rates [8]. Therefore, studies involving small groups of patients should be interpreted most cautiously. The history of evidence-based medicine has shown that seemingly simple evaluations, such as those comparing two heparin preparations, may yield contradictory results in separate trials involving the randomisation of thousands of patients (for instance, Synergy trial vs previous enoxaparin trials [9]). Therefore, small studies attempting to evaluate complex highly case-variable procedures such as AF ablation are unlikely to yield conclusive statistical results. Most AF ablation studies fail to define statistical power and are grossly underpowered to assess all-important total death risk. The implication that AF ablation substantially reduces the incidence of sudden cardiac death has no survival–statistical foundation [10].

Lack of Defining Precise Pharmacologic Protocols and Treatment with Antiarrhythmic Drug Therapy

Because so-called antiarrhythmic agents represent drugs with fundamentally different actions and toxicities, it is highly inappropriate to lump them together [11]. This is, for instance, true for verapamil, dihydropyridines, and diltiazem (only verapamil has clinically demonstrated antiarrhythmic effects). Most important, depending upon the dosages used, so-called antiarrhythmic agents may act as pro-arrhythmic agents and thereby increase mortality [11, 12]. Comparison of ablation with such drugs (particularly without specifying their dosages) is potentially very misleading. Variable, not prospectively defined drug administrations after ablation preclude an assessment of the therapeutic contribution of the invasive intervention to overall outcome [1].

Use of Non-validated Methods of Arrhythmia Detection

Remembered arrhythmia symptoms or symptoms inciting patients to perform ECG recordings with pocket recorders or to elicit shocks from implanted atrial defibrillators have not been shown to represent adequate techniques of AF detection as recorded by implanted devices [13–15]. These methods are deficient particularly because AF episodes are often nocturnal, occurring during sleep [7]. Recent studies with implanted devices confirm that up to 90% of AF episodes are not perceived by patients [13–15]. Further, 24- and 48-h continuous (Holter) recording are highly inadequate sampling techniques for the recording of infrequent and highly variable arrhythmia events, such as those encountered in patients suffering from AF.

Failure To Perform Trials with Appropriate Placebo Controls and To Give Possible Placebo Effects Serious Consideration

The inclusion of groups randomised to placebo or sham interventions is crucial in trials. For instance, comparison of two potentially toxic medications, such as chemotherapeutic or antiarrhythmic agents, without placebo comparison does not answer the important question whether these agents prolong or shorten survival. Furthermore, the lack of controls involving placebo or sham interventions precludes appraisal of placebo effects [16, 17]. Recent cardiological studies [18, 19] have re-emphasised the importance of placebo effects, extensively discussed in the surgical literature [16].

Failure To Develop Standard Techniques Necessary To Conduct Credible Multi-Centre Trials

One hallmark of the AF ablation literature is the continual proposal of new ablation procedures involving new instruments and techniques. The authors jump to new procedures before characterising long-term effects of their previous apparently abandoned procedures. For instance, long-term effects of right atrial ablation, advocated in early trials [20], remain largely uncharacterised. A similar difficulty was observed with the Maze operations for AF. Although each Maze procedure was claimed to be definitive, new improved procedures were described subsequently. Lack of developing standardised procedures largely prevents the implementation of credible multicentre studies.

Conduction of Studies Under the Exclusive Supervision of Clinicians Identifiable as Proponents of Ablation for Atrial Fibrillation

In modern trials, it is customary to assemble several neutral committees for the monitoring of patient selection, randomisation, data collection, adverse events, and outcomes. In AF ablation trials, objective monitoring by independent observers has almost always been omitted.

Variable or Absent Definition of the Term Cure of Atrial Fibrillation

In many AF ablation studies, claim of cure is made. Unfortunately, the term cure is rarely clearly defined. The outcomes of ablation procedures compared to those obtained with selected antiarrhythmic agents, such as amiodarone, sotalol, and propafenone, have yielded 1-year relapse-free survivals of the same order of magnitude (about 60% of the patients) [8]. Such apparently event-free survivals are probably only slightly better that those obtained without specific therapies. Cure after only 12 months cannot be claimed because the long-term course of AF is highly variable and may evolve over a lifetime [1]. It is disconcerting that investigators can claim cure based on subjective information, apparently not considering that the detection of AF relapses requires special diagnostic strategies [13–15].

Absent or Invalid Data on the Most Important Complications of Atrial Fibrillation, Including Stroke, Heart Failure, All-Cause Death, and Cardiovascular Death

Because AF is relatively well-tolerated, the rates of interventional complications, such as stroke, pulmonary vein stenosis, haemopericadium, and phrenic nerve paralysis, must be evaluated most carefully [21, 22]. In many AF ablation studies, no estimates of cumulative radiation dosage (fluoroscopy) are provided. It has been demonstrated that AF may be complicated by microembolic brain disease and cognitive deficits without signs of stroke [23, 24]. Therefore, absence of obvious stroke events by no means demonstrates the safety of AF ablation in terms of embolic brain injury. Unfortunately, no AF ablation study has included serial brain imaging studies and none has focused on intervention-related cognitive deficits.

Conclusions

The literature on ablation for AF has many of the features of clinical research in the era preceding evidence-based medicine and randomised trials. Many studies emanate from single centres, involve low patient numbers, and fail to provide adequate statistical analysis, including intention to treat analysis and evaluation of statistical power. As was the case with Maze operations, new procedures are continually proposed without completing satisfactory evaluations of previously proposed procedures. Very worrisome is that most studies have not involved neutral committees for the recording and supervision of severe complications.

The belief that AF ablation now represents a standard or, indeed, first-line treatment is excessively optimistic and may reflect occupational and economic factors encouraging mechanistic invasive procedures.

References

1. Pacifico A, Henry PD (2004) Ablation for atrial fibrillation: are cures really achieved? J Am Coll Cardiol 43:1940–1942
2. Kannel WB, Wolf PA, Benjamin EJ et al (1998) Prevalence, incidence, prognosis, and predisposing conditions for atrial fibrillation: population-based estimates. Am J Cardiol 82(suppl 8A):2N–9N
3. Wattigney WA, Mensah GA, Croft JB (2003) Increasing trends in hospitalization for atrial fibrillation in the United States, 1985 through 1999. Implication for primary prevention. Circulation 108:711–716
4. Pappone C, Oreto G, Rosanio S et al (2001) Atrial electroanatomic remodeling after circumferential radiofrequency pulmonary vein ablation – Efficacy of an anatomic approach in a large cohort of patients with atrial fibrillation. Circulation 104:2539–2544
5. Maggioni AP, Latini R, Carson PE et al (2005) Valsartan reduces the incidence of atrial fibrillation in patients with heart failure: results from the valsartan heart failure trial (Val-Heft). Am Heart J 149:548–557
6. Young-Xu Y, Jabbour S, Goldberg R et al (2003) Usefulness of statin drugs in protecting against atrial fibrillation in patients with coronary artery disease. Am J Cardiol 92:1379–1383
7. Ciaroni S, Cuenoud L, Bloch A (2000) Clinical study to investigate the predictive parameters for the onset of atrial fibrillation in patients with essential hypertension. Am Heart J 139:814–819
8. Nichol G, McAllister F, Laupacis A et al (2002) Meta-analysis of randomised controlled trials of the effectiveness of antiarrhythmic agents at promoting sinus rhythm in patients with atrial fibrillation. Heart 87:535–543
9. Ferguson JJ, Califf RM, Antman EM et al (2004) Enoxaparin vs unfractioned heparin in high-risk patients with non-ST-segment elevation acute coronary syndromes managed with an intended early invasive strategy: primary results of the SYNERGY randomized trial. JAMA 292:45–54

10. Pappone C, Rosanio S, Augello G et al (2003) Mortality, morbidity, and quality of life after circumferential pulmonary vein ablation for atrial fibrillation – Outcomes from a controlled nonrandomized long-term study. J Am Coll Cardiol 42:185–197
11. Pacifico A, Henry PD (1996) Class I or Class III agents for atrial fibrillation: are we asking the right question? Pacing Clin Electrophysiol 26:1613–1619
12. Waldo AL, Camm AJ, deRuyter H et al for the SWORD Investigators (2003). Effect of d-sotalol on mortality in patients with left ventricular dysfunction after recent and remote myocardial infarction. Lancet 348:6–11
13. Savelieva I, Camm AJ (2000) Clinical relevance of silent atrial fibrillation: prevalence, prognosis, quality of life, and management. J Interv Card Electrophysiol 4:369–382
14. Israel CW, Grönefeld G, Ehrlich JR et al (2004) Long-term risk of recurrent atrial fibrillation as documented by an implantable monitoring device. J Am Coll Cardiol 43:47–52
15. Strickberger SA, Ip J, Saksena S et al (2005) Relationship between atrial tachyarrhythmias and symptoms. Heart Rhythm 2:125–131
16. Cook RC, Alscher KT, Hsiang YN (2003) A debate on the value and necessity of clinical trials in surgery. Am J Surg 185:305–310
17. Wingerchuk DM, Noseworthy JH (2002) Randomised controlled trials to assess therapies of multiple sclerosis. Neurology 58:S40–S48
18. Saririan M, Eisenberg M J (2003) Myocardial laser revascularization for the treatment of end-stage coronary artery disease. J Am Coll Cardiol 41:173–183
19. Grines C, Rubanyi GM, Kleiman NS et al (2003) Angiogenic therapy with adenovirus 5 fibroblast growth factor-4 (Ad5FGF-4): a new option for the treatment of coronary artery disease. Am J Cardiol 92:21N–31N
20. Gaita F, Riccardi R, Calò L et al (1998) Atrial mapping and radiofrequency catheter ablation in patients with idiopathic atrial fibrillation - Electrophysiological findings and ablation results. Circulation 97:2136–2145
21. Bertaglia E, Stabile G (2005) Catheter Ablation for the Cure of Atrial Fibrillation (CACAF). Late-Braking Clinical Trials II, March 8, 2005. 54th Annual Scientific Session of the American College of Cardiology, Orlando, Florida
22. Saad EB, Rossillo A, Saad CP et al (2003) Pulmonary vein stenosis after radiofrequency ablation of atrial fibrillation – Functional characterization, evolution, and influence of the ablation strategy. Circulation 108:3102–3107
23. Ezekowitz MD, James KE, Nazarian SM et al (1995) Silent cerebral infarction in patients with nonrheumatic atrial fibrillation. The Veterans Affairs Stroke Prevention in Nonrheumatic Atrial Fibrillatiion Investigators. Circulation 92:2178–2182
24. Sabatini T, Frisoni GB, Barbisoni P et al (2000) Atrial fibrillation and cognitive disorders in older people. J Am Geriatr Soc 48:387–390

Long-Term Use of the Atrial and Dual Defibrillator: What Have We Learned?

J.M. MEKEL, A.S. THORNTON, D.A.M.J. THEUNS, L.J. JORDAENS

Background

Persistent atrial fibrillation represents a management problem for the physician and a condition associated with considerable morbidity. The results of anti-arrhythmic therapy are disappointing [1]. In the 1980s the rapid developments in implantable device technology, combined with the knowledge that atrial defibrillation thresholds were far lower with internal cardioversion than with transthoracic cardioversion [2] and the rationale for applying early cardioversion of atrial defibrillation to limit electrical remodelling, led to the development of the implantable atrial defibrillator or atrioverter. The first commercially available device was only capable of delivering low-energy shocks, specifically for atrial defibrillation; later, high-energy devices became available that could accomplish atrial and ventricular defibrillation. Electrode configurations are variable, with shock coils positioned in the right atrium and coronary sinus or only in the right ventricle or different combinations.

Stand-Alone Atrial Defibrillators

The InControl Metrix Atrioverter system (Guidant Corp., St Paul, Minn., USA) consists of an implantable atrial defibrillator connected to right atrial and coronary sinus defibrillation leads and a right ventricular pacing lead (Fig. 1). It is capable of delivering a maximum of 6 J of energy. This system was evaluated acutely in a study of 51 patients [3] and demonstrated the

Department of Electrophysiology, Erasmus Medical College, Rotterdam, The Netherlands

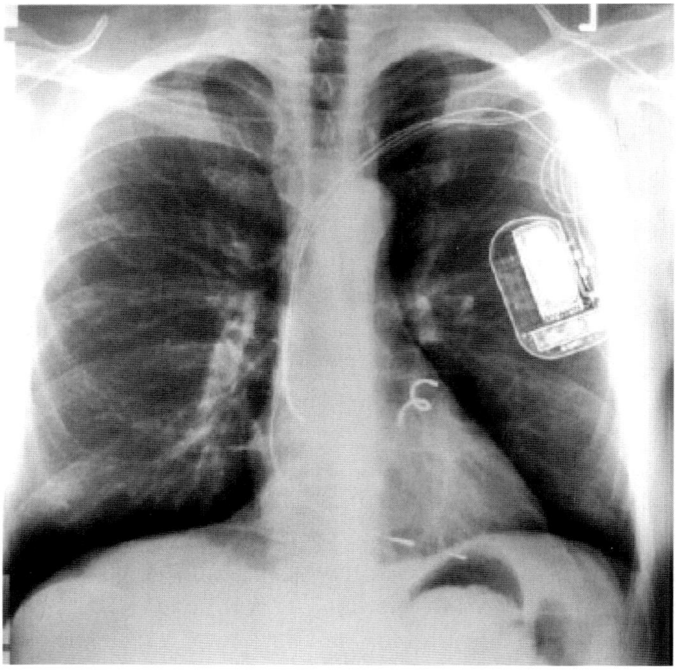

Fig. 1. Chest radiograph of a patient with an implanted atrioverter with leads in the right atrium, the coronary sinus, and the apex of the right ventricle. The right atrial and coronary sinus leads are used for arrhythmia recognition and defibrillation. The right ventricular lead is used for shock synchronisation and, if needed, ventricular pacing

capability of the device to deliver promptly and safely internal shocks for the acute treatment of recurrent episodes of atrial fibrillation. These patients were subsequently also evaluated in the ambulatory setting [4].

Dual-Chamber Defibrillators

A number of implantable cardioverter defibrillators (ICDs) capable of delivering shock therapy for atrial and ventricular tachyarrhythmias have been developed, including the Jewel AF model 7250 ICD and GEM III AT (Medtronic, Inc., Minneapolis, Minn., USA), and the Prizm AVT and Vitality AVT (Guidant Corp., St Paul, Minn., USA). In addition, these devices can deliver overdrive pacing therapy in the atrium which may obviate the need to administer a shock. The largest amount of data published has been on the Jewel AF, a dual-chamber defibrillator also capable of delivering preventive pacing therapies and atrial overdrive pacing. It delivers a maximum of 27 J of electrical energy. This device is combined with pace-sense electrodes in the right ventricle and atrium together with one ventricular and one supraventricular shocking electrode and an optional third high-voltage electrode in the coronary sinus. It may be employed as an active can device or subcutaneous patches may be added. The device uses algorithms to distinguish between atrial tachycardia, atrial fibrillation, and ventricular tachyarrhythmias. It may be programmed to deliver atrial shock therapy automatically (Fig. 2) after a variable interval or only in response to a patient-initiated request given by means of a manual activator. The former programming allows for automatic shocks to be delivered at a moment when the patient is least likely to experience it as painful, uncomfortable, or inconvenient; the latter programming allows the patient to optimise conditions for delivery of the shock, including taking a sedative or analgesic prior to shock delivery. To minimise the risk of inducing a ventricular tachyarrhythmia the device synchronises the shock with an R wave and will only deliver therapy after a relatively long R-R interval, nominally 500 ms in this device. This device was evaluated in the Worldwide Jewel AF-Only Trial [5].

Safety and Efficacy of Cardioversion of Atrial Fibrillation by Implantable Devices

In the study by the Metrix investigators [3] the device delivered a total of 670 shocks for 227 spontaneous episodes of AF in 41 patients during a mean follow-up of 259 days (2 SD = 138 days). A further 3049 shocks were delivered for induced episodes of AF during testing of the synchronisation adequacy

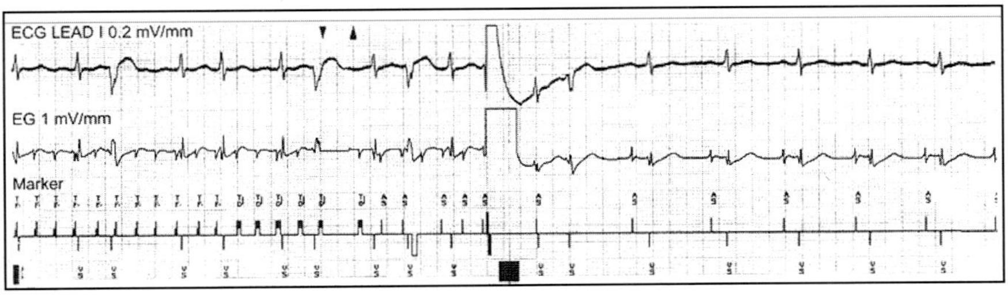

Fig. 2. Intracardiac electrogram and a marker channel showing the detection and shock termination of an episode of atrial tachycardia in a Jewel AF dual-chamber defibrillator. *TF* interval below atrial tachycardia detection interval, *TD* atrial tachycardia detection, *AS* atrial sensed event, *VS* ventricular sensed event

and atrial defibrillation threshold. There was not a single instance of ventricular arrhythmia induced by shocks delivered for atrial fibrillation, confirming that R wave synchronisation was adequately achieved by the device. It is important to note that the trial excluded patients with anything more than mild structural or ischaemic cardiac disease as well as patients with a documented episode of ventricular tachyarrhythmia. As regards efficacy, 96% of the spontaneous episodes of atrial fibrillation were successfully cardioverted by the device, but in 27% of episodes several shocks were required because of early recurrence of atrial fibrillation (ERAF). Arrhythmia recognition occurred with high specificity.

In the Worldwide Jewel AF-Only Trial [5] a total of 1036 shocks were delivered for atrial tachyarrhythmia without a single instance of induced ventricular dysrhythmia. The efficacy of delivered shocks in terminating atrial tachyarrhythmias was 86.7%. The efficacy of atrial overdrive pacing was 40%, a high percentage, explained by the fact that many episodes of atrial tachyarrhythmia started as a well-organised atrial tachycardia. The mean follow-up period was 12.6 ± 6.2 months. Based on analysis of available stored electrograms, the positive predictive accuracy of the detection algorithm was 98.9%. Fifty-four episodes of delivered therapy were inappropriate, caused by sensing of far-field signals or multiple premature atrial beats. After 1 year, 94% of the patients remained in sinus rhythm, and 91% still had atrial therapies enabled.

Again, this trial excluded patients with documented ventricular tachyarrhythmias, but moderate to severe heart disease was not an exclusion criterion (except for NYHA class IV symptoms). Of 67 episodes of ventricular tachycardia or fibrillation, 58 were successfully terminated by device intervention; the remaining 9 terminated spontaneously. The incidence of ventricular tachyarrhythmia (6.7%) was relatively high, a fact which casts doubt on the wisdom of implanting a stand-alone atrial defibrillator. However, this high incidence may have arisen from selection bias and further, a significant proportion of patients had NYHA class III symptoms and/or left ventricular ejection fraction (LVEF) of less than 35% – characteristics that in 2005 are accepted as indications for ICD implantation [6, 7]. An intriguing finding from this study is that 75% of ventricular tachyarrhythmias started during an episode of atrial tachyarrhythmia. Other studies [8] have also described a temporal relation between atrial fibrillation and ventricular tachyarrhythmia.

Anti-tachycardia pacing and shock therapy resulted in a significant reduction in the atrial tachyarrhythmia burden from a mean of 58.5 h/month to 7.8 h/month [9].

Long-Term Follow-Up of the Dual Defibrillator

Longer-term follow-up in a smaller group of patients [10] revealed a very high rate of successful device intervention, with 96% of episodes successfully terminated with a single shock. This study revealed three different patterns of atrial fibrillation recurrence, with a trend to longer duration of sinus rhythm after successful cardioversion in only a minority of patients, providing limited evidence for the concept that 'sinus rhythm begets sinus rhythm.' Timmermans et al. [11] similarly reported a decrease in the number of episodes requiring therapy and an increase in the time between episodes after 260 ± 144 days in patients implanted with the Metrix device.

Modern devices are also capable of delivering overdrive pacing in the atrium in order to terminate episodes of more organised atrial tachycardia, hopefully preventing the rhythm from degenerating into atrial fibrillation. Most can also deliver 50 Hz pacing in an attempt to convert atrial fibrillation to sinus rhythm before proceeding to shock therapy. The efficacy of these modalities is 71.3% for anti-tachycardia pacing (ATP) on atrial tachycardia and 36.2% for 50 Hz pacing for atrial fibrillation [12, 13].

Early recurrence of atrial fibrillation (ERAF) after successful ambulatory cardioversion is common [14], reaching 70% at 24 h, and is commoner with an episode duration of less than 3 h, with episodes where multiple shocks are required, and in the absence of a history of myocardial infarction.

In a long-term follow-up of 136 patients with the Metrix device [15], at a median of 40 months after implantation only 39 of 106 (37%) for whom data was available were still actively delivering therapy with the device. In 14 patients (13%) the device was being used to monitor the arrhythmia, with action taken in the event of a recurrence, either as a device-delivered or transthoracic cardioversion under the supervision of the treating physician. In 53 patients the device had either been turned off or explanted for a variety of reasons including: a rise in the defibrillation threshold, rendering the device incapable of performing successful cardioversion in 7 patients; intolerance of shocks due to frequent atrial fibrillation recurrences in 15 patients; significant bradycardia necessitating atrioventricular sequential pacing, of which this device was incapable, in 12 patients; and battery depletion in the remaining 19 patients. Of these 19 patients, 7 refused implantation of a new defibrillator due to intolerance of shocks, 9 received a second-generation dual-chamber defibrillator, 6 received a dual-chamber pacemaker (with or without preventive or therapeutic pacing algorithms) and 2 received antiarrhythmic drug therapy (in combination with a Maze procedure in 1). In 36 patients rhythm control was abandoned in favour of a strategy of rate control (including ablate-and-pace therapy in 13).

Device-Related Complications

In the study by the Metrix investigators [3] there were 8 system-related complications, including 2 cases of lead displacement. In the Worldwide Jewel AF-Only Trial [5] there were 26 system-related complications in 23 patients. Lead displacement was the commonest complication, occurring in 11 instances; 5 of these were displacements of the atrial tripolar lead, which is heavier than a standard bipolar lead. This incidence should be much less if a standard dual-coil ventricular defibrillation lead is used.

Tolerability of Delivered Shocks and Quality of Life

The tolerability of this device therapy is highly variable. Anti-tachycardia pacing is generally tolerated well, shocks less so. Nevertheless, a careful analysis of measures of quality of life in the Jewel-AF trial [16] demonstrated a convincing improvement in all subgroups of patients, with no evidence of an attenuation of this improvement in those who received shocks. Indeed, the proportion of episodes for which patients used the activator increased during the course of the study. Follow-up in this report, however, was short (6 months). In a study with a longer follow-up, Ricci et al. reported significant improvement in the quality of life and decreased hospitalisation in a group of 40 patients with the Jewel AF device implanted [17]. In one survey, acceptance of device therapy is good at 18 months after implantation [18] but does correlate with a number of patient characteristics with which the physician should be familiar, such as lower psychosocial distress, lower anxiety score, and lesser atrial fibrillation symptom burden. Automatic nighttime shocks are significantly less acceptable to patients than patient-activated shocks with pre-medication [19]. Pre-medication with sedation is preferred to that with analgesia [20].

Patient Selection

The trials conducted to date have limited the use of the atrial or dual defibrillator to patients with recurrent atrial fibrillation refractory to combination or sequential drug therapy. Patients with permanent atrial fibrillation are clearly not candidates. From the long-term follow-up data [15, 16, 18] it appears that therapy is better tolerated by patients with a lower atrial fibrillation burden.

Future of the Atrial Defibrillator

The advent of ablation techniques for atrial fibrillation [21] with good short-term and medium-term results heralds a new era in the treatment of this condition in patients with symptomatic paroxysmal or persistent atrial fibrillation in the absence of severe structural heart disease [22]. No doubt improvement in techniques with a commensurate increase in success and decrease in complications will mean this modality will be applicable in a larger group of patients, including those with more severe structural cardiac disease [23].

What then is the role for the atrioventricular defibrillator in 2005 and beyond? Patients who were previously candidates for the stand-alone atrial defibrillator, i.e. those with minimal cardiac disease but symptomatic drug-refractory paroxysmal atrial defibrillation, should nowadays have a pulmonary vein isolation procedure performed. Patients with more severe structural heart disease probably have an indication for implantation of an ICD in light of the results of the more recently published trials [6, 7]. The incorporation of atrial defibrillation modalities into ICDs (a development of the philosophy that spawned the Jewel AF device) for a select group of patients with recurrent symptomatic drug-refractory atrial fibrillation may ensure the survival of the atrial defibrillator. In particular, patients with hypertrophic obstructive cardiomyopathy, who are at risk of sudden death from ventricular tachyarrhythmias, and who can develop rapid haemodynamic deterioration with the onset of atrial dysrhythmias, may benefit remarkably from this device, especially if paced from the apex of the right ventricle with a short atrioventricular delay. A large number of patients with congenital heart disease, who are also at high risk of developing atrial and ventricular tachyarrhythmias, likewise form a particular target group.

Conclusions

Atrial and dual defibrillators held great promise when they were introduced in the 1990s.

The devices are effective and safe in selected patients. Tolerability and acceptance by patients is good in the short term but only moderate in the longer term. The complication rate is relatively low. However, advances in ablation techniques for the treatment of atrial fibrillation have limited and will continue to limit the use of implantable atrial defibrillators. In combination with ICDs they may find a continued role in a patient group that should be further defined.

References

1. Singh BN, Singh SN, Reda DJ et al (2005) Amiodarone versus sotalol for atrial fibrillation. N Engl J Med 352:1861–1872
2. Lévy S, Lauribe P, Dolla E et al (1992) A randomised comparison of external and internal cardioversion of chronic atrial fibrillation. Circulation 86:1415–1420
3. Wellens H, Lau C-P, Lüderitz B et al (1998) Atrioverter: an implantable device for the treatment of atrial fibrillation. Circulation 98:1651–1656
4. Daoud EG, Timmermans C, Fellows C et al (2000) Initial clinical experience with ambulatory use of an implantable atrial defibrillator for conversion of atrial fibrillation. Metrix Investigators. Circulation102:1407–1413
5. Gold MR, Sulke N, Schwartzman DS et al (2001) Clinical experience with a dual-chamber implantable cardioverter defibrillator to treat atrial tachyarrhythmias. J Cardiovasc Electrophysiol 12:1247–1253
6. Bardy GH, Lee KL, Mark DB et al (2005) Amiodarone or an implantable cardioverter-defibrillator for congestive heart failure. N Engl J Med 352:225–237
7. Kadish A, Dyer A, Daubert JP et al (2004) Prophylactic defibrillator implantation in patients with nonischemic dilated cardiomyopathy. N Engl J Med 350:2151–2158
8. Gronefeld GC, Mauss O, Li YG et al (2000) Association between atrial fibrillation and appropriate implantable cardioverter defibrillator therapy: results from a prospective study. J Cardiovasc Electrophysiol 11:1208–1214
9. Friedman PA, Dijkman B, Warman EN et al for theWorldwide Jewel AF Investigators (2001) Atrial therapies reduce atrial arrhythmia burden in defibrillator patients. Circulation 104:1023–1028
10. Spurrell P, Mitchell A, Kamalvand K et al (2004) Does sinus rhythm beget sinus rhythm? Long-term follow-up of the patient activated atrial defibrillator. Pacing Clin Electrophysiol 27:175–181
11. Timmermans C, Levy S, Ayers GM et al (2000) Spontaneous episodes of atrial fibrillation after implantation of the Metrix Atrioverter: observations on treated and nontreated episodes. Metrix Investigators. J Am Coll Cardiol 35:1428–1433
12. Ricci R, Pignalberi C, Disertori M et al (2002) Efficacy of a dual chamber defibrillator with atrial antitachycardia functions in treating spontaneous atrial tachyarrhythmias in patients with life-threatening ventricular tachyarrhythmias. Eur Heart J 23:1471–1479
13. Ricci R, Pignalberi C, Santini M (2003) Efficacy of atrial antitachycardia functions for treating atrial fibrillation: observations in patients with a dual-chamber defibrillator. Card Electrophysiol Rev 7:348–351
14. Schwartzman D, Musley SK, Swerdlow C et al (2002) Early recurrence of atrial fibrillation after ambulatory shock conversion. J Am Coll Cardiol 40:93–99
15. Geller JC, Reek S, Timmermans C et al (2003) Treatment of atrial fibrillation with an implantable atrial defibrillator – long term results. Eur Heart J 24:2083–2089
16. Newman DM, Dorian P, Paquette M et al (2003) Effect of an implantable cardioverter defibrillator with atrial detection and shock therapies on patient-perceived, health-related quality of life. Am Heart J 145:841–846
17. Ricci R, Quesada A, Pignalberi C et al (2004) Dual defibrillator improves quality of life and decreases hospitalizations in patients with drug refractory atrial fibrillation. J Interv Card Electrophysiol 10:85–92
18. Burns JL, Sears SF, Sotile R et al (2004) Do patients accept implantable atrial defibrillation therapy? Results from the Patient Atrial Shock Survey of Acceptance and Tolerance (PASSAT) Study. J Cardiovasc Electrophysiol 15:286–291

19. Boodhoo L, Mitchell A, Ujhelyi M et al (2004) Improving the acceptability of the atrial defibrillator: patient-activated cardioversion versus automatic night cardioversion with and without sedation (ADSAS 2). Pacing Clin Electrophysiol 27:910–917
20. Mitchell AR, Spurrell PA, Gerritse BE et al (2004) Improving the acceptability of the atrial defibrillator for the treatment of persistent atrial fibrillation: the atrial defibrillator sedation assessment study (ADSAS). Int J Cardiol 96:141–145
21. Haïssaguerre M, Jaïs P, Shah DC et al (1998) Spontaneous initiation of atrial fibrillation by ectopic beats originating in the pulmonary veins. N Engl J Med 339:659–666
22. Hocini M, Sanders P, Jaïs P et al (2004) Techniques for curative treatment of atrial fibrillation. J Cardiovasc Electrophysiol 15:1467–1471
23. Hsu LF, Jaïs P, Sanders P et al (2004) Catheter ablation for atrial fibrillation in congestive heart failure. N Engl J Med 351:2373–2383

Hybrid Therapy as an Alternative in Refractory Atrial Fibrillation: When, Why, and How?

S. SAKSENA[1], N. SKADSBERG[2]

Introduction

Hybrid therapy has been proposed for the treatment of drug-refractory atrial fibrillation (AF). The development of hybrid therapy has been going on over the past 10 years and has largely stemmed from the modest efficacy and limited patient benefits seen with a variety of monotherapies in patients with drug-refractory AF. A number of clinical studies have demonstrated that drug-refractory AF is common and that rhythm control is rarely achieved with drug strategies alone. In the AFFIRM study, drug therapy added only a modest 23% increment to the likelihood of maintaining rhythm control in patients who were started on a rhythm control strategy [1]. Similar results were seen with amiodarone in the STAF study and in the RACE study [2, 3]. As a result, non-pharmacological monotherapies such as atrial pacing and catheter ablation either of focal triggers or isolation of these foci as well as linear ablation of the atrial substrate were proposed. The last 10 years have been spent in evaluating each of these monotherapies as a suitable non-pharmacological alternative to drug therapy of AF for rhythm control. In each of these instances, there has been some success, but a substantial proportion of patients has failed to respond to the monotherapy.

Focal catheter ablation of AF triggers in patients with little or no structural heart disease has been performed in the pulmonary veins [4]. Focal ablation has had modest success; in prospective studies and recent meta-analysis this has averaged around 50–70% at most centres [5]. In a recent worldwide survey, practitioners described somewhat higher success rates at

[1]Electrophysiology Research Foundation, Warren, New Jersey; [2]Robert Wood Johnson Medical School, New Brunswick, New Jersey, USA

centres that had larger volumes of patients, but nevertheless most centres saw only modest success rates. Even these modest success rates were achieved in many centres with the concomitant use of anti-arrhythmic drugs, in a hybrid approach with the ablation procedure. In a survey of clinical practitioners, Mikelsen et al. reported a significant level of failure in the responses from clinical practitioners [6]. In view of these outcomes and the limited target patient population (i.e., the patients with little or no structural heart disease), few practitioners believe that monotherapy with focal catheter ablation can be curative in the large body of AF patients. More recently, isolation of the pulmonary veins has been attempted [7]. While isolation procedures have been associated with lesser degrees of complications such as pulmonary vein stenosis, efficacy rates have been variable. While certain centres report good results, the first prospective multi-centre study reported a 60% freedom from AF at 1 year [8]. Linear ablation of the right atrium has had low success rates, with rates of efficacy between 15% and 54% being reported, but many of these data may relate to treatment combined with anti-arrhythmic drugs [9, 10]. In a prospective clinical trial, a partial or complete response on the basis of symptoms and intermittent ECGs was obtained in approximately 50% of patients [10]. In this prospective study using a multi-electrode ablation catheter, anti-arrhythmic drugs were continued, allowing hybrid therapy with right-sided ablation and anti-arrhythmic medication. More importantly, linear ablation in the left atrium has been combined with pulmonary vein isolation in many centres. Pappone et al. reported a significantly higher success rate with this combination of an ablative compartmentalisation approachwith trigger isolation in the left atrium, but anti-arrhythmic drugs were continued in many patients [7].

Atrial pacing as monotherapy alone has had very minimal efficacy in patients with AF with and without bradycardia. In clinical trials involving patients with bradycardia–tachycardia syndrome, a small reduction in the AF burden as well as limited reduction of frequency have been reported, but in most trials AF recurs without restoration of rhythm control in most patients [11–14]. A major limitation of ablation studies has been patient symptom-based reporting of AF recurrences. Recent studies show this to be highly unreliable and vastly underestimates AF events [15].

Definition of Hybrid Therapy

In view of these less than encouraging results, hybrid therapy of AF has been investigated by us and increasingly by other selected centres. These data will be discussed here together with the electrophysiological basis for this approach. The electrophysiological mechanisms of hybrid therapy efficacy are currently being examined, and the results of hybrid therapy will be discussed in subsequent sections. Hybrid therapy in its broadest sense is taken to be a combination of pharmacological and non-pharmacological therapies using anti-arrhythmic and non-anti-arrhythmic therapies to optimise and even individualise patient management.

Electrophysiological Mechanisms Underlying Efficacy

The electrophysiological mechanisms underlying different approaches to hybrid therapy are, of necessity, dissimilar. Thus, individual combination of pharmacological and non-pharmacological techniques may target specific mechanisms to achieve efficacy for an individual patient. The combination of anti-arrhythmic drugs and pacing, anti-arrhythmic drugs and catheter ablation, and the combination of all three approaches – drugs, pacing and ablation – need to be considered individually. There is a potential for significant synergy between these approaches, and it seems that for each therapy more than one anti-arrhythmic mechanism may be operative. Thus, while we can both hypothesise synergistic mechanisms and can document efficacy of the hybrid therapy prescription, dissecting the contribution of each of the components of hybrid therapy still remains a major challenge.

Anti-arrhythmic drugs are well known to suppress ectopic activity in the AF, prolonged atrial refractoriness, and reduced conduction velocity. The use of these drugs would contribute to reduce the AF burden by reducing AF triggers, in the form of ectopic activity or atrial or atrioventricular (AV) nodal tachycardias. Anti-arrhythmic drugs can retard intra-atrial conduction and prolonged atrial refractoriness, thus affecting the initiation of atrial reentrant tachycardias that trigger or maintain AF. They also produce conduction block in patients, which may be important in alteration of sites of conduction delay or interruption of a reentrant pathway. These mechanisms could reduce the frequency with which AF events are triggered or prevent the inscription of reentrant tachycardias at the initiation or during maintenance of AF. They can terminate AF by producing either conduction block in reentry circuits or expanding the window or excitable gap that could be penetrated by ectopic beats or other mechanisms for spontaneous AF termination. Thus, anti-arrhythmic drug trials rarely examine the ability to terminate or interrupt tachycardias except for spontaneous cardioversion of AF, which occurs in a proportion of patients with various forms of cardiac disease. Patients with advanced structural heart disease or heart failure are clearly more resistant to drug therapy.

Atrial pacing can suppress atrial triggers as well as alter the depolarisation of the atrial substrate, changing its vulnerability to AF. However, many of these tachycardias are unaffected by atrial triggers and the AF burden is not resolved by this mechanism. Dual-site atrial pacing and biatrial pacing has been shown to abbreviate P wave duration and also improve the haemodynamics of left-sided AV filling. In a sub-study of the DAPPAF study, left atrial filling of the left ventricle was improved with increased atrial jet velocity, as well as AV conduction being improved by reduction of AV conduction intervals [13, 14, 16]. However, in the absence of anti-arrhythmic drugs dual-site atrial pacing has not shown any meaningful clinical effect on time to symptomatic AF recurrence. The recurrence and frequency of atrial flutter and AF is generally minimally altered by atrial pacing alone despite increasing evidence that premature beats can be reduced. In the DAPPAF study and later in the ASPECT and ATTEST trials, atrial pacing alone did not prolong the time to the first recurrence of symptomatic AF, and the addition of AF termination therapies did not alter this outcome [17–19]. However, when combined with the class I or III anti-arrhythmic drugs, overdrive dual-site atrial pacing prolonged the time to the first symptomatic AF recurrence in the DAPPAF study [16]. Thus, we hypothesised that the combination of dual-site atrial pacing and anti-arrhythmic drug therapies may have electrophysiological effects on both focal triggers and the atrial conduction, as well as on the haemodynamics affecting the atrial substrate which may have favourable anti-arrhythmic effects.

Catheter ablation can isolate triggers or ablate triggers, as well as isolate critical areas of the atrium that may be necessary for AF. Catheter ablation has also been performed in patients with structural heart disease or patients with drug-refractory AF that has not responded to any other approach. [18] Results have been reported to be favourable, but more objective endpoint data are unavailable.

Atrial ablation can be combined with pacing to reduce the frequency of triggers and alter the substrate to make it less vulnerable to AF maintenance. Pacing, in particular dual-site atrial pacing, and ablation therapy (mainly right atrial ablation) have been combined by us for the treatment of drug-refractory AF. Our recent reports included 130 patients with paroxysmal, persistent, or permanent AF followed over 10 years, most of them having significant structural heart disease [18]. Most importantly, pacing and ablation therapy can supplement each other. The Maze procedure can help ablate right atrial flutters as well as compartmentalise the right atrial substrate. Better visualisation of linear ablation by new techniques of three-dimensional mapping permits more effective compartmentalisation and flutter ablation. These compartments can be resynchronised by multi-site atrial pacing and P-wave abbreviation is observed. Dual-site right atrial pacing when performed in this fashion not only serves to resynchronise the two atrial compartments, but also has a marked anti-arrhythmic effect by pacing on both sides of a linear radiofrequency lesion, which can be extremely anti-arrhythmic with respect to reentrant tachycardias around the incised lesion. It is our contention that these effects result in prevention of persistence of AF. This has been demonstrated in our pilot studies with device datalogues showing progressive elimination of persistent AF and later symptomatic paroxysmal AF [19]. Patients are usually left with brief asymptomatic salvoes of atrial tachycardia or AF that last a few seconds or a few minutes and have no clinical importance.

Effectiveness and Safety of Hybrid Therapy

Efficacy of Hybrid Therapy

The efficacy of hybrid therapy in a variety of patient populations has now become evident (Tables 1, 2). In early pilot studies from our group in drug-refractory paroxysmal AF, we noted prolongation of the time to first day of recurrence as well as restoration of rhythm control in a significant proportion of patients. Long-term data from our studies are now available and the patient population has been expanded to include patients with persistent and permanent AF, with and without structural heart disease, and patients in whom heart failure was present with advanced left ventricular dysfunction (Fig. 1). There were no differences in outcome based on coexisting brady-

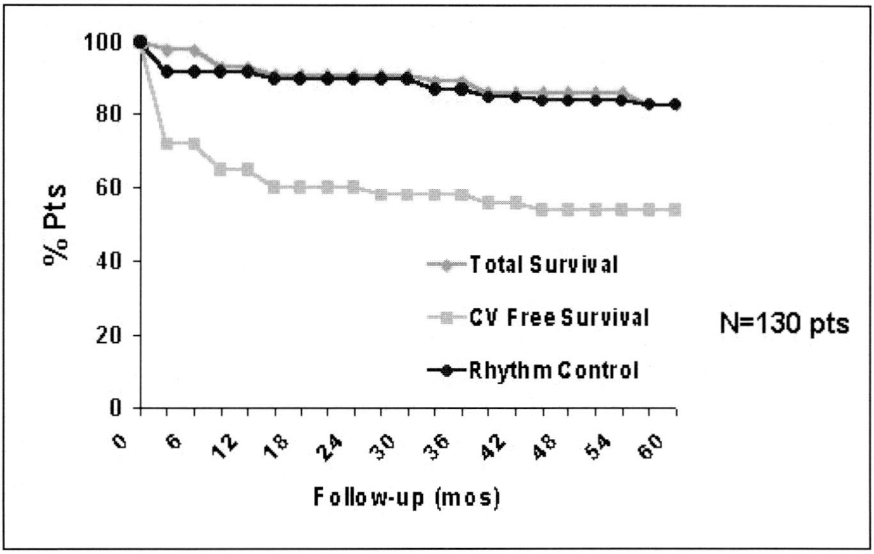

Fig. 1. Clinical outcome of a consecutive series of 130 consenting patients undergoing hybrid therapy of refractory atrial fibrillation enrolled over the period 1994-2002. Data is censored as of December 2003. *CV Free Survival* cardioversion free survival, *Rhythm control* maintenance of atrial paced or sinus rhythm with freedom from permanent AF

cardia (Fig. 2). These studies have been summarised in recent reports and will not be described in detail here [20, 21]. A tabulation of these studies is available in [21] and in Table 3. Pilot data have supported the use of this approach in even refractory permanent AF populations.

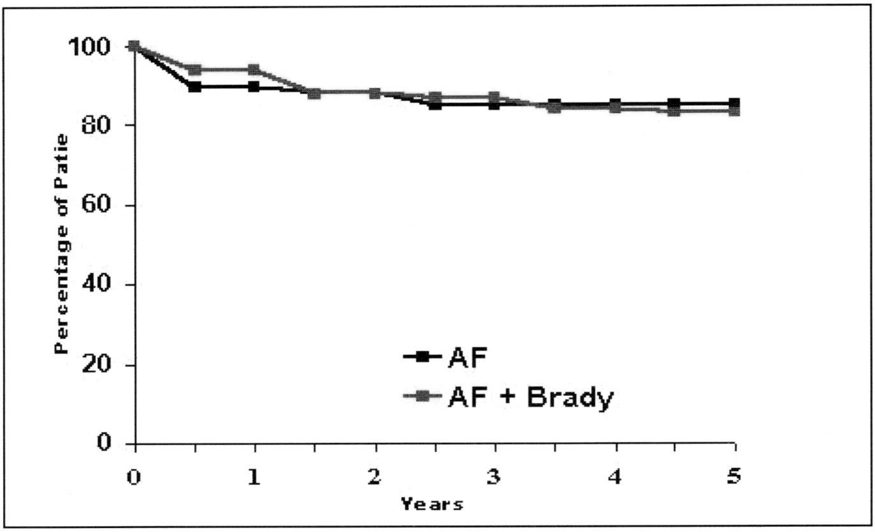

Fig. 2. Stratification of rhythm control endpoint based on the coexistence of a primary bradycardia indication for pacemaker implantation. Survival curve shows proportion of patients remaining in atrial paced or sinus rhythm free of permanent AF over an actuarial follow-up period up to five years (X axis) using a Kaplan Meier survival analysis. *AF* atrial fibrillation only, *AF + Brady* atrial fibrillation and a coexisting primary bradycardia

Table 1. Early clinical results with combination therapy: drug + ablation (data from [17])

Series	Ablation technique	Patients	Mean follow-up (months)	Rhythm control[a]	PV stenosis[b]
Garg	RA maze	PAF	12	56 (18)	None
Stabile	Tricuspid isthmus	PAF + CAF	24	58 (8)	None
Gerstenfeld	PVA	PAF 71	6	31 (23)	8.3 (angio)
Natale	PVA	PAF 293	10	86 (81)	11.5 (CT)
Kanagaratnam	PVI	PAF 71	29	83 (21)	36 (CT)
Natale	CUVA	PAF 30	12	80 (47)	3 (CT)

[a] Percentage (number) of patients
[b] Percentage of patients

Table 2. Early clinical results with combination therapy: drug + device (data from [17])

Series	Device technique	Patients	Mean follow-up (months)	% Rhythm control	% Complications
Metrix	Atrial ICD	186	9	84	6
Jewel AF	AV ICD	537	11 ±8	86	NA
Delfaut	Dual RA pacing	30	12	80	6
D'Allones	Biatrial pacing	86	33	64	15

ICD implantable cardioverter–defibrillator, *A-V* atrioventricular, *RA* right atrium, *NA* not available

Table 3. Hybrid therapy algorithms: drug + device + ablation

Series	Method	Patients	AF type	Follow-up (months)	Rhythm control
Saksena	DAP + AAD ± ABL	118	Parox/Persist	1–54 (20 ± 14)	93 pts (79%)
Prakash	DAP + AAD + TVI ABL	40	Parox AF ± A Flutter	5–56 (26 ± 14)	90% at 2 years
Saksena	DAP + AAD ± ABL ± CV	113	Parox (70)	1–81 (30 ± 23)	92% at 3 years
Filipecki	AP/ICD + RA Maze AAD	25	Persist/Perm	6–49 (17 ± 10)	75% at 18 months

DAP dual RA pacing, *AAD* anti-arrhythmic drug, *TVI* tricuspid isthmus, *ABL* ablation, *CV* cardioversion, *AP* atrial pacing, *ICD* implantable atrioventricular cardioverter-defibrillator, *Parox* paroxysmal, *Persist* persistent, *Perm* permanent, *pts* patients

Most recently we have reported on a consecutive series of patients with persistent and permanent AF in whom detailed biatrial and three-dimensional mapping was performed and hybrid therapy outcomes could be evaluated using electrogram-validated device datalogues. Rao et al. studied 47 patients with symptomatic persistent ($n = 26$) or permanent ($n = 21$) AF [22–24]. They underwent 'hybrid therapy' and were followed for 24 ± 15 months. All patients underwent linear right atrial ablation and implantation of a pacemaker or atrioventricular defibrillator capable of overdrive right atrial pacing together with therapy with previously ineffective anti-arrhythmic medication. Device datalogues were used to monitor AF recurrences (Fig. 3). Freedom from permanent AF was 97%, 90%, and 83% at 6 months and 2 and 3 years respectively. Sixteen patients (30%) had no AF recurrence after hybrid therapy. Thirty-one patients (66%) had a total of 55 AF recurrences (mean 1.8 per patient), usually in the first 6 months of therapy. These generally resolved, with 39 of the 47 patients (83%) achieving long-term rhythm control. There was a significant reduction in mean AF-related hospitalisations (from 3.5 ± 2.8 to 0.57 ± 1.1), cardioversion hospitalisations (from 3.5 ± 2.2 to 0.38 ± 0.5 per patient), and DC cardioversions (from 3.1 ± 3.9 to 0.7 ± 0.5 per patient) after hybrid therapy compared to event rates before therapy ($P < 0.05$ for all; Fig. 4). The authors concluded that hybrid therapy can establish rhythm control significantly in patients with persistent and permanent AF refractory to drugs and cardioversion therapy. This improvement is associated with a significant reduction in AF-related hospitalisations and need for cardioversion therapy.

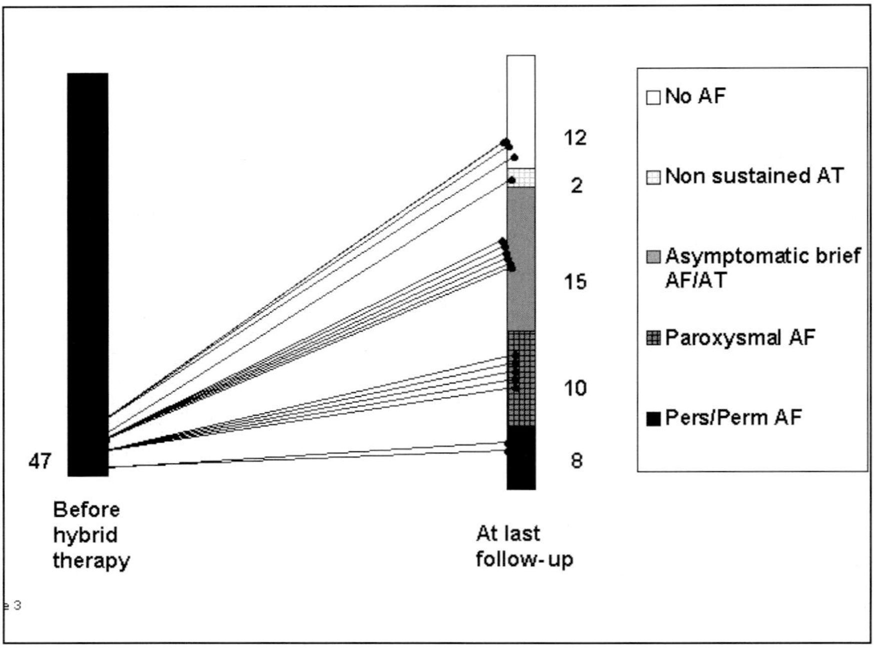

Fig. 3. Device datalogs with long term electrogram storage validating rhythm control in a cohort of patients with drug refractory persistent and permanent AF. The left panel shows the datalog electrograms showing classification of patient rhythm at initiation of hybrid therapy and the right panel shows the outcome after long term followup. *AF* atrial fibrillation, *AT* atrial tachycardia; numbers show patients in each category at end of followup

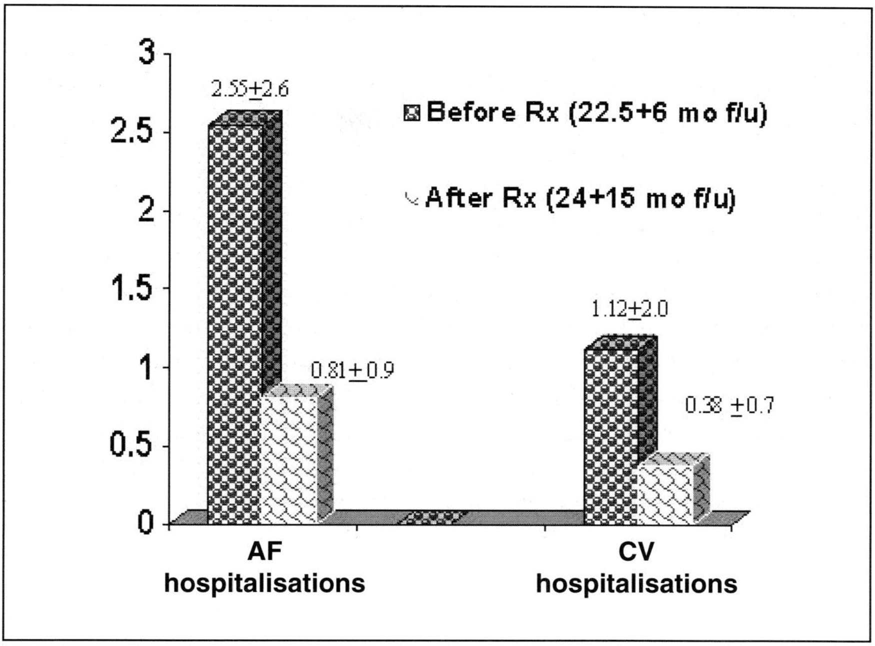

Fig. 4. Hospitalisations for atrial fibrillation and cardioversion before and after hybrid therapy. *AF* atrial fibrillation, *Cv* cardioversion, *Rx* hybrid therapy

Mechanisms of AF and Correlation with Hybrid Therapy Outcomes

For these unique patients in the study by Rao et al., biatrial mapping and AF mechanisms were available for analysis [22–24]. In the initial reported mapping data, we were able to demonstrate conclusively that biatrial mechanisms for AF were present in virtually all patients. Right atrial interventions in the form of linear ablation and dual- or single-site atrial pacing were the major form of hybrid therapy. In most patients, no targeted ablation of left atrial sites was undertaken. Yet over 80% of patients achieved excellent rhythm control. These data conclusively indicate that hybrid therapy can achieve rhythm control in refractory AF with biatrial involvement in AF.

Safety of Hybrid Therapy

Hybrid therapy has been proven safe in our long-term observational studies. There have been no procedural deaths or strokes. Complication rates average less than 2%. Long-term anti-coagulation has been withdrawn in over 25% of patients with device-documented freedom from AF for 1 year. The overall stroke incidence is 1.1% per patient year in our study population of 130 patients followed for an average of 5 years [25]. This is comparable to the stroke risk in an age-matched study population without AF.

Comparison with Therapeutic Alternatives

Alternative therapy approaches include left atrial interventions such as pulmonary vein isolation or focal ablation. There is little evidence that these offer superior rhythm control to hybrid therapy, and in fact survey data suggest much more modest efficacy [5, 6]. Long-term observational data show maintenance of efficacy based on objective device datalogues. Such data are still not available for left atrial interventions, with the usual endpoints used in ablation studies being increasingly put into question by device-based data [15]. Reports of the risks of left atrial ablation are now increasing, with major complication rates in excess of 5% [26–28]. These include mortality, stroke, symptomatic pulmonary stenosis, atrio-oesophageal fistula, etc. Hybrid therapy procedural complication rates are far lower in terms of major complications (< 2% in our experience), with no procedural deaths or stroke in over 10 years.

Finally, hybrid therapy offers ease of use, wider applicability, and shorter procedural times and radiation exposure than do prolonged ablation procedures. These advantages alone merit its use as a first line non-pharmacological alternative in refractory AF.

References

1. Wyse DG for the AFFIRM Investigators (2002) A comparison of rate control and rhythm control in patients with atrial fibrillation. N Engl J Med 347:1825–1833
2. Van Gelder IC, Hagens VE, Bosker HA et al (2002) Rate Control versus Electrical Cardioversion for Persistent Atrial Fibrillation Study Group. A comparison of rate control and rhythm control in patients with recurrent persistent atrial fibrillation. N Engl J Med 347:1834–1840
3. Carlsson J, Miketic S, Windeler J et al (2003) Randomized trial of rate-control versus rhythm-control in persistent atrial fibrillation: the Strategies of Treatment of Atrial Fibrillation (STAF) study. J Am Coll Cardiol 41:1690–1696[AQ11]
4. Haïssaguerre M, Jaïs P, Shah DC et al (1998) Spontaneous initiation of atrial fibrillation by ectopic beats originating in the pulmonary veins. N Engl J Med 339:659–666
5. Cappato R, Calkins H, Chen SA et al (2005) Worldwide survey on the methods, efficacy, and safety of catheter ablation for human atrial fibrillation. Circulation 111:1100–1105
6. Mickelsen S, Dudley B, Treat E et al (2005) Survey of physician experience, trends and outcomes with atrial fibrillation ablation. J Interv Card Electrophysiol 12:213–220
7. Pappone C, Rosanio S, Augello G et al (2003) Mortality, morbidity, and quality of life after circumferential pulmonary vein ablation for atrial fibrillation: outcomes from a controlled nonrandomized long-term study. J Am Coll Cardiol 42:185–197
8. Anonymous (2005) The CACAF Study. Late breaking clinical trials session, American College of Cardiology, Orlando, 6–9 March 2005

9. Garg A, Finneran W, Mollerus M et al (1999) Right atrial compartmentalization using radiofrequency catheter ablation for management of patients with refractory atrial fibrillation. Card Electrophysiol 10:763–771
10. Kocheril AG, Calkins H, Sharma AD et al (2005) Hybrid therapy with right atrial catheter ablation and previously ineffective antiarrhythmic drugs for the management of atrial fibrillation. J Interv Card Electrophysiol 12:189–197
11. Gillis AM, Wyse DG, Connolly SJ et al (1999) Atrial pacing periablation for prevention of paroxysmal atrial fibrillation. Circulation 99:2553–2558
12. Carlson MD, Ip J, Messenger J et al; Atrial Dynamic Overdrive Pacing Trial (ADOPT) Investigators (2003) A new pacemaker algorithm for the treatment of atrial fibrillation: results of the Atrial Dynamic Overdrive Pacing Trial (ADOPT). J Am Coll Cardiol 42:627–633
13. Padeletti L, Purerfellner H, Adler SW et al (2003) Worldwide ASPECT Investigators. Combined efficacy of atrial septal lead placement and atrial pacing algorithms for prevention of paroxysmal atrial tachyarrhythmia. J Cardiovasc Electrophysiol 14:1189–1195
14. Israel CW, Hugl B, Unterberg C et al (2001) Pace-termination and pacing for prevention of atrial tachyarrhythmias: results from a multicenter study with an implantable device for atrial therapy. J Cardiovasc Electrophysiol 12:1121–1128
15. Prakash A, Saksena S, Ziegler PD et al (2005) Dual site right atrial pacing can improve the impact of standard dual chamber pacing on atrial and ventricular mechanical function in patients with symptomatic atrial fibrillation: further observations from the dual site atrial pacing for prevention of atrial fibrillation trial. J Interv Card Electrophysiol 12:177–187
16. Saksena S, Prakash A, Ziegler P et al; DAPPAF Investigators (2002) Improved suppression of recurrent atrial fibrillation with dual-site right atrial pacing and antiarrhythmic drug therapy. J Am Coll Cardiol 40:1140–1150
17. Saksena S, Madan N (2003) Hybrid therapy of atrial fibrillation: algorithms and outcome. J Interv Card Electrophysiol 9:235–247
18. Hsu LF, Jaïs P, Sanders P et al (2004) Catheter ablation for atrial fibrillation in congestive heart failure. N Engl J Med 351:2373–2383
19. Saksena S, Mohammednia H, Madan N (2004) Long term outcome of hybrid therapy incorporating dual site right atrial pacing in patients with drug-refractory atrial fibrillation without primary bradyarrhythmias. Heart Rhythm 1:S271
20. Filipecki A, Saksena S, Lin WH (2003) Effectiveness of rhythm control in persistent or permanent atrial fibrillation with overdrive atrial pacing and antiarrhythmic drugs after linear right atrial catheter ablation. Am J Cardiol 92:1037–1044
21. Saksena S, Skadsberg ND, Rao HB et al (2005) Biatrial and three-dimensional mapping of spontaneous atrial arrhythmias in patients with refractory atrial fibrillation. J Cardiovasc Electrophysiol 16:494–504
22. Rao H, Saksena S, Mohammednia H (2004) Clinical efficacy and safety of linear right atrial ablation and implantable devices with atrial therapies for management of drug-refractory atrial fibrillation. Heart Rhythm 1:S209 (abs)
23. Rao H, Saksena S, Zaim S (2004) Arrhythmia recurrences and hospitalizations after hybrid therapy for rhythm control in drug-refractory persistent and permanent atrial fibrillation. Heart Rhythm 1:S146 (abs)
24. Madan N, Saksena S (2004) Long-term rhythm control of drug-refractory atrial fibrillation with 'hybrid therapy' incorporating dual-site right atrial pacing, antiarrhythmic drugs, and right atrial ablation. Am J Cardiol 93:569–975
25. Saad EB, Marrouche NF, Saad CP et al (2003) Pulmonary vein stenosis after cathe-

ter ablation of atrial fibrillation: emergence of a new clinical syndrome. Ann Intern Med 138:634–638

26. Nilsson B, Chen X, Pehrson S et al (2004) Acute fatal pulmonary vein occlusion after catheter ablation of atrial fibrillation. J Interv Card Electrophysiol 11:127–130
27. Pappone C, Oral H, Santinelli V et al (2004) Atrio-esophageal fistula as a complication of percutaneous transcatheter ablation of atrial fibrillation. Circulation 109:2724–2726
28. Madan N, Ibrahim E, Saksena S (2005) Withdrawal or maintenance of warfarin therapy guided by implantable device datalogs in patients with refractory atrial fibrillation: a novel application of device monitoring in recurrent atrial fibrillation. J Am Coll Cardiol 45:1079:249 (abs)

Atrial Fibrillation and Transcatheter Ablation: 'Ablate And Pace' or Pulmonary Veins Disconnection?

A. Proclemer[1], D. Pavoni[1], D. Facchin[1], M. Crosato[1], R. Ometto[1], M. Bonanno[2]

Introduction

Radiofrequency (RF) ablation of the atrioventricular node followed by pacemaker implantation, so-called ablate and pace (AP), is now a well-accepted therapy in patients with disabling or medically refractory atrial fibrillation (AF). This therapy is used in patients affected by both paroxysmal and chronic or persistent AF [1].

This review will consider first the intermediate and long-term outcomes of AP [2, 3], followed by a description of the pulmonary veins (PVs) electrical disconnection techniques, analysing in detail the immediate and intermediate outcomes and the possible complications.

Treatment of Atrial Fibrillation by Ablate and Pace

Fifteen years after its introduction into clinical practice, a substantial amount of data (long-term outcomes, identification of the best candidates for this therapy, short-term complications and those occurring during follow-up) on AP therapy for refractory AF have accumulated. The following is a synopsis of some representative studies based on large multicentre populations and meta-analyses.

Wood et al. [2] quantified the effects on the main clinical outcomes and survival with a large meta-analysis that included 21 AP studies comprising a total of 1181 patients, 97% with refractory AF and 3% with flutter or atrial tachycardia. The outcome analysis consisted of 642 patients who were enrolled in 15 studies and followed-up for a period of time that ranged from

[1]U.O. Cardiologia Ospedale S.M. Misericordia, Udine; [2]U.O. Cardiologia Ospedale S. Bortolo, Vicenza, Italy

48 days to 2.3 years. The mortality analysis included 1073 patients in 16 studies who were followed for 3 months to 2.3 years. The authors concluded that in patients with refractory atrial tachyarrhythmias AP therapy significantly decreased symptoms and the need for health care resources, while improving quality of life (QOL), ejection fraction, and exercise tolerance. Also, total and sudden mortality rates, (6.3%/year and 2%/year, respectively) were similar to, if not better than, those reported in other trials that included AF patients who did not undergo AP.

Gasparini et al. [3] reported similar results in a multicentre retrospective study that measured the long-term incidence of sudden death following treatment with AP. This study included 585 patients (mean age 66 years) with paroxysmal AF (n = 308) or chronic, symptomatic, refractory AF (n = 277), with associated organic heart disease in 71% of the patients. Mean follow up was 33.6 months; total mortality at 1 year was 4.88%, and sudden mortality 1.04% (predictive factors for these events were underlying heart disease and ejection fraction < 45%). The authors concluded that patients who had AP therapy for refractory atrial tachyarrhythmias had a lower risk of sudden death during follow-up. It was also noted that left ventricular dysfunction secondary to the underlying heart disease appeared to be the main predictive variable for such an event.

At the Mayo Clinic, Ozcan et al. [4] analysed a population of 350 consecutive patients (mean age 68 years) treated with AP between 1990 and 1998, and compared their survival to that of a subgroup of consecutive patients (mean age 67 years) treated pharmacologically for AF in the same institution, and with another subgroup (control) made up of Minnesota residents matched for age and gender. Mean follow up was 37 months and total mortality rate was 22%. The survival curve for the AP group was significantly worse than that of the control group (general population) ($P < 0.001$), while it was similar to that of the patients treated pharmacologically ($P = 0.044$). Factors predicting death, without which the observed survival would have been similar to that of the control population, were found to be history of previous myocardial infarction ($P < 0.001$), congestive heart failure ($P = 0.02$), and treatment with cardiac drugs after ablation ($P = 0.03$). Notwithstanding the limitation due to the retrospective nature of the study, the authors concluded that control of the ventricular rate and symptoms improvement in patients undergoing AP therapy did not influence negatively the prognosis and that AP was at least as safe as the traditional pharmacological treatment for AF.

Our study population consisted of 103 consecutive patients who underwent AP in our unit from January 1, 1994 to December 31, 1998 for atrial tachyarrhythmias (mean age 67 ±1 0 years; 45 males); 61% had a documented organic heart disease (14% ischaemic heart disease). At the time of the AP procedure, 13.6% of the patients were in NYHA III or IV functional class, and 14.6% had a ≤ 40% ejection fraction (EF). In terms of type of arrhythmia, AF was present in 81 patients (79%) – paroxysmal in 23%, and chronic in 56% of these patients. The indications for AP in the remaining 22 patients (21%) were atypical atrial flutter or atrial tachycardia (Table 1). Mean follow-up was 56 ± 23 months - one patient with valvular heart disease and EF 40%, experienced sudden death 17 months after AF. During follow-up, the study population showed a gradual and persistent clinical improvement; only 4.8% of the patients were in NYHA III or IV functional class at the last follow-up (Table 2, Fig. 1).

Table 1. Clinical characteristics at the moment of enrolment, of patients with atrial tachyarrhythmias treated with Ablate and Pace in Udine and Vicenza hospitals between 1994 and 1998

	Total patients (n = 103)	Alive patients (n = 86)	Dead patients (n = 17)
Sex			
Male	57	47	10
Female	83	70	13
Age when treated (years)	67 ± 10	66 ± 10	71 ± 9
Ischaemic heart disease	18	15	3
Dilated cardiomyopathy	20	13	7
Valvular heart disease	29	25	4
Hypertension	14	11	3
Hypertrophic cardiomyopathy	4	4	0
Congenital heart disease	2	2	0
No heart disease	53	47	6
Ejection fraction			
> 50%	88	80	8
40–50%	29	19	10
< 40%	33	18	5
NYHA class			
I	91	75	16
II	35	30	5
III	12	10	2
IV	2	2	0
Type of arrhythmia			
Paroxysmal atrial fibrillation	47	43	4
Chronic atrial fibrillation	57	43	14
Paroxysmal atrial flutter	14	12	2
Chronic atrial flutter	2	2	0
Paroxysmal atrial tachycardia	6	5	1
Sinus dysfunction	14	12	2
No. antiarrhythmic drugs	2.3 ± 2.0	2.5 ± 2.1	1.8 ± 1.4
Implanted PM type			
VVIR	74	56	18
DDDR	66	61	5

Table 2. Events during the follow-up period in patients with atrial tachyarrhythmias treated with Ablate and Pace in Udine and Vicenza hospitals between 1994 and 1998

	Total patients (n = 103)	Alive patients (n = 86)	Dead patients (n = 17)
Follow-up (months)	56 ± 23	55 ± 22	27 ± 18
Mortality (months from treatment)	27 ± 16		27 ± 16
Cause of death			
Heart failure	2		2
Sudden death	1		1
Other	9		9
Unknown	11		11
Ventricular fibrillation	2	1	-
Admission for heart failure	21	18	3
Heart transplantation	3	3	-
NYHA class			
I	80	68	12
II	18	14	4
III	5	4	1
IV	0	0	0
Drugs			
Oral anticoagulant (OA)	73	60	13
Antiaggregation (AG)	16	16	0
No therapy AO/AG	14	10	4

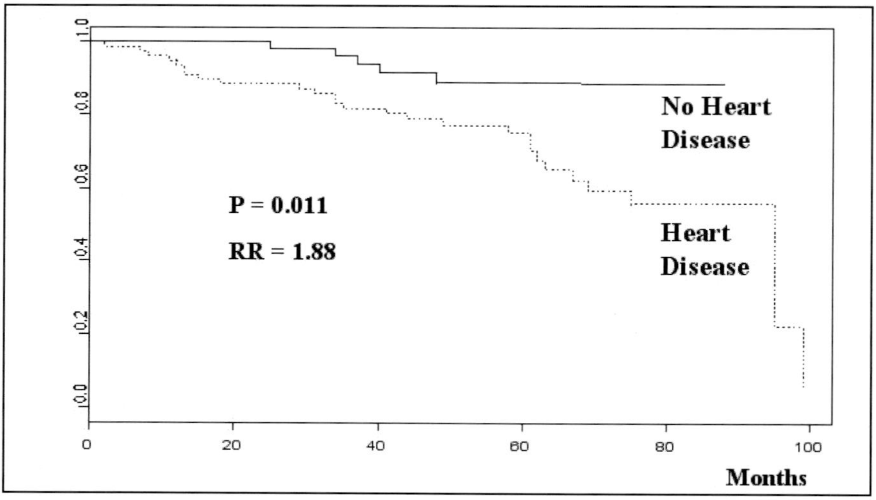

Fig. 1. Event-free survival from total mortality, cardiac arrest, heart failure in patients with or without heart disease after Ablate and Pace

Comments on the AP Therapy

As demonstrated by observational and randomised studies [3, 5–7] and a recent meta-analysis [2], AP therapy in patients with highly symptomatic or medically refractory AF results in significant short-term and medium-term improvement of the QOL main indicators, a reduction in hospital admissions, a decrease in AF-related symptoms, an increase in left ventricular function, especially in patients with reduced EF, and an increased exercise tolerance [1, 8]. These results are likely due to heart rate control and normalisation with the PM and, probably, to the reduction of the negative effects of the cardioactive drugs, such as the proarrhythmic or negative inotropic ones. In analysing the results obtained with AP therapy, it should be noted that the majority of patients presented with a major heart disease, decreased left ventricular function, a clearly enlarged left atrium, and advanced age (mean 65–70 years).

There are, however, some negative aspects to be considered, such as lifelong dependency on the PM, the nonphysiologic, electrically induced cardiac activation (right ventricular apical pre-excitation), and both the absence of preventive effects in terms of paroxysmal AF attacks and the evolution toward chronic AF due to the commonly used PMs without dedicate pacing algorithms. Moreover, a recent sub-analysis of the PA study [4] showed a significant increase in AF burden after AP therapy in patients with paroxysmal AF in spite of continued antiarrhythmic pharmacological therapy [9]. This increase has been attributed to the loss of AV and/or interventricular synchronism and to the subsequent increase in atrial wall stress, and to a neuroendocrine negative balance. Also, this study observed a slight reduction in fractional shortening in patient with a baseline value > 30% (from 39.4 to 36.4%), while in subjects with baseline values ≤ 30% before AP therapy this parameter registered a significant increase (from 27 to 33.6%).

Patients with idiopatic tachyarrhythmias showed favourable survival rates compared to those with congestive heart failure, previous myocardial infarction and need for cardioactive drug therapy. Mortality in this group of patients was, however, comparable to that of subjects with less severe AF treated only with pharmacological therapy.

The rate of sudden death seemed to be rather low both in the short-term and long-term, and mostly due to the underlying heart disease rather than the AP procedure.

In our study, the results obtained with AP remain favourable even in the long-term (mean follow-up 52 months), as demonstrated by a persistently good functional class in most of the patients and the reduced number of admissions for heart failure. The long-term complications due to cardiac pacing appear to be negligible.

Electrical Isolation/Disconnection of the Pulmonary Veins

The evidence that paroxysmal AF (PAF) in patients without heart disease or with minor structural alterations, originates, most of the time, in the PVs has opened a new era in the non-pharmacological treatment of AF [10, 11]. Increasingly numerous studies have shown that PAF attacks can be eliminated by suppressing the extra-systolic atrial triggers by RF ablation inside the PVs or by disconnecting these veins electrically by RF at the atriopulmonary junction [10, 11]. In the first case, the procedures were characterised by very long mapping times and a noticeable rate of PV stenosis, whereas in the second case the main endpoint used was the empirical elimination of all the electrical potentials inside each PV, obtained primarily during sinus rhythm or during right ventricle and coronary sinus pacing [12–15]. At the present, this procedure, defined as electrical disconnection of the PVs, is considered the most effective because it blocks, both at the entrance and at the exit, the venous impulses that could be responsible for the initiation and persistence of the AF.

Several mechanisms have been hypothesised to explain the clinical effectiveness of the electrical disconnection [16]: (1) formation of a complete, total-depth circumferential lesion with interruption of the veno-atrial connecting muscle; (2) partial damage of the veno-atrial junction fibres to make both the activation, due to an intra-venous arrhythmogenic focus, and its propagation to the adjacent atrial muscle more difficult; (3) interruption at the junction level of the re-entry pathways that initiate or maintain AF; (4) interruption of the rotors or other arrhythmogenic foci located in the left atrial posterior wall; (5) interruption/modification of the fibres and parasympathetic ganglia situated at the PV ostia, considered decisive in the AF pathogenesis in apparently healthy hearts [17]. The presumption is that the achievement of points 3 and 4 is the reason for the operative successes reported with peri-venous circumferential ablation techniques performed on larger areas.

Short-Term Results

In patients with PAF, the rate of clinical success with RF ablation aimed at atriopulmonary junction electrical disconnection varied between 60 and 80% according to the data reported by the most important laboratories (Table 3). Often, however, it is necessary to perform multiple procedures for late AF recurrences, which occur in 6–54% of patients after 30–60 days from the first procedure. Early recurrences could be due to a local, transitory pro-arrhythmic irritation. In 10% of patients with late recurrences, there can be an improvement of symptoms by using anti-arrhythmic drugs previously considered ineffective. In this case, the class 1C drugs best extend the RF ablation effectiveness, because, acting on the sodium channels, they decrease even further the already compromised conduction at the atriopulmonary junction and modify favourably the atrial substrate.

In a small number of patients it is also necessary to eliminate arrhythmogenic foci located outside the PVs. In 4–11% of such cases triggers can be found inside the superior vena cava, while in an other 10–15% AF can originate in the coronary sinus, near the crista terminalis in the right atrial posterior wall or in Marshall's vein. The electrical isolation of these structures increases the ablation efficacy by another 10–20% [18]. It must be remembered that most of the patients treated had idiopathic AF, preserved left ventricular function, and left atrial dimension at the upper limits of normal or only slightly elevated.

In patients with persistent or permanent AF, PV disconnection alone resulted in a significantly lower rates of success (40%) [13, 14]. In these cases, the complexities of the anatomofunctional substrate required the creation of other lesion lines to reduce the critical electrical mass. Additional lines between the lateral mitral ring and the left inferior PV or between the right superior and the left superior PVs, in concomitance with RF delivery inside the coronary sinus to obtain a conduction block at the level of the lateral mitral isthmus, can increase the rate of success to 60–80% depending on the study and the use of anti-arrhythmic drugs.

The Mayo Clinic group analysed the clinical-instrumental factors capable of predicting the efficacy of the PV electrical disconnection [19]. Paroxysmal

Table 3. Outcomes of ablation of paroxysmal atrial fibrillation

Author	N. of patients	No AA drugs N°	No AA drugs %	AA drugs N°	AA drugs %	Follow-up (months)
Haïssaguerre [10]	45	28	62	NA	NA	8 ± 6
Chen [11]	79	68	86	10	13	6 ± 2
Pappone [14]	179/251	148	83	4	2	10 ± 5
Gerstenfeld	41	29	70	6	15	9 ± 2
Macle/Haïssaguerre	136	90	66	20	15	9 ± 5
Marrouche	102/190	96	94	4	4	9 ± 3
Oral/Morady	58/70	41	70	NA	NA	5 ± 3
Magrum/Haines	64	42	66	NA	NA	13 ± 7
Deisenhofer	75	38	51	NA	NA	230 ± 133
Packer [19]	203	104	70	15	10	15 ± 5

AA Anti-arrhythmic

AF, AF duration, the adjunctive creation of the conduction block at the cavotricuspid isthmus level, the use of intracardiac echography and, to a lesser degree, the normal size of the left ventricle were all associated, in a univariate analysis, with significant control of AF recurrences.

The success of the electrical disconnection, however, must take into account the risk of complications related to the procedure [10–20]. These include PV stenosis, with an incidence of between 2 and 40% depending on the various experiences and the severity of the disease, cardiac tamponade (1–3%), damage to the phrenic nerve (1.2%), cerebral emboli (1–3%), and severe bradycardia (1%). The rate strictly dependent on the experience of each centre, and on the techniques used (cooled-tip catheters, RF delivery outside the PV ostium, nonfluoroscopic mapping systems, intracardiac echography). Intracardiac echography allows real-time monitoring of the position of the ablating and mapping catheters, and of the formation of microbubbles indicating parietal damage.

Intermediate-Term Results

A clear evaluation of the clinical efficacy of PV electrical disconnection as a definite treatment requires studies that compare this approach to the best pharmacological, electrical, and traditional ablative (AP) therapies. At present, only few studies have done so. Pappone et al. [20] compared the clinical outcomes of 589 patients undergoing circumferential PV ablation with electro-anatomic mapping to those of 582 patients treated with drugs. The subjects in the first group showed a higher survival rate, a decrease in co-morbidities such as cardiac insufficiency and cerebrovascular accidents, and a reduction in recurring AF. An improvement in QOL was also observed in a subgroup treated with ablation, a finding also confirmed by a recent experience at the Mayo Clinic.

Most authors, however, still feel the need for a large-scale validation of the ablation therapy and an evaluation of its economic impact.

Conclusions

At present, AP therapy in patients with paroxysmal or permanent drug refractory AF constitutes a valid alternative in the presence of major heart disease, advanced age (> 70 years), significant left atrial dilatation, important co-morbidities, and patient's preference. The high short-term success rates (95–100%), low complication rates, low incidence of sudden death (< 2%/year), the favourable comparison with a matching population, and the positive data regarding improvement in QOL suggest the validity of this therapeutic strategy in specific subgroups of patients [21].

Therapy based on PV electrical disconnection and RF suppression of extravenous arrythmogenic foci is undoubtedly a fascinating solution from the physiopathologic viewpoint. The short-term result obtained in selected patients with idiopathic AF or minor heart disease look promising, even if limited to high-level laboratories dedicated to such therapy. There is a need for randomised studies to rigorously evaluate the long-term effects of this therapy.

References

1. Kay GN, Ellenbogen KA, Giudici M (1998) The ablate and pace trial: a prospective study of catheter ablation of the AV conduction system and permanent pacemaker implantation for treatment of atrial fibrillation. J Interv Card Electrophysiol 2:121–135
2. Wood MA, Brown-Mahoney C, Kay GN et al (2000) Clinical outcomes after ablation and pacing therapy for atrial fibrillation. Circulation 101:1138–1144
3. Gasparini M, Mantica M, Brignole M et al (2000) Long-term follow-up after atrioventricular nodal ablation and pacing. PACE 23:1925–1929
4. Ozcan C, Jahangir A, Friedman PA (2001) Long-term survival after ablation of the atrioventricular node and implantation of a permanent pacemaker in patients with atrial fibrillation. N Engl J Med 344:1043–1051
5. Brignole M (2000) Ablate and pace: palliating the symptoms? Am J Cardiol 86:K4–K8
6. Brignole M, Gammage M, Jordaens L et al (1999) Report of a study group on ablate and pace therapy for paroxismal atrial fibrillation. Europace 1:8–13
7. Brignole M, Gianfranchi L, Menozzi C et al (1997) Assessment of atrioventricular junction ablation and DDDR mode-switching pacemaker versus pharmacological treatment in patients with severely symptomatic paroxysmal atrial fibrillation: a randomized controlled study. Circulation 96:2617–2624
8. Touboul P (1999) Atrioventricular nodal ablation and pacemaker implantation in patients with atrial fibrillation. Am J Cardiol 83:241D–245D
9. Willems R, Wise G, Gillis AM et al (2003) Total atrioventricular nodal ablation increases atrial fibrillation burden in patients with paroxysmal atrial fibrillation despite continuation of antiarrhythmic drug therapy. J Cardiovasc Electrophysiol 14:1296–1301
10. Haïssaguerre M, Shah D.C, Takahashi A et al (1998) Spontaneous initiation of atrial fibrillation by ectopic beats originating in the pulmonary veins. N Eng J Med 339:659–666
11. Chen SA, Tai CT, Tsai CF et al (1999) Initiation of atrial fibrillation by ectopic beats originating in the pulmonary veins. electrophysiological characteristics, pharmacological responses and effects of radiofrequency ablation. Circulation 100:1879–1886
12. Haïssaguerre M, Shah DC, Garrigue S et al (2000) Electrophysiological end point for catheter ablation of atrial fibrillation initiated from multiple pulmonary venous foci. Circulation 101:1409–1417
13. Haïssaguerre M, Shah DC, Arentz T et al (2000) Catheter ablation of chronic atrial fibrillation targeting the reinitiating triggers. J Cardiovasc Electrophysiol 11:2–10

14. Pappone C, Rosanio S, Vicedomini G et al (2001) Atrial electroanatomic remodelling after circumferential radiofrequency pulmonary vein ablation. Efficacy of an anatomic approach in a large cohort of patients with atrial fibrillation. Circulation 104:2539–2544
15. Oral H, Tada H, Ozaydin M et al (2002) Pulmonary vein isolation for paroxysmal and persistent atrial fibrillation. Circulation 105:1077–1081
16. Packer DL, Asirvatham S, Munger TM (2003) Progress in nonpharmacologic therapy of atrial fibrillation. J Cardiovasc Electrophysiol 14:S296–S309
17. Schauerte P, Scherlag BJ, Patterson E et al (2001) Focal atrial fibrillation: experimental evidence for a pathophysiologic role of the autonomic nervous system. J Cardiovasc Electrophysiol 12:592–599
18. Lin WS, Tai CT, Hsieh MH et al (2003) Catheter ablation of paroxysmal atrial fibrillation initiated by non-pulmonary vein ectopy. Circulation 107:3176–3183
19. Packer DL, Monahan KH, Peterson LA et al (2003) Predictors of successful atrial fibrillation ablation through pulmonary vein isolation. Pacing Clin Electrophysiol 26(Pt II):962
20. Pappone C, Rosanio S, Augello G et al (2003) Mortality, morbidity, and quality of life after circumferential pulmonary vein ablation for atrial fibrillation. J Am Coll Cardiol 42:185–197
21. Proclemer A, Della Bella P, Tondo C et al (1999) Radiofrequency ablation of atrioventricular junction and pacemaker implantation versus modulation of atrioventricular conduction in drug refractory atrial fibrillation. Am J Cardiol 83(10):1437-1442

HEREDITARY ARRHYTHMOGENIC SYNDROMES

Fever and Other Precipitants of Ventricular Arrhythmias in Brugada Syndrome: Do We Know How They Act?

F. Naccarella[1], C. Liying[2,5], L. ShuZheng[2], S. Sdringola Maranga[3], G. Lepera[1], F. Iachetti[1], G. Naccarelli[4], D. Corrado[6], A. Rampazzo[6], A. Nava[6], C. Felicani[1], S. Depadoa[1]

Introduction

More than 90% of sudden cardiac deaths (SCD) occur in patients with a known or previously unrecognised pre-existing coronary artery disease (CAD) or cardiomyopathy. It has become evident that SCD occurs, with sufficient frequency, in patients with an apparently normal heart, and ventricular fibrillation (VF) may represent the first clinical sign of structural heart disease that becomes manifest, only several years later, among survivors. Different causes of SCD have been documented, mainly by genetic screening and a more accurate clinical evaluation of the group of patients suffering from so-called idiopathic VF (IVF) [1–26].

Brugada syndrome [1, 5, 10, 14–16, 21–25] has been clearly shown to be one of the most frequent causes of SCD in this context, and should be differentiated from other clinical conditions or cardiac diseases [7, 13, 19, 20, 22, 26]. The purpose of the present article is: (1) to clarify the ionic alterations and electrophysiological mechanisms, underlying Brugada syndrome; (2) to verify the importance of triggering factors detected by ECG and clinical events; (3) discuss the long-term outcomes of Brugada syndrome patients and their family members.

[1]Cardiology Department, Azienda USL Città di Bologna, Bologna, Italy; [2]Cardiology Department, An Zhen Hospital, Beijing, China; [3]Cardiology Division, Hermann Memorial Hospital, Houston, TX USA; [4]NASPE-Heart Rhythm Association International Fellowship, Bologna, Italy; [5]Hershey Medical School, Hershey, PA, USA; [6]Istituto di Cardiologia, Facoltà di Medicina, Università di Padova, Padua, Italy

From Idiopathic Ventricular Fibrillation to Different Genetically Determined Arrhythmic Syndromes

The 1997 Consensus conference clearly defined the diagnostic requirements, – non-invasive and invasive, mandatory, highly recommended or elective – to evaluate patients surviving a cardiac arrest and their family members. In the wide group of IVF patients, Brugada syndrome is, today, clearly identifiable [1, 5, 10, 14–16, 21–25]. Importantly, confounding factor/s, that could account for the ECG abnormality or syncope should be carefully excluded, including atypical right bundle-branch block, left ventricular hypertrophy, early repolarisation, acute pericarditis, acute myocardial ischaemia/infarction, pulmonary embolism, Prinzmetal angina, dissecting aortic aneurysm, various central and autonomic nervous system abnormalities, Duchenne muscular dystrophy, thiamine deficiency, hyperkalaemia, hypercalcaemia, ARVDC, *pectus excavatum*, hypothermia, and mechanical compression of the right ventricular outflow tract (RVOT), such as occurs in mediastinal tumours or haemopericardium [1, 5, 10, 14–16, 21–25].

Brugada syndrome is inherited via an autosomal dominant mode of transmission. The first and only gene to be linked to Brugada syndrome is SCN5A, which encodes the alpha subunits of the sodium-channel. More than 80 mutations in SCN5A have been found, and more than 24 of them result in loss of function due to: failure of the sodium channel to express a shift in the voltage and time dependence of sodium channel current activation, inactivation, or reactivation; entry of the sodium channel into an intermediate state of inactivation from which it recovers more slowly; or accelerated inactivation of the sodium channel [5, 10]. A higher incidence of SCN5A mutations has been reported in familial than in sporadic cases [5, 10, 23–25].

A second locus on chromosome 3, close to but distinct from the SCN5A locus, was recently found and is associated with a relative benign prognosis. SCN5A mutations account for 18–30% of Brugada syndrome cases, implying that, in the remaining cases, mutations in other genes cause the disease.

Antzelevitch made the most important contribution to the understanding of the ionic changes in Brugada syndrome. Ventricular epicardial and M-cell, but not endocardial cell, action potentials display a large phase 1, due to the presence of a predominant transient outward current (I_{to}), giving rise to a spike-and-dome or notched configuration of the action potential. Important differences also exist in the magnitude of I_{to} between right and left ventricular epicardial and M-cells, with right ventricular cells displaying a much greater I_{to}. These transmural ion channel distinctions lead to a differential response of the epicardium and endocardium to sodium channel block, I_{KATP} activation, and hypercalcaemia. Heterogeneous loss of the action potential dome, within epicardium and between epicardium and endocardium, accentuates local epicardial as well as transmural dispersion of repolarisation, thus creating a vulnerable window within the epicardium and across the ventricular wall [5, 6–9, 10].

The ECG J-wave, or Osborn-wave, has long been recognised as pathognomonic of hypothermia or hypercalcaemia [4, 8]. In fact, the decrease in temperature has been shown to accentuate this transmural voltage gradient, thus increasing the amplitude of the J-wave. This effect is due to differences in the Q_{10} for the kinetics of I_{Ca} and I_{to}. A greater cooling induces a more evident slowing of I_{Ca} activation or I_{to} activation. Similarly, in Brugada syndrome, I_{KATP} activation or inhibition of I_{Na} and I_{Ca} are involved, resulting in a markedly abbreviated response in some areas of the epicardium [4–9]. Agents that block I_{to}, such as quinidine, restore the epicardial action potential and normalise the ST segment. Furthermore, a lower density of I_{to} in the female heart has been shown. This correlates with a lower propensity of female hearts to develop Brugada syndrome, despite equal transmission of the mutation in both sexes [5, 7].

Conversely, it has been demonstrated that premature inactivation of the sodium channel due to SCN5A mutation is a function of body temperature. Thus, several authors have suggested that a febrile condition could unmask Brugada syndrome and precipitate serious arrhythmic events [5, 7, 17].

Drugs Affecting STT Pattern and Mimicking Brugada Syndrome

Several drugs are able to induce Brugada-like ECG patterns, and discontinuation of these drugs is associated with reversal of the previously observed pattern. Even shortly after a direct current cardioversion, a Brugada-like pattern has been observed for several hours. The largest experience has been obtained with sodium channel blockers, which are used also as a provocative test [5, 21], and with psychotropic drugs, mainly tricyclic antidepressants [5, 18], which should be carefully administered and accurately monitored. At present time, it is not known whether some individuals are gene carriers for Brugada syndrome. Thus, the following families of drug should be carefully used:

1. Antiarrhythmic drugs, mainly sodium channel blockers, such as class IC drugs (flecainide, pilsicainide, propafenone), class IA drugs (ajmaline, procainamide, disopyramide, cibenzoline), calcium channel blockers (verapamil), beta-blockers (propranolol mainly, but also the others at toxic doses).
2. Antianginal drugs, such as calcium channel blockers (nifedipine, diltiazem, etc.), nitrates (isosorbide dinitrate, nitroglycerine), potassium channel openers (nicorandil and other analogues).

3. Psychotropic drugs, such as tricyclic antidepressant (amitriptyline, nortriptyline, desipramine, clomipramine and analogues), tetracyclic antidepressant (maprotiline), phenotiazine (perphenazine, cyamemazine), selective serotonin reuptake inhibitors (fluoxetine).
4. Other drugs, such as dimenhydrinate, cocaine, alcohol intoxication.

Factors Triggering of Arrhythmic Events

The ECG manifestations of congenital Brugada syndrome are often concealed, but can be unmasked or modulated by sodium channel blockers, a febrile state, vagotonic agents, vagotonic manoeuvres, and several other stimuli. Moreover, alpha-adrenergic agonists, beta-adrenergic blockers, tricyclic or tetracyclic antidepressants, a combination of glucose and insulin, hyperkalaemia, hypokalaemia, hypercalcaemia, alone or in combination, can be responsible as triggering factors (TF) of arrhythmic events. Alcohol and cocaine toxicity has been reported as a TF [5]. These agents may also induce acquired forms of Brugada syndrome. Superimposed acute myocardial ischaemia can mimic ST-segment elevation similar to that in Brugada syndrome. This effect is due to a depression of the calcium channel current (I_{Ca}) and activation of the ATP-sensitive potassium channel current (I_{KATP}) during ischaemia. This suggests that patients with congenital and acquired forms of Brugada syndrome are at higher risk for ischaemia-related SCD (5). VF and SCD [5] usually occur at rest, post-exercise, and at night, as confirmed by the circadian pattern of 64 VF episodes in 19 sudden unexplained nocturnal death syndrome (SUNDS) patients treated with ICDs. Circadian variation of sympathovagal balance hormones and other metabolic factors are likely to contribute to this circadian pattern. Bradycardia, resulting from altered autonomic balance, drugs, or an association of factors may contribute to the initiation of arrhythmias in these subjects, in whom a myocardial presynaptic sympathetic dysfunction has been demonstrated. Even the RVOT could be similarly affected by a sympathovagal imbalance, as shown by the difficulty in demonstrating local innervation in these areas or by the presence of localised zones of primary or secondary myocardial dysfunction (Figs. 1, 2).

Hypokalaemia has been implicated as a contributing factor in Brugada syndrome, mainly in Asia, specifically Thailand, where potassium deficiency is endemic. Furthermore, it was noted that many SUNDS victims had consumed large meals of glutinous (sticky) rice or carbohydrates for dinner before the night of death. In fact, glucose and insulin infusion could unmask the Brugada ECG.

Furthermore, Dumaine and other authors demonstrated that sodium channel inactivation can be observed with both low (< 30°C) and high

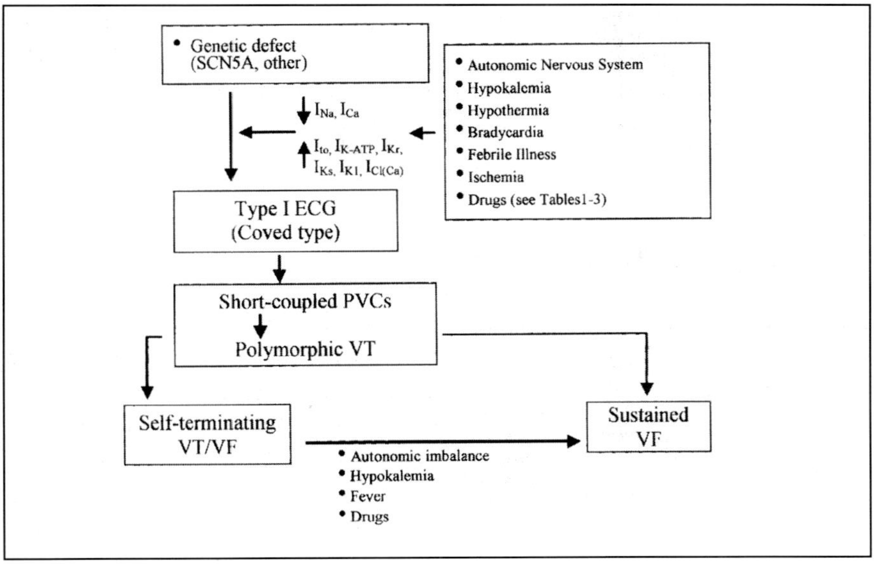

Fig. 1. Predisposing factors for ECG and arrhythmic manifestations of Brugada syndrome (modified from [5])

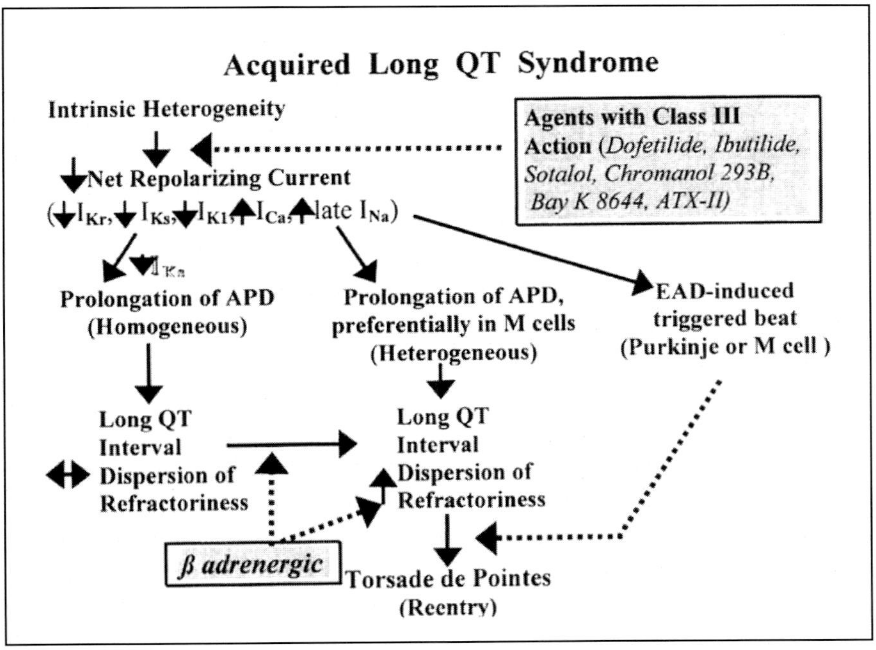

Fig. 2. Predisposing factors for ECG and arrhythmic manifestations of acquired vs congenital long QT and other catecholaminergic arrhythmic syndromes (modified from [27])

Table 1. Brugada syndrome: predisposing factors and prognostic outcomes (modified from Behlassen)

Aggravating factors:	
	Sodium channels blockers (flecainide > ajmaline > procainamide)
	Increased vagal tone (night time) or post-exercise, post-emotional, during venous puncture increased vagal tone
	Extreme beta-adrenergic blockade
	Hypercalcaemia, hypokalaemia and association of:
	Gender-related unknown or partially known factors (a more prominent Ito in men vs women
	General anaesthesia and surgery
	Tricyclic antidepressant
	Other drugs
	Fever (accelerated inactivation of sodium channels)
	Strong family history of sudden death
	Coved-type pattern in the rest ECG
	Syncopal episodes
	Racial factor?
Improving factors:	
	Moderate non-competitive exercise
	Beta-adrenergic stimulation (non-clinically useful)
	Demonstrated quinidine sulfate administration in any given patient
	No family history of sudden death
	Saddleback-type pattern in the rest ECG

(> 38°C) temperatures. While in humans severe hypothermia is rare, febrile states are very frequent and could unmask Brugada syndrome and precipitate VF. Even hot baths and hot climates, as in North-Eastern Thailand, have been claimed as precipitating factors [5].

Risk Stratification and Outcomes

Risk stratification is still the most important goal of Brugada syndrome researchers worldwide [1–5, 23–26]. Patients initially presenting with aborted SD, are at the highest risk for a recurrence (from 69% at 54 ± 54 months of observation of Brugada syndrome symptoms [5] to 26% at 22 ± 24 months, as in our own patient population) [26].

Patients presenting with syncope and a spontaneously appearing type-1 ECG have a recurrence rate of 19% at 26 ± 36 months of follow-up. An 8% occurrence of cardiac events was observed in initially asymptomatic patients. Priori presented different data [5] in a less selected patient population, as did Eckardt recently [23]. Our data are more similar to those of Brugada, since probably a more selected population was followed-up, including many families with a striking evidence of cardiac arrest and SCD occurring early in life [25].

Asymptomatic patients, at highest risk are most likely those who show type 1 ECG spontaneously, those with syncope, those with the coved type versus the saddleback type of ST-segment elevation, and those with a family history of cardiac arrest.

Combined ECG markers such as the width of the S-wave and ST-segment elevation magnitude, may be helpful in risk stratification. Other groups showed that combined ST-segment elevation and the presence of late potentials could be diagnostically useful, but the value of these combined markers remains to be tested in a prospective fashion. Data from Brugada, Corrado, and our group (Tables 2, 3) suggest that, both among symptomatic and asymptomatic patients, the inducibility of VT/VF during programmed electrical stimulation (PES) may forecast risk. However, Priori and Eckardt did not find an association between inducibility and recurrence of VT/VF [5, 23]. These differences could be due to selection bias of isolated cases versus cases with a family distribution and to non-comparable stimulation protocols.

Conclusions

In conclusion, patients at the highest risk are those who already experienced aborted SCD and those with a spontaneously abnormal type 1 ECG, even without syncope but mainly those with true syncope [1, 5, 23, 26].

Men have a 5.5-fold higher risk of SCD than women [1, 5, 23, 25]. Furthermore, recent information confirmed that a negative family history does not exclude the risk of SCD [5], while patients with an evident family distribution of SCD seem to be at higher risk [5, 24, 25].

Many old and new drugs should be avoided in Brugada patients, while patients on these therapies who show a Brugada-like ECG should be carefully evaluated and monitored.

Electrolytes imbalance should be monitored and general anaesthesia should be performed under strict control during surgery in these subjects [16].

Vagal manoeuvres, vagal stimuli, and bradycardia itself could be TF of serious events distinct from other arrhythmic syndromes, such as some forms of congenital or acquired long QT syndromes [7]; short QT syndrome [19]; familial polymorphic ventricular tachycardia; catecholaminergic VT with normal QT interval, secondary to cardiac ryanodine receptor-calcium release channel mutations [20, 22]; and arrhythmogenic right ventricular dysplasia (ARVDC) [2]. In all of these conditions, sympathetic tone, alone or in combination with other factors, is considered the most important TF of arrhythmic events (Fig. 2).

Table 2. Comparison of the published data of the five largest registries worldwide on Brugada syndrome patients and family members: part 1

	Brugada et al. Circulation 2002	Brugada et al. Circulation 2003	Priori et al. Circulation 2002	Eckardt et al. Circulation 2005	Corrado et al. Eur Heart J 2005	Naccarella et al. ECAS 2005
No. (no. men)	334 (255)	547 (408)	200 (152)	212 (152)	209 (182)	200 (152)
Index (men)		294	130 (110)	165 (132)	68	/
Aborted SCD	71	0	22	24	20	15
Syncope	73	124	34	65	41	25 (12)
Asymptomatic	190	423	144	123	148	148
Age at diagnosis, years	42 ± 16	41 ± 15	41 ± 18	45 ± 6	38.9 ± 12	39 ± 12
Brugada ECG pattern (%)						
Spontaneous	234 (70)	391 (71)	90/176 (51)	125 (59)	126 (60)	38 (90)
After class I	100 (30)	156 (29)	86 (49)	87 (41)	83 (40)	60 (61)
Family history of SCD (%)	180/334 (54)	302/547 (55)	26/130 (22)	60/212 (28)	129 (62)	37/200 (19)
Aborted SCD	23 (38)	0	NA	3 (13)	NA	15/37 (41)
Syncope	26 (39)	NA	NA	16 (25)	NA	37/200 (19)
Asymptomatic	131 (72)	NA	NA	41 (33)	NA	22/200 (11)
SCN5A (%)						
Screened index patients						
Mutation	NA	NA	130	136	28	29
	NA	NA	28 (22)	32 (24)	6/28 (21)	3/29 (10)

NA not available

Table 3. Comparison of the published data of the five largest registries worldwide on Brugada syndrome patients and family members; part 2

	Brugada et al. Circulation 2002	Brugada et al. Circulation 2003	Priori et al. Circulation 2002	Eckardt et al. Circulation 2005	Corrado et al. Eur Heart J 2005	Naccarella et al. ECAS 2005
Electrophysiological study, n (%)	252	408	86	186	68	57
Inducible	130 (52)	163 (40)	57 (66)	93 (50)	27 (40)	17/57 (30)
Aborted SCD	44/54 (83)	NA	18 (82)	15/22 (68)	19/27 (70)	12/17 (71)
Syncope	41/62(68)	NA	NA	40/65 (62)	NA	3/57 (5)
Asymptomatic	45/136 (33)	NA	NA	38/98 (39)	NA	28/57 (49)
ICD, n (%)	NA	177 (32)	NA	113 (53)	29 (14)	9/12 (75)
Follow-up, mo	33 ± 39	24 ± 33	34 ± 44	40 ± 50	3.6 ± 1.9	16 ± 25
Aborted SCD	54 ± 54	NA	NA	83 ± 66	NA	22 ± 24
Syncope	26 ± 36	NA	NA	39 ± 37	NA	26 ± 42
Asymptomatic	27 ± 29	NA	NA	34 ± 52	NA	14 ± 59
Events during follow-up, n (%)	74 (39)	45 (8)	13	9 (4)	16 (8)	21/57 (37)
Aborted SCD	44 (62)	NA	NA	4 (17)	11 (68)	15/57 (26)
Syncope	14 (19)	NA	NA	4 (6)	2 (1)	3/57 (5)
Asymptomatic	16 (8)	NA	6	1 (1)	1	2/57 (4)

NA not available

Hypokalaemia resulting from other electrolytic disorders or the use of certain drugs should be carefully controlled.

Stress testing in not useful in Brugada syndrome, unless for arrhythmias occurring in the post-exercise and recovery phases, when vagal tone is predominant or when the imbalance favours parasympathetic over sympathetic tone. Sports activities are not allowed for subjects with clearly diagnosed Brugada syndrome or for those with drug-induced abnormalities after provocative testing, even in asymptomatic subjects. Conversely, stress test and provocative manoeuvres are particularly useful and, sometimes even more useful than PES, in so-called catecholaminergic precipitated ventricular arrhythmias and in other arrhythmic syndromes, such as those mentioned above.

Twelve-lead 24-h serial Holter monitorings are more useful to assess the spontaneous variability of ST T-segment elevation, in addition to a more prominent ST T-segment elevation (coved) and bradycardia, the occurrence of non-sustained or sustained ventricular arrhythmias, and, not infrequently, atrial fibrillation or flutter. Concomitant complicating factors which are not sufficiently investigated at the time of the event may be difficult to identify later.

Acknowledgements

We thank Valentina Galletti, and Elena Seragnoli for help in preparing this paper and for assembling the figures. We thank Elena Cuomo, Director of the Service of KNOWLEDGE MANAGEMENT of Maggiore Hospital G.Laschi Library, Azienda USL Bologna, Bologna, Italy.

References

1. Anonymous (1997) Survivors of out-of-hospital cardiac arrest with apparently normal heart. Need for definition and standardized clinical evaluation. Consensus statement of the joint Steering Committees of the Unexplained cardiac arrest Registry of Europe and of the Idiopathic ventricular fibrillation Registry of the United States. Circulation 95:265–272
2. Kontny F, Dale J (1990) Self-terminating idiopathic ventricular fibrillation presenting as syncope: a 40-year follow-up report. J Int Med 227:211–213
3. Fish JM, Di Diego JM, Nesterenko V et al (2004) Epicardial activation of left ventricular wall prolongs QT interval and transmural dispersion of repolarization. Implications for biventricular pacing. Circulation 109:2136–2142
4. Fish JM, Antzelevitch C (2004) Link between hypothermia and the Brugada syndrome. J Cardiovasc Electrophysiol 15:942–944
5. Antzelevitch C, Brugada P, Borggrefe M et al (2005) Brugada syndrome. Report of the Second Consensus Conference. Circulation 111:659–670
6. Antzelevitch C, Belardinelli L, Zygmunt AC et al (2004) Electrophysiological effects of ranolazine, a novel antianginal agent with antiarrhythmic properties. Circulation 110:904–910

7. Antzelevitch C, Extramiana F (2004) Amplified transmural dispersion of repolarization as the basis for arrhythmogenesis in a canine ventricular-wedge model of short-QT syndrome. Circulation 110:3661–3666
8. Gussak H et al (1995) ECG phenomenon called the J-wave. J Electrocardiol 28:49–58
9. Yan GX, Antzelevitch C (1996) Cellular bases for the electrocardiographic J-wave. Circulation 93:372–379
10. Fish JM, Antzelevitch C (2003) Cellular and ionic bases for the sex related difference in the manifestation of the Brugada syndrome and progressive conduction disease phenotypes. J Electrocardiol 36:173–179
11. Haverkamp W, Rolf S, Eckardt L et al (2005) Long QT syndrome and Brugada syndrome. Drugs, ablation or ICD? Herz 30(2):111–118
12. Watanabe H, Chinushi M, Washizuka T et al (2005) Variable electrocardiographic effects of short term quinidine sulphate administration in Brugada syndrome. Pacing Clin Electrophysiol 28(5):372–377
13. Mohler PJ, Bennett V (2005) Ankyrin-based cardiac arrhythmias: a new class of channelopathies due to loss of cellular targeting. Curr Opin Cardiol 20(3):189–193
14. Rossenbacker T, Carroll SJ, Liu H et al (2004) Novel pore mutation in SCN5A manifests as a spectrum of phenotypes ranging from atrial flutter, conduction diseases and Brugada syndrome to sudden cardiac death. Heart Rhythm 1(5):610–615
15. Ackerman MJ, Splawski I, Makielski JC et al (2004) Spectrum and prevalence of cardiac sodium channel variance among black, white, Asian and Hispanic individuals: implications fpr arrhythmogenic susceptibility and Brugada/long QT syndrome genetic testing. Heart Rhythm 1(5):600–607
16. Santambrogio LG, Mencherini S, Fuardo M et al (2005) The surgical patients with Brugada syndrome: a four cases clinical experience. Anesth Analg 100(5):1263–1266
17. Peng J, Cui YK, Yi SD et al (2005) Fever and Brugada syndrome: report of 21 cases. Di Yi Jun Yi Da Xue Xue Bao 25(4):432–434
18. Chow BJ, Gollob M, Birnie D (2005) Brugada syndrome precipitated by a tricyclic antidepressant. Heart 91(5):651
19. Gaita F, Giustetto C, Bianchi F et al (2004) Short QT syndrome: pharmacological treatment. J Am Coll Cardiol 43:1494–1499
20. Priori S, Napolitano C, Memmi M et al (2002) Clinical and molecular characterization of patients with catecholaminergic polymorphic ventricular tachycardia. Circulation 106:69–74
21. Hong K, Brugada J, Oliva A et al (2004) Value of electrocardiographic parameters and ajmaline test in the diagnosis of Brugada syndrome caused by SCNA mutations. Circulation 110:3023–3027
22. Marks AR (2002) Clinical implications of cardiac ryanodine receptor/calcium release channel mutations linked to sudden cardiac death. Circulation 106:8–10
23. Eckardt L, Probst V, Smits JPP et al (2005) Long-term prognosis of individuals with right precordial ST-segment-elevation Brugada syndrome. Circulation 111:257–263
24. Hong K, Antzelevitch C, Brugada P et al (2004) Brugada syndrome: 12 years of progression. Acta Med Okayama 58:255–261
25. Naccarella F, Bresciani B, Lepera G et al (2005) Prospective follow-up of thirteen Brugada patients and of their families (200 members). Non-invasive evaluation and drug tests. Proceedings of the First annual congress of the European cardiac arrhythmia society. Marseille, April 10–12 2005 (in press)

26. Corrado D, Leoni L, Naccarella F et al (2003) Implantable cardioverter-defibrillator therapy for prevention of sudden death in patients with arrhythmogenic right ventricular cardiomyopathy dysplasia. Circulation 108:3084–3091
27. Camm AJ, Malik M, Yap GY (2004) Acquired long QT syndrome. Blackwell Futura Publishing, Philadelphia

Drug Challenge in Brugada Syndrome: How Valuable Is It?

T. Wichter, E. Schulze-Bahr, M. Paul, G. Breithardt, L. Eckardt

Introduction

Since its introduction as a clinical entity in 1992 [1], Brugada syndrome has been the focus of increasing interest as a relevant cause of syncope and sudden cardiac death in young and otherwise healthy subjects without structural heart disease.

The disease is characterised by ST-segment elevation in the right precordial surface ECG leads and a high incidence of otherwise unexplained syncope, polymorphic ventricular tachycardia, and sudden death in patients with structurally normal hearts. The disease is predominant in males and manifests in adolescence or early adulthood, with a mean age of approximately 40 years at the time of sudden death. Brugada syndrome is estimated to be responsible for up to 4% of all sudden deaths and 20% of sudden deaths in patients with structurally normal hearts. The true prevalence of Brugada syndrome in the general population is unknown and difficult to estimate, because ECG features may be subtle, concealed, or transient.

The disease is endemic in Southeast Asia, where ECG findings diagnostic for Brugada syndrome (type-1 ECG) were reported in up to 12/10 000 inhabitants and non-diagnostic ECG findings (type-2 and type-3 ECG) in 58/10 000 individuals [2]. In European and North American populations, Brugada syndrome and Brugada-type ECG findings are much less prevalent (approx. 5/10 000 inhabitants).

University Hospital and Medical School of Münster, Department of Cardiology and Angiology, Münster, Germany

Diagnostic Criteria

Diagnostic criteria of Brugada syndrome were recently proposed and summarised in a consensus document endorsed by the Heart Rhythm Society and the European Heart Rhythm Association [3]. The diagnosis is made in the presence of typical ECG manifestations in conjunction with clinical features, such as documented ventricular fibrillation (VF), polymorphic ventricular tachycardia (VT), unexplained syncope, a family history of sudden cardiac death at < 45 years, coved-type ECGs in family members, inducibility of VT/VF during programmed electrical stimulation, or nocturnal agonal respiration.

ECG Manifestations

In Brugada syndrome, type-1 ECG is characterised by a coved ST-segment elevation ≥ 2 mm (0.2 mV) followed by a negative T-wave in the right precordial ECG leads (V_1–V_3). Type-2 ST-segment elevation has a saddle-back appearance with a high take-off ST-segment elevation of ≥ 2 mm, a trough displaying ≥ 1 mm ST elevation, and then either a positive or biphasic T-wave (Fig. 1). Type-3 ECG shows either a saddle-back or coved ST-segment elevation of < 1 mm.

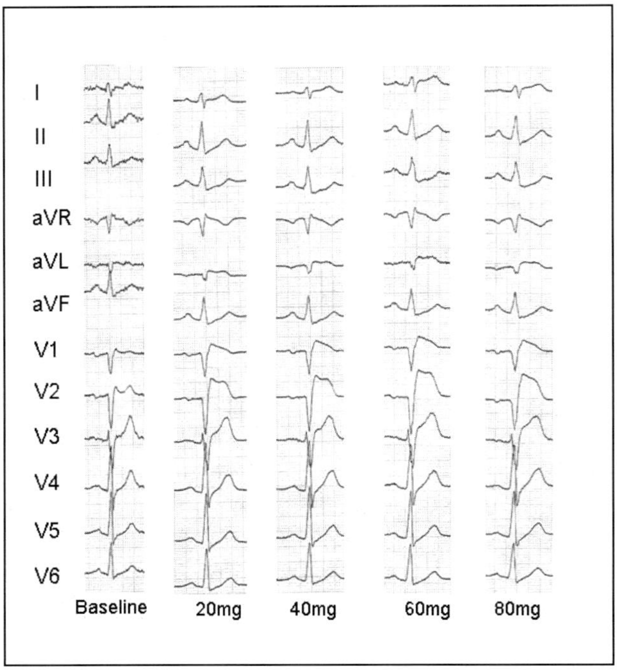

Fig. 1. 12-lead surface ECG demonstrating the dynamic transition of type-2 ECG (saddle-back type) to type-1 ST-segment elevation ('coved-type') in the right precordial leads during drug challenge with intravenous ajmaline in a patient with Brugada syndrome

Type 1 ECG is diagnostic for Brugada syndrome if it occurs spontaneously or after provocation with sodium channel blockers, vagotonic agents, or during febrile states. One or more of the above clinical criteria should also be present. Type 2 and type 3 ECG patterns are not diagnostic of Brugada syndrome unless then can be converted to a type-1 ECG after administration of sodium channel blockers. Conversion of type-3 to type-2 ST-segment elevation by drug challenge is considered inconclusive for the diagnosis of Brugada syndrome [3].

Pathophysiology of ECG Features

The ECG characteristics of Brugada syndrome are considered to result from an amplification of heterogeneities in the early phases of the action potential of cells residing in different transmural layers of the right ventricular wall.

A spike and dome (notch) morphology in epicardial (but not endocardial) layers mediated by transient outward current (I_{to}) creates a transmural voltage gradient responsible for the J-wave in the surface ECG. Accentuation of the action potential notch in the right ventricular epicardium due to rebalancing of currents active at the end of phase 1 is considered responsible for the augmented J-wave and ST-segment elevation in Brugada syndrome [4]. Pathophysiological conditions (fever, abnormal vagotonus) or inhibition of the sodium channel current (I_{Na}) with drugs such as ajmaline, flecainide, or procainamide result in further accentuation of the action potential notch and subsequent exaggeration of the J-wave and ST-segment elevation. The resulting transmural dispersion of repolarisation and refractoriness creates an arrhythmogenic substrate. Premature ventricular extrasystoles occurring during a 'vulnerable window' may then trigger circus movement reentry, ultimately leading to polymorphic VT, VF, and sudden death.

Spontaneous ECG Variations

It is well known that ECG features of Brugada syndrome may show considerable variations over time. Type-1 ST-segment elevation may not be present at all recorded ECGs but may change to type-2 or type-3 findings, or may even normalise completely [5]. The transient appearance of diagnostic ECG findings hampers the estimation of disease prevalence, the diagnostic accuracy, and risk stratification in Brugada syndrome, with important impact for patient management. In that respect, all available previous ECGs should be reviewed when Brugada syndrome is suspected. In addition, the sensitivity of ECG diagnosis may be enhanced when recording the right precordial leads in the second or third intercostals space instead of standard lead positions (fourth intercostal space) with or without the use of body surface potential mapping and or additional drug challenge [6].

Modulation of ECG Features

A variety of conditions and drugs may modulate the ECG features of Brugada syndrome [7]. Adrenergic stimulation (i.e. tachycardia, isoproterenol), parasympathetic blockers (i.e. atropine), and inhibition of the I_{to} current (i.e. quinidine) diminish ST-segment elevation.

In contrast, ECG features of Brugada syndrome are unmasked or aggravated by increased body temperature (fever), hypokalemia, parasympathetic stimulation (bradycardia, vagal triggers, edrophonium), sympathetic blockade (β-blockers, β-adrenergic blockers), inhibition of the I_{Na} current (i.e. sodium channel blockers) and others. Autonomic dysfunction with decreased adrenergic activity, potentially contributing to autonomic dysbalance and increased net vagal tone, was recently confirmed by our group with the use of quantitative radionuclide imaging (SPECT and PET) of presynaptic innervation [8, 9].

Unmasking of Brugada syndrome in response to drugs probably underlies a rebalancing of currents active at the end of phase 1 of the action potential. Vagotonic agents, I_K-ATP activators and hypokalemia achieve this by augmenting outward currents whereas sodium channel blockers, β-blockers, cocaine, antidepressants, and antihistamines such as terfenadine likely accomplish this by reducing inward currents [10, 11].

An augmentation of right precordial ST-elevation in Brugada syndrome is related to the arrhythmogenesis and increases the likelihood of spontaneous life-threatening arrhythmias. This is supported by the observation of marked ST-segment elevation just prior to or following the onset of polymorphic VT or VF. In addition, our studies with body surface potential mapping demonstrated that the area of ST-segment elevation correlates with the inducibility of VT in the absence of drug provocation [12]. These effects must be taken into consideration and several drugs that accelerate ST-segment elevation must be considered contraindicated in patients with Brugada syndrome (Table 1) [3]. However, under appropriate conditions, sodium channel blockers may be used as a diagnostic challenge to unmask typical ECG features of Brugada syndrome [5].

Table 1. Drugs inducing Brugada-like ECG patterns (adapted from [3])

Antiarrhythmic drugs
1. Sodium channel blockers
Class IC drugs (ajmaline, flecainide, propafenone, pilsicainide)
Class IA drugs (ajmaline, procainamide, disopyramide)
2. Calcium channel blockers (verapamil)
3. Beta-blockers (propranolo, metoprolol, bisoprolol, etc.)
Antianginal drugs
1. Calcium channel blockers (nifedipine, diltiazem, etc.)
2. Nitrates (isosorbite dinitrate, isosorbite mononitrate, nitroglycerine)
3. Potassium channel openers (nicorandil)
Psychotropic drugs
1. Tricyclic antidepressants (amitryptiline, nortryptiline, desipramine, clomipramine)
2. Tetracyclic antidepressants (maprotiline)
3. Phenothiazine (perphenazine, cyamemazine)
4. Selective serotonin reuptake inhibitors (fluoxetine)
Other drugs and conditions
1. Dimenhydrinate
2. Cocaine intoxication
3. Alcohol intoxication
4. Febrile state
5. Vagotonic drugs and conditions

Drug Challenge in Brugada Syndrome

Drug challenge with intravenous administration sodium channel blockers (Fig. 1) may be used for diagnostic evaluation and risk stratification in patients with Brugada syndrome, patients with unexplained syncope or cardiac arrest, or asymptomatic individuals with ECG findings suspicious for Brugada syndrome. In addition, it may be helpful in the diagnostic assessment of relatives of an index patient. Current indications for drug challenge in Brugada syndrome are summarised in Table 2.

Table 2. Drug challenge in Brugada syndrome: proposed diagnostic protocol (modified from [17])

Indications:
Aborted sudden death, polymorphic VT, or unexplained syncope in patients without structural heart disease.
Family history of Brugada syndrome, sudden cardiac death and/or recurrent syncope of unknown origin.
Suspicious non-diagnostic ECG in asymptomatic patients without structural heart disease.

Environment:
Patient in fasting, resting, and drug-free state.
Safe venous access, continuous 12-lead ECG recording, blood pressure monitoring.
Presence of physician with experience in intensive care medicine.
Advanced cardiopulmonary life-support facilities available including external defibrillator, intubation set and drugs (atropine, isoproterenol).

Drugs and dosages:

Ajmaline:	1 mg/kg over 10 min i.v.
Flecainide:	2 mg/kg (150 mg max.) over 10 min i.v.
Procainamide:	10 mg/kg over 10 min i.v.
Pilsicainide:	1 mg/kg over 10 min i.v.

Performance:
Fractionated slow intravenous drug administration up to target dose over 10 min.
Continuous ECG documentation at paper speed of 10 mm/s (one strip at 25 or 50 mm/s every 2 min).
Patient and ECG supervision and monitoring until normalisation of the ECG.

Termination criteria:
Reached target dose.
QRS prolongation ≥ 130% of baseline.
Occurrence of type-1 ECG (J-point elevation or ST-segment elevation ≥2 mm in at least one right precordial lead.
Occurrence of premature ventricular beats, ventricular tachycardia, sinus arrest or AV-block (2nd or 3rd degree).

Diagnostic Impact

The importance of pharmacologic challenge in suspected Brugada syndrome was indicated in several large series [13, 14], where 30–50% of patients showed normal ECGs at baseline and the syndrome could only be diagnosed after challenge with sodium channel blockers. In contrast, drug challenge is generally not performed in patients with a diagnostic type-1 ECG under baseline conditions, because of its limited additional diagnostic and prognostic value and its potential for proarrhythmic adverse events [3].

Because ECG changes may be transient, concealed, or absent at the time of first evaluation of a patient with Brugada syndrome, pharmacologic challenge represents an important tool in the identification of affected patients who are at potential risk of sudden death. Given that symptomatic patients at first evaluation may have a negative ECG at baseline, a false negative response to drug challenge may lead to underdiagnosis of Brugada syndrome. Therefore, the highest possible sensitivity and reproducibility of sodium channel blocker administration for pharmacologic challenge are warranted.

Hong et al. [15] recently reported the value of drug challenge with ajmaline in 71 individuals representing four families with Brugada syndrome and documented SCN5A mutations. The test was positive in 28 of 35 mutation carriers and the penetrance of disease phenotype increased from 33 to 79%. The sensitivity, specificity, and positive and negative predictive values were 80, 94, 93, and 83% respectively. Smits et al. [16] reported similar findings. Drug challenge with sodium channel blockers did not differentiate between patients with and without SCN5A mutation with regard to the magnitude of the ST-segment elevation but showed a larger increase in QRS duration and PQ intervals in SCN5A mutation carriers. Therefore, drug challenge may be helpful in identifying mutation carriers by unmasking latent conduction defects, as evidenced by prolonged HV intervals, PQ intervals, and QRS durations at baseline or after sodium channel blockade.

Our group previously reported the results of drug challenge with ajmaline in 158 patients [17]. Overall, a positive test was found in 23% of the patients, in 50% of patients with a suspicious pattern of the basal ECG, and in 45% of patients with aborted sudden death and structurally normal hearts. Nine out of 63 patients with syncope had a positive test, the majority having a family history of unexplained sudden death and a suspicious ECG at baseline. These data suggest that the test is highly effective in correctly diagnosing the syndrome in patients with the strong suspicion of having a primary electrical disease. Because of the prognostic implications, patients with survived cardiac arrest and unexplained syncope in the absence of structural heart disease should therefore undergo drug challenge for the potential unmasking of Brugada syndrome.

However, the possibility of a positive drug challenge in individuals not having the Brugada syndrome raises concern because of the potential therapeutic implications, i.e. in patients after unexplained syncope. In our previous study [17], only two of 94 patients with syncope and a normal ECG at baseline had a positive ajmaline test. Whether these are false-positive tests or very subtle manifestations of the disease will be clarified only when genetic diagnosis becomes available. Currently, the diagnostic meaning and therapeutic impact of a positive test in such patients remains unclear.

Prognostic Impact

Brugada et al. [13] reported that patients with an initial presentation of resuscitated cardiac arrest carry the highest risk of life-threatening recurrences (69% at 54 ± 54 months of follow-up), followed by patients with syncope and spontaneous type-1 ECG (19% at 26 ± 36 months of follow-up). Similar results were found by others [14, 18], however with lower event rates. While Brugada et al. [13] reported an 8% cardiac event rate in initially asymptomatic patients, Priori et al. [14] reported event rates of approximately 4%, and Eckardt et al. [18] observed a cardiac event in only one of 123 (0.8%) patients that were asymptomatic at baseline.

According to Brugada et al. [13], among asymptomatic individuals with Brugada-type ECG features, male patients with inducible VT or VF and spontaneous type-1 ECG appear to carry the highest risk. In contrast, patients in whom ST-segment elevation occurred only after provocation with sodium channel blockers appeared to be at minimal or no risk. Studies by others [14, 19] and by our own group [18] did not find a relationship between the inducibility of VT or VF during programmed electrical stimulation and the recurrence of VT or VF among either symptomatic or asymptomatic patients with Brugada syndrome. This controversy may be due to differences in patient selection, diagnostic criteria, and non-comparable or non-standardised stimulation protocols [18, 20].

In a study involving 547 patients with Brugada syndrome but no history of cardiac arrest [21], the risk of arrhythmic events in patients with a spontaneously abnormal type-1 ECG was 7.7-fold higher risk than in patients in whom diagnostic type-1 ECG developed only after drug challenge. Male gender and inducible sustained VT or VF were associated with a 5.5- and 8-fold higher risk of sudden death, respectively. A positive family history was not related to an adverse outcome when compared with sporadic cases of Brugada syndrome. This correlates well with the findings of Smits et al. [16], who did not observe differences in gender, age, family history, index event, and inducibility of VT or VF in patients with or without the presence of SCN5A mutations in Brugada syndrome.

In summary, drug challenge has a limited additional prognostic impact within the risk stratification of patients with Brugada syndrome. According to the current Consensus Report [3], symptomatic patients with type-1 ECG at baseline or after drug challenge who present with aborted sudden death should receive an ICD without additional need for electrophysiologic study (class I recommendation). A similar approach applies for patients with syncope, seizure, or nocturnal agonal respiration after exclusion of noncardiac causes of these symptoms (class IIa). In asymptomatic patients, an electrophysiologic study is recommended in patients with a spontaneous type-1

ECG (class IIa) or in patients with drug-induced type-1 ECG and a positive family history (class IIb). If VT or VF is inducible, the patient should receive an ICD. Asymptomatic patients without a family history and who develop type-1 ECG only after drug challenge should be closely followed [3]. This concept, however, remains controversial due to limited data available from controlled clinical trials or registries. It requires continuous update as more data become available in the future.

Drugs and Dosages

Drug challenge in suspected Brugada syndrome may be performed by intravenous administration of class IC sodium channel blockers, such as ajmaline (IA/IC), flecainide, propafenone, or pilsicainide. The class IA sodium channel blockers procainamide and disopyramide have been used less frequently because of their lesser potency to unmask the ECG characteristics of Brugada syndrome. The recommended dosages and infusion rates are listed in Table 2.

Intravenous ajmaline (1 mg/kg) has been reported as the most effective and most sensitive drug to unmask Brugada-type ECG features (Fig. 1). Early studies reported 100% sensitivity in selected patients [5]. In larger cohorts, the sensitivity remained high, reaching up to 90%. Further advantages of the drug include its short half-life, which allows short monitoring times after intravenous administration for drug challenge. Unfortunately, the low price and limited number of indications have led to withdrawal from the market in the majority of countries. Therefore, sodium channel blockers other than ajmaline are frequently used for drug challenge in Brugada syndrome. However, flecainide and procainamide are both less effective and less sensitive in unmasking Brugada syndrome and require longer monitoring due to prolonged effect. The reproducibility of test results with ajmaline and flecainide has been reported to be high [17, 22].

In a direct comparison of ajmaline and flecainide in 22 patients, the positive concordance of test results was 68%. Intravenous flecainide (2 mg/kg) proved less effective and failed to unmask ECG signs of Brugada syndrome produced with ajmaline (1 mg/kg) in seven of 22 patients (32%), despite equivalent changes in QRS and PQ intervals, suggesting similar effects on sodium channel current. Experimental studies in a canine model suggested that the lesser effectiveness of flecainide largely results from its more potent inhibition of I_{to} which counters the sodium-blocking effects of the drug [11]. Although the class IA drug procainamide produces does not block I_{to} at clinically relevant drug concentrations, it has proved to be less potent than class IC drugs (ajmaline, flecainide) in unmasking Brugada syndrome, probably because of a lower level of use-dependent sodium channel block [23].

An experimental model recently demonstrated that the combined block of sodium (I_{Na}) and calcium (I_{Ca}) currents by class IC sodium channel blockers and verapamil may be even more effective in unmasking Brugada syndrome than sodium channel blockade alone [24]. The addition of verapamil resulted in an enhancement of the effect of sodium channel blockers to create the Brugada phenotype. Although this concept might improve the diagnostic sensitivity of the test, caution is warranted when extrapolating these findings to clinical practice before appropriate studies provide confirmation in humans with Brugada syndrome.

Adverse Events

The most relevant adverse effects of drug challenge in Brugada syndrome relate to proarrhythmia. Nonsustained or sustained polymorphic VT or VF may occur during the test. The arrhythmias may be symptomatic and even life-threatening because they may range from frequent extrasystoles and ventricular runs to polymorphic VT and cardiac arrest due to VF [17, 22]. These arrhythmias may be difficult to terminate after administration of sodium channel blocking drugs. In addition, these drugs may provoke incessant VT or VF (possibly by conduction slowing), which may be difficult or impossible to terminate [25]. Therefore, when performing drug challenge in Brugada syndrome, appropriate safety precautions must be ensured, and criteria for termination of drug administration should be defined. Avoiding drug overdose and respecting stopping criteria can effectively prevent proarrhythmic events during drug challenge in Brugada syndrome [17].

Standardised Protocol

To provide reproducible results and to avoid procedure-related complications and adverse events, pharmacological drug challenge in Brugada syndrome should follow a standardised protocol. Such a protocol has recently been proposed by our group (Table 2) [17].

Drug challenge should be performed with the patient in a fasting, resting, and drug-free state under continuous ECG monitoring (speed of 10 mm/s, interposed with recordings at 25 or 50 mm/s at each dose step). The test should only be performed in a setting fully equipped for resuscitation (defibrillation, emergency medication, intubation, mechanical ventilation) in the presence of a physician with experience in intensive care medicine [3, 17].

Intravenous sodium channel blockers should be administered slowly and with great caution according to recommended dosage and infusion rate

(Table 2). In young and otherwise healthy individuals, the test may be performed as a bedside procedure. Particular caution should be exercised in patients with pre-existing conduction disturbance (atrial, ventricular, or both) or in the presence of wide QRS, wide P waves, or prolonged PR intervals in order to avoid complete AV block. In such patients, drug challenge with sodium channel blocker may better be performed during an electrophysiological study with temporary pacing electrodes in place to prevent complications related to conduction block [3].

Drug challenge should be stopped when the diagnostic type-1 ECG develops, the type-2 ST-segment elevation increases by ≥ 2 mm, premature ventricular beats or other arrhythmias occur, or when the QRS complex widens to ≥ 130% of baseline. Following these safety rules, proarrhythmic or other relevant complications are very unlikely and have rarely been observed. However, in case arrhythmic complications do occur, isoproterenol and sodium lactate may be effective antidotes to reverse the effect of sodium channel blockers [3, 17].

Conclusions

In patients with structurally normal hearts and unexplained syncope or cardiac arrest, Brugada syndrome is considered a frequent underlying condition. In patients with suspected Brugada syndrome but inconclusive or normal ECG findings at baseline, drug challenge with intravenous administration of sodium channel blockers according to a standardised protocol is a powerful tool to unmask diagnostic type-1 Brugada ECG features and thereby identify patients at risk of sudden death. The additional impact of drug challenge in the risk stratification algorithms of patients already diagnosed with Brugada syndrome is less well-established and requires additional studies.

Acknowledgements
This work was supported in part by grants from the Deutsche Forschungsgemeinschaft (SFB 556, projects A1 and C4), Bonn, Germany, and by the Leducq Foundation, Paris France.

References

1. Brugada P, Brugada J (1992) Right bundle branch block, persistent ST segment elevation and sudden cardiac death: a distinct clinical and electrocardiographic syndrome. A multicenter report. J Am Coll Cardiol 20:1391–1396
2. Miyasaka Y, Tsuji H, Yamada K et al (2001) Prevalence and mortality of the Brugada-type electrocardiogram in one city in Japan. J Am Coll Cardiol 38:771–774

3. Antzelevitch C, Brugada P, Borggrefe M et al (2005) Brugada syndrome: Report of the second consensus conference. Circulation 111:659–670
4. Antzelevitch C (2001) The Brugada syndrome: ionic basis and arrhythmia mechanisms. J Cardiovasc Electrophysiol 12:268–272
5. Brugada R, Brugada J, Antzelevitch C et al (2000) Sodium channel blockers identify risk for sudden death in patients with ST-segment elevation and right bundle branch block but structurally normal hearts. Circulation 101:510–515
6. Bruns HJ, Eckardt L, Vahlhaus C et al (2002) Body surface potential mapping in patients with Brugada syndrome: right precordial ST segment variations and reverse changes in left precordial leads. Cardiovasc Res 54:58–66
7. Miyazaki T, Mitamura H, Miyoshi S et al (1996) Autonomic and antiarrhythmic drug modulation of ST-segment elevation in patients with Brugada syndrome. J Am Coll Cardiol 27:1061–1070
8. Wichter T, Matheja P, Eckardt L et al (2002) Cardiac autonomic dysfunction in Brugada syndrome. Circulation 105:702–706
9. Kies P, Wichter T, Schäfers M et al (2004) Abnormal myocardial presynaptic norepinephrine recycling in patients with Brugada syndrome. Circulation 110:3017–3922
10. Antzelevitch C, Brugada P, Brugada J et al (2003) Brugada syndrome: 1992–2002. A historical perspective. J Am Coll Cardiol 41:1665–1671
11. Wolpert C, Echternach C, Veltmann C et al (2005) Intravenous drug challenge using flecainide and ajmaline in patients with Brugada syndrome. Heart Rhythm 2:254–260
12. Eckardt L, Bruns HJ, Paul M et al (2002) Body surface area of ST elevation and the presence of late potentials correlate to the inducibility of ventricular tachyarrhythmias in Brugada syndrome. J Cardiovasc Electrophysiol 13:742–749
13. Brugada J, Brugada R, Antzelevitch C et al (2002) Long-term follow-up of individuals with the electrocardiographic pattern of right bundle branch block and ST-segment elevation in precordial leads V1 to V3. Circulation 105:73–78
14. Priori SG, Napolitano C, Gasparini M et al (2002) Natural history of Brugada syndrome: insights for risk stratification and management. Circulation 105:1342–1347
15. Hong K, Brugada J, Oliva A et al (2004) Value of electrocardiographic parameters and ajmaline test in the diagnosis of Brugada syndrome caused by SCN5A mutations. Circulation 110:3023–3027
16. Smits JPP, Eckardt L, Probst V et al (2002) Genotype-phenotype relationship in Brugada syndrome: electrocardiographic features differentiate SCN5A-related patients from non-SCN5A-related patients. J Am Coll Cardiol 40:350–356
17. Rolf S, Bruns HJ, Wichter T et al (2003) The ajmaline challenge in Brugada syndrome: diagnostic impact, safety, and recommende protocol. Eur Heart J 24:1104–1112
18. Eckardt L, Probst V, Smits JPP et al (2005) Long-term prognosis of individuals with right precordial ST-segment elevation Brugada syndrome. Circulation 111:257–263
19. Kanda M, Shimizu W, Matsno K et al (2002) Electrophysiologic characteristics and implications of induced ventricular fibrillation in symptomatic patients with Brugada syndrome. J Am Coll Cardiol 39:1799–1805
20. Eckardt L, Kirchhof P, Schulze-Bahr E et al (2002) Electrophysiologic investigation in Brugada syndrome: yield of programmed ventricular stimulation at two ventricular sites with three premature beats. Eur Heart J 23:1394–1401
21. Brugada J, Brugada R, Brugada P (2003) Determinants of sudden cardiac death in patients with the electrocardiographic pattern of Brugada syndrome and no previous cardiac arrest. Circulation 108:3092–3096

22. Gasparini M, Priori SG, Mantica M et al (2003) Flecainide test in Brugada syndrome: a reproducible but risky tool. Pacing Clin Electrophysiol 26:338–341
23. Shimizu W, Antzelevitch C, Suyama K et al (2000) Effects of sodium channel blockers on ST segment, QRS duration, and corrected QT interval in patients with Brugada syndrome. J Cardiovasc Electrophysiol 11:1320–1329
24. Fish JM, Antzelevitch C (2004) Role of sodium and calcium channel block in unmasking the Brugada syndrome. Heart Rhythm 1:210–217
25. Roden DM 1994) Risks and benefits of antiarrhythmic therapy. N Engl J Med 331:785–791

Electrophysiologic Study in Brugada Syndrome: More Questions Than Answers?

C. Wolpert, C. Echternach, C. Veltmann, R. Schimpf, M. Borggrefe

Introduction

Brugada syndrome is an inherited arrhythmogenic disorder characterised by typical ECG changes in the right precordial leads and an increased risk of sudden cardiac death. Since the patient population is heterogeneous with respect to family history, symptoms, and age, there is a major focus on diagnostics and risk stratification. The prognostic value of electrophysiologic studies is controversial. Since the first reports on patients with Brugada syndrome, the data on outcome in this population at risk of sudden death has changed towards a better prognosis for asymptomatic patients. An intensified screening process and the inclusion of more sporadic and asymptomatic cases as well as younger patients is probably the main reason for this. Whereas in early reports programmed stimulation played a major role in risk prediction, in terms of a higher arrhythmia risk in the presence of inducible VT/VF, recent reports have not always confirmed these results even in larger patient populations. Therefore, the role of programmed stimulation remains unclear.

Which Stimulation Protocol Should Be Performed in Patients with Brugada Syndrome?

In the previous investigations, especially in multicentre studies, different stimulation protocols in patients with Brugada syndrome were tested [1–11]. To compare the results of programmed electrical stimulation, the following

1st Department of Medicine-Cardiology, University Hospital Mannheim, Faculty of Clinical Medicine of the University of Heidelberg, Mannheim, Germany

protocol has been suggested: stimulation at two sites (right ventricular apex and right ventricular outflow tract), three driving-cycle lengths (600, 430, 330) and 1, 2, or 3 premature extrastimuli with a minimum coupling interval of 200 ms. Nonetheless, different protocols are currently in use. For example, the driving-cycle lengths differ; some investigators use only 2 extrastimuli and others reduce the last premature-stimulus cycle length until refractoriness. This renders results of programmed electrical stimulation less comparable. Interestingly, when comparing the inducibility of sustained VT or VF between groups using a minimum cycle length of 200 ms and groups that stimulate until ventricular refractoriness, the overall amount of inducible VT/VF remains quite constant. It is even more striking that, e.g. Eckardt et al. [4] and our own group [unpublished data] found an overall VT/VF inducibility in 28/41 (67%) and 21/31 patients (68%), respectively. These results are comparable to those of other investigators who used a minimum cycle length of 200 ms but obtained a VT/VF inducibility of only 36% [4], and 31% (12/31) when restricting the coupling interval of the last extrastimulus to a minimum of 200 ms. It would therefore be desirable to follow a common protocol or to prospectively compare both protocols with respect to their predictive power of arrhythmia risk.

Are the Results of Programmed Stimulation Reproducible?

Assuming a predictive value of VT/VF inducibility, a major question is whether it is reproducible or whether there are different responses to programmed stimulation caused by various factors, such as vagal activity, sympathetic activation, sedation, hormonal status, or chance, which may lead to positive or negative results at different time points. Gasparini et al. [1] addressed this question by administering repeated programmed electrical stimulation in patients with Brugada syndrome. They demonstrated that the results remained comparable from one EP study to the other in 82% of the patients. Only the number of extrastimuli necessary for induction and the coupling interval of the premature extrastimulus varied in some patients. However, the authors also considered non-sustained VT between 6 and 30 s as inducible, which limits interpretation of the results because most physicians would consider this as non-inducible. Thus, it remains to be investigated in greater detail whether the results of programmed electrical stimulation are reproducible, since, especially in a subgroup of symptomatic patients, inducibility plays a major role in deciding whether to prophylactically implant a defibrillator.

Are Symptomatic Patients With Inducible Ventricular Arrhythmias at Higher Risk of Ventricular Fibrillation Than Patients Without Inducible VT/VF?

For symptomatic patients with Brugada syndrome, reports on the role of inducibility of VT/VF for risk stratification are controversial. In a study with 144 symptomatic patients with Brugada syndrome, Brugada et al. [9] identified VT/VF inducibility as a strong predictor of a future malignant ventricular tachyarrhythmia or sudden death. Other variables, such as family history or abnormal ECG only after therapy with class I drugs, were not predictive. In contrast, Priori [5] and co-workers did not find VT/VF inducibility to be a predictor for future arrhythmias or sudden death in a study of 86 patients who underwent programmed electrical stimulation. In a recent report by Eckardt et al. [11], inducibility also failed to predict future sudden death or VT/VF documented by an implantable cardioverter defibrillator (ICD) in 186 patients with Brugada syndrome who were followed over a mean duration of 40 ± 50 months. However, the results showed a higher likelihood of inducibility in patients with previous symptoms or aborted sudden death compared to asymptomatic patients. The mean follow-up period of 45 patients investigated by Morita et al. [3] was 38 ± 27 months. There was no significant difference between the frequency of cardiac events in symptomatic patients with induced VF (cardiac event 1.5 ± 0.1 times/year) and in those without induced VF (cardiac event 2.0 ± 1.6 times/year). One reason for the conflicting reports of Brugada et al. and other authors may be a certain selection bias, because the percentage of symptomatic patients is higher in the Brugada registry reported by Brugada et al. [8–10] Therefore, there is a strong need for further studies in more homogeneous populations in order to re-evaluate the role of programmed electrical stimulation in Brugada syndrome.

Should Programmed Stimulation Be Performed in Asymptomatic Patients and If So, When?

It is still a matter of discussion whether asymptomatic patients with a surface ECG that displays typical Brugada-like changes should undergo programmed electrical stimulation. Whereas in early reports Brugada et al. [8–10] demonstrated a significant risk of VT/VF in asymptomatic patients with inducible VT/VF, more recent reports describe a better outcome of asymptomatic patients irrespective of inducibility. Therefore, the Second Brugada Consensus Conference [12] recommended programmed electrical stimulation only for asymptomatic patients with a family history of sudden death suspected to be due to Brugada syndrome and a spontaneous abnormal ECG. If patients display the ECG only after sodium-channel-blocker challenge and no family history is present, electrophysiologic studies are not recommended. This recommendation is, at least to a certain extent questionable, since it is well known that the typical ECG pattern may transiently not be present and that it fluctuates in a significant proportion of patients, so that a typical ECG recording may be a result of chance or other influencing factors. At least in our own population, 20% of the patients with a negative index ECG display an abnormal basal ECG during repetitive recording during further follow-up [unpublished data].

Clinical Implications

Electrophysiologic studies are an important diagnostic tool in the characterisation of patients with Brugada syndrome, especially for scientific reasons. For clinical issues, its value has somewhat changed, and the new recommendations of the Brugada Consensus Conference do not require electrophysiologic studies in asymptomatic patients with a normal baseline ECG and no family history of sudden death. However, how much one can rely on single ECG recordings to say that there is no basal abnormal ECG in a patient, remains to be assessed in a larger population, because ECGs display a great amount of fluctuation. Finally, there are different stimulation protocols in use with either less or more aggressive coupling intervals, which may lead to a decreased sensitivity or specificity. The answer to the question whether there is a difference in positive or negative predictive value for sudden death risk depending on the protocol used needs to be further evaluated in comparative studies of large populations.

References

1. Gasparini M, Priori SG, Mantica M et al (2002) Programmed electrical stimulation in Brugada Syndrome: How reproducible are the results? J Cardiovasc Electrophysiol 13:880–887
2. Brugada P, Brugada R, Mont L et al (2003) Natural history of Brugada Syndrome: The prognostic value of programmed electrical stimulation of the heart. J Cardiovasc Electrophysiol 14:455–457
3. Morita H, Fukushima-Kusano K, Nagase S et al (2003) Site-specific arrhythmogenesis in patients with Brugada Syndrome. J Cardiovasc Electrophysiol 14:373–379
4. Eckardt L, Kirchhof P, Schulze-Bahr E et al (2002) Electrophysiologic investigation in Brugada syndrome: yield of programmed ventricular stimulation at two ventricular sites with up to three premature beats. Eur Heart J 23:1394–1401

5. Priori S, Napolitano C, Gasparini M et al (2002) Natural history of Brugada Syndrome: Insights for risk stratification and management. Circulation 105:1342–1347
6. Kanda M, Shimizu W, Matsuo K et al (2002) Electrophysiologic characteristics and implications of induced ventricular fibrillation in symptomatic patients with Brugada syndrome. J Am Coll Cardiol 39:1799–1805
7. Kakishita M, Kurita T, Matsua K et al (2000) Mode of onset of ventricular fibrillation in patients with Brugada syndrome detected by implantable cardioverter defibrillator therapy. J Am Coll Cardiol 36:1646–1653
8. Brugada J, Brugada R, Antzelevitch C et al (2002) Long-term follow-up of individuals with the electrocardiographic pattern of right bundle-branch block and ST-segment elevation in precordial leads V1 to V3. Circulation 105:73–78
9. Brugada P, Geelen P, Brugada R et al (2001) Prognostic value of electrophysiologic investigations in Brugada syndrome. J Cardiovasc Electrophysiol 12:1004–1007
10. Brugada J, Brugada P (1997) Further characterization of the syndrome of right bundle branch block, ST segment, and sudden cardiac death. J Cardiovasc Electrophysiol 8:325–331
11. Eckardt L, Probst V, Smits JP et al (2005) Long-term prognosis of individuals with right precordial ST-segment-elevation Brugada syndrome. Circulation 111:257–263
12. Antzelevitch C, Brugada P, Borggrefe M et al; Heart Rhythm Society; European Heart Rhythm Association (2005) Brugada syndrome: report of the second consensus conference: endorsed by the Heart Rhythm Society and the European Heart Rhythm Association. Circulation 111(5):659–670

Short QT Syndrome: How Frequent Is It and What Are Its Peculiar Features?

F. Gaita

During the last 20 or 30 years the literature on long QT has constantly increased, while short QT has been substantially ignored. Algra et al. [1], however, reported in 1992 that in a group of 6693 patients who underwent 24-h Holter monitoring a mean QTc below 400 ms was associated with a two-fold risk of sudden death compared to an intermediate QTc value (400–440 ms), and with a similar risk to a mean QTc above 440 ms.

Only recently the association of sudden death [2] and atrial fibrillation [3] with short QT interval has been recognised and short QT syndrome identified as a genetic disorder [4, 5]. In 2003 our group established the relation between short QT and sudden death with the description of two families having a short QT interval at baseline ECG and several cases of sudden death in the family history [2]. Factors that shorten QT interval include an increase in heart rate, hyperthermia, increased calcium or potassium plasma levels, acidosis, and alterations of the autonomic tone. Secondary causes of transient QT interval reduction were excluded in these patients. This alteration of the repolarisation could be documented in all available ECGs recorded at different time points and ages, with a QT interval always less than 300 ms, without significant dynamic changes during heart rate variations or on exertion. A QT interval constantly below 300 ms was proposed as the definition of short QT.

Patients with short QT syndrome present with a wide spectrum of clinical manifestations, ranging from mild symptoms, such as palpitations and dizziness, to syncope and sudden death. Sudden death may occur at any time during the life span, sometimes in children in the first months of life. Sudden

Department of Cardiology, Cardinal Massaia Hospital, Asti, Italy death is often the first clinical presentation. Syncope and palpitations with documentation of atrial fibrillation even at a young age and of ventricular extrasystoles are other symptoms related to short QT syndrome. In the observed patients non-invasive and invasive evaluation confirmed the presence of structurally normal hearts, and autopsies did not reveal any cardiac disease.

To understand how a short QT interval may be related to life-threatening arrhythmias, we have to remember that QT interval is the electrocardiographic expression of ventricular repolarisation, and there is a constant relationship between the ventricular effective refractory period (ERP) and the QT interval. On electrophysiological study these patients show very short atrial and ventricular ERPs. The duration of the refractory periods of the myocardium is known to be an important parameter for the vulnerability of the heart to fibrillation at both atrial and ventricular levels.

Sudden death in the presence of short QT interval in the described families occurred in several generations, in both male and female subjects, suggesting an autosomal dominant mode of inheritance. Ventricular repolarisation is determined by the inward sodium and calcium currents and by the outward potassium currents. The molecular substrate of short QT interval and related arrhythmic events should thus be either a factor that reduces sodium or calcium inward currents or a factor that increases potassium outward currents. Two different missense mutations in HERG (KCNH2), the gene encoding for the rapidly activating delayed rectifier potassium channel, I_{Kr}, causing a gain of function in the channel were first identified [4], and later this variety of short QT syndrome was called SQTS 1. Subsequently, congenital short QT was also linked to a mutation in KCNQ1 (KvLQT1), causing a gain of function in I_{Ks}, the slowly activating delayed rectifier potassium current [5], and this was designated SQTS 2. A mutation has been recently identified in a third gene, KCNJ2 (Kir2.1) encoding for another potassium channel, I_{K1}, causing a gain in function of the channel (SQTS 3) [6]. However, the prevalence of these mutations does not seem high, since only in two of the six families we have so far collected was a mutation in HERG found, and none showed other known mutations. It is reasonable to suppose that mutations involving other genes are present, similarly to what happens in long QT syndrome.

Analysing the data from 23 patients with a personal and/or familial history of sudden death or aborted sudden death, QT interval values up to 320 ms and QTc up to 340 ms were noted [7]. No statistically significant relationship between QT and QTc interval duration and history of sudden death was found; therefore so far it does not seem possible to establish a value of QT interval that would identify patients with short QT who are at higher risk of sudden death.

Short QT interval is easier to recognise at low heart rates; with increasing heart rates it tends to be closer to the normal values. At higher rates, however, QT values are still always below the normal values, and this makes the diagnosis possible even in infants, who typically have high heart rates. This is particularly important considering that sudden death frequently occurs in the first months of life.

Concerning the mechanism of arrhythmogenesis in short QT syndrome, it is likely that the short atrial and ventricular refractory periods observed in these patients represent the substrate of atrial and ventricular arrhythmias; in fact it is well known that the shorter the refractory periods, the shorter the wavelengths are and more likely reentry is to occur.

Because of the high incidence of sudden cardiac death and the absence of known pharmacological therapy, implantation of a cardioverter–defibrillator (ICD) is currently the treatment of first choice [2, 8]. Quinidine prolongs the QT interval and the ventricular ERP and prevents induction of ventricular arrhythmias [9, 10]; however, long-term follow-up of patients with ICD who also receive this drug is needed to clarify whether it may be an alternative to ICD implantation.

In conclusion, short QT syndrome is an arrhythmogenic genetic disorder with a high incidence of sudden death. Short QT syndrome should always be considered in the presence of a family history of sudden death, but also in patients with idiopathic atrial fibrillation and in patients with syncope and a structurally normal heart.

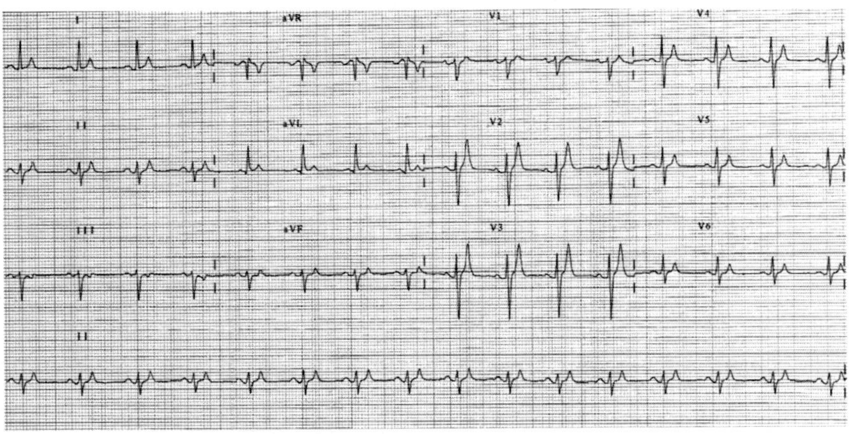

Fig. 1. Electrocardiogram of a patient with short QT syndrome. Heart rate 95 bpm, QT 220 ms, QTc 277 ms

References

1. Algra A, Tijssen JGP, Roelandt JRTC et al (1993) QT interval variables from 24 hour electrocardiography and the two year risk of sudden death. Br Heart J 70:43–48
2. Gaita F, Giustetto C, Bianchi F et al (2003) Short QT syndrome. A familial cause of sudden death. Circulation 108:965–970
3. Gussak I, Brugada P, Brugada J et al (2000) Idiopathic short QT interval: a new clinical syndrome? Cardiology 94:99–102
4. Brugada P, Hong K, Dumaine R et al (2004) Sudden death associated with short QT syndrome linked to mutations in HERG. Circulation 109:30–35
5. Bellocq C, van Ginneken A, Bezzina C (2004) Mutation in the KCNQ1 gene leading to the short QT-interval syndrome. Circulation 109:2394–2397
6. Priori SG, Pandit SV, Rivolta I et al (2005) A novel form of short QT syndrome (SQTS3) is caused by a mutation in the KCNJ2 gene. Circ Res 96:800–807
7. Giustetto C, Wolpert C, Anttonen O et al (2005) Clinical presentation of the patients with short QT syndrome. Heart Rhythm 2:S61
8. Schimpf R, Wolpert C, Bianchi F et al (2003) Congenital short QT syndrome and implantable cardioverter defibrillator. Inherent risk for inappropriate shock delivery. J Cardiovasc Electrophysiol 14:1273–1277
9. Gaita F, Giustetto C, Bianchi F et al (2004) Short QT syndrome: pharmacological treatment. J Am Coll Cardiol 43:1294–1299
10. Wolpert C, Schimpf R, Giustetto C et al (2005) Further insights into the effect of quinidine in short QT syndrome caused by a mutation in HERG. J Cardiovasc Electrophysiol 16:1–5

ICD Therapy for Short QT Syndrome: The Risk of Inappropriate Shocks and How to Avoid Them

M. Borggrefe[1], C. Wolpert[1], C. Giustetto[2], F. Gaita[2], U. Bauersfeld[3], R. Schimpf[1]

The short QT syndrome is a new congenital entity associated with familial atrial fibrillation and/or sudden death or syncope occurring in all age groups, even in newborns. The syndrome is characterised electrocardiographically by a shortened QTc interval less than 320 ms, shortened atrial and ventricular effective refractory periods, and a high percentage of inducible ventricular tachyarrhythmias during programmed electrical stimulation (Fig. 1) [1, 2]. In this genetically heterogeneous disease three different gain-of-function mutations in genes encoding for cardiac potassium channels (*KCNH2*, *KCNQ1*, and *KCNJ2*) have been identified so far [3–5]. The initial and long-term follow-up of the five initial patients with a short QT syndrome supplied with an implantable cardioverter defibrillator (ICD) will be reported below.

In two unrelated families with a short QT syndrome (SQT1) ICD devices were implanted for primary and secondary prevention [2]. The mean QT intervals were 252 ± 13 ms (QTc 287 ± 13 ms); there were two male and three female patients, mean age 38 ± 19 years. One patient, a 16-year-old adolescent, received a Marquis VR 7230 (Medtronic Inc., Minneapolis, Minn., USA) in the left subpectoral region and a tripolar pace/sense/shock electrode in the right ventricular apex with true bipolar pacing and sensing capabilities (6943 Sprint, Medtronic Inc.). The other four patients received an Atlas VR V-199 and three Photon Micro VR-194 systems (St. Jude Medical Inc., St. Paul, Minn., USA) in the left subpectoral region with true bipolar pacing and sensing (TVL-ADX 1559, RIATA 158) and two SPL leads with integrated bipolar sensing (St. Jude Medical Inc.). Each implantation covered

[1]1st Department of Medicine-Cardiology, University Hospital Mannheim, Germany; [2]Division of Cardiology, Ospedale Civile di Asti, Italy; [3]Division of Cardiology, University Children's Hospital Zurich, Switzerland

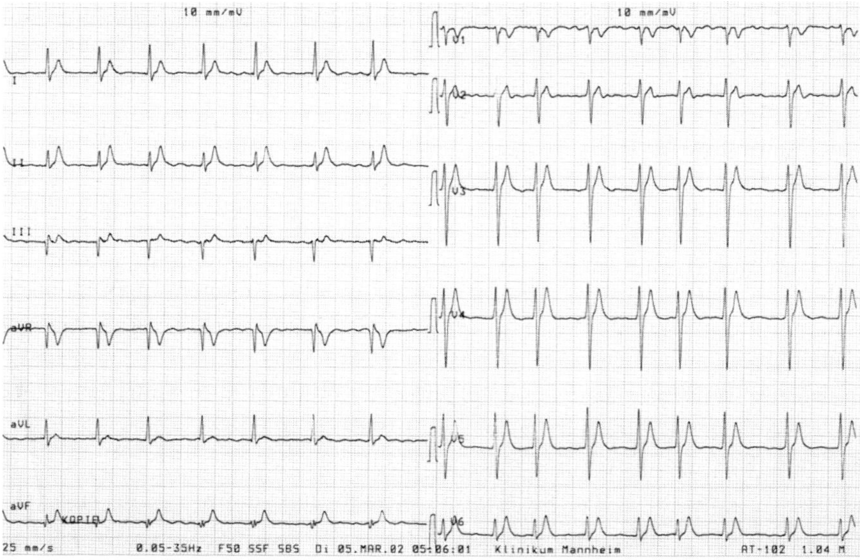

Fig. 1. ECG from a 71-year-old patient with a short QT syndrome and atrial fibrillation (QT interval 240 ms, QTc 290 ms, paper speed 25 mm/s)

a thorough measurement of lead impedances, ventricular pacing thresholds, and the verification of stable R wave signals. In addition, detailed testing of the lowest and highest ventricular sensitivity was performed, including induction of ventricular fibrillation at lowest ventricular sensitivity, which was 1.2 mV for the Medtronic device and 1.0 mV for the St. Jude Medical systems. After inappropriate shock delivery extensive manoeuvres were tested in all patients during real-time electrogram recording. These covered breathing manoeuvres, posture changes, exercise testing, and fluoroscopic exclusion of an altered lead position.

Four of the five patients received inappropriate shock deliveries 54 ± 52 days after implantation at a mean sinus rhythm cycle length of 460 ± 120 ms. The post-ventricular sensing refractory periods were 120 ms in the first patient and 125 ms in the other patients [6].

In all patients, measured standard parameters during implant such as ventricular shock impedance (54 ± 7.2 Ω), pacing threshold (0.7 ± 0.3 V/0.4 ± 0.13 ms), ventricular sensing (12 ± 4 mV) were within the normal range.

However, the first patient received two inappropriate shock deliveries only 45 min after termination of the operation due to T wave oversensing. The T wave was detected at a maximal ventricular sensitivity of 0.3 mV and double counting of the R and T wave led to inappropriate therapy. After an initial R/T wave signal ratio of 2.4:1, a reduction of the ratio to 2:1 due to slight reduction of the R wave signal was found. For future prevention of inappropriate therapies, it is necessary to assess both the calculation of the signal and algorithm and the capabilities of specific programming of the sensitivity. The sensing decay after detection of the R wave in the Medtronic algorithm is exponential. Each detected R wave induces an exponential decay starting at an amplitude of 75% of the R wave. The maximum amplitude of the decay start is the eightfold maximum programmed sensitivity. The only option to react to T wave oversensing by reprogramming is to reduce the maximum ventricular sensitivity given a stable and high R wave signal, thus elevating the start of the exponential decay. The ventricular refractory period with complete suppression of ventricular sensing is permanently programmed at 120 ms. Therefore ventricular sensitivity was reduced to 0.9 mV.

During the subsequent months further episodes of inappropriate shocks occurred (Fig. 2). The ventricular sensitivity had to be programmed to 1.2 mV, which is the maximum programmable sensitivity in the Medtronic device. To guarantee correct sensing of low-amplitude ventricular tachyarrhythmias, undersensing was excluded by an ICD test with induction of ventricular fibrillation.

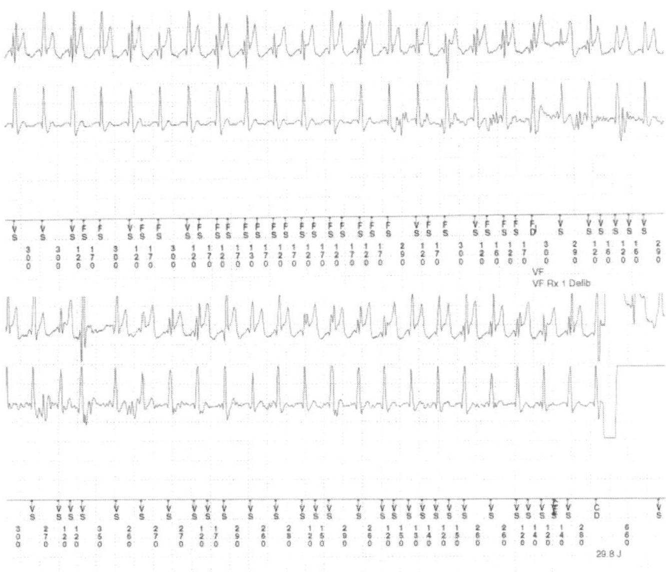

Fig. 2. Stored endocardial electrogram derived from the ventricular pace/sense/shock electrode of the patient from Fig. 1 (Marquis VR 7230; Medtronic Inc.). *First line:* Bipolar near-field electrogram between distal tip and ring of electrode; *second line:* far-field electrogram between defibrillation coil of ventricular electrode and device can; *third line:* corresponding annotation of the detected events by the ICD. *VS* Sensed ventricular events; continuous sensing of R wave and T wave before charging end of condenser (*CE*) and charge delivery (*CD*). *Fourth line:* Cycle lengths between each sensed event in numbers; double counting of R wave and T wave signals with RT time interval of 140 ms

Another patient, a 67-year-old woman, experienced one inappropriate shock delivery 4 weeks after implantation due to double counting of the R and T wave. As in the first patient, the amplitude of the T wave has increased during follow-up. The algorithms of the Atlas and Photon devices act differently to the Marquis algorithm. The algorithm integrates the QRS signal and starts a sensing decay from a programmable start threshold value (nominal 50% of the maximum amplitude of the R wave, measured in the refractory period, up to 100% of the maximum R wave amplitude). The following decay is linear, in contrast to the exponential decay from Medtronic, and the sensitivity is increased every 312 ms by 1 mV. A delay for the linear decay is programmable from 0 to 220 ms. As a third step, the maximum ventricular sensitivity can be reduced, and eventually the ventricular refractory period may be increased from 125 to 157 ms. However, the risk of underdetection or prolongation of arrhythmia detection has to be thoroughly evaluated. In this patient the maximum ventricular sensitivity was reduced to 0.5 mV. The R wave signal was stable at 17.7 mV. As a second step the start threshold value was increased from 50% to 62.5% and a decay delay of 60 ms was programmed. All manoeuvres (see above) documented correct R wave sensing. During a follow-up of 2 years so far, no further inappropriate therapies and double sensing were documented with a stable R and T wave signal.

The daughter of the previous patient, a 40-year-old woman with a short QT syndrome, experienced two inappropriate shocks due to T wave oversensing. The R wave signal was reduced to 4 mV. The patient was treated with quinidine, which previously in patients with a SQT1 syndrome showed prolongation of the QT interval into the normal range [7, 8]. The first young adolescent also received quinidine at a dosage of 1 g/day after he experienced both an episode of primary ventricular fibrillation and multiple inappropriate shocks [9]. In both patients the drug prolonged the QT interval, and although the amplitude of the T wave was unaltered after drug therapy no more inappropriate episodes occurred. One explanation could be that under drug treatment the frequency content of the T wave signal, which is calculated by the sense amplifier of the ICD, changed and the signal was no longer detected.

Finally, the last patient, a 35-year-old man, received an inappropriate discharge 53 days after implantation due to T wave oversensing. Again, a postoperative increase of the T wave amplitude was documented. As in the second reported case, an adaptation of the programming with a decay delay of 60 ms and a start threshold of 62.5% was initiated. During a follow-up of 2.5 years no inappropriate shock was documented. The other two patients did not receive inappropriate shock therapies. However, both of them were prophylactically programmed with a decay delay of 60 ms and start threshold of 62.5% as a reaction to the inappropriate therapies of the first three patients.

Although infrequent, T wave oversensing still constitutes a substantial pro-arrhythmic risk [10]. The most common causes are atrial fibrillation, sinus tachycardia, other supraventricular tachycardias, and R wave oversensing [11–16]. However, in patients with a short QT syndrome T wave oversensing may constitute a significant and inherent risk for inappropriate therapies. Shortened QT intervals and significantly elevated T wave amplitude represent a constant phenomenon. A postoperative reduction in the R wave amplitude, and in two cases increase of the T wave signal, was the reason for oversensing despite the fact that no abnormalities were observed at implant or prehospital discharge testing in any of the affected patients. During close follow-up, amplitude changes of the intracardiac R and T wave signals must be assessed. In contrast to patients with long QT syndrome, double sensing of the R and T wave should be less likely in patients with short QT syndrome as the T wave occurs early after beginning of the RR interval and the sensitivity is lowest in the early phase of the sensing algorithms after the detection of the R wave. However, the abnormal amplitude of the T wave signal and potentially the frequency content of the T wave may vary in comparison to those of normal patients and thus could pass the sense amplifier of the ICD [17].

There are different algorithms currently available which address T wave oversensing, and which vary between the manufacturers. The programming has to be adjusted based upon the specific sensing algorithm involved. A multi-programmable algorithm appears to be most suitable for preventing oversensing of short coupled high-amplitude T wave signals in patients with short QT syndrome. However, this needs to be evaluated in larger patient numbers. Another three patients who received an ICD did not experience inappropriate therapies during short-term follow-up (Guidant, Indianapolis, Ind., USA) [18, 19].

Nevertheless, irrespective of the different sensing algorithms, a prerequisite for individual adaptation of sensing parameters is a lead position which guarantees a constant and high R wave signal. This has to be balanced against correct arrhythmia detection and discrimination.

References

1. Gussak I, Brugada P, Brugada J et al (2000) Idiopathic short QT interval: a new clinical syndrome? Cardiology 94:99–102
2. Gaita F, Giustetto C, Bianchi F et al (2003) Short QT syndrome: a familial cause of sudden death. Circulation 108:965–970
3. Brugada R, Hong K, Dumaine R et al (2004) Sudden death associated with short QT syndrome linked to mutations in HERG. Circulation 109:30–35
4. Bellocq C, van Ginneken AC, Bezzina CR et al (2004) Mutation in the KCNQ1 gene leading to the short QT-interval syndrome. Circulation 109:2394–2397

5. Priori SG, Pandit SV, Rivolta I et al (2005) A novel form of short QT syndrome (SQT3) is caused by a mutation in the KCNJ2 gene. Circ Res 96:800–807
6. Schimpf R, Wolpert C, Bianchi F et al (2003) Congenital short QT-syndrome and ICD treatment: inherent risk for inappropriate shock delivery. J Cardiovasc Electrophysiol 14:1273–1277
7. Gaita F, Giustetto C, Bianchi F et al (2004) Short QT syndrome: pharmacological treatment. J Am Coll Cardiol 43:1494–99
8. Wolpert C, Schimpf R, Giustetto C et al (2005) Further insights into the effect of quinidine in short QT syndrome caused by a mutation in HERG. J Cardiovasc Electrophysiol 16:54–58
9. Schimpf R, Bauersfeld U, Gaita F et al (2005) Short QT syndrome: successful prevention of sudden cardiac death in an adolescent by implantable cardioverter defibrillator treatment for primary prophylaxis. Heart Rhythm 2:416–417
10. Pinski SL, Fahy GJ (1995) The proarrhythmic potential of implantable cardioverter-defibrillators. Circulation 92:1651–1664
11. Washizuka T, Chinushi M, Kasai H et al (2001) Inappropriate discharges from an intravenous implantable cardioverter defibrillator due to T wave oversensing. Jpn Circ J 65:685–687
12. Washizuka T, Chinushi M, Tagawa M et al (2001) Inappropriate discharges by fourth generation implantable cardioverter defibrillator in patients with ventricular arrhythmias. Jpn Circ J 65:927–930
13. Böhm A, Pinter A, Preda I (1998) QT dependent T wave sensing. Pacing Clin Electrophysiol 21:1490–1491
14. Weretka S, Michaelsen J, Becker R et al (2003) Ventricular oversensing: a study of 101 patients implanted with dual chamber defibrillators and two different lead systems. Pacing Clin Electrophysiol 26:65–70
15. Gershon YP, Kosar EM (1996) Problems in managing patients with long QT-syndrome and implantable cardioverter defibrillators: a report of two cases. Pacing Clin Electrophysiol 19:863–867
16. Weber M, Block M, Brunn J et al (1996) Inadequate therapies with implantable cardioverter-defibrillators – incidence, etiology, predictive factors and preventive strategies. Z Kardiol 85:809–819
17. Passman R (2003) Inappropriate implantable cardioverter defibrillator therapy in short QT syndrome. Old problem in a new disease. J Cardiovasc Electrophysiol 14:1278–1279
18. Bjerregaard P, Gussak I (2004) Atrial fibrillation in the setting of familial short QT interval. Heart Rhythm 1:S165 (abs)
19. Hong K, Bjerregaard P, Gussak I et al (2005) Short QT syndrome and atrial fibrillation caused by mutation in KCNH2. J Cardiovasc Electrophysiol 16:394–396

Quinidine to Treat Short QT Syndrome: A Real Alternative to ICD?

C. Giustetto

Short QT syndrome (SQTS) is a recently described familial arrhythmogenic disorder related to an accelerated repolarisation time. Patients with short QT syndrome present with a wide spectrum of clinical manifestations, ranging from mild symptoms such as palpitations and dizziness to syncope and sudden death [1]. Sudden death sometimes occurs in children in the first months of life and is often the first clinical presentation. Palpitations with documentation of atrial fibrillation occur even at a young age [2]. ECG shows QT intervals of less than 320 ms and QTc not exceeding 340 ms [3]. Physical examination, blood laboratory exams, echocardiogram, and stress test are normal. Mutations causing a gain of function in the rapidly activating delayed rectifier potassium current (I_{Kr}) [4], in the slowly activating delayed rectifier potassium current (I_{Ks}) [5], and in the cardiac inward rectifier current (I_{K1}) [6], have been described.

Due to the high incidence of sudden cardiac death and the absence of known pharmacological therapy, the placement of an implantable cardioverter–defibrillator (ICD) is presently the first-choice therapy [1, 7]. ICD implantation, however, is not feasible in every patient. For this reason we administered various anti-arrhythmic drugs to patients with short QT syndrome to evaluate whether they could prolong the QT interval into the normal range and, thus, potentially prevent symptoms and arrhythmia recurrences [8]. As the mutations found in our first families increase the activity of I_{Kr}, the first drugs we administered were the class III anti-arrhythmic agents sotalol and ibutilide, which are selective I_{Kr} blockers. However, these drugs did not prolong the QT interval. The mutation must cause the loss of

Department of Cardiology, Cardinal Massaia Hospital, Asti, Italy some of the physiological regulatory mechanisms, and I_{Kr} become insensitive to drugs that normally have a specific action on it [4]. Quinidine, however, produced a marked prolongation of the QT interval, which then entered the normal range, and of ventricular effective refractory periods, preventing induction of ventricular fibrillation. Furthermore, quinidine treatment produced the appearance of an obvious ST segment and of broader T waves [8]. The basis of the greater effectiveness of quinidine is not fully understood, but a greater affinity of quinidine for the open state of the I_{kr} channel and its ability to block I_{Ks} might explain the prolongation of the QT interval.

So far we have treated 21 patients, 10 of whom received an ICD, while 11 did not (2 because they were very young and 9 refused the implant). The 11 patients who did not receive an ICD were started on hydroquinidine, as were another 5 patients who did receive an ICD, who had symptomatic episodes of atrial fibrillation. In the patients who received hydroquinidine, QT interval lengthened from 271 ± 13 ms to 347 ± 33 ms ($P < 0.005$), and QTc changed from 297 ± 15 ms to 397 ± 25 ms ($P < 0.0005$). One of the characteristics of the short QT syndrome is the lack of dependence of QT interval on heart rate. In 3 patients who repeated a stress test during quinidine treatment, it was observed that the drug restored the heart rate dependence of the QT interval towards the normal range [9]. The HERG mutation (encoding for I_{Kr}) was found in 6 out of the 11 patients; no known mutation was found in the other 5. A repeat electrophysiological study was carried out with hydroquinidine therapy in the 9 adult patients: ventricular effective refractory period (ERP) lengthened to more than 200 ms in all of them and ventricular fibrillation was no longer inducible. The mean follow-up is 17 ± 13 months. None of the patients on hydroquinidine died, nor did any have documented or symptomatic atrial fibrillation recurrences. Two patients stopped drug therapy due to enteric side effects.

Quinidine may also be useful in the prevention of inappropriate shocks due to oversensing of the high voltage T waves in patients with ICDs [7]. However, a longer follow-up is needed to decide in favour of the effectiveness of a drug in a life-long disease.

References

1. Gaita F, Giustetto C, Bianchi F et al (2003) Short QT syndrome. A familial cause of sudden death. Circulation 108:965–970
2. Gussak I, Brugada P, Brugada J et al (2000) Idiopathic short QT interval: a new clinical syndrome? Cardiology 94:99–102
3. Giustetto C, Wolpert C, Anttonen O et al (2005) Clinical presentation of the patients with short QT syndrome. Heart Rhythm 2:S61
4. Brugada P, Hong K, Dumaine R et al (2004) Sudden death associated with short QT

syndrome linked to mutations in HERG. Circulation 109:30–35
5. Bellocq C, van Ginneken A, Bezzina C (2004) Mutation in the KCNQ1 gene leading to the short QT-interval syndrome. Circulation 109:2394–2397
6. Priori SG, Pandit SV, Rivolta I et al (2005) A novel form of short QT syndrome (SQTS3) is caused by a mutation in the KCNJ2 gene. Circ Res 96:800–807
7. Schimpf R, Wolpert C, Bianchi F et al (2003) Congenital short QT syndrome and implantable cardioverter defibrillator. Inherent risk for inappropriate shock delivery. J Cardiovasc Electrophysiol 14:1273–1277
8. Gaita F, Giustetto C, Bianchi F et al (2004) Short QT syndrome: pharmacological treatment. J Am Coll Cardiol 43:1294–1299
9. Wolpert C, Schimpf R, Giustetto C et al (2005) Further insights into the effect of quinidine in Short QT syndrome caused by a mutation in HERG. J Cardiovasc Electrophysiol 16:1–5

ICD for the Long QT Syndrome: Which Indications, Complications, and Results?

P.J. Schwartz[1,2], C. Spazzolini[1], L. Crotti[1,2]

The number of patients affected by the long QT syndrome (LQTS) who are told by their physicians that they should receive an implantable cardioverter-defibrillator (ICD) is increasing exponentially. Why? In this short essay we will try to provide an answer to this question, and we will also briefly review the data available to assess whether or not adequate information exists on the indications and results of the growing use of the ICD for patients with LQTS. While the data are what they are, the opinions expressed here are our own and reflect to a large extent the clinical experience developed by one of us in managing and treating LQTS patients during the past 35 years [1–4].

The Issue

To simplify matters we will start by stating the obvious: patients who have survived a cardiac arrest should immediately receive an ICD, in addition to traditional therapy. Thus, our entire discussion will concern patients whose only symptom has been one or more syncope episode, before or on therapy. The possibility of implanting an ICD in an asymptomatic patient is not even discussed, because in a disease whose natural history shows that 50% of patients remain asymptomatic through life *without* therapy [5], this represents, in our opinion, an aberration. Unfortunately, aberrations do occur.

A second starting point is that the evidence from multiple databases [3] that cardiac arrest/sudden death (CA/SD) as first episode may occur in up to 12% of patients with LQTS dictates the necessity to treat all LQTS patients

[1]Department of Cardiology, University of Pavia and IRCCS Policlinico S. Matteo, Pavia;
[2]Molecular Cardiology Laboratory, IRCCS Policlinico S. Matteo, Pavia, Italy

with β-blockers once they have been diagnosed as affected [3]. This rule has few exceptions, largely on the basis of the age of the patient at the time of diagnosis, and in some subgroups (e.g., LQT1) on the basis of gender.

Management and Outcome of Patients with Syncope

Having limited, on the basis of common sense, the discussion to patients with syncope, let us now examine what we know about their prognosis. What happens to a patient treated with β-blockers? Even though the genotype of the patient is usually still unknown when the first decision has to be made, it is no longer acceptable to ignore the practical consequences of genotyping or to look for excuses for being ignorant on this matter. At the present time, 70% of affected patients are positively genotyped in our laboratory (Molecular Cardiology Laboratory, Policlinico S. Matteo and University of Pavia) within 4–5 months, and the same is true in most laboratories. Furthermore, for most patients – including those who are genotype-negative – the experienced clinician can predict the genotype fairly accurately [6] on the basis of: (1) the morphology of the T wave [7, 8]; (2) the 'triggers' or conditions associated with the events [9]; and (3) the different prevalences of the different genotypes [5, 10]. Finally, our evidence that – as predicted in 1980 [11] – low penetrance exists in LQTS, and that therefore within each family several individuals may have a normal QT interval and still be mutation carriers [12], makes failure to attempt genotyping in every LQTS patient inexcusable, with significant medico-legal implications.

It is on this rational basis that one should look at the available data. In our study based on the LQTS International Registry [13], Moss et al. [14] provided data based on 869 patients treated with β-blockers. As always, data from registries and not from randomised trials have to be examined with special care. When the analysis leaves out the survivors of a cardiac arrest (who should receive an ICD in any case), the patients who were off therapy for more than 3 months, and the patients who became symptomatic in the first year of life (because they represent a subgroup at extremely high risk who should be dealt with and considered separately from the rest of the LQTS population), it turns out that mortality on β-blocker therapy was 1.6%! This is a very important figure to be considered carefully when proposing invasive therapies.

If one looks at genotyped patients, there are important data there as well. In a three-centre study, all with a high referral rate, in 157 LQT1 patients the combined incidence of CA/SD over a very long average follow-up (12 years) was only 1.2% [15]. In the study from our group based on 187 LQT1 patients the combined incidence of CA/SD was 1.1% [16]. Thus, these two major studies provide almost identical data which show beyond doubt that 98% of LQT1 patients can do very well on β-blocker therapy. It is very unlikely that a LQT1 patient who has not yet had a cardiac arrest would significantly benefit from an ICD. It is important to remember that LQT1 patients represent at least 50% of all LQTS patients.

Two large series of patients provide data on LQT2 patients. In one [9], based on 91 LQT2 patients all with symptoms, there was a combined 4% incidence of CA/SD on therapy. Of note, these were all cases of cardiac arrest and there were no sudden deaths. In the other [16], the combined incidence of CA/SD was 6.6%, but once again these events were all cardiac arrests and there were no deaths. When one looks objectively at these data one has to recognise that 93–96% of LQT2 patients do well on β-blockers even though the protection appears not as complete as for LQT1 patients.

The same two reports, on the other hand, demonstrated a relatively high incidence of CA/SD among LQT3 patients, the most uncommon of the three major genetic subgroups. This incidence of failures in the two studies was, respectively, 17% and 14%. These figures justify serious consideration for therapeutic approaches beyond β-blockers. Such additional approaches include obviously the ICDs, but not only. For LQT3 patients, one can expect a fair amount of benefit by also adding left cardiac sympathetic denervation (LCSD) [17] or the sodium channel blocker mexiletine [4, 18].

Before discussing the actual ICD data it is necessary to recall the alternative options. We presented last year updated information on the long-term results of LCSD. This 35-min operation performed without opening the chest has resulted in a more than 90% reduction in the number of cardiac events [17]. The population under study was one at extremely high risk, as documented by the number of symptomatic patients (99%), the high percentage (75%) of those with cardiac events despite β-blockers, and the extreme average prolongation of the QT interval (QTc = 543 ± 65 ms). Among the patients with syncope, there has been a 5-year mortality rate of 3% and an incidence of resuscitated cardiac arrest of 8%. LCSD also shortened QTc by an average of 40 ms, and we have found that lethal cardiac events after surgery occurred only among those patients who continued to have a QTc greater than 500 ms (Fig. 1). A very important and highly related finding was made in those patients who developed storms or who had multiple shocks following ICD implant; in this unfortunate group LCSD was able to reduce by 95% the number of shocks, thus having a dramatic impact on the quality of life of these patients and of their families (Table 1).

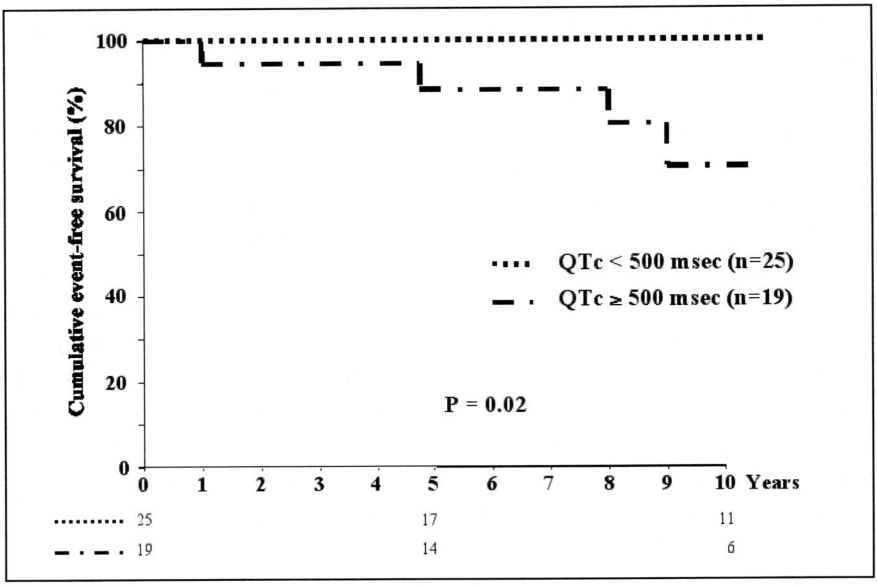

Fig. 1. Kaplan–Meier curves of event-free survival and survival according to QTc interval after left cardiac sympathetic denervation in patients with only syncope or aborted cardiac arrest before left cardiac sympathetic denervation (modified with permission from [17])

Table 1. ICD multiple shocks and left cardiac sympathetic denervation (LCSD)

Patients with LCSD post ICD	5
Follow-up ICD → LCSD	17±16 months
Follow-up post LCSD	4.1 years
Pre LCSD shocks per patient per year	29.3
Post LCSD shocks per patient per year	3.3
Reduction	95%

ICD implantable cardioverter defibrillator

Registries for ICD in LQTS

There are only two relatively large sets of data on LQTS patients who have received an ICD, those from Zareba et al. [19] on 125 patients and those from the European Registry [20], initiated by our group with the support of many European electrophysiologists, which has enrolled so far 112 patients, including most of those recently reported by Mönnig et al. [21]. The number of genotyped patients in the two series is relatively small; nonetheless, it is of interest – and probably not by chance – that there is an excess of LQT2 patients.

The available data are rather disquieting. In the two registries, only 43% and 46% of the implanted patients had had an aborted cardiac arrest, which should be the primary and main reason for implantation. In the series of Zareba et al. 35% received an ICD because of one syncope irrespectively of β-blocker therapy and 13% were mostly asymptomatic individuals who received implants because of a sudden death in the family! The latter decision was taken by physicians apparently unaware of the evidence showing that a sudden death in the family does not increase the risk of lethal events among other family members [22]; if the decision is taken not for true medical reasons but because of emotional considerations, then it is a different story. In the European Registry the number of asymptomatic patients who have had an ICD implanted is 5%. In addition, 19% of the patients received an ICD for syncope occurring prior to institution of β-blocker therapy! These data sadly show that in more than 50% of cases the ICD is implanted in patients who have not had the most appropriate indication, namely a cardiac arrest.

The number of appropriate shocks during follow-up in patients *not* implanted for cardiac arrest is a very important one. Unfortunately, we have not been able to find this number in the article by Zareba et al. In our data set this figure is 12% within an average follow-up of 3 years.

Zareba et al. [19] tried to demonstrate the beneficial effect of the ICD by comparing mortality in this group to a group of LQTS patients considered to be similar to those who received the ICD and who continued to be treated conventionally. They concluded by stating that LQTS-related deaths occurred in 1.3% vs 16% ($P = 0.07$), thus showing the superiority of the ICD vs the non-ICD therapy. As commented by others [23], these data generate numerous questions. This was a retrospective comparison in which the control (non-ICD) group was chosen by the authors among the patients in the LQTS registry. Two aspects cause concern. One is that 16% mortality in properly treated LQTS is, to say the least, an exceptionally high figure. The second is that more than half of these deaths occurred within 3 months from the moment selected retrospectively by the authors to be regarded as time zero for this statistical analysis. It seems to us that comparisons on the life expectancy of LQTS patients treated or not treated with an ICD should require a more rigorous analysis and that, once again, it should be limited to the patients without cardiac arrest about whom there seems to be an ongoing debate.

One has also to look also at the down side. In the report by Zareba et al. there were two deaths, giving an incidence of 1.6% which – interestingly, and worth remembering – is the same as that among patients without cardiac arrest in the large report by Moss et al. [14] discussed above. One patient, a child, died because of recurrent torsades-de-pointes; the other, a 21-year-old girl, committed suicide. The possibility that the suicide was related to the ICD (as previously reported for other cases) was not considered, and the statistical analysis has included only 1 LQTS-related death. In the European Registry inappropriate shocks occurred in 10% of patients and 8% had multiple repetitive discharges. Importantly, given the relatively short follow-up of 3 years, 27% of the patients underwent invasive/surgical interventions on either the generator or the leads of the ICD for a variety of reasons ranging from end-of-life of battery to lead fracture or lead dysfunction, or others.

The bottom line here is that the implantation of an ICD is not the end of the problems for many LQTS patients. This is one important reason, not to mention the significant and often devastating psychological impact, especially in young patients, for doing everything possible to limit the ICD implants to those patients who really are appropriate candidates.

Having looked at the available data, one inescapable conclusion is that too many patients receive an ICD for questionable or incorrect indications. Of the several reasons which may underlie this reality one merits attention, and this is the physician's fear of medico-legal consequences for not having implanted an ICD in a patient who subsequently develops a cardiac arrest or dies suddenly. Clearly, to recommend an ICD implies no fears about survival, it is simple and fast, and if complications do occur that is just too bad. To explain to patients or parents that non-ICD therapies, despite their high degree of efficacy, do not offer a 100% protection and a tragic event cannot be ruled out; that the potential complications of an ICD during a lifetime should be carefully weighed against the almost 100% survival; that quality of life would be impacted differently by the various options: all these considerations take a lot of time and emotional involvement by the physician, who often chooses the simplest solution. While we understand these practical reasons, our concern is that too often the final decision is made more for the physician's than for the patient's protection.

Conclusions

There is a high and in many cases inappropriate use of ICDs in patients with long QT syndrome with syncope. The pros and cons of the ICD and of the other available therapies should be clearly explained to all patients before recommending one or another.

It should be remembered that LQTS is profoundly different from most of the more prevalent conditions for which an ICD is usually recommended, and that among the special features of LQTS the tight relationship between release of catecholamines and life-threatening arrhythmias is an important one capable of initiating storms of shocks.

The wise use of the ICD in LQTS can save many lives. The unwise use of the ICD in LQTS can ruin many lives. A competent and caring physician should not be unmindful of his/her complex responsibilities toward the – usually young – LQTS patients.

Acknowledgements
The authors are grateful to Medtronic-Bakken Research Center B.V., The Netherlands, and to Guidant Italia Srl for their support of the European ICD Registry for the Long QT Syndrome. They also thanks Pinuccia De Tomasi for expert editorial support.

References

1. Schwartz PJ, Periti M, Malliani A (1975) The long Q-T syndrome. Am Heart J 89:378–390
2. Schwartz PJ (1985) Idiopathic long QT syndrome: progress and questions. Am Heart J 109:399–411
3. Schwartz PJ, Priori SG, Napolitano C (2000) The long QT syndrome. In: Zipes DP, Jalife J (eds) Cardiac electrophysiology. From cell to bedside, 3rd edn. Saunders, Philadelphia, pp 597–615
4. Schwartz PJ (2005) Management of the long QT syndrome. Nat Clin Pract Cardiovasc Med 2:346–351
5. Priori SG, Schwartz PJ, Napolitano C et al (2003) Risk stratification in the long-QT syndrome. N Engl J Med 348:1866–1874
6. Schwartz PJ, Priori SG (2004) Long QT syndrome: genotype-phenotype correlations. In: Zipes DP, Jalife J (eds) Cardiac electrophysiology. From cell to bedside, 3rd edn. Saunders, Philadelphia, pp 651–659
7. Moss AJ, Zareba W, Benhorin J et al (1995) ECG T-wave patterns in genetically distinct forms of the hereditary long QT syndrome. Circulation 92:2929–2934
8. Zhang L, Timothy KW, Vincent GM et al (2000) Spectrum of ST-T-wave patterns and repolarization parameters in congenital long QT syndrome. ECG findings identify genotypes. Circulation 102:2849–2855
9. Schwartz PJ, Priori SG, Spazzolini C et al (2001) Genotype-phenotype correlation in the long QT syndrome. Gene-specific triggers for life-threatening arrhythmias. Circulation 103:89–95
10. Splawski I, Shen J, Timothy KW et al (2000) Spectrum of mutations in long-QT syndrome genes. Circulation 102:1178–1185
11. Schwartz PJ (1980) The long QT syndrome. In: Kulbertus HE, Wellens HJJ (eds) Sudden death. M Nijhoff, The Hague, pp 358–378
12. Priori SG, Napolitano C, Schwartz PJ (1999) Low penetrance in the long QT syndrome. Clinical impact. Circulation 99:529–533
13. Moss AJ, Schwartz PJ (2005) 25th Anniversary of the international Long QT Syndrome Registry: an ongoing quest to uncover the secrets of LQTS. Circulation 111:1199–1201
14. Moss AJ, Zareba W, Hall WJ et al (2000) Effectiveness and limitations of beta-blocker therapy in congenital long-QT syndrome. Circulation 101:616–623

15. Vincent GM, Bithell C, Schwartz PJ et al (2003) Efficacy of beta-blockers in the LQT1 genotype of long QT syndrome. Circulation 108:IV–506 (abs)
16. Priori SG, Napolitano C, Schwartz PJ et al (2004) Association of long QT syndrome loci and cardiac events among patients treated with beta-blockers. JAMA 292:1341–1344
17. Schwartz PJ, Priori SG, Cerrone M et al (2004) Left cardiac sympathetic denervation in the management of high-risk patients affected by the long-QT syndrome. Circulation 109:1826–1833
18. Schwartz PJ, Priori SG, Locati EH et al (1995) Long QT syndrome patients with mutations on the SCN5A and HERG genes have differential responses to Na+ channel blockade and to increases in heart rate. Implications for gene-specific therapy. Circulation 92:3381–3386
19. Zareba W, Moss AJ, Daubert JP et al (2003) Implantable cardioverter defibrillator in high-risk long QT syndrome patients. J Cardiovasc Electrophysiol 14:337–341
20. Crotti L, Spazzolini C, De Ferrari GM et al (2004) Is the implantable defibrillator appropriately used in the long QT syndrome? Data from the European Registry. Heart Rhythm 1(Suppl):582
21. Mönnig G, Köbe J, Löher A et al (2005) Implantable cardioverter-defibrillator therapy in patients with congenital long-QT syndrome: a long-term follow-up. Heart Rhythm 2:497–504
22. Kimbrough J, Moss AJ, Zareba W et al (2001) Clinical implications for affected parents and siblings of probands with long QT syndrome. Circulation 104:557–562
23. Viskin S (2003) Implantable cardioverter defibrillator in high-risk long QT syndrome patients. J Cardiovasc Electrophysiol 14:1130–1131

How To Differentiate Right Ventricular Outflow Tract Tachycardia from Arrhythmogenic Right Ventricular Cardiomyopathy?

C. WOLPERT, C. ECHTERNACH, C. VELTMANN, R. SCHIMPF, M. BORGGREFE

Introduction

Arrhythmogenic right ventricular cardiomyopathy (ARVC) is a disease characterised by partial replacement of myocardial tissue by fibrofatty tissue. Ventricular tachycardia may originate from the diseased areas and cause haemodynamically non-tolerated ventricular tachycardia, syncope, or sudden death already in young patients.

Time of first diagnosis is usually before the age of 40 and not infrequently already in adolescence. The aetiology of ARVC varies and there are different hypotheses as to how ARVC develops [1, 2]. Among affected patients, there is a predominance of males and early reports suggested that in some cases the disease may be familial. Moreover, a number of different gene mutations in desmosomes have been identified, such as mutations in cytoskeletal proteins, plakoglobin, and desmoplakin, and both autosomal-dominant and autosomal-recessive modes of inheritance have been reported. In some patients disease is also manifested in the left ventricle [3, 4].

Right ventricular outflow tract (RVOT) tachycardia is a benign condition. In the absence of structural heart disease, it is considered to be primary electrical defect that results in ventricular extra beats, salvos, or sustained tachycardias mainly from the right ventricular outflow tract, but also infrequently from other regions in the right ventricle, above the pulmonary valve or the sinus valsalva. A variety of mechanisms have been suggested, including cAMP-triggered activity through late after-depolarisation. RVOT tachycardia is also mainly observed in young patients, predominantly females, and often

1st Department of Medicine-Cardiology, University Hospital Mannheim, Faculty of Clinical Medicine of the University of Heidelberg, Mannheim, Germany

becomes symptomatic already in young adults. When confronted with a patient with left bundle-branch-block tachycardia with inferior axis, a diagnosis of idiopathic RVOT tachycardia can be made only after exclusion of ARVC. The differential diagnosis of ARVC is based on the criteria of the Task Force of the Working Group Myocardial and Pericardial Disease of the European Society of Cardiology and of the Scientific Council on Cardiomyopathies of the International Society and Federation of Cardiology. Classification is based on electrocardiographic patterns of depolarisation and repolarisation, echocardiography, endomyocardial biopsy findings, magnetic resonance imaging results, arrhythmia history, and other criteria [5]. However, clinical presentation alone does not allow a diagnosis to be made in the majority of patients. To differentiate between ARVC and RVOT tachycardia is a clinical challenge, and an intense work up is essential to making the correct therapeutic decision.

Electrocardiogram in Sinus Rhythm

There are different signs in the surface ECG of patients with arrhythmogenic right ventricular cardiomyopathy, most strikingly, the T-wave inversion and an epsilon-wave in lead V1 or V2. In addition, a localised increase of the QRS duration of > 110 ms in leads V1–V3 or positive late potentials are signs for a potential ARVC [1, 6, 7]. However, they are not observed in every patient and especially not during early stages of the disease. Although patients with a normal ECG at rest are less likely to suffer from ARVC, in the studies of Niroomand [6] and O'Donnell [7], repolarisation abnormalities in the precordial leads varied between the two studies from 66% to 52% in patients with ARVC, and from 23% to 6% in patients with RVOT tachycardia.

The ECGs of patients with ARVC often display an incomplete right bundle-branch block or T-wave inversion in the right precordial leads, sometimes also until V4, V5. In Niroomand's study, T-wave inversion was seen in 13/15 patients (87%), while 14% of patients displayed epsilon waves [6]. O'Donnell observed positive late potentials on the signal-averaged electrogram in 78% of patients with ARVC and in none of the patients with idiopathic RVOT tachycardia.

Electrocardiogram During Ventricular Tachycardia

In patients with ARVC, the ventricular tachycardia (VT) shows a pattern of left bundle-branch block. The QRS axis is shifted to the right when the VT originates in the pulmonary infundibulum. The axis may also be shifted to the extreme left when the VT arises from the diaphragmatic wall or is located in the right ventricular apex or close to the tricuspid annulus [1, 2]. In patients with ARVC, the upstroke of the QRS complex seems to have some 'slurring' and a slew rate that is less steep. The QRS complex also appears broader. In the study by Niroomand et al., the axis during VT in ARVC was inferior in 48%, intermediate in 27%, and left/superior in 20% of patients. In contrast, in patients with idiopathic RVOT tachycardia, it was inferior in 90% and intermediate or superior in only 5% [6].

The most common clinical presentation of RVOT tachycardia is a frequent, nonsustained repetition of uniform, monomorphic VT alternating with periods of sinus rhythm. Isolated ventricular extra systoles present the same morphologic pattern as observed in tachycardia. The cycle length of sustained ventricular tachycardia commonly ranges from 140 to 180 bpm [8, 9].

Transthoracic Echocardiography

The structural major abnormalities in ARVC can be detected by echocardiography, but minor abnormalities are seen only by magnetic resonance imaging (MRI). The signs of the disease are dilation of the right ventricle, the presence of aneurysm during diastole, and dyskinetic areas in the inferobasal region. Therefore, if there is any doubt about the diagnosis after transthoracic echocardiography, the patient should undergo cardiac MRI.

Nuclear Magnetic Resonance Imaging

Patients with right ventricular tachycardia should undergo MRI before intervention in order to detect aneurysms, intramyocardial fat, or advanced wall thickening before catheter ablation, if not distinct on echocardiography or right ventricular ventriculography [10].

Electrophysiological Study

Electrophysiological studies (EPSs) may help to differentiate RVOT tachycardia due to ARVC from idiopathic RVOT-VT. In the setting of ARVC, the signals of the endocardial electrograms may be significantly altered in terms of activation delay, fragmentation, amplitude decrease, or dense scarring. These features are not likely to be found in idiopathic RVOT tachycardia patients. Some investigators have analysed the endocardial electrograms by using an electroanatomical mapping tool. Using this approach, Boulos et al. found a significant difference between patients with ARVC and those with idiopathic RVOT tachycardia [11]. They also compared the duration and amplitude of the electrogram between normal probands, patients with RVOT-VT, and patients with an ARVC, and could demonstrate that while there was no difference between normal probands and patients with an idiopathic RVOT-VT, there was a very large difference compared to ARVC patients [11]. Areas with a strong disposition to fibrofatty degeneration and therefore areas to look for fragmentation or scarring are the RVOT, the subtricuspidal base of the ventricle, and the RV-apex. Another indicator for VT in structural heart disease is repetitive inducibility by programmed stimulation and the presence of a critical coupling interval. O'Donnell found that, in contrast to idiopathic RVOT-VT patients (3%), VT was induced by extra stimulation in 82% of patients with ARVC which indicates a re-entrant mechanism [6]. Furthermore, in that study, in patients with idiopathic RVOT tachycardia there was usually only one morphology in premature beats or VT, whereas 71% of patients with ARVC presented from one to six morphologies characteristic of inducible tachycardia. Therefore, in the presence of VT pleomorphism an ARVC should be suspected. Finally, the study also noted that fragmented diastolic electrograms occurred in 82% of patients with ARVC [6].

Inducibility maybe facilitated by infusion of isoproterenol in both clinical entities and is therefore not a criterion to discriminate between the two diseases.

Triggering Factors for VT and Symptoms

Idiopathic ventricular tachycardia from the RVOT and VT in ARVC are difficult to discriminate based on circumstances of onset, because sustained tachycardia and salvos tend to be induced by stress, catecholamines, or physical exercise in both cases [1, 2, 6]. However, there is a difference in symptoms in terms of severity for the overall population. Whereas syncope is more frequent in ARVC and cardiac arrest does practically not occur in idiopathic RVOT-VT, in idiopathic VT there are more mild to moderate palpitations and dizziness due to bradycardia with bigeminus and resulting peripheral pulse deficit. In ARVC, intensive physical activity or extreme anxiety is known to cause fast and recurrent VT with a considerable risk of sudden death. Therefore, it should be absolutely avoided in those patients [1].

Conclusions

The diagnosis of an idiopathic RVOT-VT is made by exclusion of ARVC or any other structural heart disease. If there are no signs of RV myocardial changes, such as dilatation, dyskinesia, hypokinesia, or aneurysms and wall thickening, and there are no electrocardiographic signs of ARVC, the patient most likely has an idiopathic RVOT-VT. However, especially in families with a history of sudden death, close follow-up may be useful. When enough minor or major criteria are met, the patient should be risk-stratified and treatment options should be tailored to the individual, taking into consideration the risks and benefits. In some younger patients with, e.g. syncope and one other minor criterion and RVOT-VT, this decision is often very difficult and will probably remain difficult. Genetic testing should be performed in all patients with a family history in order to detect relatives at risk.

References

1. Fontaine G, Fontaliran F, Hébert JL et al (1999) Arrhythmogenic right ventricular dysplasia. Annu Rev Med 50:17–35
2. Corrado D, Fontaine G, Marcus FI et al (2000) Arrhythmogenic right ventricular dysplasia/cardiomyopathy: need for an international registry. Circulation 101:E101-E106
3. Paul M, Schulze-Bahr E, Breithardt G et al (2003) Genetics of arrhythmogenic right ventricular cardiomyoapthy-status quo and future perspectives. Z Kardiol 92:128–136
4. Gerull B, Heuser A, Wichter T et al (2004) Mutations in the desmosomal protein plakophilin-2 are common in arrhythmogenic right ventricular cardiomyopathy. Nat Genet 36:1162–1164
5. McKenna WJ, Thiene G, Nava A et al (1994) Diagnosis of arrhythmogenic right ventricular cardiomyopathy. Task force of the working group on myocardial and precardial disease of the European Society of Cardiology and the scientific council on cardiomyopathies of the International Society and Federation of Cardiology. Br Heart J 71:215–218
6. Niroomand F, Carbucicchio C, Tondo C et al (2002) Electrophysiological characteristics and outcome in patients with idiopathic right ventricular arrhythmia compared with arrythmogenic right ventricular dysplasia. Heart 87:41–47
7. O'Donnell D, Cox D, Bourke J et al (2003) Clinical and electrophysiological differences between patients with arrhythmogenic right ventricular dysplasia and right ventricular outflow tract tachycardia. Eur Heart J 24:801–810
8. Altemose G, Buxton A (1999) Idiopathic ventricular Tachycardia. Annu Rev Med 50:159–177
9. Farzaneh-Far A, Lerman B (2005) Idiopathic ventricular outflow tract tachycardia. Heart 91:136–138
10. Carlson MD, White RD, Trohman RG et al (1994) Right ventricular outflow tract ventricular tachycardia: detection of previously unrecognised anatomic abnormalities using cine magnetic resonance imaging. J Am Coll Cardiol 24:720–727
11. Boulos M, Lashevsky I, Gepstein (2005) Usefulness of electroanatomical mapping to differentiate between right ventricular outflow tract tachycardia and arrhythmogenic right ventricular dysplasia. Am J Cardiol 95:935–940

How To Diagnose and Approach Epicardial Ventricular Tachycardia

E. Sosa, M. Scanavacca

Introduction

Epicardial ventricular tachycardia (VT) is defined as VT in which the critical sites of the reentrant circuit (or the 'sites of origin') are located exclusively in the subepicardial tissue, as shown by entrainment manoeuvres or VT that is terminated within 10 s with standard radiofrequency (RF) pulses, or both. This arbitrary definition is based on data obtained in our electrophysiology (EP) laboratory. Until now, the epicardial origin of a given VT has been suspected in those patients with nonischaemic VT, a QRS complex duration longer than 200 ms (specificity of 86% and sensitivity of 69% for epicardial circuits), and a delta-wave-like pattern (sensitivity and specificity of 80% for epicardial circuits). Berruezo et al. [1] recently reported similar ECG findings. At our centre, determination of the prevalence of an epicardial circuit is based on our experience using the above-mentioned criteria obtained at the EP lab. In our initial series of 215 consecutive patients, epicardial VT was systematically identified using a percutaneous subxiphoid approach. Epicardial VTs were identified in 32% of patients with post-myocardial-infarction (MI) VT, 36% of patients with Chagas heart disease, and 25% of patients with idiopathic dilated cardiomyopathy [2].

Despite innovations in mapping techniques, the standard endocardial ablation of VT remains an enormous challenge especially in VT associated with structural heart disease. In this subset of patients, results following the use of an conventional endocardial approach have not been consistent [3, 4]. The presence of epicardial circuits has been considered as one of the reasons for the failure of endocardial ablation, and these circuits have been described

Clinical Arrhythmia and Pacemaker Units, Heart Institute – InCor –, University of São Paulo Medical School, São Paulo, Brazil in several types of cardiac disease treated by surgical and nonsurgical techniques [5, 6].

The existent of epicardial VTs has been previously reported. Littmann et al. [7], using epicardial laser photocoagulation during surgical ablation of 25 VTs in 10 patients, observed that post-MI VT may result from epicardial macroreentry. Slow conduction within the reentry circuit can be localised by epicardial mapping, and epicardial ablation interrupts epicardial post-MI VT. In patients with non-ischaemic VT, Cassidy [8] and Perlman [9] suggested that abnormal, fractionated, or late endocardial electrograms, or both, are less frequently seen in patients with dilated cardiomyopathy than in patients with post-MI VT, and the incidence of abnormal epicardial electrograms roughly equals that of abnormal electrograms. Svenson et al. [10] described the existence of epicardial circuits in post-MI VT, suggesting that they are particularly important in inferior-wall infarcts. More recently, other authors have described patients with epicardial VT [11-14].

Methods

Technique for Mapping and Ablating Epicardial VTs

Several techniques for mapping the epicardial surface of the heart in the EP laboratory by the electrophysiologist have been described. The transeptal [15] and coronary cusp approaches [16] can be useful to map specific forms of idiopathic VT, originating in the left ventricular outflow tract. Coronary veins can be used to carry out epicardial mapping, but manipulation of the catheter is limited by the anatomical distribution of these vessels [17]. To the best of our knowledge, the subxiphoid percutaneous approach to the epicardial space is the only technique currently available that allows extensive and unrestricted mapping of the epicardial surfaces of both ventricles [2, 18-23].

The Subxiphoid Percutaneous Approach

The epicardial subxiphoid percutaneous approach has been previously described in detail [2, 18]. Approaching the pericardial space is easy and can be done after positioning multipolar catheters in the coronary sinus and right ventricular apex through the femoral venous approach, and before starting anticoagulation. The pericardial space is reached by using a commercially available needle, originally developed to perform a spinal tap (Fig. 1) (epidural needle: 17 Gox 3–7/8' (9.84 cm) and 17Gox 5' (12.5 cm) TW with cm markings; Arrow International; Reading, PA]. Other types of needles can be used; however, the operator must be aware of the higher risk of perforation of the heart.

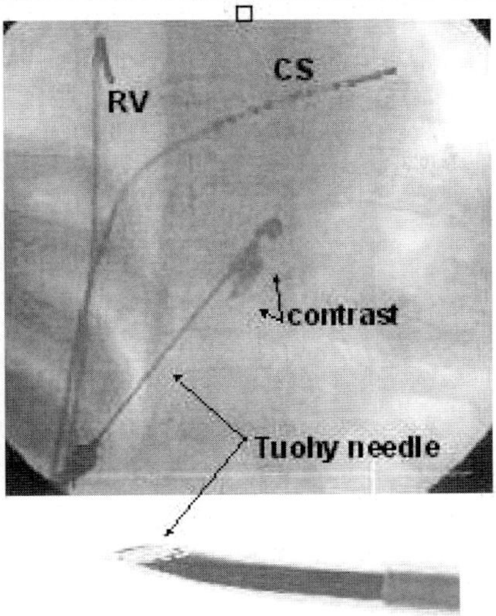

Fig. 1. Left-anterior oblique view of the heart and catheter position in coronary sinus (*CS*) and right ventricular (*RV*) apex. Observe the location of the contrast medium, injected soon after feeling heart movement, to determine whether the needle tip is pushing against or passing through the tissue

The puncture must be done at the angle between the left border of the subxiphoid process and the lower left rib. The spatial orientation of the needle will determine what portion of the ventricles will be reached. The needle usually has to point toward the left shoulder, and it must be introduced more horizontally if the target is the anterior portion of the ventricles and more vertically if the diaphragmatic portion of the heart is the area of interest. After crossing the subcutaneous tissue, needle movement should be monitored by fluoroscopy in the left anterior oblique view, 35–40° (Fig. 2). The needle must be carefully moved toward the heart silhouette until the surgeon can detect movement of the heart.

The injection of a small amount (~1 ml) of contrast demonstrates whether the needle tip is pushing against or passing through the tissue. If the diaphragm has not been reached, the contrast will be seen in the subdiaphragmatic area. When the needle reaches the pericardial sac, the contrast will spread around the heart, restricted to its silhouette (Fig. 2a). The appearance of a 'sluggish' layering of contrast medium indicates that the needle is correctly positioned in the pericardial space. A soft floppy-tipped guidewire is then passed through the hollow, an #8F introducer is advanced, and a regular ablation catheter is then introduced into the pericardial space (Fig. 2b–d).

Once the catheter is inside the pericardial space, epicardial ventricular electrograms can be readily recorded during sinus rhythm and during VT. The entire surface of the heart can be mapped and eventually ablated.

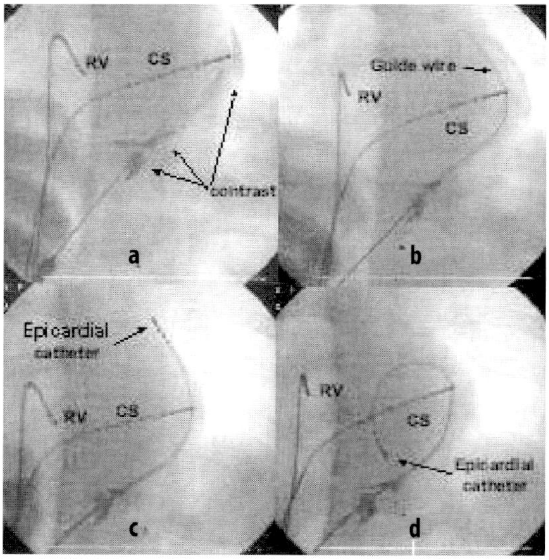

Fig. 2a–d. Left-anterior oblique views during a subxipfoid epicardial approach. **a** Note the appearance of a 'sluggish' layering of the contrast medium indicating that the needle is correctly positioned in the pericardial space. **b** A soft floppy-tipped guidewire is passed through the hollow and a #8F introducer is advanced. **c, d** Once the catheter is inside the pericardial space, the epicardial atrial and ventricular surfaces of the heart can be mapped and eventually ablated

Results

From the initial report in 1996 [18] to December 2003 [2], we have used this approach to treat 215 consecutive patients with VT. In 138 of these patients, VT was associated with Chagas disease, while 50 patients were post-inferior-MI, and 15 had VT associated with idiopathic dilated cardiomyopathy (IDCM). Twelve patients had idiopathic VT. The number of episodes of inducible VT ranged from 1.8 to 2.2. Nonmappable VT were observed in 40–44% of patients. Only one episode of endocardial VT was induced in an average of 5% of the patients, and only one episode of epicardial VT was induced in an average of 3.5% of patients. Regarding mappable VT, epicardial VT was present in 25% of IDCM-related VT, 32% of post-MI-related VT, and 36% of the episodes of VT associated with Chagas disease. Successful RF ablation (interruption and no reinduction) was obtained from the epicardium in 50% of post-MI VT patients, 60% of Chagas VT patients, and 55% of IDCM VT patients.

We are aware that, at least theoretically, critical epicardial sites could have been entrained or interrupted within 10 s from both the endocardial and the epicardial surfaces, making it difficult to demonstrate the presence of a

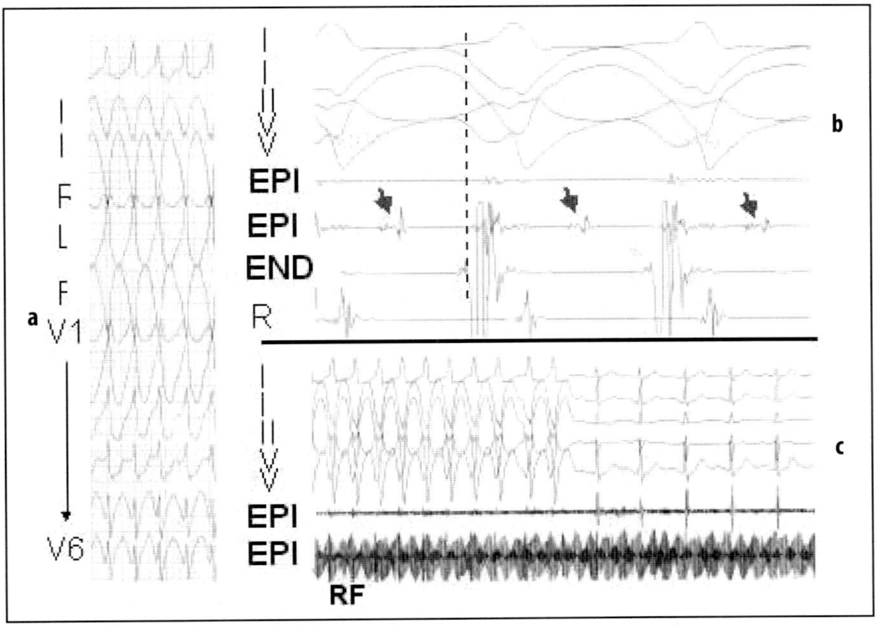

Fig. 3a–c. a 12-lead ECG during ventricular tachycardia (VT). **b** Best mid-diastolic electrogram during a recording of VT at the pericardial surface of the left ventricle. **c** Interruption of VT soon after epicardial RF delivery

truly epicardial circuit in a given case. In addition, it is not known how often this occurs. Epicardial VTs may occur in patients with idiopathic VT [22] and in those with VT associated with ischaemic [20] and non-ischaemic [6, 19] VT (Fig. 3).

Problems Related to the Subxiphoid Epicardial Approach

Puncture

Several concerns exist regarding the use of this approach. The first is related to the possibility of inducing puncture accidents. Predictable and avoidable accidents were related to a 'dry' right ventricular puncture in 4.5% of 215 consecutive patients who underwent epicardial ablation. A drainable haemopericardium containing 200 ± 98 ml of blood was observed in 7% of the patients. These predictable accidents are mostly related to the learning curve. One patient in this series had bleeding in the abdominal cavity from an injured diaphragmatic vessel, which required blood transfusion and laparotomy to control. This is an unpredictable and difficult to avoid complication.

Coronary Artery Damage

One of the main concerns during epicardial mapping and ablation is the avoidance of coronary artery damage. In this regard, d'Avila et al. [24] reported experimental data from nine mongrel dogs in which linear and single RF lesions were applied on or near the coronary artery. The authors concluded that, in an acute model, RF application delivery above the artery may result in intimal hyperplasia and thrombosis. However, susceptibility to damage was inversely proportional to vessel size, and no endothelial lesions were present in vessels with an internal perimeter > 2 mm.

The long-term effects of RF lesions on the epicardial coronary artery were analysed by Miranda el al. [25] in seven young pigs observed for a least 70 days after RF ablation. The results suggested that RF pulse delivery in the vicinity of the epicardial vessels does not provoke either MI or vascular thrombosis. The endothelium was preserved in most of the animals, but intense intimal thickening was seen in a few. The presence of fat and veins interposed between the epicardial coronary arteries and the catheter tip was related to much less intimal thickening, but the long-term significance of intimal thickening is still unknown.

Our current approach to minimise the risk of damaging the coronary vessels is to obtain an angiogram before ablation in all patients. Based on the analysis of the anatomy of the coronary arteries, safe areas for epicardial ablation can be selected. Depending on the area where the ablation site is located, another angiogram can be obtained during the procedure, immediately before starting ablation, although we do not routinely do this. As a general rule, we assume that a safe application can be delivered when the distance between the catheter tip and a visible coronary vessel is > 1 cm. However, if a putative critical site of the tachycardia circuit can only be identified close to a coronary artery despite extensive mapping, then, as in all clinical scenarios, a risk–benefit analysis should be undertaken.

RF application resulted in coronary artery occlusion of a marginal branch causing non-Q-wave MI with a CKMB peak of 35 U/l in only one of 215 consecutive patients.

Effects of Epicardial Fat on Epicardial Mapping and Ablation

The presence of epicardial fat interposed between the catheter tip and an epicardial target also deserves special mention. Depending on its location and amount, the fat tissue may reduce the efficacy of epicardial catheter ablation. D'Avila et al. [26] compared bipolar epicardial electrograms and ventricular epicardial stimulation thresholds obtained with a 4-mm ablation catheter from 44 areas without and 45 areas with epicardial fat in ten patients during open-chest surgery. The authors observed that epicardial fat thickness of up to 5 mm interposed between the ablation catheter and the epicardium does not change the amplitude and duration of the bipolar epicardial electrogram or the epicardial ventricular stimulation threshold. In areas with a layer of epicardial fat thickness > 5 mm, ventricular capture was not possible even at 10-mA pulses.

The role of epicardial fat in RF lesion formation was analysed in animal models by using standard and cooled-tip RF catheters [27]. This study suggested that fat attenuates epicardial lesion formation. The absence of blood flow in the epicardial space causes the catheter tip to heat up too quickly. The use of a cool-tipped ablation catheter allows more energy to be delivered and a larger lesion to be created despite the presence of fat interposed between the catheter tip and the epicardium. Similar results [28] could be extrapolated to epicardial cryoablation, which can create very deep lesions; however, the presence of a fat layer of > 5 mm strongly attenuates this type of lesions. These data are important and may help to explain failures during epicardial RF ablation.

Pericarditis

Another potential complication seen after epicardial catheter ablation is post-procedure pericarditis. In the experimental laboratory, animals mapped and ablated intrapericardially may develop intense postpericarditis [29], which can be eliminated by the pericardial infusion of 2 mg triamcinolone/kg at the end of the procedure. Such intense pericarditis was not seen in patients in our series. Precordial distress and pain were observed in approximately 30% of our patients; however, pericardial effusion was minimal and the symptoms were easily controlled with regular anti-inflammatory drugs. All 29 patients in our series who had more than one epicardial procedure, ranging from 1 week to 10 months after the first procedure, were free of pericardial effusion, neither were pericardial adhesions present.

Pericardial Adhesions

Postoperative pericardial adhesions may represent a limitation of the percutaneous transthoracic epicardial approach. In our series, five patients had monomorphic VT 7–10 years after open-chest surgery [23]. The ejection fraction was around 40%. Despite the presence of postoperative adhesions, all patients underwent the endocardial and epicardial approach simultaneously. Pericardial puncture was directed to the inferior wall of the heart, where pericardial adhesions are thought to be less important than in the anterior wall. The pericardial space was entered in all patients. Fourteen VTs were induced, and eight VTs were unmappable. Three of six mappable VTs were successfully ablated from the endocardium, and two were successfully ablated from the epicardium.

Phrenic Nerve Injury

Injury of the phrenic nerve is a rare complication of endocardial atrial RF ablation. The phrenic nerves course through the upper chest, medial to the mediastinal pleura, and the apex of the right or left lung. The right phrenic nerve lies laterally to the right brachiocephalic vein and the superior vena cava. The left phrenic nerve courses along the lateral aspect of the transverse arch of the aorta. The two nerves subsequently pass anteriorly to their respective pulmonary hila and then inferiorly in a broad vertical plane along the margin of the heart, between the fibrous pericardium and the mediastinal pleura. While the application of RF pulses in the lateral aspect of the heart silhouette can theoretically induce phrenic nerve injury [30-32], we have never observed this complication. Nonetheless, we are aware that the incidence of this complication could be underestimated because unilateral diaphragmatic paralysis usually does not cause significant shortness of breath unless other underlying pulmonary disease is present.

For prevention of phrenic nerve injury, high output pacing (15 mA, 5-ms pulse duration) at the eventual ablation site (theoretically near the phrenic course) before RF delivery and even during RF application may be of use. This is not a problem at our centre, because usually we do not apply many pulses to ablate epicardial VT.

When To Perform the Epicardial Approach?

This question has not been answered, and it depends on the preference of the electrophysiologist. It is not clear whether one should use the epicardial approach only after an endocardial failure or only when the ECG of a patient with clinical VT suggests an epicardial origin of VT. As a matter of fact, the simultaneous approach may have several advantages, such as reduction in cost, better chance of mapping and ablating all inducible VTs, and an opportunity to acquire more expertise with the technique.

Conclusions

Epicardial VT may occur in ischaemic, non-ischaemic, and idiopathic VT. Truly subepicardial VT can preferentially be ablated from the epicardial surface. The percutaneous subxiphoid approach to the pericardial space is easy and can be done safely in the EP laboratory by an electrophysiologist. This approach may improve the results of the catheter ablation procedure.

References

1. Berruezo A, Mont L, Nava S et al (2004) Electrocardiographic recognition of the epicardial origin of ventricular tachycardias. Circulation 109(15):1842–1847
2. Berruezo A, Mont L, Nava S (2005) Epicardial mapping and ablation technique to control ventricular tachycardia. J Cardiovasc Electrophysiol 16:449–452
3. Klein LS, Shih HT, Hackett FK et al (1992) Radiofrequency catheter ablation of ventricular tachycardia in patients without structural heart disease. Circulation 85:1666–1674
4. Stevenson WG (2005) Catheter ablation of monomorphic ventricular tachycardia. Curr Opin Cardiol 20(1):42–47
5. Svenson RH, Littmann L, Gallagher JJ et al (1990) Termination of ventricular tachycardia with epicardial laser photocoagulation: a clinical comparison with patients undergoing successful endocardial photocoagulation alone. J Am Coll Cardiol 15:163–170
6. Swarup V, Morton JB, Arruda M et al (2002) Ablation of epicardial macroreentrant ventricular tachycardia associated with idiopathic nonischemic dilated cardiomyopathy by a percutaneous transthoracic approach. J Cardiovasc Electrophysiol 13(11):1164–1168
7. Littmann L, Svenson RH, Gallagher JJ et al (1991) Functional role of the epicardium in postinfarction ventricular tachycardia. Observations derived from computerized epicardial activation mapping, entrainment, and epicardial laser photoablation. Circulation 83(5):1577–1591
8. Cassidy DM, Vassallo JA, Miller JM et al (1986) Endocardial catheter mapping in patients in sinus rhythm: relationship to underlying heart disease and ventricular arrhythmias. Circulation 73(4):645–652
9. Perlman RL, Miller J, Kindwall KE (1990) Abnormal epicardial and endocardial electrograms in patients with idiopathic dilated cardiomyopathy: relationship to arrhythmias. Circulation 82 (Suppl III):III-708 (abs)
10. Svenson RH, Littmann L, Gallagher JJ et al (1990) Termination of ventricular tachycardia with epicardial laser photocoagulation: a clinical comparison with patients undergoing successful endocardial photocoagulation alone. J Am Coll Cardiol 15:163–170
11. Brugada J, Berruezo A, Cuesta A et al (2003) Nonsurgical transthoracic epicardial radiofrequency ablation: an alternative in incessant ventricular tachycardia. J Am Coll Cardiol 41(11):2036–2043

12. Soejima K, Stevenson WG, Sapp JL et al (2004) Endocardial and epicardial radiofrequency ablation of ventricular tachycardia associated with dilated cardiomyopathy: the importance of low-voltage scars. J Am Coll Cardiol 43(10):1834–1842
13. Hsia HH, Marchlinski FE (2002) Characterization of the electroanatomic substrate for monomorphic ventricular tachycardia in patients with nonischemic cardiomyopathy. Pacing Clin Electrophysiol 25:1114–1127
14. Ouyang F, Bansch D, Schaumann A et al (2003) Catheter ablation of subepicardial ventricular tachycardia using electroanatomic mapping. Herz 28:591–597
15. Sosa E, Scanavacca M, d'Avila A (2002) Catheter ablation of the left ventricular outflow tract tachycardia from the left atrium. J Interv Card Electrophysiol 7(1):61–63
16. Hachiya H, Aonuma K, Yamauchi Y et al (2000) Successful radiofrequency catheter ablation from the supravalvular region of the aortic valve in a patient with outflow tract ventricular tachycardia. Jpn Circ J 64(6):459–463
17. de Paola AA, Melo WD, Tavora MZ et al (1998) Angiographic and electrophysiological substrates for ventricular tachycardia mapping through the coronary veins. Heart 79(1):59–63
18. Sosa E, Scanavacca M, d'Avila A et al (1996) A new technique to perform epicardial mapping in the electrophysiology laboratory. J Cardiovasc Electrophysiol 7(6):531–536
19. Sosa E, Scanavacca M, D'Avila A et al (1999) Radiofrequency catheter ablation of ventricular tachycardia guided by nonsurgical epicardial mapping in chronic Chagasic heart disease. Pacing Clin Electrophysiol 22(1 Pt 1):128–130
20. Sosa E, Scanavacca M, d'Avila A et al (2000) Nonsurgical transthoracic epicardial catheter ablation to treat recurrent ventricular tachycardia occurring late after myocardial infarction. J Am Coll Cardiol 35(6):1442–1449
21. Sosa E, Scanavacca M, d'Avila A (2001) Transthoracic epicardial catheter ablation to treat recurrent ventricular tachycardia. Curr Cardiol Rep 3(6):451–458
22. Sosa E, Scanavacca M, d'Avila A et al (2000) Nonsurgical transthoracic mapping and ablation in a child with incessant ventricular tachycardia. J Cardiovasc Electrophysiol 11(2):208–210
23. Sosa E, Scanavacca M, D'Avila A et al (2004) Nonsurgical transthoracic epicardial approach in patients with ventricular tachycardia and previous cardiac surgery. J Interv Card Electrophysiol 10(3):281–288
24. d'Avila A, Gutierrez P, Scanavacca M et al (2002) Effects of radiofrequency pulses delivered in the vicinity of the coronary arteries: implications for nonsurgical transthoracic epicardial catheter ablation to treat ventricular tachycardia. Pacing Clin Electrophysiol 25(10):1488–1495
25. Miranda RC (1999) Estudo dos efeitos das aplicações de radiofrequencia sobre as artérias coronárias, grandes artérias da base, esôfago e brônquio de suínos. Tese (doutorado) – São Paulo, Brazil
26. d'Avila A, Dias R, Scanavacca M et al (2002) Epicardial fat tissue does not modify amplitude and duration of the epicardial electrograms and/or ventricular stimulation threshold. Eur J Cardiol 23:109 (abs)
27. d'Avila A, Houghtaling C, Gutierrez P et al (2004) Catheter ablation of ventricular epicardial tissue: a comparison of standard and cooled-tip radiofrequency energy. Circulation 109(19):2363–2369
28. d'Avila A, Holmvang G, Houghtaling C et al (2004) Focal and linear endocardial and epicardial catheter-based cryoablation of normal and infarcted ventricular tissue. Heart Rhythms 1, issue 1S

29. d'Avila A, Scanavacca M, Sosa E et al (2003) Pericardial anatomy for the interventional electrophysiologist. J Cardiovasc Electrophysiol 14:422–430
30. Rumbak M, Chokshi SK, Abel N et al (1996) Left phrenic nerve paresis complicating catheter radiofrequency ablation for Wolf-Parkinson-White syndrome. Am Heart J 132:1281–1285
31. Durante-Mangoni E, Vecchio D, Ruggiero G (2003) Right diaphragm paralysis following cardiac ablation for inappropriate sinus tachycardia. PACE 26:783–784
32. Lee BK, Choi KJ, Kim J et al (2004) Right phrenic nerve injury following electrical disconnection of the right superior pulmonary vein. PACE 27:1444–1446

SUDDEN DEATH: PREDICTION AND PREVENTION

Predicting the Sudden Death in the Athlete

D. Corrado, C. Basso, M. Schiavon, G. Thiene

Introduction

Atherosclerotic coronary artery disease accounts for the vast majority of sudden deaths (SDs) in the middle-aged and older population. Several epidemiologic studies have assessed the relationship between physical exercise and the risk of sudden coronary death in this age group, in which physical activity can be regarded as a 'two-edged sword' [1–3]. The available evidence indicated that there is an increased risk of acute coronary events in persons who do not exercise regularly. Instead, habitual sport activity may offer protection over the long-term from the overall risk of acute myocardial infarction and sudden coronary death. Regular exercise is deemed to prevent the development and progression of atherosclerotic coronary artery disease by promoting favourable effects on lipid metabolism and weight reduction and by enhancing the stability of coronary artery plaques and myocardial electrical activity [4–6]. Therefore, although exercise is a potential trigger of acute coronary events in adults, regular physical activity offers protection over the long-term against pathologic cardiovascular events.

In contrast, little is known about the risk of SD in younger people engaged in competitive sports [7–10]. Whether sport activity in this age group provides health benefits as in adults or instead enhances the risk of SD remains to be established.

Department of Cardiology and Institute of Pathological Anatomy, University of Padua and Center for Sports Medicine, USLL 16, Padua, Italy

Enhanced Cardiovascular Risk in Young Athletes

We recently examined the incidence and causes of SD in the athletic and non-athletic young population (12–35 years old) of the Veneto Region of Italy in order to establish the impact of sport activity on the risk of SD in this age group. From 1979 to 1999, there were 300 cases of SD in adolescents and young adults, producing an overall cohort incidence rate of 1 per 100 000 persons per year. Fifty-five SDs occurred among athletes (2.3 per 100 000 per year) and 245 among non-athletes (0.9 per 100 000 per year), with an estimated relative risk of SD from all causes of 2.5 (1.8–3.4; $P < 0.0001$). The relative risk of SD among athletes vs non-athletes was 1.95 (1.3–2.6; $P = 0.0001$) for men and 2 (0.6–4.9; $P = 0.15$) for women.

The rates of SD by cardiovascular diseases were 2.1 in 100 000 athletes per year, compared with 0.7 in 100 000 non-athletes per year (RR 2.8, CI 1.9–3.7; $P < 0.001$). The estimated RR of cardiovascular SD was 2.0 for male athletes (CI 1.4–2.8; $P = 0.0001$) and 2.6 for female athletes (CI 0.8–6.4; $P = 0.06$). The cardiovascular causes producing the highest risk of sport-related SD were anomalous origin of the coronary artery from the wrong coronary sinus (RR = 79), arrhythmogenic right ventricular cardiomyopathy (ARVC) (R.R. = 5.4), and premature coronary artery disease (R.R. = 2.6).

By Poisson multivariate regression analysis, the estimated RRs of sports activity for total SD and cardiovascular SD were 1.95 and 2.1, respectively, while the estimated RRs of male gender were 2.5 and 2.8, respectively. The interaction between sports involvement and gender, for both total and cardiovascular SD, was not significant.

Our study of the Veneto region was the first to quantify the hazard of physical exercise in adolescents and young adults. The major finding was that competitive sport activity is associated with a 2.5-fold increase in the risk of total SD and a 2.8-fold increase in the risk of cardiovascular SD in young individuals. Sports is not itself the cause of the enhanced mortality, but it triggers SD in those athletes who are affected by cardiovascular conditions, such as ARVC, premature coronary artery disease, and anomalous coronary artery origin, each of which predisposes to life-threatening ventricular arrhythmias during physical exercise.

Risk of Sudden Death During Sports: Role of Age and Gender

The assessment of the precise frequency with which SD occurs in young athletes during organised competitive sports encounters a number of practical obstacles and results in limitations mostly related to retrospective analysis. Studies in the United States probably resulted in underestimation of the true prevalence of sports-related SD, since they relied on reporting from individual schools and institutions, or on media accounts. Van Camp et al. [11], in a nationally based survey, estimated the prevalence of SD in high school and college athletes from the United States to be 0.4/100 000 athlete-years. Estimated rates in male athletes (age 13–24 years, mean 16.9 ± 2.0) were 0.66/100 000 high-school-athlete-years and 1.45/100 000 college-athlete-years, while the estimated rates in female athletes (age 14–22 years, mean 16.2 ± 2.4) were 0.12/100 000 high-school-athlete-years and 0.28/100 000 college-athlete-years. However, the methodology employed in that study was largely dependent on news media accounts, with their inherent limitations. Maron et al. [12] estimated the prevalence of cardiovascular SD in competitive high school athletes (age range 13–19, mean 16 years) from Minnesota to be 0.35/100 000 sports participations and 0.46/100 000 individual participants annually (0.77/100 000 male athletes).

In the Veneto region, the incidence of SD by all causes was 2.3 per 100 000 athlete-years and that of SD from cardiovascular diseases was 2.1 per 100 000 athlete-years. The reasons for the higher mortality rates found in the present study compared with those reported by Maron et al. may include: (1) our prospective vs their retrospective analysis; (2) different underlying pathologic conditions, which, in part, reflect differences in ethnic and genetic factors; (3) participation at a higher level of intensity among Italian competitive athletes; (4) the higher mean age in our series of athletes (mean age 23 years) compared with high school and college participants in the USA (mean age 16 years). In this regard, it is noteworthy that the development of phenotypic manifestations and arrhythmias associated with a risk of SD during sports, including cardiomyopathies, premature coronary artery disease, ion channel diseases (such as Brugada syndrome), and progressive cardiac conduction disease (such as Lenègre disease), is age-dependent and occurs during young adulthood [13–17]. Therefore, the risk of fatal events in high school and college participants in the USA is lower and may explain the differences with the Italian estimates.

Moreover, in the Veneto study, SDs of young competitive athletes showed a clear gender predilection, with striking male predominance (male to female ratio of 10:1). This predominance of fatal events in male athletes is consistent with the findings of previous surveys of the deaths of these athletes and has been explained as being due to the fact that females participate less commonly in competitive sports programs than male. Accordingly, the prevalence of sports participation of young females in the Veneto region study was only 25% of that of young males. However, male gender was itself an independent risk for SD in athletes. Males are usually exposed to generally more intensive training and greater levels of intensity during athletic competition than females. Moreover, in the age range of competitive sports, males have a higher prevalence and/or phenotypic expression of potentially lethal cardiac diseases, such as hypertrophic cardiomyopathy, ARVC, and premature coronary artery disease [14–17].

Cardiovascular Causes of Sudden Death in Young Athletes

ARVC and premature coronary artery disease are the most common pathologic backgrounds underlying SD in young athletes in the Veneto region of Italy [8–10]. Previous studies in the United States showed a higher prevalence of other pathologic conditions, such as hypertrophic cardiomyopathy, anomalous coronary arteries, and myocarditis [7, 11]. This discrepancy may be explained by several factors. There have been no previous studies comparable to that of the Veneto region that have prospectively investigated a consecutive series of SDs in young people living in a well-defined geographic area and comprising a homogeneous ethnic group. Therefore, the previously reported causes may have been influenced by the unavoidable limitations in patient selection arising from retrospective analysis. Moreover, with studies of large series, autopsy investigation is usually carried out by multiple examiners, including local pathologists and medical examiners. In the present study, to obtain a higher level of confidence in the results, morphological examination of all hearts was performed by the same team of experienced cardiovascular pathologists according to a standard protocol. Comparison between previous studies and the present one with regard to the prevalence of ARVC among the causes of SD in young people and athletes is limited by the fact that ARVC is a clinico-pathologic condition that has been only recently discovered [13]. ARVC is rarely associated with cardiomegaly and usually spares the left ventricle, so that affected hearts may be erroneously diagnosed as normal hearts. In the past, therefore, a number of SDs in young people and athletes, in which the routine pathologic examination disclosed a normal heart, may, in fact, have been due to an unrecognised ARVC. The high incidence of ARVC in our series may also be due to a genetic factor in the population of the Veneto region [18, 19], although ARVC cannot be considered as a peculiarly 'Venetian disease,' since there is growing evidence that it is ubiquitous, still largely underdiagnosed at clinical and post-mortem investigations, and accounts for significant arrhythmic morbidity and mortality worldwide [20]. Finally, the pre-participation screening of young people who plan to take part in competitive athletic activity, which has been in practice in Italy for more than 20 years, has changed the natural prevalence of the pathologic background of sports-related SD. For example, we recently demonstrated that SD from hypertrophic cardiomyopathy in young competitive athletes was successfully prevented by identification and disqualification of affected athletes at pre-participation screening [9]. As a consequence of this process, other cardiovascular conditions, such as ARVC and premature coronary artery disease, have come to account for a greater proportion of all SDs in Italian athletes.

Mechanisms of Sudden Death in Young Athletes

Previous studies showed that sudden cardiac death is usually the result of an interaction between structural abnormalities of the heart and transient acute abnormalities. The mechanisms of SD in the Veneto region series of young competitive athletes included exercise-related acute myocardial ischaemia, sympathetic stimulation, and abrupt haemodynamic changes leading to life-threatening ventricular arrhythmias. In this study, the cardiovascular conditions most likely to cause sport-related SD were anomalous origin of coronary artery from the wrong coronary sinus (RR = 79) and ARVC (R.R. = 5.4). The pathophysiology of cardiac arrest in athletes with anomalous coronary arteries has been related to abrupt ventricular fibrillation precipitated by exercise-related myocardial ischaemia. This, in turn, is the result of aortic expansion that compresses the anomalous vessel against the pulmonary trunk, increases the acute angulation of the coronary take-off, and aggravates the slit-like shape of the lumen [21, 22]. The propensity for ARVC to precipitate effort-dependent sudden cardiac arrest is still unclear. Physical exercise may acutely increase right ventricular afterload and cavity enlargement, which in turn, may elicit ventricular arrhythmias by stretching the diseased right ventricular myocardium [23]. Alternatively, a 'denervation supersensitivity' of the right ventricle to catecholamines has been proposed [24]. Sympathetic nerve trunks may be damaged and/or interrupted by fibrofatty replacement in the right ventricle, which distinctively progresses from the epicardium to the endocardium, resulting in a denervation supersensitivity to catecholamines. Arrhythmogenic mechanisms in the denervated supersensitive myofibers include dispersion of refractoriness and reentry, triggered activity, or both. Recently, in a subgroup of patients with familial ARVC, a cardiac ryanodine receptor (RYR2) missense mutation leading to abnormal calcium release from the sarcoplasmic reticulum was identified [25]. It is noteworthy that wall mechanical stress, like that induced by right ventricular volume overload during exercise, is expected to exacerbate cardiac ryanodine channel dysfunction. Therefore, a potential arrhythmogenic mechanism of sport-related cardiac arrest in patients with ARVC is triggered activity due to late after-depolarisations, which are provoked by intracellular calcium overload and enhanced by adrenergic stimulation [26].

Conclusions

In adults, regular physical exercise offers protection against coronary events and SD. Conversely, sport activity is associated with a significantly higher rate of SD in adolescents and young adults. Sports does not enhance mortality per se; rather, it acts as a trigger of cardiac arrest in those athletes with silent cardiovascular conditions, mostly cardiomyopathy, premature coronary artery disease, and congenital coronary anomalies, each of which predisposes to life-threatening ventricular arrhythmias during physical exercise. These results should not discourage young people from participating in sports, but point to the need for an extensive and accurate pre-participation screening strategy aimed at early identification and disqualification of those subjects affected by cardiovascular diseases associated with the risk of SD.

References

1. Curfman GD (1993) The Health benefits of exercise. A critical reappraisal. New Engl J Med 328:574–576
2. Curfman GD (1993) Is exercise beneficial- or hazardous- to your heart? New Engl J Med 239:1730–1731
3. Maron BJ (2000) The paradox of exercise. New Engl J Med 343:1409–1411
4. Hambrecht R, Niebauer J, Marburger C et al (1993) Various intensities of leisure time physical activity in patients with coronary artery disease: effects on cardiorespiratory fitness and progression of coronary atherosclerotic lesions. J Am Coll Cardiol 22:468–477
5. Gordon DJ, Rifkind BM (1989) High-density lipoprotein – the clinical implications of recent studies. N Engl J Med 321:1311–1316
6. Hull SS Jr, Vanoli E, Adamson PB et al (1994) Exercise training confers anticipatory protection from sudden death during acute myocardial ischemia. Circulation 89:548–552
7. Maron BJ, Roberts WC, McAllister MA et al (1980) Sudden death in young athletes. Circulation 62:218–229
8. Corrado D, Thiene G, Nava A et al (1990) Sudden death in young competitive athletes: clinico-pathologic correlations in 22 cases. Am J Med 89:588–596
9. Corrado D, Basso C, Schiavon M et al (1998) Screening for hypertrophic cardiomyopathy in young athletes. New Engl J Med 339:364–369
10. Corrado D, Basso C, Rizzoli G et al (2003) Does sports activity enhance the risk of sudden death in adolescents and young adults? J Am Coll Cardiol 42:1959–1963
11. Van Camp SP, Bloor CM, Mueller FO et al (1995) Non-traumatic sports death in high school and college athletes. Med Sci Sports Exerc 27:641–647
12. Maron BJ, Gohman TE, Aeppli D (1998) Prevalence of sudden cardiac death during competitive sports activities in Minnesota high school athletes. J Am Coll Cardiol 32:1881–1884
13. Thiene G, Nava A, Corrado D et al (1988) Right ventricular cardiomyopathy and sudden death in young people. N Engl J Med 318:129–133
14. Corrado D, Fontaine G, Marcus FI et al (2000) Arrhythmogenic right ventricular dysplasia/cardiomyopathy. need for an international registry. Circulation 101:e101

15. Corrado D, Basso C, Poletti A et al (1994) Sudden death in the young: is coronary thrombosis the major precipitating factor? Circulation 90:2315–2323
16. Maron BJ, Shirani J, Poliac LC et al (1996) Sudden death in young competitive athletes. Clinical, demografics, and pathological profiles. JAMA 276:199–204
17. Antzelevitch C, Brugada P, Borggrefe M et al (2005) Brugada syndrome: report of the second consensus conference. Circulation 111:659–670
18. Nava A, Thiene G, Canciani B et al (1988) Familial occurrence of right ventricular dysplasia: a study involving nine families. J Am Coll Cardiol 12:1222–1228
19. Rampazzo A, Nava A, Danieli GA et al (1994) The gene for arrhythmogenic right ventricular cardiomyopathy maps to chromosome 14q23–q24. Hum Mol Genet 3:959–962
20. Corrado D, Basso C, Thiene G et al (1997) Spectrum of clinicopathologic manifestations of arrhythmogenic right ventricular cardiomyopathy/dysplasia: a multicenter study. J Am Coll Cardiol 30:1512–1520
21. Basso C, Maron BJ, Corrado D et al (2000) Clinical profile of congenital coronary artery anomalies with origin from the wrong aortic sinus leading to sudden death in young competitive athletes. J Am Coll Cardiol 35(6):1493–1501
22. Corrado D, Thiene G, Cocco P et al (1992) Non-atherosclerotic coronary artery disease and sudden death in the young. Br Heart J 68:601–607
23. Douglas PS, O'Toole ML, Hiller WDB et al (1990) Different effects of prolonged exercise on the right and left ventricles. J Am Coll Cardiol 15:64–69
24. Wichter T, Hindricks G, Lerch H et al (1994) Regional myocardial sympathetic dysinnervation in arrhythmogenic right ventricular cardiomyopathy. Circulation 89:667–683
25. Tiso N, Stephan DA, Nava A et al (2001) Identification of mutations in the cardiac ryanodine receptor gene in families affected with arrhythmogenic right ventricular cardiomyopathy type 2 (ARVD2). Hum Mol Genet 10:189–194
26. Priori SG, Napolitano C, Tiso N et al (2000) Mutations in the cardiac ryanodine receptor gene (hryr2) underlie catecholaminergic polymorphic ventricular tachycardia. Circulation 103:196–200

New Markers of Sudden Cardiac Death: Genetic Variables

N. El-Sherif, G. Turitto, V. Lakireddy

Conventional Risk Stratification for Sudden Cardiac Death

All recently completed as well as ongoing sudden cardiac death (SCD) primary implantable cardiovertor defibrillator (ICD) prophylaxis trials have addressed patients with one or more conventional risk factors for SCD (Fig. 1). The electrophysiologic surrogates for SCD, including measures of myocardial conduction disorders, dispersion of repolarisation, and autonomic imbalance, are based on sound scientific evidence. Although it is acknowledged that the positive predictive power of a risk stratifier in a clinical trial is closely related to the duration of follow-up, the majority of conventional risk stratifiers of SCD have a relatively low positive predictive value, which would preclude their wide application as guidelines for ICD implantation in patients known to be at risk for SCD. This is not to mention the impracticality of their use for risk stratification in the general asymptomatic public. This has prompted the search for new approaches for risk stratification and management of SCD based on recent insights gained from advances in molecular biology and genetics.

Familial Clustering of SCD

In the last several years, there has been an accumulating body of research evidence suggesting that there are molecular, genetic, biophysical, and biochemical indicators of SCD [1, 2]. One recent clue of the role that genetic factors may play in SCD has been evidence of 'family clustering' of SCD victims.

Cardiology Division, Department of Medicine, State University of New York, Downstate Medical Center, and New York Harbor VA Health Care Center, Brooklyn, New York, USA

Conventional Risk Stratifiers of SCD

Electropysiologic Surrogates	Functional Contractile Surrogates
*Measures of myocardial conduction disorder	*NYHA Class
SAECG, EPS	* LVEF
*Measures of dispersion of repolarisation	* LV mass
QT dispersion, TWA	* Peak 0_2 consumption
*Measures of autonomic imbalance	* Brain natriuretic peptide
Resting heart rate, HRV, BRS	

Fig. 1. Risk stratification for sudden cardiac death. *BRS* baroreceptor sensitivity, *EPS* electrophysiologic study, *HRV* heart rate variability, *LV* left ventricle, *LVEF* left ventricle ejection fraction, *NYHA* New York Heart Association, *SAEGC* signal-average electrocardiogram, *TWA* T wave alternans

Population studies have reported that familial clustering of SCD events is an important independent factor in multifactorial analyses of SCD risk. This may be related to shared environmental or genetically transmittable abnormalities. Evidence favouring a focus on genetic factors was presented in recent epidemiologic studies suggesting not only that familial risks for SCD appear substantial, but that they are statistically distinct and separable from familial risks of myocardial infarction (MI) [3-5]. In one study [4], a parental history of SCD increased the relative risk of SCD to 1.8 after adjustment for conventional coronary artery disease (CAD) risk factors, but it did not elevate the risk for deaths coded as nonsudden. In a small subset of individuals in whom there was a history of both maternal and paternal SCD events, the relative risk for SCD in offspring was increased to 4.

The Autonomic System and Enhanced Susceptibility to SCD

Autonomic neural influences, especially increased adrenergic and decreased cholinergic activity, can modulate susceptibility to SCD. Resting heart rate has been shown to be an independent risk factor for SCD in middle-aged men[6]. There are also data showing the heritability of heart rate variation [7]. Adrenergic agonists are known to trigger ventricular arrhythmias, and the diurnal patterns of their circulating levels are similar to those of SCD events[8]. Polymorphic variations in β1- and β2-adrenergic receptors have been noted in patients with dilated cardiomyopathy [9] and have been reported to influence mortality in heart failure patients[10]. β1- and β2 adrenergic receptor subtype effects have been implicated in the inherited lethal ventricular arrhythmias in German Shepherd dogs [11]. Recent association between plasma nonesterified fatty acids and SCD may be related to increased adrenergic tone or the effect on ion channel and transporters [12]. Furthermore, mental stress was found to be associated with lateralisation of mid-brain activity, resulting in imbalanced activity in right and left cardiac sympathetic nerves and increased dispersion of repolarisation, predisposing to arrhythmia [13].

Cardiac Gene Mutations and Enhanced Susceptibility to SCD

Invaluable insight into the role of genetic mutations and SCD has come from studies of mutations of sarcolemmal ion-channel genes involved in myocardial excitability and transcellular conduction, such as the long QT syndrome [14] and the Brugada syndrome [15], as well as of genes that modulate or modify intracellular calcium, such as those involving the cardiac ryanodine receptor/calcium release channel RyR2 [16] and CASQ2 [17] in catecholaminergic polymorphic ventricular tachycardia (VT). The discovery of literally hundreds of different mutations in the genes that cause the phenotypic long QT syndrome [14], for example, raised the possibility that silent polymorphism or mutations of cardiac genes may be more prevalent in the asymptomatic general public and may contribute to enhanced susceptibility to arrhythmogenesis and SCD under specific circumstances. Such circumstances can include hypokalaemia-induced long QT syndrome [18] and proarrhythmic responses to drugs [19–21]. For example, one report demonstrated that a polymorphism in the gene for MiRP-1 (T8A), estimated to occur in 1.6% of the population, was associated with a proarrhythmic response to the antibiotic Bactrim due to a blunted I_{Kr} current in response to the sulfamethoxazole component of the drug [19]. In another report, a variant allele of the cardiac sodium-channel gene SCN5A (Y1102) was found to be widespread among African Americans (13%) and African Caribbeans (19%), whereas it is not found in either Asians or whites. This polymorphism was associated with prolongation of the QT interval and drug-induced arrhythmias [21]. The extent to which polymorphism of cardiac ion channels explains proarrhythmic responses to drugs is unknown. However, the interaction of silent genetic alterations with more general physiologic states, such as enhanced catecholamine drive, and pathologic states, such as acute ischaemia, remains to be determined. Moreover, the role of modifier genes (gene–gene interaction) is beginning to be appreciated. In general, genotype–phenotype correlation studies show significant variability in the phenotypic expression of the disease among affected individuals with identical causal mutations. Overall, causal mutations account for a fraction of the variability of phenotypes, and genetic background, referred to as the modifier genes, plays a significant role. Modifier genes are not involved in the genesis of the disease but modify the severity of the phenotypic expression. The final phenotype is the result of interactions among causal genes, modifier genes, and environmental factors. Modifier genes have been investigated in cardiac diseases, such as hypertrophic cardiomyopathy [22] and heart failure [23]. Identification of modifier genes will complement the results of studies of causative genes and could enhance genetic-based diagnosis, risk stratification, and implementation of preventive and therapeutic measures of SCD.

Coronary Artery Disease and SCD Cascade

The majority of SCD occurs in patients with atherosclerotic CAD (65–85%) (Fig. 2) [24]. However, there is considerable evidence that traditional markers of CAD, such as hypertension obesity, smoking, diabetes, and lipid abnormalities, are not specific enough to identify patients at high risk for SCD [25]. Patients with similar risk factors for CAD may suffer from SCD or nonfatal ischaemic events. The reason for this difference is not clear. Exciting evidence has been acquired recently in genetic studies of CAD and MI. One disease-causing gene for CAD and MI has been identified as MEF2A, which is located on chromosome 15q26.3 and encodes for a transcriptional factor with high level of expression in coronary endothelium [26]. Approximately 1–2% of CAD patients may carry an MEF2A mutation. Several other susceptibility genes have been identified using genome-wide association studies or genome-wide linkage studies [26]. There is a new understanding of the cascade that relates the distal events of atherosclerosis to the proximal event of SCD. New risk markers for SCD in CAD are likely to cluster under factors that may directly facilitate the development of acute coronary syndromes, specifically those factors that may facilitate transient triggering events, including plaque rupture, enhanced thrombogenesis, and coronary artery spasm [1, 2]. There is significant new data showing correlation between SCD and (1) markers of plaque vulnerability, such as heritable alterations of specific matrix metalloproteinases [27]; (2) markers of enhanced thrombogenesis, such as increased D-dimer, increased apo-B, and decreased apo-A1 [28], and polymorphism in platelet glycoprotein receptors [29]; (3) genetic variations that predispose to vasospasm, such as variations in the vascular endothelial nitric-oxide synthetase (eNOS) system [30, 31]; and (4) markers of inflammatory response, such as C-reactive protein (CRP) [32]. Recent

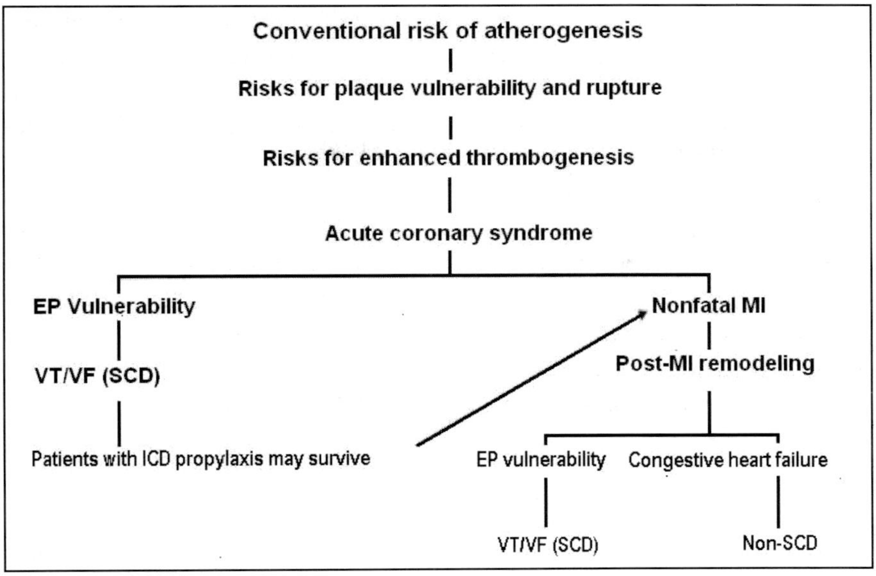

Fig. 2. Coronary artery disease and sudden cardiac death (SCD) cascade. *EP* electrophysiologic, *ICD* implantable cardioverter defibrillator, *MI* myocardial infarction, *VF* ventricular fibrillation, *VT* ventricular tachycardia

studies have shown that CRP directly suppresses endothelial progenitor cell survival, differentiation, and function, key components of angiogenesis and the response to chronic ischaemia [33].

Diabetes, CAD, and Risk of SCD

Cardiovascular disease is the leading cause of death in individuals with type-2 diabetes, which affects about 15 million Americans [34]. This is compatible with the 'common soil' hypothesis, which postulates that both diabetes and cardiovascular disease have common genetic and environmental antecedents, i.e. 'they spring from the same soil' [35]. There is evidence that diabetes is a significant risk factor for SCD but not for nonfatal MI [36]. The increased risk of death and mortality rates associated with diabetes are compounded by the fact that many diabetic individuals are unaware that they suffer from the metabolic syndrome. Recent strong evidence has shown that the elevated risk for cardiovascular disease starts to increase long before the onset of clinical diabetes, confirming the so-called ticking clock hypothesis [37]. The incidence of impaired glucose tolerance and diabetes may be as high as 39% and 31%, respectively, in patients admitted with acute MI [38]. Recent studies have documented increased inflammation, neovascularisation, and intraplaque haemorrhage in human diabetic atherosclerosis [39]. Peroxisomal proliferator-activated receptors (PPARs) are now considered the nuclear transcriptional regulators of atherosclerosis [39]. Recent experimental studies have documented plaque stabilisation with PPAR-gamma agonists, a group of medications holding great promise in the treatment of diabetic atherosclerosis [39]. Due to the vulnerability of diabetic patients to plaque rupture and acute MI, a question of considerable importance is whether patients with CAD, diabetes, or prediabetes, and relatively preserved LV systolic function (LVEF $\geq$ 35%) can benefit from primary ICD prophylaxis.

Post-MI Remodelling and Electrophysiologic Vulnerability

A key electrophysiologic alteration in post-MI remodelled heart is down-regulation of K^+ gene expression and K^+ currents, resulting in spatially heterogeneous prolongation of action potential duration and increased dispersion of refractoriness [40, 41]. It has long been recognised that cardiac hypertrophy from whatever cause is consistently associated with down-regulation of K^+ channel genes and K^+ currents. However, recent studies have shown that in the post-MI heart this down-regulation occurs early and may be dissociated from the slower time course of post-MI remodelled hypertrophy [42]. Therefore, it is not surprising that the post-MI heart is more sensitive to hypokalaemia and the proarrhythmic effects of drugs that depress K^+ currents, especially I_{Kr} blockers. Some pharmacologic interventions that have been shown to reduce the incidence of SCD in post-MI patients, such as magnesium [43] and spironolactone [44], may act by countering the effects of low K^+.

SCD and Systolic Dysfunction

A decreased left ventricular systolic function (LVEF < 35%) recently has become the main arbiter for primary ICD prophylaxis of SCD. Although the exact mechanisms involved in the strong correlation between decreased LV systolic function and increased incidence of SCD are not clearly defined, it is recognised that one way to combat SCD is to try to halt or improve the deterioration in LV function. The mechanism(s) for the transition from compensated to decompensated heart failure is under intensive investigation, and it is clear that multiple factors are involved [45]. Some of the more important mechanisms are the role of continuous loss of cardiomyocytes to apoptosis in the noninfarcted myocardium, the negative consequences of remodelling of the interstitial matrix, down-regulation of the β-adrenergic receptor–G-protein–adenylyl cyclase pathway, down-regulation of the L-type calcium current, and alterations in calcium-regulated excitation–contraction coupling [45]. Recent years have seen significant advances in the treatment of ventricular systolic dysfunction and heart failure. The therapeutic armamentarium includes not only pharmacologic agents, but also electrical and surgical devices. In addition to the cornerstone drugs for heart failure, such as digoxin, diuretics, ACE inhibitors, and beta-blockers, new agents, such as the aldosterone receptor antagonist spironolactone, the endothelin antagonist bosentan, the vasopeptidase inhibitor omapatrilat, tumour necrosis factor-α, and the brain natriuretic peptide (BNP) nesiritide, have been investigated in multicentre trials with varying results [46]. For example, BNP level was shown to be a strong predictor of SCD in patients with chronic heart failure [47]. A recent study showed that patients with low plasma BNP, measured at the convalescent phase after acute MI, have an extremely low incidence of SCD [48]. In contrast, elevated BNP had a better predictive power among those with preserved LV function (LVEF $>$ 40%) [48]. Thus, measurement of BNP may have utility as a risk stratifier for primary ICD prophylaxis. Electrical devices, including biventricular pacemakers, in selected groups of patients can improve LVEF and mortality [49]. Furthermore, surgical procedures, such as passive external support, have been shown in experimental studies to reverse remodelling, with reduced systolic wall stress and improved adrenergic signalling [50]. The success of LV assist devices [51] has shown that even in an advanced stage of heart failure the remodelling process can be reversed. with significant improvement of ventricular function. Finally, clinical research has demonstrated that gene transfer is a potential therapeutic option to restore diseased cardiomyocytes and rescue the failing heart [52].

Conclusions

The immediate future goals for risk stratification and management of SCD can be summarised as follows [53]:

1. Identification of novel clinical, biochemical, and genetic markers for SCD and assessment of the functional consequences of sequence variants identified in human genetic studies, as well as relevant environmental–genetic interactions.
2. Determination of the heritability of genetic risk factors for SCD, as well as the factors involved in ethnic-specific differences in risk of SCD.
3. Identification of a battery of a relatively limited number of incrementally cumulative low- to intermediate-risk variants and development of a 'signature' combination of clinical, biochemical, and genetic markers of SCD.

However, we should not be surprised that the positive predictive value of some of the new risk factors, similar to conventional risk factors, will be relatively low, especially if they are applied to large populations that are at low risk. In fact, the true value of risk stratification of SCD in the future may be to identify low-risk populations that do not warrant prophylactic intervention with therapy with demonstrated efficacy, e.g. the ICD. One approach is to target patients who receive an ICD for primary prophylaxis per approved criteria and concomitantly conduct studies within those cohorts to attempt to identify low-risk patients.
4. Identification of novel pharmacologic and nonpharmacologic approaches for risk modification and prevention of SCD. A prime example is the recent interest in clinical prevention of SCD by *n*-3 polyunsaturated fatty acids. Although the relatively new diet–heart hypothesis that underlies this therapeutic modality has yet to catch the attention of the clinical community at large, experimental and clinical evidence points to the validity of this approach [54].
5. Wider collaboration among different academic and industrial institutions by sharing research results and resources, such as clinical data, blood, and other tissues from biorepository centres. The ultimate goal is to identify novel methods for risk stratification, risk modification, and prevention of SCD that can be applied to the general public at large.

References

1. Spooner PM, Albert C, Benjamin EL et al (2001) Sudden cardiac death, genes, and arrhythmogenesis: Consideration of new population and mechanistic approaches from a National Heart Lung, and Blood Institute Workshop, part I. Circulation 103:2361–2364
2. Spooner PM, Albert C, Benjamin EL et al (2001) Sudden cardiac death, genes, and arrhythmogenesis: Consideration of new population and mechanistic approaches from a National Heart, Lung, and Blood Institute Workshop, part II. Circulation103:2447–2452
3. Friedlander Y, Siscovick DS, Weinmann S et al (1998) Family history as a risk factor for primary cardiac arrest. Circulation 97:155–160
4. Jouven X, Desnos M, Guerot C et al (1999) Predicting sudden death in the population: The Paris Prospective Study I. Circulation 99:1978–1983
5. Friedlander Y, Siscovick DS, Arbogast P et al (2002) Sudden cardiac death and myocardial infarction in first degree relatives as predictors of primary cardiac arrest. Atherosclerosis 162:211–216
6. Jouven X, Zureik M, Desnos M et al (2001) Resting heart rate as a predictive risk factor for sudden death in middle aged men. Cardiovasc Res 50:373–378
7. Singh JP, Larson MG, O'Donnell CJ et al(1999) Heritability of heart rate variability: The Framingham Heart Study. Circulation 99:2251–2254
8. Muller JE (1999) Circadian variation and triggering of acute coronary events. Am Heart J 137(Pt 2)51–58

9. Podlowski S, Wenzel K, Luther HP et al (2000) Beta 1-adrenoceptor gene variations: A role in idiopathic dilated cardiomyopathy? J Mol Med 78:87–93
10. Liggett SB, Wagoner LE, Craft LL (1998) The lle164 beta2-adrenergic receptor polymorphism adversely affects the outcome of congestive heart failure. J Clin Invest 102:1534–1539
11. Sosunov EA, Gainullin RZ, Moise NS et al (2000) Beta1, and beta2-adrenergic receptor subtype effects in German shepherd dogs with inherited lethal ventricular arrhythmias. Cardiovasc Res 48:211–219
12. Jouven X, Charles MA, Desnos M et al (2001) Circulating nonesterified fatty acid level as a predictive risk factor for sudden cardiac death in the population. Circulation 104:756–761
13. Critchley HD, Taggart P, Sutton PM et al (2005) Mental stress and sudden cardiac death: asymmetric midbrain activity as a linking mechanism. Brain 128:75–85
14. Splawski I, Shen J, Timothy KW et al (2000) Spectrum of mutations in long QT syndrome genes. KVLQT1, HERG, SCN5A, KCNE1, and KCNE2. Circulation 102:1178–1184
15. Priori SG, Napolitano C, Gasparini M et al (2000) Clinical and genetic heterogeneity of right bundle branch block and ST-segment elevation syndrome: A prospective evaluation of 52 families. Circulation 102:2509–2515
16. Priori S, Napolitano C, Memmi M et al (2002) Clinical and molecular characterization of patients with catecholaminergic polymorphic ventricular tachycardia. Circulation 106:69–74
17. Lahat H, Pras E, Olender T et al (2001) A missense mutation in a highly conserved region of CASQ2 is associated with autosomal recessive catecholamine-induced polymorphic ventricular tachycardia in Bedouin families from Israel. Am J Hum Genet 69:1378–1384
18. Kubota T, Shimizu W, Kamakura S et al (2000) Hypokalemia-induced longQTsyndrome with an underlying novel missense mutation in S4-S5 linker of KCNQ1. J Cardiovasc Electrophysiol 11:1048–1054
19. Sesti F, Abbott GW, Wei J et al (2000) A common polymorphism associated with antibiotic-induced cardiac arrhythmia. Proc Natl Acad Sci USA 97:10613–10618
20. Napolitano C, Schwartz PJ, Brown AM et al (2000) Evidence for a cardiac ion channel mutation underlying drug-induced QT prolongation and lifethreatening arrhythmias. J Cardiovasc Electrophysiol 11:691–696
21. Splawski I, Timothy KW, Tateyama M et al (2002) Variant of SCN5A sodium channel implicated in risk of cardiac arrhythmia. Science 297:1333–1336
22. Marian J (2002) Modifier genes for hypertrophic cardiomyopathy. Curr Opin Cardiol 17:242–252
23. Le Corvoisier P, Park HY, Carlson KM (2003) Impact of genetic polymorphism in heart failure prognosis. Arch Mal Coeur Vaiss 96:197–206
24. Anonymous (2000) Heart disease and stroke statistics, 2001 Update. Dallas, TX, American Heart Association
25. Braunwald E (1997) Shattuck Lecture Cardiovascular medicine at the turn of the millennium: Triumphs, concerns and opportunities. N Engl J Med 377:1360–1369
26. Wang Q (2005) Advances in the genetic basis of coronary artery disease. Curr Atherosclerosis Rep 7(3):235–241
27. Gnasso A, Motti C, Irace C (2000) Genetic variation in human stromelysin gene promoter and common carotid geometry in healthy male subjects. Arterioscler Thromb Vasc Biol 20:1600–1605
28. Moss AJ, Goldstein RE, Marder VJ et al (1999) Thrombogenic factors and recurrent

coronary events. Circulation 99:2517–2522
29. Weiss EJ, Bray PF, Tayback M et al (1996) A polymorphism of a platelet glycoprotein receptor as an inherited risk factor for coronary thrombosis. N Engl J Med 334:1090–1094
30. Nakayama M,Yasue H,Yoshimura M et al (1999) T786→C mutation in the 5'-flanking region of the endothelial nitric oxide synthase gene is associated with coronary spasm. Circulation 99:2864–2870
31. Wang XL, Sim AS,Wang MX et al (2000) Genotype dependent and cigarette specific effects on endothelial nitric oxide synthase gene expression and enzyme activity. FEBS Lett 471:45–50
32. Albert CM, Ma J, Rifai N et al (2002) Prospective study of C-reactive protein, homocysteine, and plasma lipid levels as predictors of sudden cardiac death. Circulation 105:2595–2599
33. Verma S, Kuliszewski AM, Szmitko PE et al (2004) C-reactive protein attenuates endothelial progenitor cell survival, differentiation, and function: further evidence of a mechanistic link between C-reactive protein and cardiovascular disease. Circulation 109:2058–2067
34. American Diabetes Association: diabetes facts and figures, 2000. Available from http://www.diabetes.org
35. Stern MP (1995) Diabetes and cardiovascular disease, the 'common soil' hypothesis. Diabetes 44:396–374
36. Balkau B, Jouven X, Ducimetiere P et al (1999) Diabetes as a risk of factor for sudden death. Lancet 354:1968–1969
37. Hu FB, Stampfer MJ, Haffner SM et al (2002) Elevated risk of cardiovascular disease prior to clinical diagnosis of type 2 diabetes. Diabetes Care 25:1129–1134
38. Haffner SM (2002) Glucose-intolerance testing in acute myocardial infarction. Lancet 359:2127–2128
39. Moreno PR, Fuster V (2004) New aspects in the pathogenesis of diabetic atherothrombosis. J Am Coll Cardiol 44:2293–3000
40. Qin D, Zang ZH, Caref EB et al (1996) Cellular and ionic basis of arrhythmias in post infarction remodeled ventricular myocardium. Circ Res 79:461–473
41. Gidh-Jain M, Huang B, Jain P et al (1996) Differential expression of voltage-gated K+ channel genes in left ventricular remodeled myocardium after experimental myocardial infarction. Circ Res 79:669–675
42. Huang B, Qin D, El-Sherif N (2000) Early down-regulation of K^+ channel genes and currents in the post infarction heart. J Cardiovasc Electrophysiol 11:1252–1261
42. Gyamlani G, Parikh G, Kulkani AG (2000) Benefits of magnesium in acute myocardial infarction. Timing is crucial. Am Heart J 139:e2
44. Pitt B, Zannad F, Remme WJ et al (1999) The effect of spironolactone on morbidity and mortality in patients with severe heart failure. N Engl J Med 341:709–717
45. Lorell BH (1997) Transition from hypertrophy to failure. Circulation 96:2824–2827
46. Carson P (2001) Current reviews of heart failure trials. Cardiology 7:27–32
47. Berger R, Huelsmon M, Strecker K et al (2002) β-type natriuretic peptide predicts sudden death in patients with chronic heart failure. Circulation 105:2392–2397
48. Tapanainen JM, Lindgren KS, Makikallio TH et al (2004) Natriuretic peptides as predictors of non-sudden and sudden cardiac death after acute myocardial infarction in the beta-blocking era. J Am Coll cardiol 43:757–763
49. Bradley DJ, Bradley EA, Baughman KL et al (2003) Cardiac resynchronization and death from progressive heart failure: A meta-analysis of randomized controlled trials. JAMA 289:730–740

50. Saavedra WF, Tunin RS, Paolocci N et al (2002) Reverse remodeling and enhanced adrenergic reserve from passive external support in experimental dilated heart failure. J AmColl Cardiol 39:2069–2076
51. Frazier OH, Benedict CR, Radovancevic B et al (1996) Improved left ventricular function after chronic left ventricular unloading. Ann Thorac Surg 62:675–682
52. Hajjar RT, del Monte F, Matsui T et al (2000) prospects for gene therapy of heart failure. Circ Res 86:616–621
53. El-Sherif N, Turitto G (2003) Risk stratification and management of sudden cardiac death: A new paradigm. J Cardiovasc Electrophysiol 14:1113–1119
54. Leaf A, Kang JX, Xiao Y-F et al (2003) Clinical prevention of sudden cardiac death by n-3 polyunsaturated fatty acids and the mechanism of prevention of arrhythmias by n-3 fish oils. Circulation 107:2646–2652

Sudden Arrhythmic Death: Which Genetic Determinants?

G.A. Danieli

Introduction

Sudden cardiac death (SCD) is a serious health problem in developed countries. Estimates of the incidence of SCD in human populations are still imprecise For example, Myerburg and Spooner [1] pointed out that the frequently cited estimate of 250 000–300 000 SCDs per year in the US is solely based on the assumption that about 50% of 600 000 cardiovascular deaths occurred suddenly. In a 30-year population-based study conducted in Olmsted County, Minnesota, the reported rate of SCD among subjects age 20–40 was 8.7/100 000 in men and 4.1/100 000 in women [2]. More recently, in England, the incidence of unexpected SCDs in healthy people age 16–64 was estimated at 11/100 000/year [3]. While these two studies produced data of the same order of magnitude, the estimate of SCD in humans remains far from being fixed.

Heterogeneity of Determinants of Sudden Death

Sudden death is defined as a natural but unexpected fatal event occurring within 1 h from the manifestation of symptoms in an apparently healthy subject [4]. Deaths recorded as 'sudden' are frequently the ultimate outcome of complex and progressive diseases that developed over a long period of time; these encompass many different clinical and aetiological phenotypes. Terminal arrhythmogenesis may be a result of the interplay between several different processes, including atherosclerosis and thrombosis, defects in

Laboratory of Human Molecular Genetics and Genomics, Department of Biology, University of Padua, Padua, Italy

electrogenesis and propagation, influences of the sympathetic and parasympathetic systems, ischaemia, and poor vascular control. For these reasons, in people over 60, a fatal event should be considered 'relatively unexpected', whereas a fatal event is definitely 'unexpected' in teenagers and in young adults, although a small percentage of them may carry concealed forms of affections predisposing to SCD.

In a prospective study carried out in Venice (Italy) from 1979 to 1996 on sudden deaths among young athletes and non-athletes (under 35 years of age), 49 of 269 sudden deaths (18%) were recorded among athletes. The most frequent causes of such deaths were: arrhythmogenic right ventricular cardiomyopathy (22.4%), atherosclerotic coronary artery disease (18.4%) and anomalous origin of coronary artery (12.2%). Among non-athletes, the most frequent causes of sudden death were: atherosclerotic coronary artery disease (16.4%), mitral valve prolapse (9.5%), and diseases of the conduction system (9.1%) [5].

In the same study, in a cohort of 33 735 athletes less than 35 years of age, 1058 subjects were excluded from competitive sports for medical reasons, 58.7% of which involved cardiovascular vulnerabilities. Of these, rhythm and conduction defects accounted for 38.3%, hypertension for 27.1%, and valvular defects for 21.7 [5].

It is clear from these data that SCD is a very heterogeneous category that includes events due to several different causes, ranging from severe myocardial ischaemia to severe conduction defects, to malignant arrhythmias.

More recently, the delineation of a subset of SCDs, sudden arrhythmic deaths (SADs), was proposed, characterised by the *sudden* occurrence of fibrillation or of potentially lethal ventricular tachy- or bradyarrhythmias as a cause of death [6]. Although this novel category is probably phenotypically more homogeneous, it undoubtedly still comprises a heterogeneous group of diseases, since early triggers of lethal arrhythmias or fibrillation may differ from patient to patient and may be due to different genetic determinants.

Genes Involved in the Increased Risk of Sudden Arrhythmic Death

The role of genes in SCD was outlined by Spooner et al. in two key reports [7, 8].

In the cohort of SCDs studied by Behr et al. [3], 41% of SCDs in the 16–64 age group were reported as unexplained, since cardiac pathological findings were normal and toxicological tests were negative. However, subsequent cardiologic assessment of 104 first-degree relatives of 32 SCD subjects revealed the presence of an inherited cardiac disease in seven families (22%): four families carried a long QT syndrome; one a non-structural cardiac electrophysiological disease; one had myotonic dystrophy, and one hypertrophic cardiomyopathy.

More recently, 43 consecutive families were investigated [9] in which more than one person suffered SCD at less than 40 years of age. Molecular genetic analysis was conducted to confirm the diagnosis, and all studied relatives underwent resting/exercise ECG and Doppler echocardiography. An inherited disease and likely cause of death was identified in 17 of 43 families (40%). Twelve families showed primary electrical disease: catecholaminergic polymorphic ventricular tachycardia (5 families), long-QT syndrome (4 families), Brugada syndrome (2 families), and long-QT/Brugada syndrome (1 family). Furthermore, there were three families with inherited arrhythmogenic right ventricular cardiomyopathy, one family with hypertrophic cardiomyopathy, and one family with familial hypercholesterolaemia. After molecular genetic analysis, which was successful in ten families, 151 pre-symptomatic disease carriers (8.9 per family) were identified.

The percentage of inherited cardiac diseases among victims of SAD is probably higher than presently estimated. Actually, thorough clinical investigation of relatives of such individuals is still rather infrequent; moreover, when molecular genetic tests are done, only a small fraction of the genes potentially involved in predisposition to SAD are screened.

In the last 10 years, mutations in a series of genes were shown to cause different forms of cardiomyopathy, and it was demonstrated that cardiomyopathy per se is a risk factor for SCD or SAD. A list of genes in which pathogenic mutations were recorded in human cardiomyopathies, far from being complete, is reported in Table 1.

Moreover, in the last decade, mutations in genes encoding different cardiac sarcolemmal Na and K ion channel subunits, listed in Table 2, have also been described. Such mutations increase the propensity to SCD, due to defective cell depolarisation and repolarisation. A recent review [10] outlined that a single clinical phenotype may be caused by different genetic substrates and, conversely, that a single gene may cause very different phenotypes acting through different pathways.

Mutations in the cardiac ryanodine receptor (RYR2) have been associated with both arrhythmogenic right ventricular cardiomyopathy type 2 [11] and catecholaminergic ventricular tachycardia [12]. This has led to the novel concept that monogenic arrhythmic disorders are linked to defects in myocardial Ca^{2+} handling [13]. Later, it was reported that LQT4 , associated with a high risk of SAD after exercise and emotional stress, is due to mutation of the gene encoding ankyrin-B. Ankyrin B appears to be involved in positioning of sarcolemmal voltage-gated Na+ channel, Na+/K+ ATPase, NCX and SR inositol 1,4,5-triphosphate Ca^{2+} release channels; therefore, mutations in AKK2 (ankyrin B) result in defective intracellular Ca^{2+} handling [14]. However, it is also known that TNNT2, mutations in which cause cardiomyopathy hypertrophic (CMH), associated with a high risk of SAD,

Table 1. List of genes in which pathogenic mutations were recorded in human cardiomyopathies

Disease	Locus	I	Gene	OMIM
CMH1	14q12	AD	MYH7 (myosin H chain)	192600
CMH2	1q32	AD	TNNT2 (troponin T)	115195
CMH3	15q22.1	AD	TPM1 (a-tropomyosin)	115196
CMH4	11p11.2	AD	MYBPC3	115197
CMH7	19q13.4	AD	TNNI3 (troponin I)	191044
CMH8	3p	AD	MYL3 (myosin L chain)	160790
CMH9	2q24.3	AD	TTN (Titin)	188840
CMH	14q12	AD	MYH6 (myosin H chain)	160710
CMH	20q13.3	AD	MYLK2	606566
CMH	15q14	AD	ACTC (actin)	102540
CMH	12q23-q24.3	AD	MYL2 (myosin L chain)	160781
CMH/WPW	7q36	AD	PRKAG2	600858
CMH	9q34	AD	GSN (gelsolin)	137350
CMH	Xq22	XR	GLA (a-galactosidase)	301500
CMD1A	1q21.2	AD	Lamin A/C	115200
CMD1D	1q32	AD	TNNT2 (troponin T)	601494
CMD1G	2q31	AD	TTN (titin)	604145
CMD1I	2q35	AD	DES (desmin)	604765
CMD1L	5q33-q34	AR	SGCD (d-sarcoglycan)	606685
CMD3A	Xq28	XR	G4.5 (?)	300069
CMD	14q12	AD	MYH7 (myosin H chain)	160760
CMD	14q11.2-q12	AD	TNNT2 (troponin T)	191045
CMD	15q14	AD	ACTC (actin)	102540
CMD	15q22.1	AD	TPM1 (atropomyosin	191010
CMD	Xq28	XR	G4.5	302060
CMD	6p24	AR	DSP (desmoplakin)	605676
CMD	Xp21	XR	DYS (dystrophin)	300376
CMD	9q13	AR	FRDA (frataxin)	229300
CMD	18cen-q12.3	AD	TTR (transthyretin)	176300
CMD	Xp21.1	XR	XK (McLeod)	314850
CMD	17q25.2-q25.3	AR	GAA (acid maltase)	232300
ARVD1	14q23-q24	AD	TGFbeta3	107970
ARVD2	1q42-q43	AD	RYR2 (ryanodine receptor)	600996
ARVD8	6p24	AD	DSP (desmoplakin)	605676
ARVD9			PKP2 (plakophilin2)	
ARVD-NAXOS	17	AR	JUP (plakoglobin)	188840

Table 2. Genes encoding different cardiac sarcolemmal Na and K ion channel subunits

Gene	Locus	I	Disease	OMIM
KCNQ1	11p15.5	AD	LQT1	192500
KCNH2	7q35-q36	AD	LQT2	152427
SCN5A	3p21	AD	LQT3 - BRUGADA	603830
KCNE1 (MINK)	21q22.1-q22.2	AD	LQT5	176261
KCNE2 (MIRP1)	21q22.1-q22.2	AD	LQT6	603796
KCNQ1/KCNE1	11p15.5/21q21.2 - q22.2	AR	JLNS1	220400
KCNJ2	17q23.1 – q24.2	AD	ANDERSEN-TAWIL	170390

plays a fundamental role in dynamic Ca^{2+} buffering during the cardiac cycle; therefore, the link between myocardial calcium signalling and cardiac arrhythmias is increasingly evident [15]. It would not be surprising that mutations in additional, still unidentified genes encoding proteins involved in intracellular Ca^{2+} handling might predispose to SCD.

Identification of Causative Mutations in Sudden Arrhythmic Death

As shown by Tan et al. [9], identification of causative mutations in patients with SAD is very important for pre-symptomatic detection of at-risk family members. In centres with experience in diagnosing inherited cardiac disease, clinical assessment and genetic testing should be offered to families of victims of SAD. However, detecting causative mutations in SAD is not easy at all, even in the presence of a previous and well-established clinical diagnosis.

Ideally, only DNA sequencing of an entire gene (exons, introns, and UTRs) and of its promoter region, coupled with a method for detecting large deletions would assure a detection rate close to 100%. In practice, in most laboratories, mutation screening involve only the coding sequences. Denaturing high-performance liquid chromatography (DHPLC) has a detection rate of over 95%, but for several genes, such as RYR2, the screening protocol must involve also DNA sequencing of those exons for which the DHPLC detection rate is poor [16].

Restriction of mutation screening to coding sequences, detection rates lower than 100%, and with genetic heterogeneity significantly reduce the expected detection rate of a given gene. In fact, in most laboratories, genetic analysis identifies disease-causing mutations in 68% of patients with LQT syndrome, 20% of patients with Brugada syndrome, 32% of patients with PVA (CPVT+ARVD2), and about 50% of patients with arrhythmogenic right ventricular cardiomyopathy.

While nonsense mutations are always pathogenic, a missense mutation identified in a patient or in a victim of SAD must be considered as putative causative mutations until a very large number of control subjects from the same population are shown to be negative for the specific variation. In this situation, information on a 'putative causative mutation' should be used with extreme prudence when dealing with genetic testing of relatives of an index case.

An important and still open problem is how to evaluate individual risk in asymptomatic probands. When the pathogenic mutation is detected in a relative, it is almost impossible to predict whether or not the mutation will cause the same clinical phenotype observed in the index case. Differences in environmental factors and individual genetic background may produce significant variations in the clinical phenotype caused by the same pathogenic mutation. Non-pathogenic variability in genes involved in a specific function related to excitation-contraction coupling (e.g. intracellular Ca^{2+} handling) and their independent assortment at each meiosis are expected to produce wide clinical variability even within the same family.

Last but not least, identifying the causative mutation in a patient with SAD lacking previous diagnosis is a very difficult task. Results of accurate autopsies may help in selecting which genes should be screened first, but the genetic heterogeneity of most cardiac diseases predisposing to SAD always makes identification of the causative mutation a long, expensive, and often frustrating work.

Perspectives

The genetic heterogeneity of SAD is very large. Although several genes have been identified in which pathogenic mutations predispose to SAD, a number of additional genes involved in this susceptibility have escaped detection. Table 3 reports a short list of inherited arrhythmic disorders in which the involved gene(s) remains to be identified.

The positional candidate approach, which has proven successful in many instances in human molecular genetics, relies on the collection of DNA samples from large three-generation families, in which thorough clinical assessment of each individual should be available. Unfortunately, such families are extremely rare.

An alternative approach based on genome-wide association study was recently proposed [6]. According to this study design, appropriately matched patients and controls are subject to genome-wide single nucleotide polymorphism (SNP) genotyping by DNA chips; SNP allele frequencies are compared in order to identify regions associated with disease. Such regions are then

Table 3. A short list of inherited arrhythmic disorders in which the involved gene(s) is unknown

Disease	Locus	OMIM
Atrial fibrillation with bradyarrhythmia	?	163800
Atrial tachyarrhythmia with short PR interval	?	108950
Cardiac conduction defect with sudden death	?	115080
Progressive familial heart block, type I,I	19q13.2-q13.3	604559
Progressive familial heart block, type II	?	140400
Ventricular fibrillation, paroxysmal familial	3p21	603829

scanned for known functional elements, and cross-species comparisons are used to identify unknown regulatory elements. At the end, functional elements are directly sequenced to identify causal variants. This design is very attractive, although its success is strictly dependent on the appropriate selection of patients and of controls. The recent introduction of DNA chips for typing up to 10 000 SNP per individual assay makes this perspective feasible and interesting.

Due to rapid progress in our knowledge of mutations predisposing to SAD, the feasibility of screenings for detecting at-risk subjects is being discussed. The problem of preventive screening is particularly relevant when dealing with young athletes [17–19].

At the present, mutation screening for the genes MYH7, MYBPC3, TNNT2, TNNT3, SCN5A, RYR2, DSP, and PKP2, most frequently involved in SAD, would cost over $800 per person; this would make the perspective of screening unrealistic, even if it were restricted to teenagers involved in competitive sports. However, further development of dedicated DNA chips for analysis of selected groups of genes is likely to change this perspective in the next future.

References

1. Myerburg RJ, Spooner PM (2001) Opportunities for sudden death prevention: Directions for new clinical and basic research. Cardiovasc Res 50:177–185
2. Shen WK, Edwards WD, Hammil SC et al (1995) Sudden unexpected non-traumatic death in 54 adults: a 30 year population-based study. Am J Cardiol 76:148–152
3. Behr E, Wood DA, Wright M et al (2003) Cardiological assessment of first-degree relatives in sudden arrhythmic death syndrome. Lancet 362:1457–1459
4. Goldstein S (1982) The necessity of a uniform definition of sudden coronary death. Witnessed death within 1 hour of the onset of acute symptoms. Am Heart J 103:156–159

5. Corrado D, Basso C, Schiavon M, Thiene G. (1998) Screening for hypertrophic cardiomyopathy in young athletes. N Engl J Med 339:364–369
6. Arking DE, Chugh SS, Chakravarti A, Spooner PM (2004) Genomics in sudden cardiac death. Circ Res 94:712–723
7. Spooner PM, Albert C, Benjamin EJ et al (2001) Sudden cardiac death, genes and arrhythmogenesis. Part I. Circulation 103: 2361–2364
8. Spooner PM, Albert C, Benjamin EJ et al (2001) Sudden cardiac death, genes and arrhythmogenesis. Part II. Circulation 103:2447–2452
9. Tan HL, Hofman N, van Langen IM et al (2005) Sudden Unexplained Death. Heritability and Diagnostic Yield of Cardiological and Genetic Examination in Surviving Relatives. Circulation 112:207–213
10. Priori SG, Napolitano C (2004) Genetics of cardiac arrhythmias and sudden cardiac death. Ann N Y Acad Sci 1015:96–110
11. Tiso N, Stephan DA, Nava A et al (2001) Identification of mutations in the cardiac ryanodine receptor gene in families affected with arrhythmogenic right ventricular cardiomyopathy type 2 (ARVD2). Hum Mol Genet 10:189–194
12. Priori SG, Napolitano C, Tiso N et al (2001) Mutations in the cardiac ryanodine receptor gene (hRyR2) underlie catecholaminergic polymorphic ventricular tachycardia. Circulation 103:196–200
13. Scoote M, Williams AJ(2002) The cardiac ryanodine receptor (calcium release channel): emerging role in heart failure and arrhythmia pathogenesis. Cardiovasc Res 56:359–372
14. Mohler PJ, Schott JJ, Gramolini AO et al (2003) Ankyrin-B mutation causes type 4 long-QT cardiac arrhythmia and sudden cardiac death. Nature 421: 634–639
15. Scoote M, Williams AJ (2004) Myocardial calcium signalling and arrhythmia pathogenesis. Biochem Biophys Res Commun 322:1286–1309
16. Bagattin A, Veronese C, Bauce B et al (2004) Denaturing HPLC-based approach for detecting RYR2 mutations involved in malignant arrhythmias. Clin Chem 50:1148–1155
17. Borjesson M, Nylander E (2005) Sudden cardiac death in athletes is usually caused by undiagnosed heart disease. Cardiac screening of young athletes under discussion. Lakartidningen 102:560–563
18. Maron BJ (2005) How should we screen competitive athletes for cardiovascular disease? Eur Heart J 26:428–430
19. Wike J, Kernan M (2005) Sudden cardiac death in the active adult: causes, screening, and preventive strategies. Curr Sports Med Rep 4:76–82

Brain Natriuretic Peptide as a Predictor of Sudden Cardiac Death

H.V. Huikuri

Introduction

Atrial natriuretic peptide (ANP) and brain natriuretic peptide (BNP) are vasoactive peptide hormones with natriuretic, diuretic, and vasodilator activity [1–3]. They have emerged as important candidates in the development of diagnostic and prognostic tools for cardiovascular diseases [3, 4]. An association between elevated levels of natriuretic peptides (NP) and increased mortality has been established in patients with heart failure [5, 6] as well as in patients with acute coronary syndromes [7, 8]. Moreover, previous studies have further extended the role of BNP measurements to risk stratification of the general population [9–11].

Prediction of sudden cardiac death (SCD) after an acute myocardial infarction (AMI) is still a challenge. Several methods of prediction have been proposed [12–20], but none of them, except the measurement of left ventricular systolic function, is in routine clinical use in screening patients for candidacy for anti-arrhythmic therapy such as implantation of a cardioverter–defibrillator [17]. New methods of risk stratification are therefore urgently needed.

BNP and Sudden Cardiac Death

At least two studies have assessed the role of BNP in predicting SCD [18, 19]. A study among patients with chronic heart failure specifically addressed the value of BNP measurement in the prediction of SCD [18]. Berger et al. [18]

Division of Cardiology, Department of Internal Medicine, University of Oulu, Finland

studied 452 patients with a left ventricular ejection fraction of less than 35%. Forty-four patients suffered sudden death during a mean follow-up time of 592 ± 387 days. Univariate risk factors of sudden death were log BNP level ($P = 0.006$), log N-terminal ANP level ($P = 0.003$), left ventricular ejection fraction (LVEF; $P = 0.005$), log N-terminal BNP level ($P = 0.006$), systolic blood pressure ($P = 0.01$), high endothelin level ($P = 0.03$), and NYHA class ($P = 0.04$). In the multivariate model, log BNP level was the only independent predictor of sudden death ($P = 0.0006$). Using a cutoff point of log BNP < 2.11 (130 pg/ml), Kaplan–Meier sudden-death-free survival rates were significantly higher in patients below (99%) compared with patients above (81%) this cutoff point ($P = 0.0001$).

Tapanainen et al. [19] studied 521 patients with a recent AMI. During a mean follow-up of 43 ± 13 months 16 patients (3.1%) suffered SCD. On univariate analysis, high levels of all measured peptides and low EF predicted the occurrence of non-sudden cardiac death ($P < 0.001$ for all). Peptides and EF also predicted the occurrence of SCD ($P < 0.05$), with elevated BNP (> 23.0 pmol/1) being the most powerful predictor of SCD [hazard ratio (HR) 4.4, 95% confidence interval (CI), 1.4 to 13.8, $P = 0.01$]. After adjusting for clinical variables, only elevated BNP (HR 3.9, 95% CI, 1.2 to 12.3, $P = 0.02$) and low EF (< 0.40%; $P = 0.03$) remained as significant predictors of SCD.

The main implication of these studies is that the measurement of BNP can be used to identify the 'low risk' patients who may not need further risk stratification and may not benefit from prophylactic cardioverter-

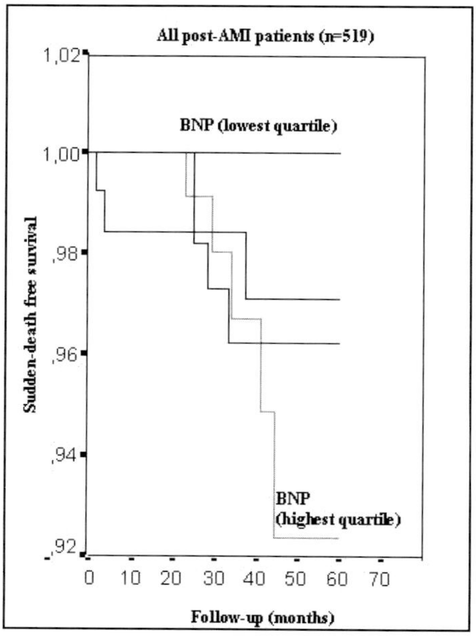

Fig. 1. Kaplan–Meier survival curves: sudden-death-free survival among patients after acute myocardial infarction (post-AMI patients) in relation to plasma brain natriuretic peptide (BNP) level (by quartile)

defibrillator implantation despite depressed left ventricular function. For example, in the re-analysis of the study by Tapanainen et al. there were no SCDs among the patients with the lowest BNP quartile even when they had an EF of less than 35% (Figs. 1–3). Elevated BNP also had a predictive power among patients with preserved left ventricular function (EF > 40%) (relative

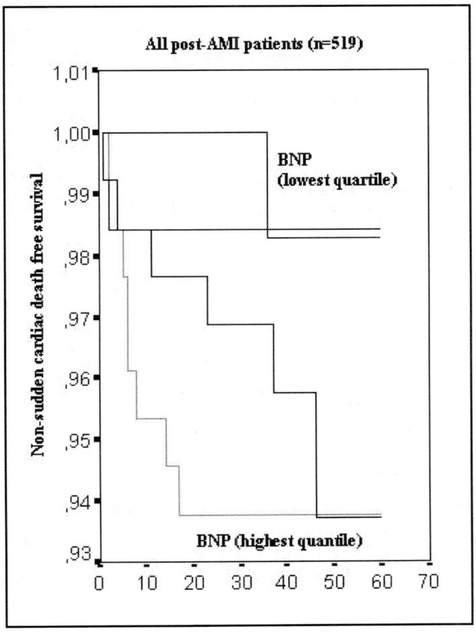

Fig. 2. Kaplan–Meier survival curves: non-sudden-cardiac-death-free survival among post-AMI patients in relation to plasma brain natriuretic peptide (BNP) level (by quartile)

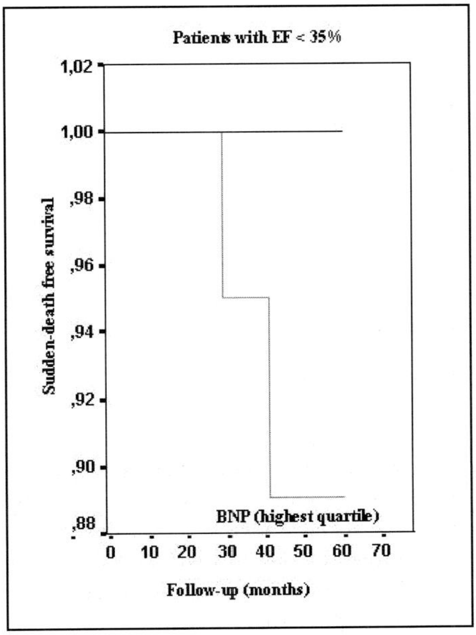

Fig. 3. Kaplan–Meier survival curves: sudden-death-free survival among post-AMI patients with an ejection fraction (EF) less than 35% (highest quartile only)

risk 3.9, 95% CI, 1.0–16.5, $P = 0.05$). Patients with an EF below 40% also accounted for the highest cumulative number of SCD events. Prediction and prevention of SCD among the large number of survivors of AMI who have preserved left ventricular function will be important in future efforts aimed at reducing the overall burden of premature SCD. Measurement of BNP may have clinical value in this respect.

Prediction of SCD After AMI

Several risk markers, such as autonomic markers, the signal-averaged electrocardiogram (ECG), and T-wave alternans, have been extensively studied as predictors of SCD after AMI [12–14, 19–21]. Most of the studies have suggested that these variables provide information on the risk of subsequent SCD and arrhythmia events [12–14, 21]. However, the majority of these observational studies were performed in the era before optimised medical therapy. For example, in the Autonomic Tone and Reflexes After Myocardial Infarction (ATRAMI) study, which showed that autonomic markers predict sudden death, only around 20% of patients were receiving β-blocking therapy [12]. Similarly, in studies showing that T-wave alternans after AMI predicts SCD, only 13% of patients were receiving β-blocking medication [14, 21]. Our previous analyses of the same population as in the present study suggested that arrhythmia risk variables such as autonomic markers, signal-averaged ECG, and T wave alternans lose some of their predictive power among post-AMI patients with optimised β-blocking therapy [19, 20]. In the light of these findings, the present observations suggest that elevated BNP may have some potential value in the prediction of SCD among current post-AMI populations.

Elevated BNP and Risk of SCD

There may be several reasons why BNP provides more specific information on the risk of SCD than do the other peptides or even the measurement of LV systolic function. Both ANP and N-terminal ANP are more closely related to atrial volume loading, whereas BNP secretion from the ventricles is increased during progressive HF [22, 23] and is released from the ventricles in response to increased pressure, stretch, and hypertrophy [24]. Ventricular stretch, hypertrophy, and fibrosis can have significant influences on the electrophysiological properties of the heart via mechano-electrical feedback [25–28]. Thus, BNP may be an indirect marker of the mechanical factors predisposing a person to the onset and perpetuation of life-threatening arrhythmias. This is also supported by an observation that BNP specifically predicted the occurrence of SCD late after the index event. It is possible that elevated BNP is a marker of LV remodelling occurring late after AMI, which then predisposes to sudden arrhythmic death.

Clinical Implications

A significant proportion of post-AMI patients, even with adequate treatment, are still at high risk of dying during the first few years after the AMI. The prediction and prevention of SCD is of particular importance, because recent large-scale randomised trials have documented the mortality benefit from prophylactic cardioverter-defibrillator implantation in certain high-risk subgroups of patients [17]. The data from two studies suggest that BNP level should be included as one of the risk variables in future studies comparing the various indexes as predictors of SCD.

References

1. Levin ER, Gardner DG, Samson WK (1998) Natriuretic peptides. N Engl J Med 339:321–328
2. Richards AM, McDonald D, Fitzpatrick MA et al (1988) Atrial natriuretic hormone has biological effects in man at physiological plasma concentrations. J Clin Endocrinol Metab 67:1134–1139
3. DeLemos JA, McGuire DK, Drazner MH (2003) B-type natriuretic peptide in cardiovascular disease. Lancet 362:316–332
4. Ruskoaho H (2003) Cardiac hormones as diagnostic tools in heart failure. Endocr Rev 24:341–356
5. Cowie MR, Mendez GF (2002) BNP and congestive heart failure. Prog Cardiovasc Dis 44:293–321
6. Anand IS, Fisher LD, Chiang YT et al (2003) Val-HeFT Investigators. Changes in brain natriuretic peptide and norepinephrine over time and mortality and morbidity in the Valsartan Heart Failure Trial (Val-HeFT). Circulation 107:1278–1283
7. Jernberg T, Stridsberg M, Venge P et al (2002) N-terminal pro brain natriuretic peptide on admission for early risk stratification of patients with chest pain and no ST-segment elevation. J Am Coll Cardiol 40:437–445
8. Morrow DA, de Lemos JA, Sabatine MS et al (2003). Evaluation of B-type natriuretic peptide for risk assessment in unstable angina/non-ST-elevation myocardial infarction: B-type natriuretic peptide and prognosis in TACTICS-TIMI 18. J Am Coll Cardiol 41:1264–1272
9. McDonagh TA, Cunningham AD, Morrison CE et al (2001) Left ventricular dysfunction, natriuretic peptides, and mortality in urban population. Heart 2001 86:21–26
10. Wallen T, Landahl S, Hedner T et al (1997) Brain natriuretic peptide predicts mortality in the elderly. Heart 77:264–267
11. Wang TJ, Larson MG, Levy D et al (2004) Plasma natriuretic peptide levels and the risk of cardiovascular events and death. N Engl J Med 350:655–663

12. La Rovere M, Bigger J Jr, Marcus F et al (1998). Baroreflex sensitivity and heart-rate variability in prediction of total cardiac mortality after myocardial infarction. ATRAMI (Autonomic Tone and Reflexes After Myocardial Infarction) Investigators. Lancet 351:478–484
13. El Sherif N, Denes P, Katz R et al (1995) Definition of the best prediction criteria of the time domain signal-averaged electrocardiogram for serious arrhythmic events in the postinfarction period. The Cardiac Arrhythmia Suppression Trial/Signal-Averaged Electrocardiogram (CAST/SAECG) Substudy Investigators. J Am Coll Cardiol 25:908–914
14. Ikeda T, Saito H, Tanno K et al (2002) T-wave alternans as a predictor for sudden cardiac death after myocardial infarction. Am J Cardiol 89:79–82
15. The Multicenter Post-Infarction Research Group (1983) Risk stratification and survival after myocardial infarction. N Engl J Med 309:331–336
16. Bigger JJr, Fleiss J, Kleiger R et al (1984) The relationships among ventricular arrhythmias, left ventricular dysfunction, and mortality in the 2 years after myocardial infarction. Circulation 69:250–258
17. Huikuri HV, Castellanos A, Myerburg RJ (2001) Sudden death due to cardiac arrhythmias. N Engl J Med 345:1473–1482
18. Berger R, Huelsman M, Strecker K et al (2002) B-type natriuretic peptide predicts sudden death in patients with chronic heart failure. Circulation 105:2392–2397
19. Tapanainen JM, Still AM, Airaksinen KEJ et al (2001) Prognostic significance of risk stratifiers of mortality, including T wave alternans, after acute myocardial infarction: results of a prospective follow-up study. J Cardiovasc Electrophysiol 12:645–652
20. Huikuri HV, Tapanainen JM, Lindgren K et al (2003) Prediction of sudden cardiac death after myocardial infarction in the beta-blocking era. J Am Coll Cardiol 42:652–658
21. Ikeda T, Sakata T, Takami M et al (2000) Combined assessment of T-wave alternans and late potentials used to predict arrhythmic events after myocardial infarction. A prospective study. J Am Coll Cardiol 35:722–730
22. Yasue H, Yoshimura M, Sumida H et al (1994) Localization and mechanism of secretion of B type natriuretic peptide in comparison with those of A-type natriuretic peptide in normal. Circulation 90:195–203
23. Luchner A, Stevens TL, Borgeson DD et al (1998) Differential atrial and ventricular expression of myocardial BNP during evolution of heart failure. Am J Physiol 274:H1684-H1689
24. Chen HH, Burnett JC (2000) Natriuretic peptides in the pathophysiology of congestive heart failure. Curr Cardiol Rep 2:198–205
25. Hansen DE, Craig CS, Hondeghem LM (1990) Stretch-induced arrhythmias in the isolated canine ventricle. Evidence for the importance of mechanoelectrical feedback. Circulation 81:1094–1095
26. Kowey PR, Friechling TD, Sewter J et al (1991) Electrophysiological effects of left ventricular hypertrophy. Effect of calcium and potassium channel blockade. Circulation 83:2067–2075
27. Reiter MJ, Synhorst DP, Mann DE (1988) Electrophysiological effects of acute ventricular dilatation in the isolated rabbit heart. Circ Res 62:554–562
28. Zabel M, Koller BS, Sachs F (1996) Stretch-induced voltage changes in the isolated beating heart: importance of the timing of stretch and implications for stretch-activated ion channels. Cardiovasc Res 32:120–130

Non-Esterified Fatty Acids as Markers of Sudden Death

R.F. Pedretti, M. Ambrosetti, A. Laporta, S. Masnaghetti, R. Raimondo, M. Salerno, F. Santoro, R. Vaninetti, S. Sarzi Braga

Introduction

Epidemiological studies on the low mortality rate of Greenland Inuits from ischaemic heart disease led to the suggestion that despite the high total fat intake of Eskimos, this low mortality rate was due to the abundance of *n*-3 polyunsaturated fatty acids (PUFA) from seafood in their diet [1–6]. The *n*-6 class of PUFA is derived largely from vegetable oils while the *n*-3 class is derived primarily from fish oils in today's diet. Both classes are necessary for health and must be obtained from our diets. Linoleic acid (C18:2*n*-6), the parent PUFA of the *n*-6 class, is adequately present in the usual diet of today and can be elongated and desaturated in our bodies. In the chloroplasts of green leaves, algae, and phytoplankton, linoleic acid can be desaturated to create α-linolenic acid (C18:3*n*-3), the parent of the *n*-3 class of PUFA. It is largely through ingestion of marine phytoplankton that the *n*-3 fatty acids enter the food chain and become abundant in marine foods. A few vegetable oils, notably canola oil and linseed oil, contain α-linolenic acid, which our bodies can also elongate and desaturate to form eicosapentaenoic acid (EPA) (C20:5*n*-3) and docosahexaenoic acid (DHA) (C22:6*n*-3), using and competing in the process with the *n*-6 fatty acids for the same enzymes. The above hypothesis-initiated research by many investigators into possible anti-atherogenic effects of *n*-3 PUFA. Much has been learned regarding physiological and biochemical changes induced by this class of essential fatty acids that could have potential anti-atherogenic effects; nevertheless, controversy persists in the current literature regarding the clinical evidence for beneficial effects from fish ingestion (the major dietary source of *n*-3 fatty acids) on

Division of Cardiology, IRCCS Fondazione Salvatore Maugeri, Scientific Institute of Tradate, Tradate (Varese), Italy

the development of coronary artery disease.

The possibility that *n*-3 PUFA (including α-linolenic acid) may reduce the risk of sudden cardiac death is based on evidence from some prospective and case–control studies [7–13]. Suggested mechanisms to explain these findings do not centre on lipid or blood pressure lowering or on anti-thrombotic effects, but on a specific stabilising effect of *n*-3 PUFA on the myocardium itself.

Anti-arrhythmic Effect of n-3 PUFA: Evidence from Studies in Animals

Animal experiments found that *n*-3 PUFA may have a significant and strong anti-arrhythmic effect. Initial studies by McLennan et al. showed that a 12-month diet including *n*-3 PUFA prevented ventricular fibrillation in rats during coronary occlusion and during reperfusion of ischaemic myocardium [14]. Investigators showed also that a diet based on *n*-6 PUFA had a relative protective effect, while a diet with saturated fatty acids increased the incidence of the arrhythmias. Further studies showed that the anti-arrhythmic effect of *n*-3 PUFA was greater in older animals (more susceptible to sudden death) and was present not only when the diet was long-term but also when it was short-term. Moreover, after a diet based on *n*-3 and *n*-6 PUFA, the ventricular fibrillation threshold in a monkey animal model was higher than after a standard diet or one rich in saturated fatty acids [15]. Furthermore, the use of *n*-3 PUFA was associated with lower inducibility of ventricular fibrillation by programmed stimulation in this animal model during acute myocardial ischaemia [16]. Finally, an intravenous infusion of *n*-3 PUFA in conscious exercising dogs with a prior anterior myocardial infarction, just before occlusion of the left circumflex coronary artery, slowed heart rate and prevented life-threatening ventricular arrhythmias that invariably occurred in these susceptible animals [17, 18].

Anti-arrhythmic Effect of n-3 PUFA: Possible Mechanisms

The mechanisms of anti-arrhythmic effects of *n*-3 PUFA are as yet undefined, but many hypotheses have been advanced. Changes in the phospholipid composition of cell membrane induced by n-3 PUFA may be one mechanism. Cell membrane function is closely related to its phospholipid composition, and supplementation with *n*-3 PUFA results in an increase of EPA and DHA and a complementary reduction of arachidonic acid levels [19, 20–22]. These changes in the phospholipid composition of the membrane cell can modify the fluidity of the membrane itself, which is a main determinant of enzyme and receptor function [19].

A second possible effect of *n*-3 PUFA may be related to possible competition with arachidonic acid for the metabolic synthesis of eicosanoids [23–25]. High levels of EPA may induce a reduction of the production of TXA_2, which has potential pro-arrhythmic as well as vasoconstrictor and pro-thrombotic effects, and an increase of the PGI_2/TXA_2 ratio, which may contribute to the anti-arrhythmic effect of *n*-3 PUFA [26–31].

Some interesting experimental findings also suggest that only the free fatty acid form of PUFA exerts the anti-arrhythmic effect. It is possible that free fatty acids that originate from the *n*-3 PUFA that are incorporated into the membranes of the myocytes become available during acute myocardial ischaemia in order to exert anti-arrhythmic activity [32, 33].

Finally, concerning the capability of *n*-3 PUFA to modulate the ionic channels of the myocyte membranes, experimental findings support an inhibitory effect of *n*-3 PUFA on the sodium and calcium currents as well as on the function of enzymatic systems, as a consequence of the changes in the membrane fluidity [34–39]. In addition, a possible effect of *n*-3 PUFA on receptors may contribute to the suppression and prevention of malignant arrhythmias [40, 41].

The Omega-3 Index: A New Risk Factor for Death from Coronary Artery Disease?

Recent evidence from GISSI Prevenzione Trial suggests that supplementation with 850 mg/day of *n*-3 PUFA (that is EPA and DHA) can reduce the risk of coronary heart disease (CHD) by 25% and sudden cardiac death by about 45% in survivors of myocardial infarction [9]. The American Heart Association now recommends about 1.0 g/day EPA + DHA to reduce risk of death from coronary artery disease in the secondary prevention setting [42]. In addition, for individuals without known disease (primary prevention), the American Heart Association recommends the consumption of at least two, preferably oily, fish meals per week [42]. This amount of fish would provide about 500 mg EPA + DHA per day.

Since red blood cell (RBC) membranes reflect cardiac membrane *n*-3 PUFA content, Harris and von Schacky proposed that the content of EPA + DHA in RBC membranes (expressed as a percentage of total fatty acids) may be considered as a new risk factor for death from coronary artery disease, especially sudden cardiac death [43]. This marker has been called the 'Omega-3 Index'. Harris and von Schacky conducted a randomised, prospective, double-blind trial to determine the effects of relatively small intakes of *n*-3 PUFA on the Omega-3 Index [43]. Subjects were randomised to receive 0 (placebo), 0.5, 1.0, and 2.0 g EPA + DHA per day for 5 months following a 1-month placebo run-in period. Subjects were instructed to completely avoid consumption of oily fish for the duration of the study but otherwise to make no changes in their diets. There were no differences among the four treatment groups at baseline. For the placebo group ($n = 22$), levels decreased slightly but significantly ($P < 0.001$). The index rose from 4.7% ± 0.9% to 7.9% ± 1.7% in the 0.5 g/day group ($n = 22$; $P < 0.001$) to 9.9% ± 2.9% with 1 g/day ($n = 9$; $P < 0.001$) and to 11.6% ± 2.4% with 2 g/day ($n = 4$; $P = 0.02$). To link the Omega-3 Index with risk estimated in several published studies, the authors compared plasma phospholipid EPA + DHA and whole blood long-chain omega-3 fatty acids [EPA + DHA plus docosapentanoic acid (DPA)] to the Omega-3 Index in a random set of 65 (phospholipids study) and 38 (whole blood study) fasting blood samples. Correlation coefficients between the Omega-3 Index and whole blood omega-3 fatty acids and plasma phospholipids EPA + DHA were both greater than 0.9.

Concerning the relationship between the Omega-3 Index and risk for coronary artery death, in 3 United States studies the Omega-3 Index (or biomarkers convertible into it) was related to risk. Siscovick et al. obtained blood from 80 adults experiencing primary cardiac arrest in the Seattle area and from 108 healthy matched controls [10]. The patients did not have known CHD at the time of their events. The Omega-3 Index was determined from these samples and related to risk for primary cardiac arrest. The multivariate-adjusted odds ratios for primary cardiac arrest in the highest Omega-3 Index quartile were about 10% of that in the lowest quartile (95% confidence interval, 0.1 to 0.4). The mean Omega-3 Index in the highest quartile was 6.5% with a range of 5.5% to 10.9%. Levels in the lowest quartile (highest risk) averaged 3.3% with a range of 2.0% to 4.0%. Albert et al. utilised data from the Physicians' Health Study (PHS) [11]. In this study, 14 916 healthy male physicians were screened for a wide variety of risk factors and provided baseline blood samples between 1982 and 1984. Over the next 17 years, 94 men experienced sudden cardiac death. Whole blood long-chain omega-3 fatty acids (i.e. percentage of total fatty acids as EPA + DHA + DPA) in these cases was compared to that of 184 age and smoking status-matched controls. As in the Seattle study, risk of sudden cardiac death was reduced by about 90% in those subjects with the highest blood EPA + DHA levels compared with those with the lowest levels. To help define the target Omega-3 Index, the whole blood values from the PHS were converted into this parameter using the following equation: Omega-3 Index (%) = Plasma (%) EPA + DHA x 0.97 + 3.43

Transformation of the data revealed that the average Omega-3 Index for the highest quartile was 6.9% with a range of 6.1% to 10.1%. Levels in the lowest quartile were about 3.8% with a range of 2.4% to 4.5%. The third study to examine the relationship between a blood measure of omega-3 fatty acids and risk of CHD death was reported by Lemaitre et al. utilising data from the Cardiovascular Health Study [44]. These investigators found a strong, protective relationship between (in this case) serum phospholipid EPA + DHA and risk for fatal ischaemic heart disease.

The only *n*-3 PUFA intervention trial that followed clinically meaningful coronary artery disease endpoints in which the Omega-3 Index was assessed was SCIMO [45]. This was a randomised, placebo-controlled, prospective trial in which quantitative coronary angiography was utilised to follow the effects of EPA + DHA supplementation on plaque progression and regression in 223 coronary heart disease patients over 2 years. In this trial *n*-3 PUFA supplementation (3 g EPA + DHA/day for 3 months followed by 1.5 g/day for 18 months) resulted in a slower rate of disease progression ($P = 0.04$) and a trend toward cardiovascular events (6.25% vs 1.8%, $P = 0.1$). The Omega-3 Index increased from a baseline value of 3.4% to 8.3% ($P < 0.05$) after 2 years on trial.

Harris and von Schacky also analysed the meaning of the Omega-3 Index estimated from EPA + DHA in secondary prevention trials [43]. The first study was the Diet and Reinfarction Trial (DART) [7]. In this study, 2033 men were randomised to either receive or not receive advice to increase their oily fish intake to about 300 g/week. After 2 years of follow-up, those receiving the fish advice experienced a 29% reduction in all-cause mortality and a 32% decrease in ischaemic heart disease mortality compared to controls. The authors estimated an intake of 2.5 g of EPA per week (357 mg/day). Assuming that EPA contributes about 40% of the total EPA + DHA in oily fish, the intake in this study was about 900 mg/day. The Gruppo Italiano per lo Studio della Sopravvivenza nell'Infarto miocardico Prevenzione study tested the effects of EPA + DHA supplementation on death from CHD [9]. Patients ($n = 11\ 324$) receiving modern cardiac pharmacotherapy were randomised to receive 850 mg/day of EPA + DHA, 300 mg/day of vitamin E, both, or neither (the unsupplemented control group). After 3.5 years of follow-up, the group given just the EPA + DHA ($n = 2836$) experienced a 20% reduction in all-cause mortality, a 35% decrease in cardiac death, and a 45% reduction in sudden death (all $P < 0.01$) compared to the control group ($n = 2828$). These effects became statistically significant within 3–4 months of randomisation. Thus, similar intakes of EPA + DHA in the DART and the GISSI-P study resulted in similar protection. The results of the dose-ranging study performed by Harris and von Schacky would suggest that intakes of about 900 mg/day of EPA + DHA would produce an Omega-3 Index of about 9.5% [43]. Based upon their data as presented above, the authors were able to make an informed estimate of the Omega-3 Indexes associated with low and high risk for death from CHD. They found that the average Omega-3 Index associated with the lowest risk for death from CHD was about 8%, whereas the index associated with the highest risk was lower than 4%.

In their discussion, the authors emphasised that there are several requirements that a potential risk factor or marker must meet to be clinically useful. The Omega-3 Index fulfils many of these. The epidemiological data, both between and within populations, as well as from prospective studies, are quite consistent. A relationship between membrane EPA + DHA levels and risk of sudden cardiac death is biologically plausible. Currently, the most likely mechanism by which they appear to operate is via a reduction in myocardial susceptibility to lethal arrhythmias. In addition, EPA + DHA may enhance plaque stability, and may be anti-atherosclerotic via a variety of other mechanisms.

The most important question to be asked of a putative risk factor is whether changing the risk factor alters disease outcomes. The intervention trials described above suggest that EPA + DHA fulfil this critical criterion as well. Moreover, modifiable risk factors (cholesterol, blood pressure, smoking, etc.) have a practical value that unmodifiable ones (age, gender, family history) lack. The Omega-3 Index can be quickly and easily increased simply by consuming more long-chain omega-3 fatty acids. The rationale for measuring the Omega-3 Index consists in the fact that it is difficult to know exactly how much EPA + DHA one is actually consuming from fish. The EPA + DHA content of a serving of any given fish is unknown. EPA + DHA content by species present average levels that can vary markedly depending on season, maturity, the fish's diet, post-catch processing, and cooking methods. Even if the omega-3 intake were known, each person is metabolically unique, with idiosyncrasies in digestion, absorption, tissue distribution, and cellular metabolism. Individual variations in the in vivo conversion of α-linolenic acid (the plant-derived omega-3 fatty acid) into EPA and DHA as well as other dietary variables (e.g. kilocalories, omega-6 fatty acids) can also influence tissue EPA + DHA levels. These factors conspire together to produce different levels in people who all consume the same amount of EPA + DHA. Consequently, knowledge of baseline levels will guide the physician's recommendations; not surprisingly, low baseline values may require a larger dose than a high baseline value. Therefore, the Omega-3 Index may be useful for assessing both baseline risk and a change in risk as a function of intake.

Conclusions

Low levels of EPA and DHA are independently associated with increased risk of death from coronary heart disease, especially with sudden cardiac death. In randomised secondary prevention trials, fish or fish oil have been demonstrated to reduce total and CHD mortality. RBC fatty acid composition reflects long-term intake of EPA and DHA. RBC EPA and DHA levels may be considered a new risk factor for death from CHD. This potential new risk factor, the Omega-3 Index, seems to be inversely associated with risk for CHD mortality. An Omega-3 Index of 8% or greater was associated with the greatest cardioprotection, whereas an index of 4% or less was associated with the least. Thus, the Omega-3 Index may represent a novel, physiologically relevant, easily modified, independent, and graded risk factor for death from CHD that could have significant clinical utility.

References

1. Bang HO, Dyerberg J, Nielsen AB (1971) Plasma lipid and lipoprotein pattern in Greenlandic West-coast Eskimos. Lancet 1:1143–1145
2. Bang HO, Dyerberg J (1980) The bleeding tendency in Greenland Eskimos. Dan Med Bull 27:202–205
3. Bang HO, Dyerberg J, Sinclair HM (1980) The composition of the Eskimo food in north western Greenland. Am J Clin Nutr 33:2657–2661
4. Dyerberg J, Bang HO, Stofferesen E et al (1978) Eicosapentaenoic acod and prevention of thrombosis and atherosclerosis? Lancet 2:117–119
5. Dyerberg J, Bang HO, Hjorne N (1975) Fatty acid composition of the plasma lipids in Greenland Eskimos. Am J Clin Nutr 28:958–966
6. Dyerberg J, Bang HO (1979) Hemostatic function and platelet polyunsaturated fatty acids in Eskimos. Lancet 2:433–435
7. Burr ML, Fehily AM, Rogers S et al (1989) Diet and reinfarction trial (DART): design, recruitment, and compliance. Eur Heart J 10:558–567
8. Singh RB, Niaz MA, Sharma JP et al (1997) Randomized, double-blind, placebo-controlled trial of fish oil and mustard oil in patients with suspected acute myocardial infarction: the Indian experiment of infarct survival – 4. Cardiovasc Drug Ther 11:485–491
9. Anonymous (1999) Dietary supplementation with n-3 polyunsaturated fatty acids and vitamin E after myocardial infarction: results of the GISSI-Prevenzione trial. Gruppo Italiano per lo Studio della Sopravvivenza nell'Infarto miocardico. Lancet 354:447–455
10. Siscovick DS, Raghunathan TE, King I et al (1995) Dietary intake and cell membrane levels of long-chain n-3 polyunsaturated fatty acids and the risk of primary cardiac arrest. JAMA 274:1363–1367
11. Albert CM, Hennekens CH, O'Donnell CJ et al (1998) Fish consumption and risk of sudden cardiac death. JAMA 279:23–28
12. Hu FB, Stampfer MJ, Manson JE et al (1999) Dietary intake of alpha-linolenic acid and risk of fatal ischemic heart disease among women. Am J Clin Nutr 69:890–897
13. Rissaben T, Voutilainen S, Syyssonen K et al (2000) Fish oil-derived fatty acids, docosahexaenoic acid and docosapentaenoic acid, and the risk of acute coronary events: the Kuopio Ischaemic Heart Disease Risk Factor Study. Circulation 102:2677–2679
14. McLennan PL, Abeywardena MY, Charnock JS (1988) Dietary fish oil prevents ventricular fibrillation following coronary artery occlusion and reperfusion. Am Heart J 116:709–717
15. McLennan PL, Abeywardena MY, Charnock JS (1989) The influence of age and die-

tary fat in an animal model of sudden cardiac death. Aust N Z J Med 19:1–5
16. McLennan PL, Bridle TM, Abeywardena MY et al (1992) Dietary lipid modulation of ventricular fibrillation threshold in the marmoset monkey. Am Heart J 123:1555–1561
17. Billman GE, Hallaq H, Leaf A (1994) Prevention of ischemia-induced ventricular fibrillation by omega 3 fatty acids. Proc Natl Acd Sci USA 91:4427–4430
18. Billman GE, Kang JX, Leaf A (1997) Prevention of ischemia-induced cardiac sudden death by n-3 polyunsaturated fatty acids in dogs. Lipids 32:1161–1168
19. Charnock JS (1994) Lipids and cardiac arrhythmia. Prog Lipid Res 33:355–385
20. Spector AA, Mathur SN, Kaduce TL et al (1980) Lipid nutrition and metabolism of cultured mammalian cells. Prog Lipid Res 19:155–186
21. Spector AA Yorek MA (1985) Membrane lipid composition and cellular function. J Lipid Res 26:1015–1035
22. Spector AA (1999) Essentiality of fatty acids. Lipids 34(suppl):S1-S3
23. Moncada S, Needleman P, Bunting S et al (1976) Prostaglandin endoperoxide and thromboxane generating systems and their selective inhibition. Prostaglandins 12:323–335
24. Moncada S, Gryglewski R, Bunting S et al (1976) An enxyme isolated from arteries transforms prostaglandin endoperoxides to an unstable substance that inhibits platelet aggregation. Nature 263:663–665
25. Hamberg M, Samuelsson B (1974) Prostaglandin endoperoxides. Novel trasnsformations of arachidonic acid in human platelets. Proc Natl Acad Sci USA 71:3400–3404
26. Knapp HR, Reilly IA, Alessandrini P et al (1986) In vivo indexes of platelet and vascular function during fish-oil administration in patients with atherosclerosis. N Engl J Med 314:937–942
27. Knapp HR, Salern N Jr (1989) Formation of PGI3 in the rat during dietary fish oil supplementation. Prostaglandins 38:509–521
28. Knapp HR (1989) Omega-3 fatty acids, endogenous prostaglandins, and blood pressure regulation in humans. Nutr Rev 47:301–313
29. Fischer S, Weber PC (1984) Prostaglandin I3 is formed in vivo in man after dietary eicosapentaenoic acid. Nature 307:165–168
30. Kelley DS, Rudolph IL (2000) Effect of individual fatty acids of omega-6 and omega-3 type on human immune status and role of eicosanoids. Nutrition 16:143–145
31. James MJ, Gibson RA, Cleland LG (2000) Dietary polyunsaturated fatty acids and inflammatory mediator production. Am J Clin Nutr 71:343S-348S
32. Nair SS, Leitch JW, Falconer J et al (1997) Prevention of cardiac arrhythmia by dietary (n-3) polyunsaturated fatty acids and their mechanism of action. J Nutr 127:383–393
33. Nair SS, Leitch JW, Garg ML (1999) Specific modifications of phosphatidylinositol and nonesterified fatty acid fractions in cultured porcine cardiomyocytes supplemented with n-3 polyunsaturated fatty acids. Lipids 34:697–704
34. Kang JX, Leaf A (1996) Evidence that free polyunsaturated fatty acids modify Na+ channels by directly binding to the channel proteins. Proc Natl Acad Sci USA 93:3542–3546
35. Hallaq H, Smith TW, Leaf A (1992) Modulation of dihydropyridine-sensitive calcium channels in heart cells by fish oil fatty acids. Proc Natl Acad Sci USA 89:1760–1764
36. Xiao YF, Kang JX, Morgan JP et al (1995) Blocking effects of polyunsaturated fatty

acids on Na+ channels of neonatal rat ventricular myocytes. Proc Natl Acad Sci USA 92:1100–1104

37. Garrat JC, McEnvoy MP, Owen DG (1996) Blockade of two voltage-dependent potassium channels, mKv1.1 and mKv1.2, by docosahexaenoic acid. Eur J Pharmacol 314:393–396
38. Xiao YF, Gomez AM, Morgan JP et al (1997) Suppression of voltage-gated L-type Ca_2^+ currents by polyunsaturated fatty cids in adult and neonatal rat ventricular myocytes. Proc Natl Acad Sci USA 94:4182–4187
39. Negretti N, Perez MR, Walker D et al (2000) Inhibition of sarcoplasmatic reticulum function by polyunsaturated fatty acids in intact, isolated myocytes from rat ventricular muscle. J Physiol 523(Pt 2):376–375
40. Skuladottir GV, Johannson M (1997) Inotropic response of rat heart papillary muscle to alpha 1-and beta-adrenoreceptor stimulation in relation to dietary n-6 and n-3 polyunsaturated fatty acids (PUFA) and age. Pharmacol Toxicol 80:85–90
41. de Jonge HW, Dekkers DH, Bastiaanse EM et al (1996) Eicosapentaenoic acid incorporation in membrane phospholipids modulates receptor-mediated phospholipase C and membrane fluidity in rat ventricular myocytes in culture. J Mol Cell Cardiol 28:1097–1108
42. Kris-Etherton PM, Harris WS, Appel LJ (2002) Fish consumption, fish oil, omega-3 fatty acids, and cardiovascular disease. Circulation 106:2747–2757
43. Harris WS, von Shacky C (2004) The Omega-3 Index: a new risk factor from death for coronary artery disease? Prev Med 39:212–220
44. Lemaitre RN, King IB, Mozaffarian D et al (2002) n-3 Polyunsaturated fatty acids, fatal ischemic heart disease and non-fatal myocardial infarction in older adults. The Cardiovascular Health study. Am J Clin Nutr 76:319–25
45. von Schacky C, Angerer P, Kothny W et al (1999) The effect of dietary n-3 fatty acids on coronary atherosclerosis. A randomized, double-blind, placebo-controlled trial. Ann Intern Med 130:554–562

Value of Angiotensin-Converting Enzyme Inhibitors to Prevent Sudden Death

G. Fabbri, A.P. Maggioni

The renin–angiotensin system plays a major role in the pathogenesis and progression of atherosclerosis, and the value of angiotensin-converting enzyme inhibitors (ACE-I) in reducing mortality rates and major cardiovascular events in patients with chronic heart failure, asymptomatic left ventricular systolic dysfunction, and in those with acute myocardial infarction (MI) has been established by multiple randomised clinical trials [1–3]. The clinical indications for ACE-I have also been clearly defined in patients at high risk of cardiovascular events or diabetes [4].

The systematic overview of trials of early ACE-I therapy in acute MI shows that the benefit in terms of mortality reduction is generally consistent among patients with different baseline characteristics and underlying risk. In addition, most of the benefit from this treatment occurs during the first few days, when mortality is high [5]. The reduction in mortality at 30 days was small but highly significant – 7% (SD 2–11%, $P < 0.004$), corresponding to the avoidance of an average of five deaths per 1000 patients treated for 1 month.

ACE-I have been shown to improve prognosis not only when started early after MI but also when administered some time after MI. A significant reduction in total mortality was found in nearly 6000 patients with signs or symptoms of heart failure or left ventricular systolic dysfunction randomised to receive ACE-I starting 3–16 days after the MI [6–8]. In the Survival and Ventricular Enlargement (SAVE) study, patients were randomised (captopril/placebo) after infarction and showed a 19% reduction in mortality in

ANMCO Research Center, Florence, Italy

the captopril group with an average follow-up of 42 months. Mortality reduction was 22% in the Trandolapril Cardiac Evaluation (TRACE) study and 27% in the Acute Infarction Ramipril Efficacy (AIRE) trial [2]. Further, the SAVE and other studies have demonstrated a significant reduction in the risk of re-infarction in patients treated with ACE-I, from 13.2% to 10.8%.

The reduction in total mortality is, in these trials, mostly due to a reduction in death due to cardiovascular causes. A substantial proportion of cardiovascular mortality is constituted by sudden death, but it would be difficult to achieve sufficient power in a single trial testing the effect of ACE-I on this mode of death, so none has ever been carried out. In the TRACE trial [7], trandolapril treatment was associated with a significant 24% reduction in sudden death (RR 0.76; 95% CI 0.59 to 0.98); in the Vasodilator–Heart Failure Trial II (V-HeFT II), comparing enalapril with hydralazine-isosorbide dinitrate combination therapy in patients with symptomatic heart failure, sudden deaths were significantly reduced by 42% with ACE-I [9], while in the Studies of Left Ventricular Dysfunction Treatment (SOLVD-T) study the reduction in deaths classified as being due to arrhythmia was insignificant (RR 0.90, 95% CI 0.83 to 1.31) [10]. The overview of the trials of ACE-I involving patients with congestive heart failure showed a nonsignificant trend toward a reduction in sudden death (OR 0.91, 95% CI 0.73 to 1.12), with therapy reducing mainly deaths due to progressive heart failure [1].

A meta-analysis of randomised clinical trials of ACE-I in patients with MI and heart failure or left ventricular systolic dysfunction, with treatment starting within 14 days of the index event and at least 6 weeks' follow-up, showed a significant reduction in cardiovascular mortality and sudden death [11]. Fifteen trials were included in the meta-analysis, with a total of 15 104 patients; the results showed a reduction in total mortality from 16.8% to 14.4% (OR 0.83, 95% CI 0.71 to 0.97), cardiovascular death was reduced from 14.7% to 12.5% (OR 0.82, 95% CI 0.69 to 0.97).

Sudden cardiac death was classified in 96% of the cases by an endpoints committee and in the remaining cases was defined as 'sudden unexpected collapse without documentation of arrhythmia or collapse due to intractable ventricular tachycardia/fibrillation' by the authors of the paper. Among cardiovascular deaths, sudden death accounted for 36.8% in ACE-I-treated patients and in 39.8% in untreated patients; the reduction was significant (OR 0.80, 95% CI 0.70 to 0.92). Two large post-MI trials were not included in the analysis: GISSI-3 and ISIS-4, the first because it was not placebo-controlled and lisinopril was prescribed for only 42 days, and the second on the grounds of the duration of the trial (35 days) and because mode of death was not recorded [12, 13]. However, in the GISSI-3 study, ACE-I had a significant protective effect on sudden death (OR 0.81, 95% CI 0.72 to 0.89), and in the ISIS-4 there was a similar impact on total mortality.

More recent studies have shown the benefit of ACE-I in reducing cardiovascular events in high-risk individuals without heart failure or left ventricular dysfunction [4, 14]. In a report from the Heart Outcomes Prevention Evaluation (HOPE) study, unexpected death (defined as death occurring within 24 h of the onset of symptoms without clinical or post-mortem evidence of other identifiable causes), documented arrhythmic death, and non-fatal cardiac arrest were combined in a composite end point to examine the effect of ramipril on sudden death in these high-risk patients. An Events Adjudication Committee reviewed all main outcomes of the study [15]; the common definition of sudden death as death within 1 h from the onset of symptoms was not used because many of the deaths were not witnessed. After more than 4 years of follow-up, the composite end point was significantly reduced by 21% in the patients randomised to receive ramipril (RR 0.79, 95% CI 0.64 to 0.98). Recently, the EUROPA trial reported a reduction with perindopril, although not significant, in the risk of cardiac arrest (RR 0.54, 95% CI 0.20 to 1.47) in patients with a risk profile similar to that of participants in HOPE. Table 1 summarises the reduction in sudden death in the above-mentioned trials. The mechanisms by which the ACE-I reduce sudden death are not fully delineated. These drugs, in addition to their effect on blood pressure, have several cardioprotective effects: modulation of neurohormonal activation with reduction of circulating norepinephrine and angiotensin II [16], restoration of balance between myocardial oxygen supply and prevention of recurrent MI [4, 6, 10], attenuation, and reversal of the remodelling process that may lead to a reduction in life-threatening arrhythmias [17]. Other mechanisms such as the reduction in potassium depletion or the increase in prostacyclin synthesis may be involved in these effects of ACE-I on the incidence of sudden death. The fact that, in the HOPE study, the divergence of curves occurs after 2 years of treatment tends to support the idea that the effect of ramipril is mainly due to preventing remodelling and to reducing myocardial ischaemia.

In conclusion, data from high-risk patients and from patients with MI indicates that ACE-I are associated with a significant reduction in sudden death. There are two limitations to the reports: first, the definition and ascertainment of sudden death are not uniform among the trials, and, second, the publication bias, common to all meta-analyses. However, because sudden cardiac death was not the primary end point of the studies, the fact that a study was negative with respect to sudden death is less likely to have influenced the possibility of publication.

Table 1. Reduction in sudden death with ACE-I in heart failure, myocardial infarction, and high-risk patients

Trial	No. of patients	Patients' characteristics	Treatment	OR/RR	95% CI
TRACE	1749	WMI < 2, EF < 35%	Trandolapril	0.76	0.59–0.98
SOLVD-T	2569	NYHA II–III, EF ≤ 35%	Enalapril	0.90	0.73–1.13
Overview HF patients	7105	-	-	0.91	0.73–1.12
Overview MI patients	15 104	-	-	0.80	0.70–0.92
GISSI 3	19 394	MI (< 6 weeks)	Lisinopril	0.81	0.72–0.89
HOPE	9297	High risk without LV systolic dysfunction	Ramipril	0.79	0.64–0.98
EUROPA	12 218	Stable coronary artery disease	Perindopril	0.54	0.20–1.47

HF heart failure, *MI* myocardial infarction, *WMI* wall motion index, *EF* ejection fraction, *NYHA* New York Heart Association class, *LV* left ventricular

References

1. Garg R, Yusuf S (1995) Overview of randomized trials of angiotensin-converting enzyme inhibitors on mortality and morbidity in patients with heart failure. Collaborative Group on ACE Inhibitor Trials. JAMA 273:1450–1456
2. Flather MD, Yusuf S, Kober L et al (2000) Long term ACE-inhibitor therapy in patients with heart failure or left ventricular dysfunction: a systematic overview of data from individual patients. ACE-Inhibitor Myocardial Infarction Collaborative Group. Lancet 355:1575–1581
3. Latini R, Tognoni G, Maggioni AP et al (2000) Clinical effects of early angiotensin converting enzyme inhibitor treatment for acute myocardial infarction are similar in the presence and absence of aspirin: systematic overview of individual data from 96 712 randomized patients. Angiotensin Converting Enzyme Inhibitor Myocardial Infarction Collaborative Group. J Am Coll Cardiol 35:1801–1807
4. The Heart Outcomes Prevention Evaluation Study Investigators (HOPE) (2000) Effects of angiotensin converting enzyme inhibitor, ramipril, on cardiovascular events in high risk patients. N Engl J Med 342:145–153
5. Anonymous (1998) Indications for ACE inhibitors in the early treatment of acute myocardial infarction: systematic overview of individual data from 100 000 patients in randomized trials. ACE Inhibitor Myocardial Infarction Collaborative Group. Circulation 97:2202–2212

6. Pfeffer MA, Braunwald E, Moye LA et al on behalf of the SAVE investigators (1992) Effect of captopril on mortality and morbidity in patients with left ventricular dysfunction after myocardial infarction: results of the Survival and Ventricular Enlargement Trial. N Engl J Med 327:669–677
7. Torp-Pedersen C, Kober L for the TRACE Study Group (1999) Effect of the ACE inhibitor trandolapril on life expectancy of patients with reduced left ventricular function after acute myocardial infarction. Lancet 354:9–12
8. The Acute Infarction Ramipril Efficacy (AIRE) Study Investigators (1993) Effect of ramipril on mortality and morbidity of survivors of acute myocardial infarction with clinical evidence of heart failure. Lancet 342:821–828
9. Cohn JN, Johnson G, Ziesche S et al (1991) A comparison of enalapril with hydralazine-isosorbide dinitrate in the treatment of chronic congestive heart failure. N Engl J Med 325:303–310
10. Anonymous (1991) Effect of enalapril on survival in patients with reduced left ventricular ejection fraction and congestive heart failure. The SOLVD Investigators. N Engl J Med 325:293–302
11. Domanski MJ, Exner DV, Craig BB et al (1999) Effect of angiotensin converting enzyme inhibition on sudden cardiac death in patients following acute myocardial infarction. A meta-analysis of randomized clinical trials. J Am Coll Cardiol 33:598–604
12. Anonymous (1994) GISSI-3: effects of lisinopril and transdermal glycerol trinitrate singly and together on 6-week mortality and ventricular function after acute myocardial infarction. Gruppo Italiano per lo Studio della Sopravvivenza nell'Infarto Miocardico. Lancet 343:1115–1122
13. Anonymous (1995) ISIS-4 a randomized factorial trial assessing early oral captopril, oral mononitrate and intravenous magnesium sulphate in 58 050 patients with suspected acute myocardial infarction. ISIS-4 (Fourth International Study of Infarct Survival) Collaborative Group. Lancet 345:669–685
14. Fox KM, EURopean trial On reduction of cardiac events with Perindopril in stable coronary Artery disease Investigators (2003) Efficacy of perindopril in reduction of cardiovascular events among patients with stable coronary artery disease: randomised, double-blind, placebo-controlled, multicentre trial (the EUROPA study). Lancet 362:782–788
15. Teo KK, Mitchell LB, Pogue J et al (2004) Effect of ramipril in reducing sudden deaths and non fatal cardiac arrest in high-risk individuals without heart failure or left ventricular dysfunction. Circulation 110:1413–1417
16. Grassi G, Cattaneo BM, Seravalle G et al (1997) Effects of chronic ACE inhibition on sympathetic nerve traffic and baroreflex control of circulation in heart failure. Circulation 96:1173–1179
17. Pognizd S (1994) Focal mechanisms underlying ventricular tachycardia during prolonged ischemic cardiomyopathy. Circulation 90:1441–1458

Value of Non-antiarrythmic Drugs in Preventing Sudden Cardiac Death: Aldosterone Antagonists

L. Sahiner, A. Oto

Introduction

Sudden cardiac death remains as an important public health problem, even in industrialised countries, despite the considerable improvement in emergency medical services and the introduction of new therapeutic strategies. Sudden cardiac death (SCD) is responsible for 50% of the mortality from cardiovascular disease [1]. In many cases, SCD may be the first manifestation of coronary artery disease. It is the most common cause of death due to ischaemic heart disease among the adult population under 65 years of age, and survival rates after out-of-hospital cardiac arrest remain low. It has been shown in clinical trials that, compared to the administration of antiarrhythmic drugs, implantable cardioverter defibrillators (ICD) significantly reduce mortality due to SCD. This treatment option has added a new dimension to the prevention and management of SCD. Besides antiarrhythmic drugs and ICDs, there are other drugs that have an indirect but nonetheless important role in preventing SCD. Although these medications do not have a direct electrophysiologic action, they prevent SCD by affecting basic neurohumoral, ischaemic, biochemical, and fibrotic mechanisms that may cause ventricular tachyarrhythmias. Aldosterone antagonists are an example of non-antiarrhythmic drugs that have been shown to reduce the incidence of SCD in clinical trials.

Cardiovascular Effects of Aldosterone

Following its discovery in the early 1950s, the endocrine actions of aldosterone have been extensively studied and documented [2–5]. Aldosterone's

Hacettepe University School of Medicine, Department of Cardiology, Ankara, Turkey main endocrine function is the regulation of sodium and potassium, and volume homeostasis. The activity of the hormone is mediated through sodium reabsorption and potassium excretion in the distal renal tubules and collecting ducts. Its release from the adrenal cortex is stimulated by increased levels of serum potassium, angiotensin II, adrenocorticotropic hormone (ACTH), and by sodium depletion [6–8]. Aldosterone regulates extracellular volume and electrolyte balance via mineralocorticoid receptors on renal tubular epithelial cells.

In addition to renal tubular epithelial cells, mineralocorticoid (MR) receptors are present in various non-renal locations [9], mainly, heart [10, 11], brain tissue [12], and the vasculature [13]. This finding suggests that aldosterone has local effects at different tissue levels. In animal studies, aldosterone biosynthesis was also shown in myocardium [11], brain [12] and vascular smooth muscle cells [14]. Aldosterone synthesis at extra-adrenal sites seems to be regulated by the same factors that regulate adrenal synthesis, and many of the negative effects of aldosterone are mediated by MR receptors in these non-renal sites. For example, increased local production of aldosterone and angiotensin converting enzyme (ACE) have been detected in the ventricles of patients with heart failure. It has been shown that aldosterone contributes to cardiovascular toxicity in humans independent of the effects of angiotensin II, and a correlation exists between aldosterone concentration and cardiovascular morbidity and mortality. In the Cooperative North Scandinavian Enalapril Survival Study (CONSENSUS), significantly greater mortality at 6 months was shown in patients who had baseline aldosterone concentration above the median values [15].

In patients with heart failure, overproduction of aldosterone leads to an inappropriate increase in sodium and water retention. This fluid and sodium retention produces a volume overload that further impairs the ability of the heart to pump adequate amount of blood to peripheral tissues. With the reduction of forward blood flow, a generalised systemic vasoconstriction occurs that impairs renal blood flow. Eventually, a vicious circle is formed in which the release of angiotensin II from the kidneys leads to a further rise in aldosterone and volume overload.

Aldosterone increases the risk of ventricular arrhythmias by increasing renal potassium and magnesium excretion [16]. Because of the negative effect of this electrolyte imbalance, aldosterone increases the risk of SCD in patients with heart failure and in post-myocardial-infarction (MI) patients. In patients with congestive heart failure, the kaliuretic and magnesiuretic effects of aldosterone can be reverted by aldosterone receptor antagonists, which may explain the preventive effects of these drugs on SCD. Aldosterone has also been demonstrated to have proarrhythmogenic effects on rabbit cardiomyocytes by increasing sodium influx and Na/K pump activity [17].

An animal study showed that aldosterone exposure increased calcium current in adult rat cardiomyocytes, an effect that was inhibited following aldosterone blockade by spironolactone [18].

It has been shown in various animal models and clinical studies that aldosterone causes cardiovascular injury, independent of its effects on blood pressure – the so-called mechanical effects of aldosterone. Aldosterone causes vascular inflammation and fibrosis in animal models. The mechanisms through which aldosterone causes cardiac and vascular fibrosis have been investigated in many studies. Aldosterone increases vascular angiotensin (AT)1 receptor binding [19]. It also increases AT1 receptor density and mRNA accumulation in rat heart [20]. Thus, aldosterone may, at least in part, exert its adverse effects on cardiac remodelling by potentiating the effects of angiotensin II. Moreover, aldosterone has been shown to have a direct profibrotic action by increasing collagen production by cardiac fibroblasts [21, 22]. It also increases plasminogen activator inhibitor-1 (PAI-1) expression, which promotes fibrosis [23, 24]. In an animal study in normotensive rats, aldosterone infusion for 24 h led to increased cardiomyocyte apoptosis [25]. Since necrotic myocytes serve as stimuli for fibrosis in myocardium [26], increased apoptosis and myocardial necrosis may be another mechanism to explain aldosterone-mediated cardiac fibrosis.

Propeptide of type III collagen (PIIINP) is a serum marker of collagen synthesis. In the Randomised Aldactone Evaluation Study (RALES), serum PIIINP levels were significantly reduced in a group of patients treated with spironolactone [27]. In a study by Modena, 46 post-MI patients were randomised to spironolactone or to placebo. After a 1-year follow-up, serum PIIINP levels were found to be lower in the treatment arm [28]. These data suggest that aldosterone exerts an adverse remodelling effect on myocardium and promotes cardiac fibrosis. Increased myocardial fibrosis may act as a substrate for the genesis of life-threatening ventricular arrhythmias.

Aldosterone has also been shown to have proatherogenic actions and it promotes endothelial dysfunction [29]. Possible mechanisms that may be involved in aldosterone's effect on endothelial function include aldosterone-induced reduction of NO levels and a reduction in the generation of oxygen free radicals [30, 31]. Patients with heart failure who were treated with spironolactone for 1 month had an increased endothelium-dependent forearm blood-flow response to acetylcholine [32]. Aldosterone induces vascular inflammation and fibrinoid necrosis of the small arteries and arterioles, leading to a reperative fibrotic process. An inverse relation between aldosterone and large-artery compliance in late-stage heart failure patients has also been suggested [33]. Together with its hypertensive effects, aldosterone increases the occurrence of ischaemic events by promoting endothelial dysfunction, perivascular fibrosis, and a decrease in arterial compliance. This constitutes a suitable background for the progression of heart failure and the occurrence of arrhythmic SCD.

Experimental studies suggest that aldosterone has autonomic effects, independent of the actions of angiotensin II. Aldosterone blunts the baroreceptor heart-rate response to noradrenaline infusion and increases sympathetic nervous system activity [34]. It modulates parasympathetic tone and results in reduced heart rate variability (HRV) parameters. Reduced HRV is associated with increased mortality and a higher incidence of SCD in heart failure [35]. Aldosterone has also been shown to block extraneuronal noradrenaline uptake [36]. All of these actions of aldosterone can predispose to arrhythmias and SCD.

In a study conducted in rats, aldosterone blockade by canrenone (active metabolite of spironolactone) was found to attenuate left ventricular (LV) remodelling, improve LV systolic and diastolic function, reduce interstitial and perivascular fibrosis, decrease myocardial norepinephrine content, and increase the ventricular fibrillation threshold [37]. A study by Ramires et al. showed that addition of spironolactone to standard therapy in patients with congestive heart failure due to idiopathic or ischaemic dilated cardiomyopathy reduces the frequency of ventricular premature complexes and episodes of non-sustained ventricular tachycardia [38]. Aldosterone blockade has also been shown to reduce vascular collagen turnover, improve HRV, and reduce heart rate, especially in the early morning hours [35]. The latter finding is particularly noteworthy as it suggests that blocking the action of aldosterone reduces the incidence of ischaemia in the early-morning, when sudden death is 2.5 times more common in patients with heart failure. Addition of spirondactone to conventional treatment decreases QT dispersion [39] and has positive effects on HRV [40].

The 'Aldosterone Escape' Phenomenon

Despite the lowering of angiotensin II activity, ACE inhibitors completely block aldosterone production. In fact, a progressive rise in aldosterone levels under ACE inhibitor therapy has been demonstrated in clinical studies. This finding, termed 'aldosterone escape,' may be explained by ATII production independent of ACE activity (so-called angiotensin escape), ACE production that is not inhibited by ACE inhibitors, and ATII-independent aldosterone production. MacFadyen and colleagues reported that in patients with symptomatic heart failure who were on ACE inhibitor therapy aldosterone suppression failed in 38% of cases [41]. In the Randomised Evaluation of Strategies for Left Ventricular Dysfunction (RESOLVD) pilot study, aldosterone levels were significantly lower after 17 weeks in both treatment arms (candesartan and enalapril); however, levels returned almost to baseline in all three groups by the 43rd week [42]. In another study, conducted in a smaller sample of heart failure patients, 11 of 34 patients had elevated serum aldosterone levels in spite of complete ACE inhibition [43]. These data, together with knowledge of the correlation between serum aldosterone levels and mortality in heart failure patients, constitute the rationale for more specific blockade of aldosterone action in addition to ACE inhibition in patients with heart failure.

Sudden Cardiac Death and Aldosterone Receptor Antagonists: What We Have Learned from Recent Trials

Two important landmark studies have shown the clinical benefits of aldosterone receptor antagonists, RALES [44] (Randomised Aldactone Evaluation Study) and EPHESUS (Eplerenone Post-Acute Myocardial Infarction Heart Failure Efficacy and Survival Study) [45].

RALES was a randomised double-blind study that enrolled 1663 patients with severe heart failure, a LV ejection fraction below 35%, and who were being treated with ACE inhibitor, digitalis, and diuretics. Patients were randomly assigned to receive 25 mg spironolactone or placebo to assess the primary end-point of death from all causes. The trial was stopped early, after a mean follow-up of 24 months, because of the significant beneficial effect of spironolactone. There was a 30% reduction in the risk of death among patients in the spironolactone group. Importantly, spironolactone reduced the risk of death from progressive heart failure and SCD. The authors suggested that the preventive effect of spironolactone on SCD was related to decreased potassium loss and increased myocardial uptake of norepinephrine in response to the drug. The potential of spironolactone in preventing myocardial fibrosis was also suggested to have a role in reducing the risk of SCD, as myocardial fibrosis is well-known to predispose patients to reentry ventricular arrhythmias. One of the criticisms of the RALES study was that only 11% of the patients were on beta-blocker therapy. Since some of the beneficial effects of beta-blockers and spironolactone are produced by similar mechanisms, it is unclear whether spironolactone would still have a beneficial effect if the majority of patients were also on beta-blocker therapy. A substudy of RALES, published later, implicated a potential link between the antifibrotic effects of spironolactone and decreased mortality [27]. In this study, serum levels of PIIINP, which is a marker of collagen turnover, were significantly reduced by spironolactone and this predicted decreased mortality.

Eplerenone is a new, competitive antagonist of aldosterone that has a higher degree of selectivity for the mineralocorticoid receptor. EPHESUS was conducted as a double-blind, placebo-controlled study to evaluate the effect of eplerenone on mortality and morbidity among post-MI patients with additional complications of LV dysfunction and heart failure. The 6632 patients participating in the study were randomly distributed to eplerenone and placebo arms in addition to optimal medical therapy. After 16 months of follow-up, eplerenone was found to reduce risk of death from any cause by 15%. It also reduced cardiovascular deaths and hospitalisations due to cardiovascular events. Interestingly, eplerenone decreased the rate of SCD by 21%. In contrast to RALES, 75% of the patients in EPHESUS were on beta-blocker therapy.

In EPHESUS, a large part of the reduction in cardiovascular mortality was due to a 21% reduction in the rate of SCD. The authors postulated that this important beneficial effect was due, in part, to a positive effect of aldosterone on electrolyte (especially potassium and magnesium) balance. Other proposed mechanisms were reduction of coronary vascular inflammation and interstitial fibrosis, reduction of oxidative stress, improvement in endothelial function, attenuation of platelet aggregation, improvement in ventricular remodelling, reduction of sympathetic tonus, and improvement in HRV and norepinephrine uptake.

Conclusions

Based on these data, we can conclude that although aldosterone antagonists are non-antiarrhythmic drugs, they have a significant preventive effect on SCD. The available data have focused particularly on the patients with low ejection fraction and congestive heart failure. New studies are needed to expand the indications to use aldosterone antagonists to prevent SCD. Potential mechanisms by which these drugs prevent SCD include prevention of aldosterone-induced cardiac and arterial fibrosis, improvement in arterial compliance, reduction of the adverse effects of aldosterone on cardiac remodelling, improvement of endothelial function and NO activity, improvement in the autonomic nervous system function via a reduction in sympathetic nervous system tonus, improvement in HRV and baroreflex sensitivity, and an increase in myocardial norepinephrine uptake By decreasing urinary excretion of potassium and magnesium, aldosterone antagonists also aid in protecting against life-threatening ventricular arryhthmias.

References

1. Zipes DP, Wellens HJ (1998) Sudden cardiac death. Circulation 98:2334–2351
2. Tan LB, Schlosshan D, Barker D (2004) Fiftieth anniversary of aldosterone: from discovery to cardiovascular therapy. Int J Cardiol 96(3):321–333
3. Tait JF, Simpson SAS, Grundy H (1952) The effect of adrenal extract on mineral metabolism. Lancet 1(3):122–129
4. Funder JW (1993) Aldosterone action. Annu Rev Physiol 55:115–130
5. Booth RE, Johnson JP, Stockland JD (2002) Aldosterone. Adv Physiol Educ 26:8–20
6. Quinn SJ, Williams GH (1988) Regulation of aldosterone secretion. Annu Rev Physiol 50:409–426
7. Fanestil DD (1969) Mechanism of action of aldosterone. Annu Rev Med 20:223–232
8. Fanestil DD, Park CS (1981) Steroid hormones and the kidney. Annu Rev Physiol 43:637–649
9. Lombes M, Oblin ME, Gasc JM et al (1992) Immunohistochemical and biochemical evidence for a cardiovascular mineralocorticoid receptor. Circ Res 71:503–510
10. Lombes M, Alfaidy N, Eugene E et al (1995) Prerequisite for cardiac aldosterone action. Mineralocorticoid receptor and 11 beta-hydroxysteroid dehydrogenase in the human heart. Circulation 92:175–182
11. Silvestre J-S, Robert V, Heymes C et al (1998) Myocardial production of aldosterone and corticosterone in the rat. Physiological regulation. J Biol Chem 273:4883–4891
12. MacKenzie SM, Clark CJ, Fraser r et al (2000) Expression of 11ß-hydroxylase and aldosterone synthase genes in the rat brain. J Mol Endocrinol 24:321–328
13. Takeda Y, Miyamori I, Inaba s et al (1997) Vascular aldosterone in genetically hypertensive rats. Hypertension 29:45–48
14. Hatakeyama H, Miyamori I, Fujita T et al (1994) Vascular aldosterone. Biosynthesis and a link to angiotensin II-induced hypertrophy of vascular smooth muscle cells, J Biol Chem 269:24316–24320
15. Swedberg K, Eneroth P, Kjekshus J et al (1990) Hormones regulating cardiovascular function in patients with severe congestive heart failure and their relation to mortality. CONSENSUS Trial Study Group. Circulation 82(5):1730–1736
16. Tsuji H, Venditti FJ Jr, Evans JC et al (1994) The associations of levels of serum potassium and magnesium with ventricular premature complexes (the Framingham Heart Study). Am J Cardiol 74(3):232–235
17. Milhailidou A, Buhagiar K, Rasmussen H (1998) Na^+ influx and Na^+-K^+ pump activation during short-term exposure of cardiac myocytes to aldosterone. Am J Physiol 274:C175–C181
18. Benitah J, Vassort G (1999) Aldosterone upregulates $Ca2^+$ current in adult rat cardiomyocytes. Circ Res 85:1139–1145
19. Ullian ME, Walsh LG, Morinelli TA (1996) Potentiation of angiotensin II action by corticosteroids in vascular tissue. Cardiovasc Res 32:266–273
20. Robert V, Heymes C, Silvestre JS et al (1999) Angiotensin AT1 receptor subtype as a cardiac target of aldosterone: role in aldosterone-salt-induced fibrosis. Hypertension 33:981–986
21. Brilla CG, Zhou G, Matsubara L et al (1994) Collagen metabolism in cultured adult rat cardiac fibroblasts: response to angiotensin II and aldosterone. J Mol Cell Cardiol 26:809–820
22. Fullerton MJ, Funder JW (1994) Aldosterone and cardiac fibrosis: in vitro studies. Cardiovasc Res 28:1863–1867

23. Brown NJ, Kim KS, Chen YQ et al (2000) Synergistic effect of adrenal steroids and angiotensin II on plasminogen activator inhibitor-1 production. J Clin Endocrinol Metab 85:336–344
24. Loskutoff DJ, Quigley JP (2000) PAI-1, fibrosis, and the elusive provisional fibrin matrix. J Clin Invest 106:1441–1443
25. De Angelis N, Fiordaliso F, Latini R et al (2002) Appraisal of the role of angiotensin II and aldosterone in ventricular myocyte apoptosis in adult normotensive rat. J Mol Cell Cardiol 34:1655–1665
26. Goldspink DF, Burniston JG, Tan LB (2003) Cardiomyocyte death and the ageing and failing heart. Exp Physiol 88:447–458
27. Zannad F, Alla F, Dousset B et al (2000) Limitation of excessive extracellular matrix turnover may contribute to survival benefit of spironolactone therapy in patients with congestive heart failure: insights from the randomized aldactone evaluation study (RALES). Rales Investigators. Circulation 102(22):2700–2706
28. Modena MG, Aveta P, Menozzi A et al (2001) Aldosterone inhibition limits collagen synthesis and progressive left ventricular enlargement after anterior myocardial infarction. Am Heart J 141:41–46
29. Keidar S, Kaplan M, Pavlotzky E et al (2004) Aldosterone administration to mice stimulates macrophage NADPH oxidase and increases atherosclerosis development: a possible role for angiotensin-converting enzyme and the receptors for angiotensin II and aldosterone. Circulation 109:2213–2220
30. Ikeda U, Kanbe T, Nakayama I et al (1995) Aldosterone inhibits nitric oxide synthesis in rat vascular smooth muscle cells induced by interleukin-1ß. Eur J Pharmacol 290:69–73
31. Rajagopalan S, Duquaine D, King S et al (2002) Mineralocorticoid receptor antagonism in experimental atherosclerosis. Circulation 105:2212–2216
32. Farquharson A, Struthers AD (2000) Spironolactone increases nitric oxide bioactivity, improves endothelial vasodilator dysfunction, and suppresses vascular angiotensin 1/angiotensin II conversion in patients with chronic heart failure. Circulation 101:594–597
33. Duprez D, DeBuyzere M, Rietzschel E et al (1998) Inverse relationship between aldosterone and large artery compliance in chronically treated heart failure patients. Eur Heart J 19:1371–1376
34. Yee KM, Struthers AD (1998) Aldosterone blunts the baroreflex response in man. Clin Sci 95:687–692
35. MacFayden RJ, Barr CS, Struthers AD (1997) Aldosterone blockade reduces vascular collagen turnover, improves heart rate variability and reduces early morning rise in heart rate in heart failure patients. Cardiovasc Res 35:30–34
36. Weber MA, Purdy RE (1982) Catecholamine-mediated constrictor effects of aldosterone on vascular smooth muscle. Life Sci 30:2009–2017
37. Cittadini A, Monti MG, Isgaard J et al (2003) Aldosterone receptor blockade improves left ventricular remodeling and increases ventricular fibrillation threshold in experimental heart failure. Cardiovasc Res 58(3):555–564
38. Ramires FJ, Mansur A, Coelho O et al (2000) Effect of spironolactone on ventricular arrhythmias in congestive heart failure secondary to idiopathic dilated or to ischemic cardiomyopathy. Am J Cardiol 85(10):1207–1211
39. Akbulut M, Ozbay Y, Ilkay E et al (2003) Effects of spironolactone and metoprolol on QT dispersion in heart failure. Jpn Heart J 44(5):681–692
40. Korkmaz ME, Muderrisoglu H, Ulucam M et al (2000) Effects of spironolactone on heart rate variability and left ventricular systolic function in severe ischemic heart

failure. Am J Cardiol 86(6):649–653

41. MacFadyen RJ, Lee AF, Morton JJ et al (1999) How often are angiotensin II and aldosterone concentrations raised during chronic ACE inhibitor treatment in cardiac failure? Heart 82:57–61
42. McKelvie RS, Yusuf S, Pericak D et al (1999) Comparison of candesartan, enalapril and their combination in congestive heart failure. Randomized Evaluation of Strategies for Left Ventricular Dysfunction (RESOLVD) Pilot Study. The RESOLVD Pilot Study Investigators. Circulation 100:1056–1064
43. Jorde UP, Vittorio T, Katz SD et al (2002) Elevated plasma aldosterone levels despite complete inhibition of the vascular angiotensin-converting enzyme in chronic heart failure. Circulation 106, pp 1055–1057
44. Pitt B, Zannad F, Remme WJ et al (1999) The effect of spironolactone on morbidity and mortality in patients with severe heart failure. Randomized Aldactone Evaluation Study Investigators. N Engl J Med 341(10):709–717
45. Pitt B, Remme W, Zannad F et al for Eplerenone Post-Acute Myocardial Infarction Heart Failure Efficacy and Survival Study Investigators (2003) Eplerenone, a selective aldosterone blocker, in patients with left ventricular dysfunction after myocardial infarction. N Engl J Med 348(14):1309–1321

After DEFINITE, SCD-HeFT, COMPANION: Do We Need to Implant an ICD in All Patients With Heart Failure?

D.S. Cannom

Recent clinical trials of implantable cardioverter defibrillators (ICD) suggest that up to 50% of the deaths in patients with left ventricular systolic dysfunction (LVSD) secondary to coronary artery disease (CAD) are sudden or arrhythmic in nature [1]. This incidence is lower in heart failure (HF) due to non-ischaemic aetiologies. As LVSD and symptom severity progress, overall mortality increases, yet the percentage of deaths classified as sudden decreases. In more recent clinical trials using angiotensin converting enzyme (ACE) inhibitors and β-blockers, New York Heart Association (NYHA) class II patients have an annual mortality of 6% with approximately 60% of these deaths sudden. However, NYHA class IV patients have an annual mortality of approximately 20% with only around 30% of these deaths sudden [2].

Attempts at identifying which patients with HF are at an increased risk of sudden cardiac death (SCD) have met with limited success. To date, there is still no single best measurement to identify which HF patients will die from an arrhythmia rather than progressive LVSD. Simple clinical markers such as greater age, degree of LVSD, and severity of HF predict overall mortality but have low specificity for the mode of death. Syncope has been reported to be one specific clinical marker associated with increased SCD [3–5]. High-frequency ventricular ectopy does indicate a worse prognosis, yet controversy remains as to whether this is predictive of the mode of death rather than a reflection of the degree of LVSD [6, 7]. Inducibility of ventricular tachycardia (VT)/ventricular fibrillation (VF) during electrophysiology testing (EPS) has a low sensitivity in patients with non-ischaemic or dilated cardiomyopathy (DCM). It does predict an increased risk of SCD in ischaemic cardiomyopathy (CM), but does not predict overall mortality [8, 9].

Good Samaritan Hospital, Los Angeles, CA, USA

The results of the recently completed ICD trials – including Multicenter Automatic Defibrillator Implantation Trial (MADIT) I and II, Defibrillators in Nonischemic Cardiomyopathy Treatment Evaluation (DEFINITE), Sudden Cardiac Death in Heart Failure (SCD-HeFT) and Comparison of Medical Therapy, Pacing and Defibrillation in Heart Failure (COMPANION) – clearly establish a survival advantage for selected patients with HF who receive an ICD. The largest HF trial is COMPANION, which enrolled patients based on both advanced HF status (NYHA class III and IV) and a low EF: both a survival benefit and reduced congestive heart failure (CHF) hospitalisation for cardiac resynchronisation therapy (CRT) and ICD therapy in combination was clearly seen. In less advanced heart failure (NYHA class I and II), the most important risk stratifier seems to be ejection fraction rather than CHF status (see below).

The Role of the ICD in Preventing SCD in Patients with CAD

Three well-designed primary prevention trials in patients with reduced EF and CAD support a role for the ICD in patients with low EF [10–12]. MADIT I and the Multicenter Unsustained Tachycardia Trial (MUSTT) examined patients with CAD, EF below 40%, and inducible VT/VF at EPS. MADIT I reported a 54% mortality reduction, with most of the benefit seen in patients with a history of HF (approx. 40% of patients), EF below 26%, or left bundle branch block (LBBB) [10]. MUSTT showed a 27% risk reduction in SCD solely attributed to use of the ICD and not anti-arrhythmic drug therapy [11]. Approximately two-thirds of the enrolled patients were either NYHA class II or III. MADIT II evaluated patients with CAD and EF below 30% and did not require inducibility of VT/VF by EPS. The ICD produced a 31% risk reduction in overall mortality, with the majority of the benefit occurring in patients with a QRS duration greater than 120 ms [12]. Approximately 60% of the patients were either NYHA class II or III.

The DEFINITE and SCD-HeFT Trials

Previous small studies examining the role of prophylactic ICDs among patients with DCM did not define the role of the ICD. The Amiodarone versus Cardioverter Study (AMIOVIRT) reported no mortality difference among patients with DCM and asymptomatic non-sustained ventricular tachycardia (NSVT) [13]. Similarly, the German Cardiomyopathy Trial (CAT) was stopped when interim statistical analysis suggested the impossibility of any mortality difference emerging between ICDs and medical therapy among patients with DCM diagnosed within 12 months of enrolment [14].

The neutral results of these studies were due to inadequacy of the sample size and the absence of a requirement for symptomatic heart failure, which in turn contributed to lower than expected event rates. In contrast, the recently reported Defibrillators in Nonischemic Cardiomyopathy Treatment Evaluation (DEFINITE) trial, which randomised 458 patients with DCM, left ventricular ejection fraction below 35%, and asymptomatic NSVT to receive ICD or conventional medical therapy, demonstrated a 34% reduction in all-cause mortality in ICD patients, but that did not reach statistical significance [15]. A post-hoc analysis of NYHA class III patients showed a 67% relative reduction in all-cause mortality, again showing that patients with left ventricular dysfunction and more advanced HF symptoms are most likely to benefit from ICD therapy, as in MADIT I and COMPANION.

The hypothesis of SCD-HeFT was to determine, by intention-to-treat analysis, whether either ICD or amiodarone reduces all-cause mortality compared with placebo in patients with ischaemic or dilated cardiomyopathy, NYHA class II–III HF and left ventricular ejection fraction of 35% or less [16]. Event estimates were based on an estimated 10% per year all-cause mortality rate in the control arm at a minimum follow-up of 2.5 years. A total of 2521 patients were enrolled between 16 September 1997 and 18 July 2001 at 148 sites in North America and New Zealand. Follow-up terminated on 31 October 2003 yielding a median (25th, 75th percentile) follow-up duration of 40.8 (29.7, 53.0) months. This long follow-up duration exceeds that of any prior study of ICDs or drug therapy for prevention of SCD.

Fifty-two percent of enrolled patients had an ischaemic cardiomyopathy, 48% had a DCM, 70% were NYHA class II and 30% were class III. A high standard for optimal medical management of HF was maintained, which countered a historical criticism of earlier ICD trials. At last follow-up, 87% of patients were taking either an ACE or angiotensin receptor blockade (ARB), 78% were taking β-blockers, 80% were taking diuretics, and 31% were taking spironolactone. There were no important differences in relation to baseline demographic variables, substrate, NYHA class, or medical therapy among treatment groups, with the exception of slightly more β-blocker use in class II (71%) than in class III (64%) patients.

The primary result of SCD-HeFT was a significant reduction in all-cause mortality with ICD therapy compared to amiodarone or placebo. Five-year all-cause mortality was 35.8% in the placebo group, 34.1% in the amiodarone group, and 28.9% in the ICD group (Fig. 1). Thus, ICD therapy conferred a 23% relative reduction in all-cause mortality [hazard ratio (95% confidence interval) 0.77, $P = 0.007$]. This difference in mortality emerged within 18 months of enrolment and was sustained throughout follow-up. The majority of deaths were cardiac (68%, similarly distributed among treatment groups), and the mortality benefit of ICD therapy was due entirely to a reduction in

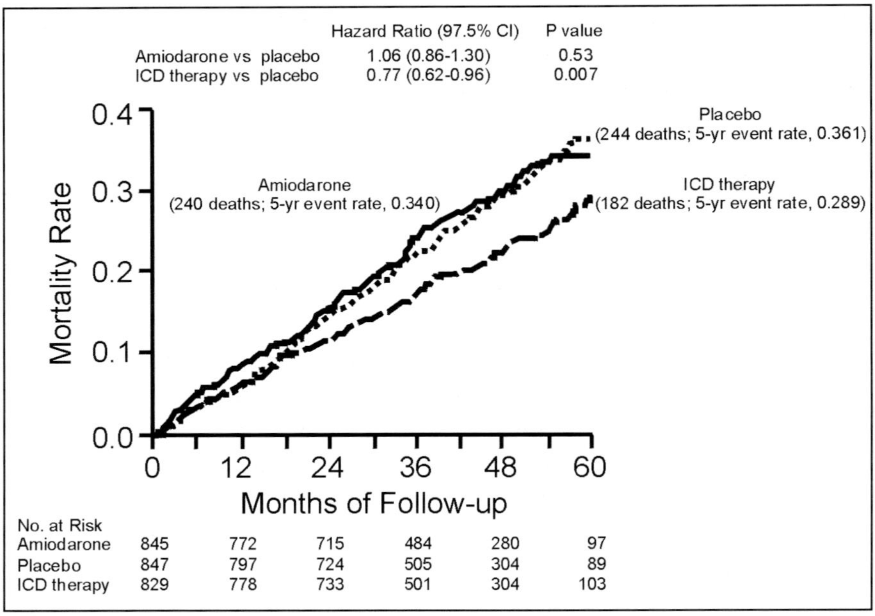

Fig. 1. The Kaplan–Meier estimates of death from any cause in the SCD-HeFT trial. Note the 5-year reduction in mortality by the ICD of 23% compared to either placebo or amiodarone. This difference was noted irrespective of the cause of the cardiomyopathy (ischaemic or dilated) but was limited to NYHA class II patients only. *CI* confidence interval

arrhythmic deaths (39% in the placebo arm vs 20% in the ICD arm).

The mortality reduction among patients with ischaemic cardiomyopathy approximates that observed in MADIT II and serves to validate the findings of that study. More importantly, the equivalent mortality reduction among patients with DCM demonstrates that the primary prevention mortality benefits of ICD therapy seen in ischaemic cardiomyopathy are identical to those seen in DCM populations.

There were many peculiarities in the SCD trial design but, although present, they do not distract from the overall results. Defibrillation threshold testing (DFT) testing was minimal, and if DFTs under 30 J could not be obtained, the device was still implanted. Also, the device was programmed as a 'shock only' device without any of the benefits of anti-tachycardia pacing programmed 'on.' Finally, the hazard ratio for those patients with a left ventricular ejection fraction over 30% (285 patients) was 1.08. The hazard ratio for patients with ejection fractions equal to or under 30% (1390 patients) was 0.73. Thus, there was no benefit of the ICD in patients with an ejection fraction between 30% and 35%. The benefit of ICD therapy was greater in patients with a QRS duration greater than or equal to 120 ms (hazard ratio 0.67). This finding was also noted in the MADIT II trial. While there was a significant reduction in mortality in patients with NYHA class II disease (7.9% at 5 years), patients with NYHA class III CHF had no apparent reduction in the risk of death (hazard ratio of ICD vs placebo 1.16) (Fig. 2).

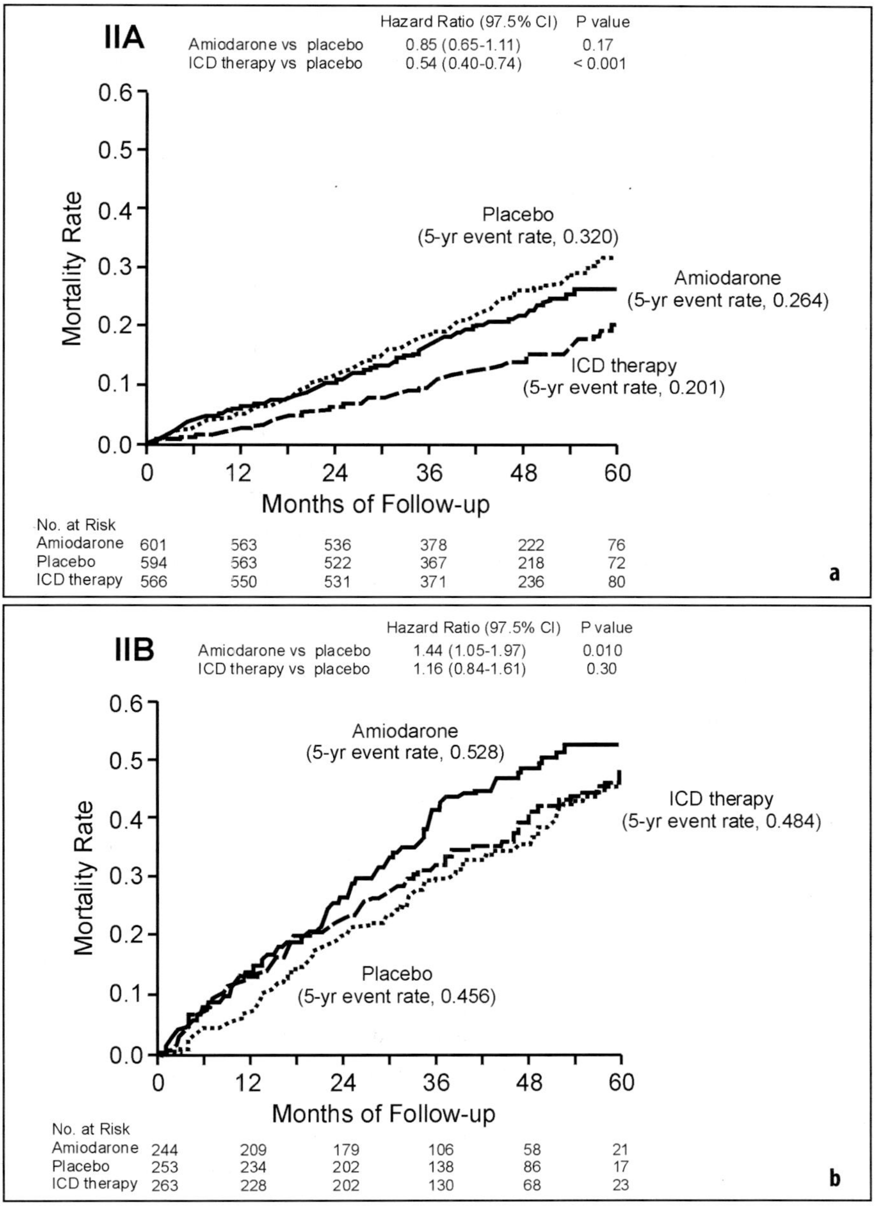

Fig. 2a, b. The Kaplan–Meier estimates of death from any cause for the prespecified subgroups of NYHA class II (**a**) and class III (**b**) in the SCD-HeFT trial. There was no apparent risk reduction of death in ICD therapy in class III patients compared with placebo (HR 1.16)

Despite this finding, the authors state in the discussion that 'we do not believe that the unanticipated subgroup effect will be found as a sufficient basis for withholding ICD therapy from patients in NYHA class III.' Recently presented data from SCD-HeFT showed that in surviving patients NYHA class actually improved over time for the surviving population within each treatment group [17]. This occurred despite the associated mortality in each arm. One possible explanation for this finding is that more intense pharmacological therapy improved these patients and that their actual CHF status was misclassified at enrolment due to under-treatment with CHF medication. An opposite finding was noted in MADIT II patients, 30% of whom had progression of their CHF over time: the role of right ventricular pacing is being evaluated as a possible cause of this deterioration.

Heart failure is probably not as relevant a way to select patients as the presence of a low ejection fraction alone. Of course most of these low ejection fraction patients will have HF. But the inconsistency of benefit from the ICD across studies (e.g. the differences in benefit in class III patients between DEFINITE and SCD-HeFT) reinforces the importance of a low ejection fraction rather than an attempt to categorise HF which depends upon a subjective interpretation of patient symptoms. Other causes of HF, e.g. diastolic dysfunction and a high ejection fraction, would not qualify a patient for an ICD. Medicare has recently agreed to fund the SCD-HeFT indications in a broad decision which includes all patients with an ejection fraction below 35% due to either an ischaemic or a non-ischaemic cause and irrespective of NYHA HF studies or QRS duration (Centers for Medicare and Medicaid Services memo accessible at http://www.cms.hhs.gov/mcd/viewdraftdecisionmemo.asp?d=139).

The COMPANION Trial

The COMPANION trial expanded the earlier studies of CRT that analysed only functional endpoints. These earlier trials, including those with an ICD, were intended primarily for US Food and Drug Administration approval for a specific device. However, the COMPANION trial was a serious scientific trial designed by some of the top experts in the HF and ICD world. Its design features and endpoints were chosen to clarify whether CRT alone or in combination with an ICD will improve mortality and morbidity in HF patients.

The COMPANION enrolment criteria included patients in NYHA class III or IV HF, with normal sinus rhythm, QRS duration 120 ms or more, a PR interval of 150 ms or more, left ventricular ejection fraction 35% or less, and left ventricular end-diastolic dimension 60 mm or more [18]. Enrolled patients were required to be taking optimal pharmacological therapy (OPT) including a β-blocker for at least 3 months, a diuretic, ACE inhibitor or ARB, and spironolactone for 1 month. Furthermore, patients had to have a history of a hospitalisation for HF in the year before enrolment. Patients were randomised in a 1:2:2 strategy to OPT alone, OPT with CRT, or OPT with CRT-D (CRT + ICD). The primary endpoint of the trial was the time to all-cause mortality or all-cause hospitalisation. A secondary endpoint was all-cause mortality.

The first patient was enrolled in the trial on 20 January 2000. On 18 November 2002, the Data and Safety Monitoring Board recommended that the Steering Committee stop enrolment because a target number of primary endpoints had been reached, and the primary endpoint and efficacy boundaries had been crossed. Therefore, enrolment was stopped on this date.

The randomisation was very consistent across all three groups. More than 80% of the patients were in NYHA class III rather than class IV HF. Also, the mean ejection fraction of the enrolled population was between 20% and 22%, which is only slightly lower than that of MADIT II (which was 23%). QRS duration averaged 158–160 ms, with approximately 70% of the patients having LBBB rather than right bundle branch block (RBBB). Despite the fact that the use of β-blockers and ACE inhibitors was required for enrolment, only 70% of the population was on ACE inhibitors, and 66–68% were on β-blockers at the time of randomisation. This demonstrates the difficulty in maintaining patients on these drugs even in a carefully controlled research environment.

The main reason that the primary endpoint of the COMPANION trial was met was the very high event rate (68%) in the OPT group. Both CRT and CRT-D reduced the primary endpoint (hospitalisation for CHF or death) by 20% ($P = 0.008$ for CRT and 0.007 for CRT-D). Although only 1600 patients were enrolled, the high event rate in the OPT group allowed the primary endpoint to be successfully reached.

The endpoint of greatest interest to the electrophysiology community was the effect of CRT-D on the secondary endpoint of all-cause mortality. The 12-month mortality in the OPT group was 19% and was double that at 24 months. CRT alone reduced 1-year mortality by 24% ($P = 0.06$), and CRT-D reduced the 1-year mortality by 43% ($P = 0.003$) compared to OPT (Fig. 3).

It is important for the clinician to appreciate that only 54–59% of the patients in this trial (depending on which arm is being considered) had an ischaemic cardiomyopathy. It also appears that the CRT benefit was equal for NYHA class III and class IV patients. QRS width affected survival, with the greatest benefit for those patients with the widest QRS (locker use was associated with a significantly more favourable outcome.

On the basis of these data, there is now scientific evidence to support the concept that CRT-D reduces HF mortality. The COMPANION trial showed

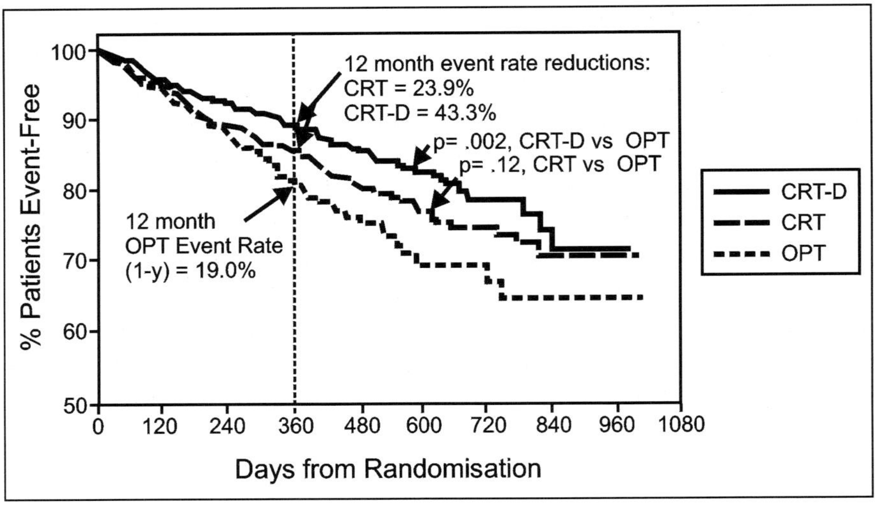

Fig. 3. The Kaplan–Meier estimates of the time to the secondary endpoint of death from any cause in the COMPANION trial. The 12-month rates of death from any cause (the secondary endpoint) were 19% in the pharmacological-therapy group, 15% in the pacemaker group, and 12% in the pacemaker–defibrillator group

that two-thirds of this effect can be attributed to CRT alone, whereas one-third is attributable to the ICD. Thus, all patients considered for CRT in 2005 are candidates for a back-up ICD as well.

Conclusions

Few, if any, technological breakthroughs in clinical electrophysiology have reached broad acceptance as quickly as the ICD and CRT. The impact of these devices on patients with end-stage HF has been an important clinical adjunct to routine background medical therapy. This field has changed so rapidly that the clinician still wrestles with the problems of how far to extend prophylactic ICD therapy to the HF population and which patients should be selected for CRT therapy and, in turn, for CRT-D therapy. A North American Society of Pacing and Electrophysiology (NASPE) Consensus Conference on Resynchronization Therapy for Heart Failure held in 2002 noted that although much progress has been made, there are many issues that still must be resolved [19]. These include the long-term benefit of device therapy, the need for further evolution of the devices themselves to assure successful implantation, studies to help optimise programmability, identification of the patient population most likely to benefit, and the importance of the economic and ethical ramifications.

One of the major challenges for the next few years is to ascertain whether we can extend the indications for CRT by implanting these devices in patients with CAD, a low ejection fraction (in the 30% range), a wide QRS (> 120 ms), and in NYHA class I or II. Such a study is MADIT CRT, which will test the hypothesis that these high-risk patients who receive CRT will subsequently have a reduced rate of HF or all-cause mortality. This important protocol was initiated in October 2004 and will enrol 1700 patients over 2 years. A similar study called Biventricular Pacing to Inhibit HF Progression (BLOCK-HF) will evaluate the potential benefit of CRT on HF progression. There are important design differences between MADIT CRT and BLOCK-HF, although both seek to answer the question as to whether CRT benefits patients before they progress to NYHA class III or IV HF. Trials such as these will further enhance our knowledge and ability to treat SCD in HF.

References

1. Cleland JG, Chattopadhyay S, Khand A et al (2002) Prevalence and incidence of arrhythmias and sudden death in heart failure. Heart Fail Rev 7:229–242
2. MERIT-HF Study Group (1999) Effect of metoprolol CR/XL in chronic heart failure: metoprolol CR/XL randomised intervention trial in congestive heart failure Lancet 353:2001–2007
3. Middlekauf HR, Stevenson WG, Stevenson LW et al (1993) Syncope in advanced heart failure: high risk of sudden death regardless of origin of syncope. J Am Coll Cardiol 21:110–116
4. Fruhwald FM, Eber B, Schumacher M et al (1996) Syncope in dilated cardiomyopathy is a predictor of sudden cardiac death. Cardiology 87:177–180
5. Fonarow GC, Feliciano Z, Boyle NG et al (2000) Improved survival in patients with nonischemic advanced heart failure and syncope treated with an implantable cardioverter defibrillator. Am J Cardiol 85:981–985
6. De Maria R, Gavazzi A, Carioli A et al (1992) Ventricular arrhythmias in dilated cardiomyopathy as an independent prognostic hallmark. Italian Multicenter Cardiomyopathy Study (SPIC) Group. Am J Cardiol 69:1451–1457
7. Teerlink JR, Jalaluddin M, Anderson S et al (2000) Ambulatory ventricular arrhythmias in patients with heart failure do not specifically predict an increased risk of sudden death. Circulation 101:40–46
8. Sager PT, Choudhary R, Leon C et al (1990) The long-term prognosis of patients with out-of-hospital cardiac arrest but no inducible ventricular tachycardia. Am Heart J 120:1334–1342
9. Buxton AE, Lee KL, DiCarlo L et al (2000) Electrophysiologic testing to identify patients with coronary artery disease who are at risk for sudden death. N Engl J Med 342:1937–1945
10. Moss AJ, Hall WJ, Cannom DS et al (1996) Improved survival with an implanted defibrillator in patients with coronary artery disease at high risk for ventricular arrhythmia. N Engl J Med 335:1933–1940
11. Buxton AE, Lee KL, Fisher JD et al (1999) A randomized study of the prevention of sudden death in patients with coronary heart disease. N Engl J Med 341:1882–1890

12. Moss AJ, Zareba W, Hall et al (2002) Prophylactic implantation of a defibrillator in patients with myocardial infarction and reduced ejection fraction. N Engl J Med 346:877–883
13. Strickberger SA, Hummel JD, Bartlett TG et al (2003) Amiodarone vs implantable defibrillator: randomized trial in patients with nonischemic cardiomyopathy and asymptomatic nonsustained ventricular tachycardia – AMIOVIRT. J Am Coll Cardiol 41:1707–1712
14. Bansch D, Antz M, Boczor S et al (2002) Primary prevention of sudden cardiac death in idiopathic dilated cardiomyopathy: The Cardiomyopathy Trial (CAT). Circulation 105:1453–1458
15. Kadish A, Dyer A, Daubert JP et al (2004) Prophylactic defibrillator implantation in patients with nonischemic dilated cardiomyopathy. N Engl J Med 351:2151–2158
16. Bardy GH, Lee KL, Mark DB et al for Sudden Cardiac Death in Heart Failure Trial (SCD-HeFT) Investigators (2005) Amiodarone or an implantable cardioverter-defibrillator for congestive heart failure. N Engl J Med 352:225–237
17. Bardy GH, Lee KL, Boehmer JP et al (2005) The progression of congestive heart failure over the course of the sudden cardiac death in heart failure trial (SCD- HeFT). Heart Rhythm 2:S39
18. Bristow MR, Saxon LA, Boehmer J et al (2004) Cardiac resynchronization therapy with or without an implantable defibrillator in advanced chronic heart failure. N Engl J Med 350:2140–2150
19. Saxon LA, De Marco T (2005) Resynchronization therapy for heart failure. Available at: http://www.hrsonline.org/professional_education_categories/articles (accessed 19 January 2005)

Health Care Systems: How to Resolve the Dilemma Between Clinical Needs and Limited Resources?

M. Brignole, S. Nisam

Magnitude of the Problem

Are the appropriate indications for ICDs (based on clinical evidence) limited by health care system resources? An overview of the number of ICD (including CRT-D) implants and their costs in USA, Europe, and Italy in 2003 and 2004 is provided in Tables 1 and 2. ICD therapy accounts for only a small percentage of the total expenditure of health care systems, and there are large numbers of appropriate patients who do not receive ICDs, although the annual incidence of implants is increasing. The number of patients receiving ICDs (or CRT-Ds) has increased ten-fold over the last 10 years in Europe and in the USA [1]. In Italy, the implantation rate in 2003 increased by 45% compared to the rate in 2002 and by a further 23% in 2004 compared to 2003 (Tables 3, 4). Nevertheless, the total expenditure for ICDs (which includes device costs plus implantation and follow-up) still remains a modest percentage of total health expenditures. Furthermore, the number of patients who could benefit from this therapy is miniscule compared to the general population. For example, in Europe, in 2004, about 40 000 patients received ICDs, and the associated in-patient expenditures, amounted to € 0.6 billion, accounting for 0.2% of total in-patient expenditures. Similarly in Italy, in 2004, about 8000 patients received ICDs/CRT-Ds, and the in-patient expenditures for these were € 0.13 billion, accounting for 0.3% of total in-patient expenditures. Figure 1 compares the expenditure for ICDs with those of other accepted therapies in the USA in 2000. The cost of ICD was four-fold lower than that for PTCA or CABG and 15-times lower than that for antibiotics.

Centro Aritmologico, Dipartimento di Cardiologia, Ospedali del Tigullio, Lavagna (Genua), Italy; Guidant Corporation, Brussels, Belgium

Table 1. Number of ICDs (and CRT-Ds) and their in-patient costs in 2003 (source: Guidant)

	ICDs/CRT-Ds (implants/million inhabitants)	ICDs/CRT-Ds (total number implanted)	Estimated costs (Euros)
USA	280	70 000	2.3 billion
Europe	60	22 500	0.6 billion
Italy	110	6 400	0.1 billion

ICD Implantable Cardioverter defibrillator, *CRT-D* cardiac resynchronisation therapy plus defibrillator

Table 2. Number of ICDs (and CRT-Ds) and their in-patient costs in 2004 (source: Guidant)

	ICDs/CRT-Ds (implants/million inhabitants)	ICDs/CRT-Ds (total number implanted)	Estimated costs (Euros)
USA	320	80 000	2.6 billion
Europe	100	36 000	1.0 billion
Italy	146	8163	0.13 billion

ICD Implantable Cardioverter defibrillator, *CRT-D* cardiac resynchronisation therapy plus defibrillator

Table 3. Number of ICDs/CRT-Ds and revenues in Italy in 2003 (source: personal communication)

ICDs:	Number (Euros)	Revenues	Number difference (%) compared to 2002	Revenue difference (%) compared to 2002
Single chamber (VR-VVI)	2584	32 583 699	42.3%	34.1%
Dual-chamber	1947	29 900 243	16.4%	12.6%
CRT-D	1846	29 761 657	90.7%	85.0%
Total ICDs	6377	92 245 599	43.1%	37.8%
Leads	6605	9 566 921	28.0%	20.6%
Total ICD/CRT-D revenues	-	101 812 520	-	36.0%

ICD Implantable Cardioverter defibrillator, *CRT-D* cardiac resynchronisation therapy plus defibrillator

Table 4. Number of ICDs/CRT-Ds and revenues in Italy in 2004 (source: personal communication)

ICDs:	Number (Euros)	Revenues	Number difference (%) compared to 2002	Revenue difference (%) compared to 2002
Single chamber (VR-VVI)	2795	32 640 921	8.2%	0.2%
Dual-chamber	2523	36 402 528	29.6%	21.7%
CRT-D	2845	44 137 047	54.1%	48.3%
Total ICDs	8163	113 180 496	28%	22.7%
Leads	8806	11 375 480	33.3%	18.9%
Total ICD/CRT-D revenues	-	124 555 976		22.3%

ICD Implantable Cardioverter defibrillator, *CRT-D* cardiac resynchronisation therapy plus defibrillator

Thus, by considering the global health care system, it is clear that the impact of ICD therapy on total health care expenditures is modest. The main reason that so much attention has been given to the costs of ICD therapy, compared to other established therapies, is that the upfront costs of the device (and implantation) are high. Whether these initial costs are reasonable when considered over the lifetime of the patient is the important issue that is addressed in this article.

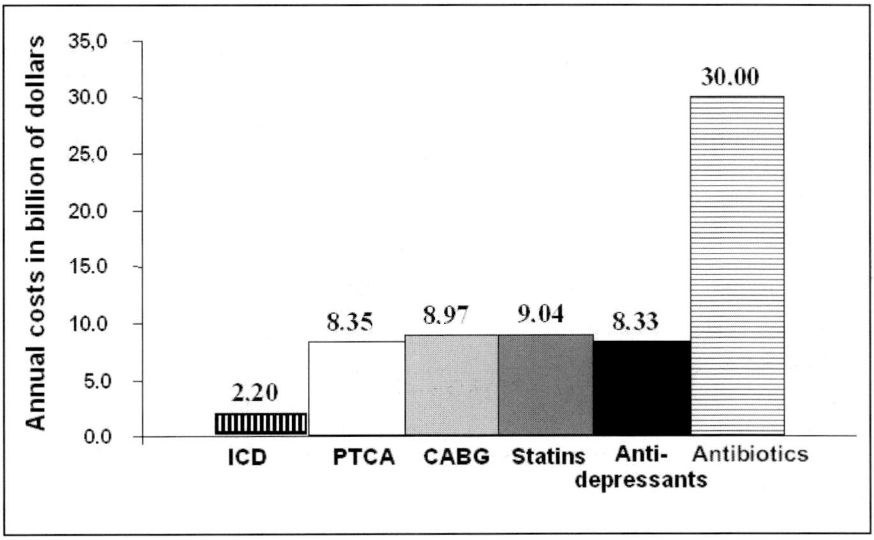

Fig. 1. Comparison between some therapies

Different Perspectives

While it cannot satisfy all the individual demands made upon it, the primary objective of a health care system is to provide a homogeneous level of assistance based on the priorities of the patient population. Correct evaluation of those priorities requires consideration of the scientific, objective, and reproducible criteria for the best allocation of available economic resources. Because of its ethical implications (i.e., 'how to improve the health status of the citizens'), the decision cannot be left exclusively to the prescribing specialist but must involve all stakeholders of the national health system. Although their perspectives differ (Table 5), the common goal is to improve citizens' health.

Table 5. Different perspectives

Stakeholder	Direct objective	Notes
Doctor of the national health care system	No profit, but budgeting	Possible conflict between the obligation to provide the best therapy and that of limiting the consumption of public resources (efficiency/efficacy ratio); possible conflict with profit issues
Doctor outside of the national health care system	No profit, no budget	Obligation to provide the best therapy; possible conflict with profit issues
ICD companies	For profit	Interest in producing high-quality devices and providing technical support, and in re-reinvesting profits in research & development, clinical support, trials, etc.
Administrator of the health care system, professional	For budget	Obligation to provide efficient health care
Administrator of the health care system, elected member	For consent	Obligation to fulfil the perceived needs of patients
Patient (and family)	For him-/herself	Interest in maintaining his/her own health

The Perspective of the Clinical Cardiologist: Evidence-Based Medicine and Guidelines

The solution appears simple and easy to apply in clinical practice: 'Follow the recommendations of the guidelines.' Indeed, a major objective of the guidelines is to enunciate clearly *which patients are appropriate for which therapies* according to the rules of evidence-based medicine. Guidelines mean nothing, if clinicians do not adhere to them, so much of the guidelines process also aims at increasing the appropriate implementation of particular therapies – on the basis of evidence-based-medicine – for appropriately selected patients. Further objectives of the guidelines include improving the quality of interventions, the clinical outcome of the patients, and the cost/efficacy ratio, and should help authorities in the allocation of resources. With the advent of evidence-based medicine, doctors have been induced to abandon empirical medicine, based on 'logical' or 'common belief,' and to move towards 'evidence of efficacy' [2]. Also, the use of ICDs must be based on the guidelines established by the leading international medical societies, following their careful review of all available data. Adoption of the standards defined by the scientific community is the best method to avoid both 'overuse' ('inappropriateness') and 'underuse' ('malpractice'). A doctor has the ethical obligation to adopt a confirmed therapy in the interest of his/her patients and, conversely, to be aware of the legal implications of not doing so.

Whether the recommendations of the guidelines are affordable and within the limitations of available resources is an obviously critical decision, but it cannot be made by the clinical cardiologist alone. There are other decision-makers, starting with the cardiologist-manager, who have the responsibility to put guidelines in the proper economic context within the health system and the clinical governance of health. Going from these principles to the specific case of ICD therapy, we have provided evidence that, in Italy and western Europe, resources are sufficient to permit the guidelines to be implemented. It is the right of the clinical cardiologist to make use of these resources; it is an obligation not to abuse them.

From the Perspective of the Cardiologist-Manager: Evidence-Based Health Care and Guidelines

The objective of a health system is to establish scientific, objective and reproducible criteria for optimal allocation of the available economic resources [3]. To accomplish this, we need objective methods of measurement in order to define priorities. All of the critical factors can be measured and compared, and the decision on the cost-effectiveness of a therapy must be based on the evidence of such measurements. The most useful methods are the number needed to treat (NNT) and the cost-effectiveness. Regarding the use of ICDs, the results of ICD therapy vs other therapies must be analysed.

The NNT is a normalised measurement of clinical efficacy and efficiency that allows comparison of different treatments. In the case of ICDs, the NNT is the number of patients that must receive an ICD implant in order to demonstrate prolonged survival by 1 year in one patient. The importance of the NNT is that it is easy to understand in clinical practice and is unrelated to the difference in costs of therapy among different countries [4]. Some examples of NNTs are listed in the Tables 6 and 7. Comparison of the data in these tables shows that ICD therapy, when used according to the recommendations of the guidelines, is more effective than many other established therapies. For example, ICD therapy for patients fitting the MADIT II criteria has an NNT of 11 (at 3 years of follow-up), which compares quite favorably with Captropril (SAVE), which has an NNT of 20, also at 3 years of follow-up. The NNT for ICD therapy remains favourable even when it is compared with therapies in which a softer end-point, namely, morbidity instead of mortality, is used (Table 7). As explained below, the NNT for ICDs improves 'dramatically with time of follow-up,' which illustrates the importance of evaluating ICD cost-effectiveness after several years of follow-up, not simply at the mean time elapsed when a particular study has ended [5]. This is precisely the reason why studies with shorter duration of follow-up give misleadingly higher NNT values; for example, in the AVID/CIDS/CASH meta-analysis, the 1-year follow-up time is far too short, and as demonstrated by Salukhe et al., longer follow-up in those trials would have shown a much lower NNT [5]. Moreover, NNT has no meaning for patient cohorts considered *contra-indicated* for ICDs on the basis of negative trials, such as CABG-Patch, DINAMIT and BEST_ICD. These trials simply showed that patients requiring revascularisation and those within 40 days of myocardial infarction are considered not appropriate candidates for ICDs.

'Cost-effectiveness' is the ratio of the *difference* in cost of ICD therapy compared to an alternative (e.g., amiodarone) divided by the *prolongation* of life achieved by ICD vs the alternative therapy. The cost-effectiveness ratio is expressed as cost/year life saved [4]. Some examples are listed in Tables 8 and 9. ICD therapy, especially when used for primary prevention, has a more favourable cost-effectiveness than many other commonly established therapies, for example compared to hospital dialysis or 2-vessel CABG surgery (Table 8) [6, 7]. In general, the duration of follow-up of the ICD studies has been shorter than that of others, which were interrupted, mainly for ethical reasons, at the time when the benefit became manifest. A recent study [5], in which the results of eight randomised trials were pooled together and the predicted effect was calculated at 1, 2, and 3 years of follow-up, showed that the benefit of ICD therapy increases with the duration of follow-up, at least for the first 3 years, without an increase of costs. For example, the NNT to save a year of life is seven-fold higher after 1 year than after 3 years of fol-

Table 6. Number needed to treat (*NNT*) to save one life for some established therapies based on the results of randomised controlled trials. Negative studies have resulted in ICDs (and other active therapies that have been tested) contraindicated or found to be not useful for patients (see text for further explanation)

Trial	Therapy	Duration	NNT
MUSTT	ICD: primary prevention	5	3
MADIT	ICD: primary prevention	2.4	4
MADIT 2	ICD: primary prevention	3	11
SCD-HeFT	ICD: primary prevention	5	14
DEFINITE	ICD: primary prevention, DCM	2	29
AVID	ICD: secondary prevention	3	9
AVID, CASH, CIDS meta-analysis	ICD vs amiodarone	1	29
CABG-PATCH	ICD post by-pass	4	NA
DINAMIT	ICD post-AMI	2.5	NA
BEST-ICD	ICD post-MI	1.5	NA
COMPANION	ICD + CRT	1	14
CARE-HF	CRT	2.5	10
CASS	CABG, left main artery	5	6
CASS	CABG, 3 vessels, EF < 50%	5	11
CASS	CABG, 3 vessels, EF > 50%	5	NA
Zwolle RCT	Primary PTCA vs thrombolysis	7	10
Primary PCI meta-analysis	Primary PTCA vs thrombolysis	1	25
FRISC 2	PTCA-CABG, unstable angina, ACS	0.5	100
TIME	PTCA-CABG, stable angina	0.5	NA
ACME	PTCA, stable angina	0.5	NA
Amiodarone meta-analysis	Amiodarone	2	37
SAVE	Captopril, heart failure	3	20
SOLVD	Enalapril, heart failure	4	22
CIBIS 2	Bisoprolol, heart failure	1	23
MERIT	Carvedilol, heart failure	1	26
ISIS 2	Streptokinase, AMI	2	24
Hypertension meta-analysis	Antihypertensive drugs (various)	5	NA
4S	Simvastatin (secondary prevention)	6	28
HPS	Simvastatin (primary and secondary prevention)	5	59

NA Not applicable

Table 7. NNT needed to avoid some composite end-points for some established therapies based on the results of some randomised controlled trials

Trial	Therapy	End-point	Duration (years)	NNT
FRISC 2	PTCA-CABG in ACS	Death, non-fatal AMI	0.5	37
TACTICS	PTCA-CABG in ACS Tn+	Death, non-fatal AMI, hospitalisation	0.5	11
TIME	PTCA-CABG, stable angina	Death, non-fatal AMI, hospitalisation	0.5	3
ACME	PTCA, stable angina	Angina	0.5	6
HPS	Simvastatin	Coronary artery disease, stroke, revascularisation	5	18
Hypertension meta-analysis	Antihypertensive drugs (various)	Stroke, coronary events	5	125

Table 8. Costs per year of life saved for some established therapies (adapted from [6])

Intervention	Cost/year life saved (1999) (Euro)
Pacemaker implant	1860
Beta-blockers in survivors of high risk acute myocardial infarction	3400
Simvastatin in a 70-year-old man with cholesterol blood level of 309 mg/dl	4300
Pravastatin for secondary prevention of chronic coronary artery disease in a man with 2 risk factors	9770
CABG (3-vessels disease) vs medical therapy	13 700
ICD in asymptomatic chronic coronary artery disease, depressed EF and non-sustained ventricular tachycardia	14 200
Streptokinase therapy for acute myocardial infarction	24 000
CABG 3-vessel disease vs PTCA	26 500
Home dialysis	26 700
tPA vs streptokinase for AMI at 1 year	37 000
In-hospital haemodialysis	61 700
CABG (2-vessels disease) vs medical therapy	85 300

Table 9. Costs per year of life saved of some established therapies (adapted from [7])

Intervention	Cost/year life saved (1999) (US dollars)
PTCA (chronic coronary artery disease, 1 vessel)	88 944
Cardiac transplant	43 087
Hypertension (diastolic 95–104 mmHg)	40 753
Primary PTCA	31 244
ICD (no pre-implant EPS)	16 555

low-up. The cost-effectiveness ratio remains acceptable also when compared with therapies that have a combined end-point of mortality and morbidity. For example, in several studies on the effects of statins, the cost per patient per year free from death, non-fatal myocardial infarction, or stroke was € 51 400 for the study AFCAPS/TexCAPS, € 26 013 for WORSCOPS, € 9970 for CARE, € 8028 for LIPID and € 6695 for 4S [8].

In addition to the need to be aware of the effectiveness of a particular therapy, the optimal use of economic resources (efficiency) is a major objective of any health care manager. For any therapy, the rule must be to provide the appropriate therapy at the lowest price. The price of an ICD varies considerably, up to two-fold or three-fold, from one model to another. This means, for example, that relatively lower priced, simple models can be used for many (most) patients, reserving the more expensive ICDs with more sophisticated features for those patients needing such features. This approach allows more efficient use of available resources.

Other Issues Outside the Competency of the Cardiologist That Need To Be Considered

There are several other issues that are outside the strict professional competency of the cardiologist that, nonetheless, need to be explored. These are political and ethical issues that are at the base of a global health care strategy. For example:

1. Who has the right to decide or control what is the 'right' price of an ICD or any other therapy?
2. In the health care system, do open markets and competition exist?
3. Or, conversely, is some kind of political control of prices justified?
4. Who should make the decision regarding the maximum affordable cost to save 1 year of life?

5. How should the latent conflicts of interest between industry and scientific societies be resolved [2]?
6. How should the latent conflicts of interest between industry and the authors of clinical practice guidelines be resolved [9]?

Discussion and Perspectives

ICDs, largely due to their proven efficacy as a life-saving therapy, have created quite a dilemma for health care providers. On the one hand, following years of prospective, controlled, clinical trials, the evidence base (number of positive studies) in support of ICD therapy is stronger than for *any other medical therapy* [10, 11]. On the other hand, the up-front costs are high, and–precisely due to the proven clinical efficacy of ICDs–the numbers of patients receiving this therapy is increasing rapidly. There could be as much as a ten-fold increase in the number of implants during the next 10–15 years (corresponding to a prudent epidemiological estimate of 400 000 patients needing an ICD according to the present indications, as recently updated by the European Society of Cardiology [12]). Even were this to occur, the corresponding expenditures would account for only 2% of total in-patient expenditures (since the cost of ICD therapy currently is 0.2% of global in-patient expenditures).

Looked upon in another way, even with this increase in patients, the number receiving ICDs would represent 0.1% of the European population (source: OECD Health Database 2004, Guidant estimates). In Italy, in 2004, ICDs were prescribed for about 8000 patients, about 0.01% of the overall Italian population; even with a five-fold increase in the number of implants during the next 5–10 years (which corresponds to a prudent epidemiological estimate of 40 000 patients needing an ICD according to the present indications), the expenditure would account for 1.5% of total in-patient expenditures and would be prescribed to 0.05% of the Italian population.

In conclusion, at least for Italy and Western countries, the dilemma between clinical needs and limited resources can reasonably be solved. Therefore, the use of ICDs should not be decided upon based on economic reasoning, but only by the appropriateness of the indications.

References

1. Camm AJ, Nisam S (2000) The utilization of the implantable defibrillator—a European enigma Eur Heart J 21:1998–04
2. Priori S, Klein W, Bassand JP (2003) Medical practice guidelines. Separating science from economics. Eur Heart J 24:1962–1964

3. Cartabellotta A (1996) Evidence-based medicine: the cultural response to the new hospital payment system. The Italian Group on Evidence-Based Medicine (GIMBE) Epidemiol Prev 20:301–303
4. Sackett D, Richardson WS, Rosenberg W et al (1998) Evidence-based medicine. Churchill Livingston, Edinburgh
5. Salukhe T, Dimopoulos K, Sutton R, et al (2004) Life-years gained from defibrillator implantation. Circulation 109:1848–1853
6. Brown RE, Henderson RA, Koster D, Simoons M (2002) Cost effectiveness of eptifibatide in acute coronary syndromes; an economic analysis of Western European patients enrolled in the PURSUIT trial. The Platelet IIa/IIb in unstable Angina: Receptor Suppression Using Integrilin Therapy. Eur Heart J 23:50–58
7. Kupersmith et al (1995) Cost-effectiveness of some therapeutic interventions. Prog Cardiovasc Dis; 37: 307–346
8. van Hout BA, Simoons ML (2001) Cost-effectiveness of HMG coenzyme reductase inhibitors; whom to treat? Eur Heart J 22:751–761
9. Choudhry NK, Stelfox HT, Detsky AS (2002) Relationships between authors of clinical practice guidelines and the pharmaceutical industry JAMA; 287: 612–617
10. Nanthakumar K, Epstein AE, Kay GN et al (2004) Prophylactic implantable cardioverter-defibrillator therapy in patients with left ventricular systolic dysfunction: a pooled analysis of 10 primary prevention trials. J Am Coll Cardiol 44:2166–2172
11. Desai AS, Fang JC, Maisel WH et al (2004) Implantable defibrillators for the prevention of mortality in patients with nonischaemic cardiomyopathy: a meta-analysis of randomized controlled trials. JAMA 292:2874–2879
12. K. Swedberg, Cleland G, Dargi H et al (2005) ESC Guidelines. http://www.escardio.org/knowledge/guidelines/Chronic%20Heart%20failure%20Slide-set%202005, last access May 19, 2005

Cost-Effectiveness and Aspects of Health Economics in Primary Prevention: What Is the Case of Dilated Cardiomyopathy?

G. Boriani, M. Biffi, C. Martignani, C. Valzania, I. Diemberger, M. Ziacchi, D. Saporito, P. Artale, M. Bertini, C. Rapezzi, A. Branzi

Existing Evidence on Treatment With Electrical Devices in Heart Failure/Left Ventricular Dysfunction

Heart failure (HF) is increasing in prevalence in Western societies, and currently affects about 6.5 million people in Europe. In patients with HF or left ventricular dysfunction, there is a substantial risk of sudden cardiac death. Although important advances have been made in pharmacological therapy for HF, its effects on mortality and morbidity are limited with regard to sudden death prevention. Attention is therefore increasingly being focused on the role of implantable devices in HF: implantable cardioverter defibrillator (ICD), cardiac resynchronisation therapy (CRT), and combination devices (CRT-D).

Three key studies (SCD-HeFT, COMPANION, and CARE-HF) provided compelling evidence that ICD and CRT-D devices should be considered in specifically selected patients with HF of either ischaemic or non-ischaemic aetiology [1–3]. In clinical practice, these patients comprise a sizeable proportion of patients requiring medical care for HF.

SCD-HeFT was a multicentre double-blind study designed to test the effect of an ICD versus amiodarone or placebo in a broad population of HF patients [1]. Among the 2521 patients included, 70% were in NYHA class II and the remainder in class III. All had an LVEF $\leq$ 35%. Similar numbers of participants had HF of ischaemic (52%) or non-ischaemic origin (48%). All the patients were on optimised medical treatment and were randomised to placebo, amiodarone, or a conservatively programmed single-lead ICD. Over

Institute of Cardiology, University of Bologna, Azienda Ospedaliera S.Orsola-Malpighi, Bologna, Italy a 3-year follow-up, amiodarone had no beneficial effect on survival. In contrast, ICD therapy decreased the risk of death (the primary endpoint) by 23% ($P = 0.007$). In total, 17% of ICD recipients died, compared with 22% of those receiving placebo and 24% of those receiving amiodarone. Importantly, the ICD was beneficial regardless of whether HF was ischaemic or non-ischaemic. A subgroup analysis of SCD-HeFT suggested that the ICD significantly improved survival only in NYHA class II patients. The authors noted that this finding conflicted with those of MADIT II and DEFINITE, and should not be taken as a basis for withholding ICD therapy from patients in NYHA III.

COMPANION was a multicentre randomised study that included 1520 patients in NYHA class III or IV with impaired left ventricular function (LVEF ≤ 35%) [2]. Importantly, each patient also had a wide QRS (QRS duration ≥ 120 ms). Patients were randomised to optimal pharmacological therapy alone, CRT alone, or CRT-D. In a follow-up of 12 months, the primary endpoint (all-cause mortality plus all-cause hospitalisation) was reduced by 19% ($P = 0.014$) with CRT and by 20% ($P = 0.01$) with CRT-D. The risk of the combined secondary endpoint of death from or hospitalisation for HF was significantly reduced by 34% ($P < 0.002$) with CRT and by 40% with CRT-D ($P < 0.001$). The additional secondary endpoint of all-cause mortality was significantly reduced by 24% (0.059). NYHA class, the distance walked in 6 min, and quality of life were also significantly improved by CRT or CRT-D.

Most recently, the CARE-HF trial has confirmed and clarified on 813 patients the findings of COMPANION with regard to CRT [3]. The inclusion criteria of CARE-HF were NYHA class III or IV with LVEF ≤ 35%, and evidence of dyssynchrony (QRS duration ≥ 120 ms). The study compared optimised medical treatment with optimised medical treatment plus CRT. In contrast to COMPANION, CARE-HF did not include treatment with CRT-D. Over a mean follow-up of 29 months, compared with optimised treatment alone, CRT reduced the primary endpoint of death from any cause or any unplanned hospitalisation for a major cardiovascular event by 37%. Only 39% of patients treated with CRT reached this endpoint compared with 55% of those receiving optimised medical treatment ($P < 0.001$). CARE-HF provided an answer to the question whether CRT alone saves lives. Indeed, CRT significantly reduced the principal secondary endpoint of all-cause mortality by 36%, compared with optimised medical treatment alone ($P < 0.002$). The benefits of CRT were similar in patients with ischaemic and non-ischaemic disease. It is noteworthy, however, that 35% of the deaths in the CRT limb of CARE-HF were sudden, suggesting that including ICD back-up would have been more effective, in view of the known ability of ICD to reduce the incidence of sudden death.

Efficacy of Cardioverter-Defibrillators in Non-ischaemic Cardiomyopathy

Randomised clinical trials on the role of ICD in patients with left ventricular dysfunction/heart failure have included a variable proportion of patients without prior myocardial infarction, affected by so-called non ischaemic cardiomyopathy. However, no single prospective randomised controlled trial on ICD therapy in non-ischaemic cardiomyopathy has provided conclusive evidence of a reduction in mortality. Moreover, although up to 30% of deaths occurring in non-ischaemic cardiomyopathy have the characteristics of sudden death, the electrophysiological mechanism leading to sudden death in this subset of patients is poorly understood [4]. In these trials, a lower than anticipated mortality in the control group and systematic underpowering of the trials may have been the reason for failure to demonstrate ICD benefit.

A meta-analysis of randomised controlled trials studied 1854 patients with non-ischaemic cardiomyopathy enrolled in five primary prevention trials. Pooled analysis suggested a significant reduction in total mortality among patient randomised to ICD (or CRT-D in COMPANION) vs medical therapy (RR = 0.69, 95% CI 0.55–0.87, P = 0.002). Assuming a mortality of approximately 7% per year (averaged control group mortality of the five trials) and a 33% relative risk reduction, the absolute risk reduction for all-cause mortality is approximately 2% for year, with a NNT (number needed to be treated) = 25 at 2 years (compared with a NNT around 18 for ischaemic cardiomyopathy) [4].

From Scientific Evidence to Evidence-Based Clinical Practice: The Issue of Costs

The evidence from randomised controlled trials indicates that serious clinical consideration should be given to device therapy (in addition to optimal medical therapy) in all patients in NYHA classes III–IV with an LVEF $\leq$ 35%, regardless of the aetiology of their HF, also including patients with non-ischaemic cardiomyopathy. Selection of the most appropriate device depends on the patient's medical need and the physician's judgement. Device therapy offers substantial benefits in addition to those achieved by optimal medical therapy.

Incorporation of this evidence into national and international guidelines and reimbursement policies should result in more patients receiving potentially life-saving device therapy. In the USA, as noted above, Medicare coverage for CRT and ICD implantation has already been extended to include the patient categories covered by COMPANION and SCD-HeFT. This evidence-based approach, if translated into current clinical practice, has the potential to improve the survival of patients affected by HF.

The ICD has traditionally been seen as an expensive form of treatment, with high up-front costs due to the device itself and the implant (followed over time by maintenance costs for device replacement). Since the ICD first appeared in clinical practice, the indications for use of ICDS have broadened dramatically, from a few selected patients with previous cardiac arrest to a large cohort of patients with heterogeneous underlying heart diseases, identified as subjects at high risk of sudden death [5–8]. Transvenous implantation has markedly decreased the hospitalisation costs and has contributed to widespread use of ICD systems. Despite marked price reductions in the last decade, the cost issue continues to limit full acceptance and application of ICD therapy, especially as regards increased use for primary prevention of sudden death [5–9].

There are various methods to assess the economic implications of a medical intervention: cost-benefit analysis, cost-effectiveness analysis, and cost-utility analysis. Moreover, economic analysis of medical interventions must also take into consideration controlled trials, and effectiveness is the actual decrease in disease that is achieved when the intervention is applied over a large, non-homogeneous population.

Cost-effectiveness analysis aims at evaluating the cost of any therapeutic intervention related to the possible benefits [5–9]. The cost of a therapy is the sum of direct costs (initial cost of therapy, costs to maintain therapy, and costs caused by unfavourable effects or by complications) and of indirect costs paid by the patient's family or by the community. The efficacy of a particular treatment is defined as the mean number of years survived by means of a therapy to an adverse event. Usually, incremental cost-effectiveness analysis is considered when two new therapeutic strategies are compared. The cost-effectiveness ratio is often expressed in dollars per year of life saved ($/YLS). In the literature [5], a treatment is considered valid if the cost-effectiveness ratio ranges between 0 and 20 000 $/YLS, convenient if the cost-effectiveness ratio ranges between 20 000 and 40 000 $/YLS, and borderline if the cost-effectiveness ratio ranges between 40 000 and 60 000 $/YLS. It is considered unfavourable if the cost-effectiveness ratio ranges between 60 000 and 100 000 $/YLS, and absolutely unfavourable above 100 000 $/YLS. It is evident that the cost-effectiveness ratio can greatly change depending on the type of population in treatment. The identification of high-risk patients ('patient targeting') seems to be the most important issue to reach a favourable cost-effectiveness ratio.

Use of ICDs in selected patients (or subgroups of patients) at high-risk of sudden death has often generated cost-effectiveness estimates that are comparable with or lower than other accepted treatments, including renal dialysis, which costs about 50 000–60 000 $/YLS [5]. In Fig. 1 the cost-effective-

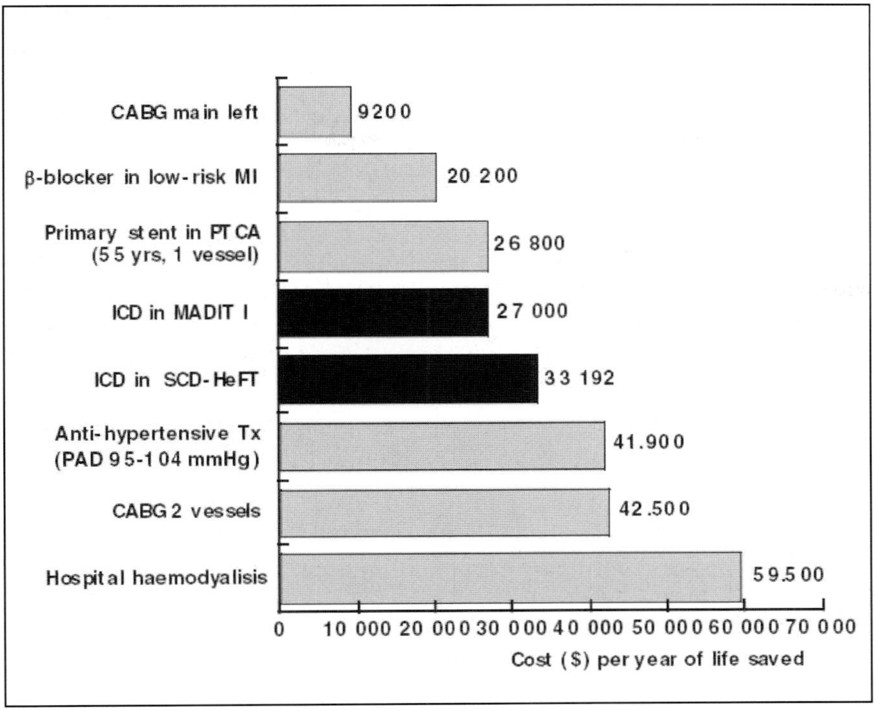

Fig. 1. Cost-effectiveness estimates (in dollars per year of life saved) for a series of widely used medical treatments compared to cardioverter-defibrillator (ICD) in MADIT I and SCD-HeFT indications. *CABG* Coronary artery by-pass graft, *MI* myocardial infarction, *Tx* treatment, *ICD* implantable cardioverter-defibrillator

ness of a series of treatments currently used in clinical practice is compared to some cost-effectiveness data related to ICDs in MADIT and SCD-HeFT trials, respectively.

In the general view, however, cost-effectiveness evaluations on ICDs have revealed a broad range of cost-effectiveness ratios, ranging from economically attractive to very expensive values. Recent randomised trials have provided less attractive ratios than those derived from the initial modeling studies [5–9]. A further source of variability is the time horizon within which cost-effectiveness is estimated. When Hlatky and Bigger [7] projected the results of all the trials published until 2001 to gauge the full gain in life expectancy, they obtained a cost-effectiveness ratio of 31 500 $/YLS, in line with what is currently considered fully acceptable in Western countries.

Another important variable regards the ICD setting (primary/secondary prevention of sudden death). For primary prevention of sudden death, the economic analysis of SCD-HeFT estimated a favourable cost-effectiveness value of 33 192 $/YLS (data were obtained by a model that considered a 2.4-year increase in life expectancy in favour of ICD therapy) [10].

An important limitation of currently available ICD cost-effectiveness estimates is the lack of data on long-term benefits. It should be noted that none of the randomised controlled trials was specifically conceived for assessing cost-effectiveness as one of the primary end-points [7, 8]. Prospective studies specifically designed to evaluate cost-effectiveness over time could be extremely valuable for health-care systems, especially in the case of non-ischaemic cardiomyopathy.

Reduced implantation costs is another way of making ICD therapy more economically feasible. The possibility of implanting a single-chamber ICD on an outpatient basis was explored in the SCD-HeFT trial [1]. The results showed that this approach was associated with a favorable cost-effectiveness value of 33192 $/YLS [10]. Further evaluations are required to assess which patients are candidates for this type of procedure.

Further long-term evaluation of the cost-effectiveness and cost-utility of ICDs could also provide a basis for identifying subsets of patients for whom the implant can be considered affordable within the context of current prices and prevailing economic constraints. Such evaluations could readily be reviewed to take advantage of any price cuts.

A further economic issue regards the use of ICDs to provide cardiac resynchronisation therapy in the HF setting [11–13]. The problem is particularly interesting, because ICDs are of proven efficacy in terms of quality of life as well as reduced morbidity and mortality, as validated by prospective controlled studies [11–13].

Conclusions

The low risk of ICD implantation and the evidence that these devices successfully terminate life-threatening ventricular tachyarrhythmias have prompted the use of ICDs in the primary prevention of sudden death in specific clinical conditions associated with a substantially increased risk of sudden arrhythmic death, including non-ischaemic cardiomyopathy. Despite continuing price reductions, cost is likely to remain a major determinant of the complete acceptance and implementation of ICD therapy. Therefore, the problem of how broadened evidence-based indications for implantation can be translated into the 'real world' remains to be addressed and resolved, considering currently available economic resources. Cost-effectiveness analysis provides the most appropriate tool for weighing costs against benefits for both ICD and CRT-D and should be directed towards specifically defined subsets of patients, including those with non-ischaemic cardiomyopathy.

References

1. Bardy GH, Lee KL, Mark DB et al (2005) Amiodarone or an implantable cardioverter-defibrillator for congestive heart failure. N Engl J Med 352:225–237
2. Bristow MR, Saxon LA, Boehmer J et al (2004) Cardiac resynchronization therapy with or without an implantable defibrillator in advanced chronic heart failure. N Engl J Med 350:2140–2150
3. Cleland JG, Daubert JC, Erdmann E et al (2005) The effect of cardiac resynchronization on morbidity and mortality in heart failure. N Engl J Med 352:1539–1549
4. Desai AS, Fang JC, Maisel WH et al (2004) Implantable defibrillators for the prevention of mortality in patients with nonischemic cardiomyopathy: a meta-analysis of randomized controlled trials. JAMA 292:2874–2479
5. Boriani G, Biffi M, Martignani C et al (2001) Cost-effectiveness of implantable cardioverter-defibrillators. Eur Heart J 22:990–996
6. Boriani G, Biffi M, Martignani C et al (2003) Cardioverter-defibrillators after MADIT II: the balance between weight of evidence and treatment costs. Eur J Heart Failure 5:419–425
7. Hlatky MA, Bigger JT (2001) Cost-effectiveness of the implantable cardioverter defibrillator? Lancet 357:1817–1818
8. Boriani G, Biffi M, Martignani C (2005) Long-term efficacy of cardioverter-defibrillators: implications for cost-effectiveness. Circulation 111:e26
9. Essebag V, Eisenberg MJ (2003) Expanding indications for defibrillators after myocardial infarction: risk stratification and cost effectiveness. Card Electrophysiol Rev 7:43–48
10. Mark DB (2004) Cost-effectiveness of ICD therapy in the Sudden Death in Heart Failure Trial (SCD-HeFT). Presented at the Late Breaking Trials session of the Annual Meeting of the American Heart Association, November 10, 2004, New Orleans, LA, USA
11. Boriani G, Biffi M, Martignani C et al (2004) Cardiac resynchronization by pacing: an electrical treatment of heart failure. Int J Cardiol 94:151–161
12. Auricchio A, Abraham WT (2004) Cardiac resynchronization therapy: current state of the art: cost versus benefit. Circulation 109:300–307
13. McAlister FA, Ezekowitz JA, Wiebe N et al (2004) Systematic review: cardiac resynchronization in patients with symptomatic heart failure. Ann Intern Med 141:381–390

Public Access Defibrillation: How Widespread Is It and What Are the Short-Term and Long-Term Results?

A. CAPUCCI, D. ASCHIERI, G.Q. VILLANI

Public access to defibrillation means making automated external defibrillators available in public and/or private places where large numbers of people gather or people who are at high risk of heart attacks live. The automated external defibrillator is a computerised medical device that can check a person's heart rhythm. It can recognise a potentially lethal rhythm that requires a shock and it can advise the rescuer when a shock is needed. The automatic external defibrillator uses voice prompts, lights, and text messages to tell the rescuer the steps to take. The concept of public access defibrillation is based on deductive reasoning. Early defibrillation improves outcome from cardiac arrest due to ventricular defibrillation (VF) [1–4]. The increased availability of automatic external defibrillators should result in earlier defibrillation, leading to better outcome from cardiac arrest. This concept has not been still proved prospectively.

Public access defibrillation dates from 1986, when the first defibrillator for public use became available. However, the concept failed to gain support for several reasons, particularly the lack of acceptance by physicians. Such devices were available through prescription, but few were prescribed despite family acceptance being reasonable, particularly in high-risk families. Cost and reimbursement also slowed acceptance. Current enthusiasm for public access defibrillation has been spurred by recent breakthroughs in automatic external defibrillator technology. Portable defibrillators can be deployed in two ways in the community: (1) in the vehicles of emergency personnel, such as police officers, who are otherwise not equipped with advanced life-support equipment or a defibrillator; or (2) in fixed locations, such as casinos,

Cardiology Department, Guglielmo da Saliceto Hospital, Piacenza, Italy

airports, health clubs, office buildings, shopping malls, or government offices. The ideal primary outcome would be 30-day survival with intact neurological function [5]. However, it may be impractical to use this as an outcome, because individual consent would be needed to examine patients and medical records. Because informed consent may be difficult to obtain after resuscitation from sudden cardiac arrest, information about functional outcomes will be missing for some patients. If this information is missing for a large number of patients or is preferentially missing for patients enrolled in one intervention arm or the other, then the results of the study may be biased. As an alternative, a primary outcome of 30-day survival could be supplemented by information about hospital discharge status.

Results of Public Access Defibrillation

An important report from Seattle, Washington, examined 'public' location in cardiac arrest [6]. These investigators again confirmed that most cardiac arrests occur in the home (76%); only 16% occur in public sites. The most common public location for cardiac arrest was Seattle Tacoma Airport, where seven cardiac arrests occurred each year. Penitentiaries were the second most common location. Shopping malls had an average of 0.7 arrests each year, and sporting arenas 0.4 each year during major events. Other, less frequent locations included hotels, government offices, schools, and churches.

The clinical situations in which the defibrillator has been shown to have the greatest efficacy to date are airports and casinos [7, 8]. These two settings are similar to each other in several ways. In both, large numbers of dedicated workers are present in a relatively small geographic area, and large numbers of people who could experience sudden cardiac arrest are in daily proximity to the defibrillator. In the studies conducted in these settings, 40% or more of individuals experiencing cardiac arrest survived; this is a far higher percentage than that typically achieved anywhere else outside of a hospital.

Results of defibrillator deployment and use in other situations may have less benefit. The Public Access Defibrillation (PAD) [9] trial was a multi-centre study in which community-based training was employed in 'high-risk' settings. The settings included facilities with more than 250 persons aged over 50 years on site for most of the day, or sites where a cardiac arrest had occurred within the past 2 years. A total of 1260 facilities were included. The community sites were mostly recreation, shopping, and entertainment facilities. Sites were randomised to have rescuers trained in CPR alone or rescuers trained in CPR and defibrillator use. Approximately 20 000 lay volunteers were trained, representing almost 10 volunteers per available defibrillator. The primary endpoint of the study was survival to hospital discharge. More cardiac arrests occurred in the CPR–defibrillator locations ($n = 129$) than in the CPR alone locations ($n = 103$). Twenty-nine patients in the CPR-defibrillator group survived to hospital discharge, compared with only 15 in the CPR alone group ($P = 0.042$). The survival rate in the CPR–defibrillator group was 22.5%. The PAD study showed that fixed-location defibrillators were useful even though the survival benefit seen was far more modest than in previous smaller, uncontrolled studies.

Recently, findings from Culley et al. [10] suggested a greater benefit from the use of public access defibrillation. In an observational study performed in Seattle, Washington, 475 defibrillators were deployed under emergency medical service (EMS)-guided surveillance. The majority of the devices were placed in areas such as shopping malls, but use of a defibrillator by mobile police was also included. Over 1% of cardiac arrests were treated with a defibrillator (1.33%), and survival to hospital discharge was a remarkable 50%. However, preliminary results in Seattle are backed by the best emergency medical response system in the world and thus may be difficult to reproduce elsewhere.

Defibrillators as Part of a Mobile EMS System

Defibrillators have also been used as an adjunct to EMS response systems. In this approach, emergency workers such as police and fire workers are equipped with defibrillators in the absence of other advanced cardiac life-support equipment and are dispatched in parallel with ambulances to cardiac arrests. Two large trials have examined the efficacy of this approach [11, 12]. Myerburg et al. [11] established such a system in Dade County, Florida, comparing outcomes of patients treated with defibrillators against the outcomes of historical controls in a non-randomised study. They found that response times to defibrillation were decreased by the dual deployment system and that survival to hospital admission was more likely among patients treated with rapid defibrillation. Unfortunately, 61% of patients in the study presented with non-shockable rhythms, and therefore, no significant improvement in survival to hospital discharge was demonstrated.

Results similar to those in the Myerburg study but less significant were obtained in a prospective randomised trial performed in the Netherlands [12]. A witnessed cardiac arrest occurred in 469 subjects who were then randomised to receive a routine EMS response or a dual dispatch system response that included a police-equipped defibrillator. Although survival to hospital admission was higher in the police defibrillator-equipped group, survival to hospital discharge was 15% in the control group and 18% in the police group, a difference that was not significant.

Based on data from these two studies, it appears that providing rescue workers with vehicle-equipped defibrillators improves response times but not long-term outcomes. The reason for this disappointing dichotomy is not yet completely clear. It may be that improvements in existing defibrillator algorithms or in post-arrest treatment will be needed before defibrillator use can demonstrate significant outcome improvement.

However, better results in respect of short- and long-term survival have been obtained in other studies. In our study, too, Piacenza Progetto Vita, police equipped with automatic external defibrillators and conventional EMS responders are simultaneously deployed to possible cardiac arrests [13]. Policemen and lay responders were trained to use automatic external defibrillator on a brief defibrillation training course without CPR instruction. While survival to hospital admission was higher in the EMS group, survival rate to hospital discharge was significantly higher in the lay volunteers group (43.7%) than in the EMS group (16.6%) ($P < 0.01$). Neurologically intact survival rate was also higher in PPV-treated than in EMS-treated patients. These patients were long-term survivors (more than 1 year). Only two patients died within 1 year, from non-cardiac causes (ictus and pulmonary cancer). The only intervention with a public defibrillator positioned in a fixed place (main city square) was recorded after 5 years from the beginning of the project, and was successfully.

White et al. of the Mayo Clinic in Rochester, Minnesota, reported their findings on police-initiated defibrillation [14]. The Rochester police department were equipped with automatic external defibrillators, on the reasoning that the police often arrive first at an emergency, and some of these could include cardiac arrest. Forty-one of 108 patients having a cardiac arrest were first shocked by the police. Spontaneous circulation was restored without additional advance cardiac life support in 14 patients (34%). These patients were long-term survivors. Among patients in whom spontaneous circulation could not be restored before arrival of the paramedics and who needed further advanced cardiac life support, only 22% were long-term survivors. The survival rate when police deliver the first shock is 49%, compared with 43% when paramedics initiate early defibrillation.

Mosesso et al. [15] reported on a similar type of project in the suburbs of Pittsburgh, Pennsylvania. A historical control was used from a time when the police were not equipped with automatic external defibrillators. The time from emergency call to delivery of the first shock was 11.8 min during the control period. After the police were equipped with automatic external defibrillators that time dropped to 8.7 min ($P < 0.0001$). Restoration of spontaneous circulation improved from 36% to 52% ($P < 0.03$), and survival more than doubled from 6% to 14% ($P = 0.10$).When the police arrived first during the control years, only 3% of patients with cardiac arrest survived. A survival rate of 26% has been achieved since the police were issued with automatic external defibrillators ($P < 0.05$).

In 1991 Qantas Airlines became the first major operational airline to deploy automatic external defibrillators on overseas flights. Several airlines had trialled such strategies, but none continued them. O'Rourke and Donaldson reported on 5 years' experience of the Qantas automatic external defibrillator programme [16]. Automatic external defibrillators were used 87 times: in 47 cases for monitoring – typically in patients with chest pain or palpitations – and in 40 for cardiac arrests. Twenty-two cardiac arrests occurred in the aircraft, while 18 occurred in the airport terminal. Six cardiac arrests in the aircraft were due to VF. Five of the six patients were successfully defibrillated with automatic external defibrillators, and two of six were long-term survivors with excellent neurological function. A major problem was uncovered when these initial data were reviewed, namely that most cardiac arrests in the aircraft were discovered early in VF. Cardiac arrest in airport terminals (18 of 40 cases) have a different pattern. Fifteen of these 18 patients had VF: each of the 15 was successfully defibrillated with the device. Four of these 15 patients were neurologically intact, long-term survivors.

Further support for a beneficial effect on survival of early defibrillation in the community is given by the data of the prospective cohort study conducted in Olmstead County [17, 18]. All patients who had an out-of-hospital cardiac arrest between November 1990 and December 2000, after implementation of a local early defibrillation program, were followed to determine long-term survival and quality of life. Of the 200 patients with an out-of-hospital cardiac arrest with ventricular fibrillation, 145 (72%) survived to hospital admission with spontaneous circulation, 84 (42%) survived to hospital discharge, and 79 (40%) were neurologically intact at discharge. Long-term survival was seen in 60 patients (30%). For the purposes of the analysis, patients with significant neurological impairment at discharge were considered non-survivors. The mean length of follow-up was 4.8 years (standard deviation 3.0 years). The expected 5-year survival rate (79%) was identical to that among age-, sex- and disease-matched controls. The long-term survival and quality of life of patients resuscitated from a cardiac arrest has been demonstrated to be similar to that of control subjects from the general population.

Conclusions

There is no question but that early defibrillation will save lives. Despite the existence of well-developed emergency medical services with rapid-response advanced life support capabilities, survival rates following out-of-hospital VF have remained low. Generally, these poor resuscitation rates are attributed to delays in the performance of basic cardiopulmonary resuscitation by bystanders or delays in defibrillation.

The appropriateness of having defibrillators available in public places such as schools, apartment buildings, and offices is becoming clear. The PAD trial has demonstrated that training and equipping volunteers to attempt early defibrillation within a structured response system can increase the number of survivors to hospital discharge after out-of-hospital cardiac arrest in public locations. In airports, aeroplanes, casinos, and other high-risk locations, public use of external defibrillators should be strongly supported. In addition, efforts by private individuals to obtain defibrillators for homes and businesses seem justified. Dual EMS systems incorporating defibrillators have also shown good improvements in outcomes compared to EMS alone. In our opinion, public access defibrillation is here to stay.

References

1. Haskell WL (1978) Cardiovascular complications during exercise training of cardiac patients. Circulation 57:920–924
2. Cummins RO (1989) From concept to standard-of-care? Review of the clinical experience with automated external defibrillators. Ann Emerg Med 18:1269–1275
3. Stults KR, Brown DD, Schug VL et al (1984) Prehospital defibrillation performed by emergency medical technicians in rural communities. N Engl J Med 310:219–223
4. Eisenberg MS, Bergner L, Hallstrom A (1979) Paramedic programs and out-of-hospital cardiac arrest. I: factors associated with successful resuscitation. Am J Public Health 69:30–38
5. Nichol G, Hallstrom AP, Kerber R et al (1998) American Heart Association report on the second public access defibrillation conference, April 17–19, 1997. Circulation 97:1309–1314
6. Becker LB, Ostrander MP, Barrett J et al (1991) Outcome of CPR in a large metropolitan area: where are the survivors? Ann Emerg Med 19:179–186
7. Caffrey SL, Willoughby PJ, Pepe PE et al (2002) Public use of automated external defibrillators. N Engl J Med 347:1242–1247
8. Valenzuela TD, Roe GN, Clark LL et al (2000) Outcomes of rapid defibrillation by security officers after cardiac arrest in casinos. N Engl J Med 343:1206–1209
9. Hallstrom AP, Ornato JP, Weisfeldt M et al (2004) Public-access defibrillation and survival after out-of-hospital cardiac arrest. Public Access Defibrillation Trial Investigators. N Engl J Med 351:637–646
10. Culley LL, Rea TD, Murray JA et al (2004) Public access defibrillation in out-of-hospital cardiac arrest: a community-based study. Circulation 109:1859–1863
11. Myerburg RJ, Fenster J, Velez M (2002) Impact of community-wide police car deployment of automated external defibrillators on survival from out-of-hospital cardiac arrest. Circulation 106:1058–1064
12. Waalewijn RA, de Vos R, Tijssen JG et al (2001) Survival models for out-of-hospital cardiopulmonary resuscitation from the perspectives of the bystander, the first

responder, and the paramedic. Resuscitation 51:113–122
13. Capucci D, Aschieri MF, Piepoli MF et al (2002) Tripling survival from sudden cardiac arrest via early defibrillation without traditional education in cardiopulmonary resuscitation. Circulation 106:1065–1070
14. White RD, Asplin BR, Bugliosi TF et al (1996) High discharge survival rate after out-of-hospital ventricular fibrillation with rapid defibrillation by police and paramedics. Ann Emerg Med 28:480–485
15. Mosesso VN Jr, Davis EA, Auble TE et al (1998) Use of automated external defibrillators by police officers for treatment of out-of-hospital cardiac arrest. Ann Emerg Med 32:200–207
16. O'Rourke MF, Donaldson E (1997) The first five years of the Quantas cardiac arrest program. J Am Coll Cardiol 29:404 (abs)
17. Mahapatra S, Bunch TJ, White RD et al (2005) Sex differences in outcome after ventricular fibrillation in out-of-hospital cardiac arrest. Resuscitation 65:197–202

In-Hospital Cardiac Arrest: How to Improve Survival?

M. Santomauro[1], A. Borrelli[1], C. Riganti[2], C. Liguori[1], E. Febbraro[1], M. D'Onofrio[3], N. Monteforte[1], S. Buonerba[1], M. Chiariello[1]

A cardiac problem is often the substrate for cardiac arrest (CA) (Table 1), but other diseases may be the underlying cause of sudden death, which in 75% of cases is due to ventricular fibrillation (VF) or ventricular tachycardia (VT), in 20% to bradyarrythmia, and in 5% to atrioventricular dissociation [1–5]. In Italy, CA strikes more than 60 000 people/year, with a 10% overall mortality, 20% of which occurs in people with no signs of disease at all [1]. The chance of survival in case of CA strictly depends on the rapidity of intervention and on the correct execution of four basic, but fundamental steps – the 'chain of survival' [2]. The very first step is activation of the emergency system, in case the patient is unconsciousness (of course, this step involves activating local emergency services). This is immediately followed by step 2, basic cardiopulmonary resuscitation, also known as basic life support (BLS) [3], which consists of a sequence of chest compressions and artificial ventilation. Defibrillation, the third step, is the only therapy able to stop VF/VT, the main cause of death in CA, while advanced cardiopulmonary resuscitation or advanced cardiac life support (ACLS) is the last step. Since its discovery, external defibrillation has been the cornerstone of emergency cardiac care (ECC) and the principal intervention in most successful resuscitations from full cardiac arrest.

A large body of out-of-hospital research [4, 6–9] shows that the rapidity of defibrillation is the most important determinant of survival in CA due to shockable arrhythmia.

Even though most CAs occur outside hospitals, the problem is still a major concern inside the hospital. In Italian hospitals, 85% of patients hospi-

[1]Department of Cardiology, University 'Federico II', Naples; [2]Health Management, University 'Federico II', Naples; [3]Intensive Care Unit, University 'Federico II', Naples, Italy

Table 1. Heart disease that may cause sudden cardiac death in patients less than 30 years and in those older than 30 years. The most frequent disease that causes sudden death in patients ≤ 30 years is hypertrophic cardiomyopathy (50%), while the incidence of coronary artery disease is about 3–20%. In patients older than 30 years, the incidence of coronary artery disease is about 85%

Causes of sudden death < 30 years	%	Causes of sudden death > 30 years	%
Aortic stenosis	3–18	Coronary artery disease	85
Eisenmenger syndrome	15	Cardiomyopathy	10
Congenital cardiomyopathy	10	Valve disease	3
Hypertrophic cardiomyopathy	1–50	Electrical alternations	2
Right ventricular dysplasia	0–26		
Mitral prolapse	1–24		
Coronary artery disease	3–20		

talised in general medicine divisions die of sudden death, while mortality is less than 10% for patients hospitalised in intensive care units. Survival rates of CA patients outside critical care units remains about 15% at best, and survival is consistently lower in general units than in critical care areas [10–15]. Explanations for this lack of progress usually involve comorbidity and unwitnessed arrests among patients in general units [14–20].

Defibrillation, in Italian hospitals, often occurs very late and not easily, as a result of either inadequate means, i.e. defibrillators, or the presence of architectural and institutional barriers, which may obstruct intervention. A defibrillator sometimes is available only in specific divisions of the hospital, and in some cases it is useless for technical reasons or due to the lack of experience of the staff. Furthermore, most of the time, intervention is carried out by a medical team from departments other than the cardiology department or the emergency room, and usually with a lengthy delay, which becomes even longer if, in the meanwhile, cardiopulmonary resuscitation (CPR) has not been carried out. General-medicine nurses are in the most difficult position of anyone involved in the resuscitation effort. They are expected to respond immediately to unanticipated crises, unlike members of the emergency team, who have time to collect their wits while in transit to the scene. More importantly, several factors preordain the almost certain failure of attempts by general-medicine nurses to initiate basic CPR and defibrillation. Administering basic CPR has been shown to be difficult for all levels of health care providers, even in non-stressful classroom simulations [21, 22], so that in an actual in-hospital cardiac arrest administering CPR is even harder and thus takes longer. Furthermore, in the emotionally stressful setting of an actual arrest, several preparatory steps must be taken: acquiring a respiratory barrier device, bringing a crash cart with cardiac board to the scene, and placing the cardiac board under the patient (a two-person task) [23, 24]. Starting ventilations, chest compressions, and defibrillation requires the coordinated actions of at least two people, because the use of pocket masks and most other barrier devices makes effective one-person CPR almost impossible. Given these obstacles, effective CPR is rarely initiated before the emergency team arrives [25]. Therefore, expecting general-medicine nurses to carry out an excessively complex and difficult task in an emergency situation may cause a state of 'learned helplessness' and increased dependence on the emergency team.

Early defibrillation programs can improve survival rates significantly by shortening the time from arrest to defibrillation. Improving the speed of in-hospital defibrillation may produce even better results (Table 2).

The purpose of an in-hospital emergency service is to decrease and prevent sudden death due to CA and to avoid the onset of its complications, e.g. brain damage, kidney failure, in patients inside the entire hospital. The onset of complications vs recovery from CA are strictly related to the time of intervention, and it is well-known that survival chances decrease by 10% per minute [6], and brain damage occurs after 4–5 min of anoxia. In order to shorten intervention time and to avoid complications, the following is needed:

1. Information and sensitisation of the staff
2. Hospital staff training in CPR and defibrillation techniques
3. The presence of a hospital notification system for in-hospital emergencies

Table 2. Percentage of survival with and without immediate basic life support with defibrillation (BLS-D). Percent survival is strictly related to the immediate administration of BLSD. If BLSD does not occur immediately, and the advanced cardiac life support (ACLS) team arrives within 7–10 min of the cardiac event, survival is about 20%. If BLSD does not occur immediately and the ACLS team arrives later than 10 min after the cardiac event, survival is very low (2–8%) and is associated with irreversible brain damage. The gold standard is early activation of the ACLS team and immediate BLS-D, which leads to a survival rate of 80–90%

Action	Survival (%)
Early activation of ACLS team	
No immediately BLS-D (7–10 min)	20
Early activation of ACLS team	
No immediately BLS-D (> 10 min)	2–8 + brain damage
Early activation of ACLS team	
BLS-D immediately	80–90

4. Selection and creation of an operative team
5. Rational positioning of emergency trolleys inside the hospital
6. Standard procedures for all staff
7. Creation of a quality control system
8. Creation of a specific coordination centre for dealing with in-hospital emergencies
9. Retraining of the staff

The Naples Heart Project will try to achieve all nine goals, through instructional materials, courses, and the creation of permanent in-hospital emergency team.

The Naples Heart Project [26, 27] began on July 2001, and since then it has created about 835 first responders among the hospital staff, 440 of whom are physicians (fully trained or still in training), 310 nurses, and 85 members of the administrative staff. Our primary purpose is to train all general-medicine nurses, physicians, and other working staff which amounts to more than 3000 people, in BLS and defibrillation (BLS-D). To meet this goal, we have organised courses [11] combining theory and practice, so that the participants can develop psychomotor abilities and automatic response patterns which guarantee that the rescuer provides the best possible aid. Both the instructional material and the courses emphasise the rational basis of the 'chain of survival' and train participants in basic CPR and defibrillation techniques courses. A practical part is intended to make the rescuer feel more comfortable when aiding the victim. The courses are tailored with respect to material, duration, and final examination according to the participants, with the easiest and safest interventional approaches taught to non-medical personnel. All courses are held during one day. The course for administrative staff is 6 h in duration and is equally divided between theory and practice. Participants are trained to use a semiautomatic defibrillator, without a monitor for ECG, and with a voice system that guides the rescuer through the steps of the 'chain of survival.' Semiautomatic defibrillators are the only ones that non-medical personnel are allowed to use, as specified by Monteleone's Law, passed on April 3, 2001 [7]. Courses for nurses (Fig. 1) are 8 h long, contain more information on physiopathology of CA, and provide training in all BLS techniques and on defibrillator usage. The courses for physician are 10 h long and provide more detailed information on the physiopathology, epidemiology, and specific patterns of CA. For all groups, biphasic wave defibrillators [8] are used, as they require less energy than monophasic defibrillators and have a comparable effectiveness at a lower energy level. All the three groups take a final test, consisting of basic questions and without the requirement to interpret an ECG. Even though all participants have shown interest in the theory and practice, not all achieved a good grade at the final test. We had to re-enrol 40 candidates in another ses-

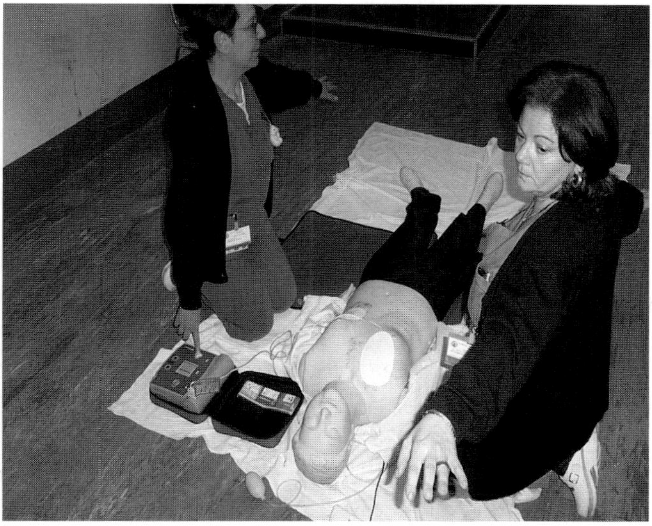

Fig. 1. Naples Heart Project BLSD first-responder course. Basic life support with defibrillation (BLS-D) training of nurses

sion and then re-test them, but positive results were achieved the second time. Since no one practices either BLS techniques or the use of defibrillators daily (with some exception), the course is repeated at least once a year and will be offered on a continual basis, including retraining after 1 year, for all the personnel.

The Naples Heart Project training centre also provides support for ACLS courses, with the goal of creating a team that offer ACLS anytime and anywhere in the hospital. ACLS courses are held over two 8-h days, during which physicians are trained in using manual defibrillators with external pacing capacity, administering drugs for the treatment of tachyarrhythmias and bradyarrhythmias, and airway intubation.

As of this writing, several sessions with 25 participants per day have been organised. The number of participants has increased from July 2001 to May 2003 (Figs. 2, 3).

The Naples Heart Project was based on a feasibility study of in-hospital emergency services. The study evaluated and analysed: type of institution, departmental and institutional dislocation, internal practicability (architectural features and preferential behaviours), staff number and distribution, presence of an emergency notification system, and instruments available. The aim is to find the best solution in order to make the chain of survival as fast and effective as possible, in every place, moment, and condition in the hospital.

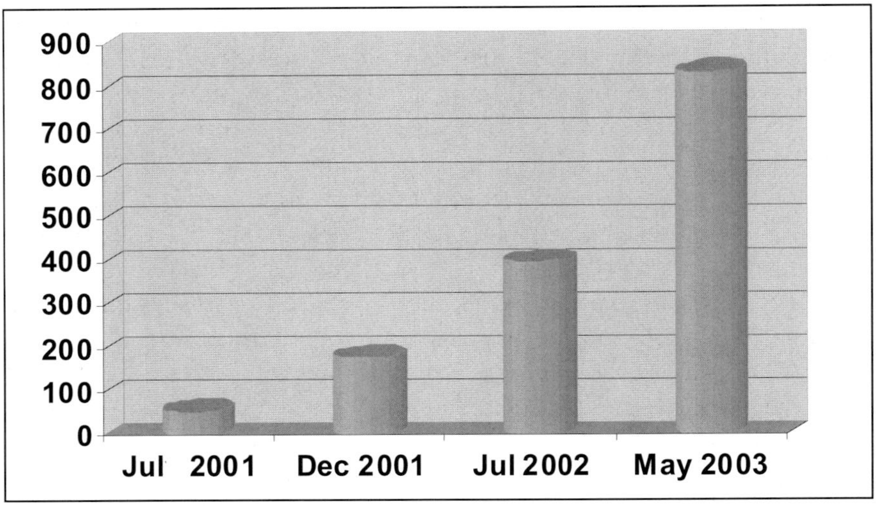

Fig. 2. Naples Heart Project BLSD first responders. The project began on July 2001, and since then it has already created about 835 BLS-D first responders among the hospital staff. Of these, 440 are specialist physicians and physicians in training, 310 are nurses and 85 are in the administrative staff

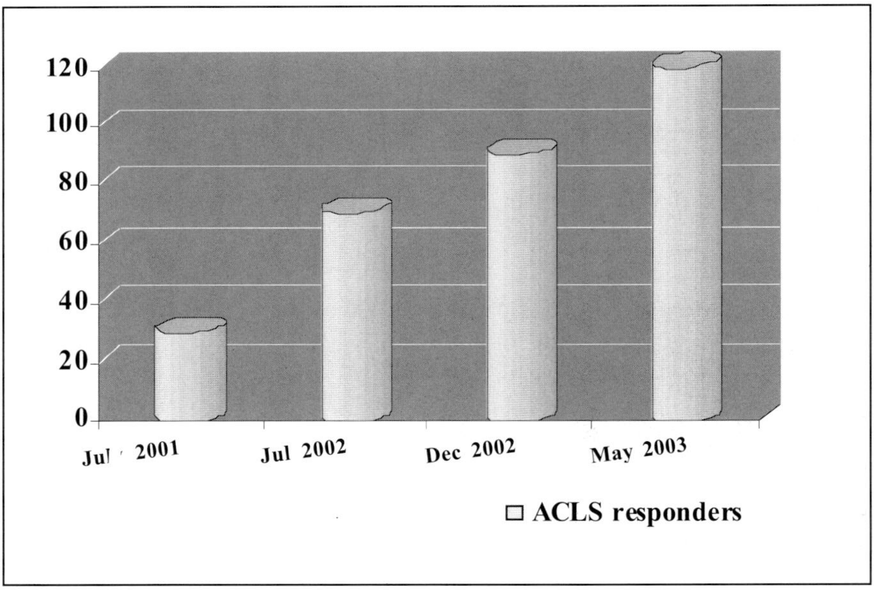

Fig. 3. Naples Heart project ACLS responders. The project's training centre provides ACLS courses in order to create an ACLS team able to respond anytime and anywhere in the hospital. Currently, 120 ACLS responders have been trained

University 'Federico II' General Hospital has about 1200 beds and is divided into separate and independent institutes. Everyday, several thousand people, including patients, physicians, technical and administrative staff, visitors, and students spend time in the general hospital. It is therefore necessary that anyone inside the general hospital is familiar with all the hospital emergency programs. In order to make this possible, we have created a brochure of the hospital emergency services, for patients and visitors, to be distributed in waiting rooms and at the main entrance. In addition, posters have been placed in every institute; meetings and conferences directed to potential BLSD providers, i.e. physicians, nurses, administrative and technical staff, have been organised. We are also planning to install a series of road signs (Fig. 4) throughout the hospital providing directions to the nearest defibrillation point.

The project also provides a rational distribution of semiautomatic defibrillators and accompanying materials, in order to have a defibrillator and a fully organised trolley for emergencies available on all floors, so that the delay due to access and transport of material is greatly decreased; furthermore it has been proposed to periodically check the emergency trolleys and other materials and to keep a checklist.

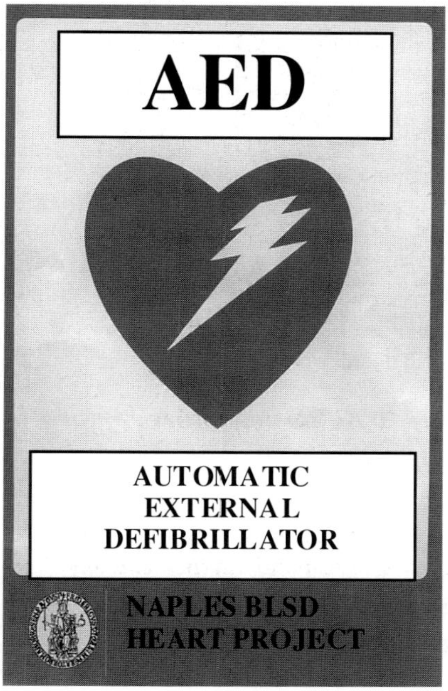

Fig.4. Defibrillation point. The Naples Heart Project provides a series of road signs throughout the hospital providing directions to the nearest defibrillation point

The project will be administered and coordinated by an in-hospital emergency system leader, who is charged with mediating contacts between the emergency team, training centre, and BLSD and ACLS providers on the one hand, and the emergency coordination group (composed of a general manager, a medical manager, and a nursing manager) on the other.

In conclusion, an in-hospital emergency has to be dealt with not as a chaotic chain, but like an organised procedure with standard protocols familiar to all staff. It is therefore necessary to organise training following a well-defined program with a fixed term; training courses must provide theoretical and practical knowledge for responding to emergency situations.

The Naples Heart Project, consisting of courses for BLS-D and ACLS responders (physicians, nurses, and staff in the general hospital), is close to achieving this goal. It is the first project of its kind in Italy, and it lays the basis for the development of a medical emergencies culture able to cope with both in and out of hospital scenarios.

References

1. Anonymous (1988) Vital statistics of the United States, 1988. National Center for Health Statistics, 2A, Hyattsville, MD, USA
2. Cummins RO, Ornato JP, Thies WH, Pepe PE (1991) Improving survival from sudden cardiac arrest: the 'chain of survival' concept. A statement for health professionals from the Advanced Cardiac Life Support Subcommittee and the Emergency Cardiac Care Committee, American Heart Association. Circulation 83(5):1832–1847
3. Anonymous (1992) Guidelines for cardiopulmonary resuscitation and emergency cardiac care, I: introduction. JAMA 268:2172–2183
4. Myerburg RJ, Kessler KM, Zaman L et al (1982) Survivors of prehospital cardiac arrest. JAMA 247:1485–1490
5. Bayes de Luna A, Coumel P, Leclercq JF (1989) Ambulatory Sudden Cardiac Death : Mechanism of production of fatal arrythmya on the basis of data from 157 cases. Am Heart J 117:151–159
6. Grotta JC (1996) The importance of time. In: proceedings of the national Symposyum on rapid identification and treatment of acute stroke. The national Institute of Neurological disorders and stroke, pp 1–9
7. Stoddard FG (1996) Public Access Defibrillation comes of age. Currents. Winter 7:1–3
8. Kerber R, Becker L, Bourland J et al (1997) Automatic external defibrillators for public access defibrillation: recommendation for specyfing and reporting arrythmya analysys, algorithm performance, incorporating new wave forms, and enhancing safety. Circulation 95:1677–1682
9. Capucci A, Aschieri D, Piepoli Mf et al (2002) Tripling survival from sudden cardiac arrest via early defibrillation without traditional education in cardiopulmonary resuscitation. Circulation 106(9):1065–1070
10. Skrifvars MB, Castren M, Kurola J, Rosenberg PH (2002) In-hospital cardiopulmonary resuscitation: organization, management and training in hospitals of different

levels of care. Acta Anaesthesiol Scand 46(4):458–463
11. Anonymous (2000) Guidelines 2000 for Cardiopulmonary Resuscitation and Emergency Cardiovascular Care. Part 6: advanced cardiovascular life support: section 4: devices to assist circulation. The American Heart Association in collaboration with the International Liaison Committee on Resuscitation. Circulation 102(8 Suppl):I105–I111
12. Handley JH, Monsieurs KG, Bossaert LL (2001) European Resuscitation Council Guidelines 2000 for adult Basic Life Support. Resuscitation 48:199–205
13. Monsieurs KG, Handley JH, Bossaert LL (2001) European Resuscitation Council Guidelines 2000 for Automated External Defibrillation. Resuscitation 48:207–209
14. McGrath PB (1987) In-house cardiopulmonary resuscitation-after a quarter of a century. Ann Emerg Med 11:1365–1368
15. Dans PE,Nevin KL, Seidman CE, McArthur JC (1985) Inhospital CPR 25 years later: why has survival decreased? South Med J 78:1174–1178
16. Tunstall-Pedoe H, Bailey L, Chamberlain DA et al (1992) Survey of 3765 cardiopulmonary resuscitations in British hospitals (the BRESUS study: methods and overall results). BMJ 304:1347–1351
17. Lazzam C, McCans JL (1991) Predictors of survival of in-hospital cardiac arrest. Can J Cardiol 7(3):113–116
18. Bedell SA, Delbanco EF, Cook EF, Epstein FH (1983) Survival after cardiopulmonary resuscitation in the hospital. N EngI J Med 309:569–576
19. Hershey CO, Fisher L (1982) Why outcome of cardiopulmonary resuscitation in general wards is poor. Lancet 1:31–34
20. Grauer K, Cavallaro D (1993) ACLS-A comprehensive review. Mosby Lifeline, St. Louis
21. Berden HJ, Hendrick JM, van Doornen JP et al (1993) A comparison of resuscitation skills of qualified nurses and ambulance nurses in The Netherlands. Heart Lung 22(6):509–515
22. Flesche C, Neruda B, Breuer S, Tarnow J (1994) Basic cardiopulmonary resuscitation skills: a comparison of ambulance staff and medical students in Germany. Resuscitation 28:S25 (abs)
23. Kaye W, Mancini ME, Giuliano KK et al (1995) Strengthening the in-hospital chain of survival with rapid defibrillation by first responders using automated external defibrillators: training and retention issues. Ann Emerg Med 25(2):163–168
24. Brown J, Latimer-Heeter M, Marinelli A et al (1995) The first 3 minutes: code preparation for the staff nurse. Orthop Nurs 14(3):35–40
25. Brenner BE, Kauffman J (1995) Response to cardiac arrests in a hospital setting: Delays in ventilation. Circulation 92:i–761 (abs)
26. Santomauro M, Ottaviano L, Borrelli A et al (2002) Organization Project for Precocious Semiautomatic in Hospital Defibrillation (heart project). Progress in Clinical Pacing, Roma, December 3–6, 2002, p 46
27. Santomauro M, Ottaviano L, Borrelli A et al (2003) Sudden cardiac death prevention through hospital early defibrillation Naples experience. PACE 26:S186

CARDIAC RESYNCHRONISATION THERAPY: INDICATIONS AND RESULTS

Usefulness of Conventional Transthoracic Echocardiography in Selecting Heart Failure Patients Likely to Benefit from Cardiac Resynchronisation Therapy

M.V. Pitzalis, R. Romito, M. Iacoviello

Beneficial effects of cardiac resynchronisation therapy (CRT), including reverse remodelling, improvement in ejection fraction, and decrease in mitral regurgitation as well as clinical improvements in exercise tolerance, quality of life, and hospitalisation rate, have been well documented [1–4], supporting the routine use of CRT as a worthwhile therapeutic option for patients with severe heart failure and left intraventricular conduction delay (QRS duration > 120 ms) who remain symptomatic despite receiving 'optimal' medical treatment. However, not all patients have subjective and/or objective responses to CRT [5, 6]. Given the complexity of the procedure and the associated costs, there is a need for parameters other than QRS duration that could prospectively identify the patients who would benefit most [7].

The beneficial effects of CRT are due to the fact that it corrects dyssynchrony resulting from inter- and intraventricular conduction delay, thus counteracting its negative haemodynamic effects. Left ventricular conduction delay induces a particular pathophysiological condition in which abrupt anterior septal motion, occurring at the time of decreasing right ventricular volume with pulmonary ejection [8], is associated with delayed contraction of the postero-lateral left ventricular wall. This condition increases wall stress during systole and oxygen demand. Moreover, the asynchrony between the septum and the lateral wall impairs the coaptation of mitral leaflets, thus favouring mitral regurgitation. Finally, tricuspid valve opening and right ventricular filling occur much earlier than mitral valve opening and left ventricular filling, thus contributing to early diastolic displacement of the septum into the left ventricle, a reduced septal contribution to ejection fraction,

Institute of Cardiology, University of Bari, Bari, Italy

and a loss of left ventricular function. All of these consequences of asynchrony can contribute, albeit to different extents, to left ventricular remodelling.

On the basis of these considerations, CRT should be offered to those patients with heart failure in whom a consistent degree of asynchrony can be detected. This is why echocardiographic parameters have been investigated. Doppler-echocardiographic-derived measures of asynchrony have the advantage of being non-invasive and can therefore be used for patient selection before the decision of implanting the device is taken. The standard Echo-Doppler measures of left ventricular asynchrony can be easily assessed and do not require complex and sophisticated software. The interventricular mechanical delay (IVMD) is assessed by calculating the difference between the left and the right pre-ejection period, i.e. the time occurring between QRS and the beginning of, respectively, aortic and pulmonary flow. In the MIRACLE study no correlation was found between IVMD and haemodynamic improvement [9]. Recently, the Cardiac Resynchronisation–Heart Failure (CARE-HF) trial has demonstrated the efficacy of CRT in reducing death from any cause or unplanned hospitalisation for a major cardiovascular event hazard ratio (HR) 0.63; 95% confidence interval (CI) 0.51–0.77; $P < 0.001$] [4]. The enrolment criteria were the presence of severe heart failure (NYHA class III or IV), left ventricular ejection fraction (LVEF) below 35%, a left ventricular end-diastolic dimension (LVEDD) greater than 30 mm (indexed to height), and QRS duration greater than 120 ms. The originality of this trial was that patients with a QRS of less than 150 ms were also required to present two of three additional echo-Doppler criteria for dyssynchrony: an aortic pre-ejection delay of more than 140 ms, an IVMD greater than 40 ms, and delayed activation of the postero-lateral left ventricular wall. After CRT, IVMD was significantly reduced by -21 ms (25–18 ms, $P < 0.001$) after three months. Moreover, patients with an IVMD of 49.2 ms or greater showed a greater risk reduction (HR 0.50; 95% CI 0.36–0.70) in comparison with those with an IVMD of less than 49.2 ms (HR 0.77; 95% CI 0.58–1.02).

We recently proposed a monodimensional echocardiographic measure of left ventricular asynchrony [6, 10]. It is evaluated by calculating the shortest interval between the maximum posterior displacement of the septum and the maximum displacement of the left posterior wall using a short axis view at papillary muscle level (septal-to-posterior wall motion delay, SPWMD; Fig. 1). Our data demonstrated that the intra- and inter-observer reproducibility of this is very high [6]. Moreover a SPWMD greater than 130 ms was more accurate in predicting short-term reverse remodelling than was QRS duration [6]. Finally, the presence of a long SPWMD was associated in the long term with further haemodynamic improvement and a better out-

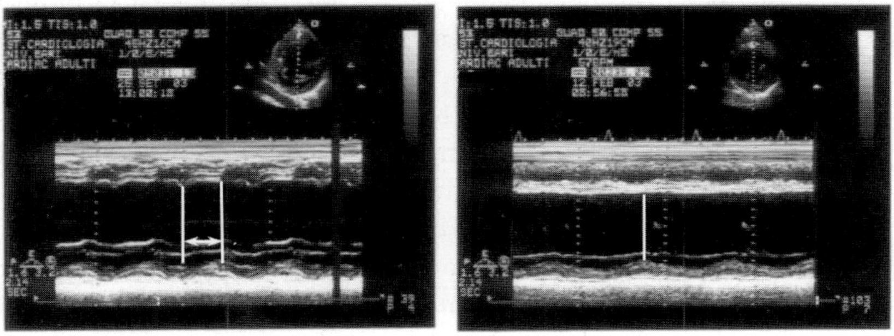

a SPWMD: 280 msec b SPWMD: 0 msec

Fig. 1. Monodimensional short-axis-view echocardiographic image taken at the level of the papillary muscles. The septal-to-posterior wall motion delay was calculated by measuring the shortest interval between the maximum posterior displacement of the septum and that of the posterior wall (**a**). When no displacement of the septum is observed, SPWMD should be considered zero (**b**). *SPWMD* septal-to-posterior wall motion delay

come in terms of heart failure worsening [10]. After 6 months, improvement in LVEF was evident in 22/28 patients (79%) with baseline SPWMD greater than 130 ms and in only 2/23 patients (9%) with SPWMD smaller than 130 ms ($P < 0.0001$). There was a significant linear correlation between SPWMD and LVEF improvement ($r = 0.69$, $P < 0.001$). Multivariate Cox regression analysis showed that SPWMD was significantly and independently associated with heart failure progression (hospitalisation or death due to worsening of heart failure) during a median follow-up of 14 months (HR for 10 ms increase in SPWMD: 0.91; 95% CI: 0.83–0.99; $P < 0.05$).

A long SPWMD is the required marker to ensure a benefit from exciting the postero-lateral wall and thus inducing more effective, synchronous intraventricular contractions. When baseline evaluation reveals a prolonged SPWMD, CRT guarantees an improved clinical outcome, but some patients with a shorter delay may also benefit from the device, which indicates the possible value of other echocardiographic methods of identifying asynchrony or other pacing methods [7]. Moreover, it has been observed that the calculation of the SPWMD cannot be obtained if the septum is akinetic after extensive anterior infarction or if the maximal posterior motion is not well defined [7]. However, SPWMD could have some advantages over the other suggested predictive parameters, since it represents a reliable measure of left ventricular asynchrony that can be obtained on a large scale using monodimensional echocardiography and can therefore be proposed as a simple parameter for patient screening.

It is mandatory that the measurement we have suggested is taken using the short axis view. When the delay is recorded from the parasternal long axis view at the level of basal segments (bs-SPWMD), it offers different information from that obtained using SPWMD. There are several reasons explaining this difference. Myocardial motion is complex and results from translational, rotational, and deformational movements that become even more complicated in the presence of wall motion abnormalities such as those occurring in the presence of akinesia or left bundle branch block. The ability to catch these movements is different when short or long axis views are under evaluation. Furthermore, left ventricular activation in patients with heart failure and left bundle branch block is complex [11] and variable [12]. Left ventricular conduction delay is the result of either an area of conduction block (due to scarred tissue or functional) or slow but homogeneous myocardial propagation. In particular, basal segments of the left ventricle show a pattern of activation that is different from that of the mid areas. Therefore, it is not surprising that the calculation of dyssynchrony between basal segments is different from that taken at the level of the mid areas. This is particularly evident when a block in the conduction is present (unfortunately, ECG cannot give any information on the type of conduction abnormality). The long axis evaluation of dyssynchrony is also burdened by the fact that it is difficult to define accurately which area e.g. lateral, postero-lateral) is being visualised and that a correct monodimensional approach (i.e. perpendicular to the long axis of the ventricle) is often difficult to obtain. Moreover, basal segments are tied to the fibrous skeleton of the heart, and therefore their movements are strongly influenced in variable and unpredictable ways by those of the aortic root as well as the mitral annulus. Finally, a parameter intended to evaluate synchrony or dyssynchrony in the transverse plane must be calculated where the myocardial fibres have a mainly circular course (i.e. at mid rather than basal level).

In conclusion, the routine use of echocardiographic assessment of ventricular asynchrony in patients with severe heart failure, LBBB, and a wide QRS interval would make it possible to avoid implanting the device in those whose cardiac function is unlikely to improve.

References

1. Cazeau S, Leclercq C, Lavergne T et al for Multisite Stimulation in Cardiomyopathies (MUSTIC) Study Investigators (2001) Effects of multisite biventricular pacing in patients with heart failure and intraventricular conduction delay. N Engl J Med 344:873–880

2. Abraham WT, Fisher WG, Smith AL et al; MIRACLE Study Group; Multicenter InSync Randomized Clinical Evaluation (2002) Cardiac resynchronization in chronic heart failure. N Engl J Med 346:1845–1853
3. Bristow MR, Saxon LA, Boehmer J et al; Comparison of Medical Therapy, Pacing, and Defibrillation in Heart Failure (COMPANION) Investigators (2004) Cardiac-resynchronization therapy with or without an implantable defibrillator in advanced chronic heart failure. N Engl J Med 350:2140–2150
4. Cleland JG, Daubert JC, Erdmann E et al; Cardiac Resynchronization-Heart Failure (CARE-HF) Study Investigators (2005) The effect of cardiac resynchronization on morbidity and mortality in heart failure. N Engl J Med 352:1539–1549
5. Reuter S, Garrigue S, Barold SS et al (2002) Comparison of characteristics in responders versus nonresponders with biventricular pacing for drug-resistant congestive heart failure. Am J Cardiol 89:346–350
6. Pitzalis MV, Iacoviello M, Romito R et al (2002) Cardiac resynchronization therapy tailored by echocardiographic evaluation of ventricular asynchrony. J Am Coll Cardiol 40:1615–1622
7. Bax JJ, Ansalone G, Breithardt O et al (2004) Echocardiographic evaluation of cardiac resynchronization therapy: ready for routine clinical use? A critical appraisal. J Am Coll Cardiol 44:1–9
8. Grines CL, Bashore TM, Boudoulas H et al (1989) Functional abnormalities in isolated LBBB. The effect of interventricular asynchrony. Circulation 79:845–853
9. St John Sutton MG, Plappert T, Abraham WT et al (2003) Effect of cardiac resynchronization therapy on left ventricular size and function in chronic heart failure. Circulation 107:1985–1990
10. Pitzalis MV, Iacoviello M, Romito R et al (2005) Ventricular asynchrony predicts a better outcome in patients with chronic heart failure receiving cardiac resynchronization therapy. J Am Coll Cardiol 45:65–69
11. Auricchio A, Fantoni C, Regoli F et al (2004) Characterization of left ventricular activation in patients with heart failure and left bundle-branch block. Circulation 109:1133–1139
12. Fung JW, Yu CM, Yip G et al (2004) Variable left ventricular activation pattern in patients with heart failure and left bundle branch block. Heart 90:17–19

Three-Dimensional Echocardiography: Which Role for CRT Patients?

P. Nihoyannopoulos

Heart failure is a major health problem reaching epidemic proportions in the industrialised world, and is associated with substantial mortality and morbidity rates. It is estimated that it affects 1–2% of the population and accounts for approximately 5% of all medical admissions. Despite major advances in medical therapy during recent years, heart failure still represents a serious and steadily expanding public health and financial threat. Cardiac resynchronisation therapy (CRT) has been introduced as an adjuvant treatment and has since developed rapidly. However, 30% of patients fail to benefit from CRT when electrical asynchrony as described by the QRS complex width is used as the sole criterion for selection. This has generated an interest in the mechanical aspect of the ventricular dyssynchrony and its superiority in describing the left ventricular dysfunction [1].

Atrioventricular (AV) dyssynchrony can be assessed from conventional echocardiography by evaluating the duration of mitral inflow. Interventricular dyssynchrony can be evaluated by assessing the extent of interventricular mechanical delay (IVMD), defined as the time difference between the left and right ventricular pre-ejection intervals. An IVMD of 40 ms or greater is considered indicative of interventricular dyssynchrony.

M-mode echocardiography may be useful for assessing intraventricular dyssynchrony from the parasternal short-axis view by measuring the septal-to-posterior wall motion delay (SPWMD). A cut-off value of 130 ms was proposed as a marker of intraventricular dyssynchrony. However, frequently the SPWMD cannot be obtained, either because the septum is akinetic following extensive anterior infarction or because the maximal posterior

Hammersmith Hospital, Imperial College, London, United Kingdom motion is ill-defined. In addition, it is often not possible to obtain perpendicular M-mode section images of the proximal left ventricle.

Tissue Doppler imaging (TDI) allows measurement of peak systolic velocity of different regions of the myocardium and timing of peak systolic velocity in relation to electrical activity (QRS complex). Based on these variables, TDI can provide accurate information on electromechanical coupling, and also assess inter- and intraventricular dyssynchrony. In addition, information on diastolic function can be obtained. Yu et al. [2] used TDI to assess intraventricular dyssynchrony in 88 normal individuals, 67 patients with heart failure and a narrow QRS complex (≤ 120 ms), and 45 with a wide QRS complex (> 120 ms). In this study, 12 sample volumes were placed in the myocardium, and for each sample the time from onset of QRS complex to peak systolic velocity was measured.

Novel echocardiographic techniques such as colour-coded tissue Doppler and real-time 3D echocardiography (RT3DE) may provide more effective guidance in identifying heart failure patients who are likely to respond positively to CRT. RT3DE provides a powerful tool for the qualitative and quantitative assessment of the left ventricle. This modality can provide information on global as well as regional left ventricular dimensions, wall thickness, and function without being limited by the inherent geometrical assumptions of conventional echocardiographic methods. The clinical use of RT3DE has been established and it has been validated against angiography, radionuclide angiography, and cardiac magnetic resonance imagin (CMRI) for the assessment of volumes and ventricular function. Recent technological advances have allowed the manufacturing of novel sophisticated matrix-array transducers, which offer fast acquisition of high-quality datasets in real time. At the same time, the development of new dedicated semi-automatic software enables the investigator to perform more accurate measurements. This has further improved inter- and intraobserver agreement as well as the repeatability of this method, while strong correlation between RT3DE and CMR in volumetric measurements has been convincingly demonstrated.

Mechanical asynchrony can occur between two or more of the 16 myocardial regions described by the American Society of Echocardiography (ASE) from basis to apex. While tissue Doppler techniques have been extensively used to assess dyssynchrony, the limited spatial resolution using tissue Doppler, usually confined to the basal myocardial segments, together with the variable algorithms used by several manufacturers, make tissue Doppler imaging impractical for routine use in the identification of patients who might benefit from CRT.

RT3DE, on the other hand, offers ideal spatial resolution involving the entire left ventricle from base to apex and can therefore be invaluable in the assessment of mechanical asynchrony. With the additional generation of three-dimensional regional volume–time curves, accurate measurement of regional function and synchronicity in one cardiac cycle can be performed. Regional time differences enable the identification of the most delayed regions, even when these are located in the most distal left ventricular regions and the apex. This technique could offer precise mapping of the mechanical asynchrony, which may be important in selecting heart failure patients who would benefit from CRT. Furthermore, by providing the electrophysiologist with regional temporal information, it could prove to be very effective in the identification of the most delayed site and thus pacing of the most delayed region.

The Dyssynchrony Index has been proposed to correlate with the ejection fraction. Moreover, the correlation between QRS width and the Dyssynchrony Index further empowers previous findings that mechanical rather than electrical synchrony offers a finer analysis of the anomalies amenable to resynchronisation.

References

1. Bax JJ, Ansalone G, Breithtardt OA et al (2004) Echocardiographic evaluation of cardiac resynchronization therapy: ready for routine clinical use? A critical appraisal. J Am Coll Cardiol: 44:1–9
2. Yu CM, Lin H, Zhang Q (2003) High prevalence of left ventricular systolic and diastolic asynchrony in patients with congestive heart failure and normal QRS duration. Heart 89:54–60

Upgrading From Right Ventricular to Biventricular Pacing: When, Why, and How?

R. Cazzin, G. Paparella

Introduction

The incidence of conduction delay in patients with congestive heart failure is approximately 30% [1], and patients with left-bundle-branch block (LBBB) have a worse survival rate than those with heart failure alone [2]. Ventricular dyssynchrony results in regional motion abnormalities of the left ventricular wall that produce a deterioration of cardiac performance.

Right ventricular apical pacing induces a left ventricular conduction pattern similar to LBBB, with a QRS vector directed upward and posteriorly. On echocardiography, chronic right ventricular apical pacing produces geometric changes that appear similar to those associated with intrinsic LBBB: shortening of ventricular filling time, reduction of ventricular d_P/d_t, and a prolonged duration of mitral regurgitation with detrimental effects on systolic and diastolic function [3]. Some reports [4, 5] have suggested that cardiac asynchrony due to LBBB is greater than dyssynchrony due to right ventricular pacing, because a larger portion of the myocardium is prematurely activated.

Cardiac resynchronisation, in which biventricular pacing reduces the intraventricular dyssynchrony of the left ventricle, is a new therapeutic option for patients who have drug-refractory end-stage heart failure [6, 7]. Many controlled prospective trials have shown that this therapeutic approach provides clinical and haemodynamic benefits in patients with advanced heart failure, severe left ventricular dysfunction, and ventricular asynchrony [8, 9]. The role of right ventricular apical pacing in treating patients with heart conditions is unclear, as is whether upgrading to biven-

U.L.S.S. 10 'Veneto Orientale', Unità Operativa Cardiologica, Portogruaro (Venice), Italy

tricular pacing in these patients would provide clinical and haemodynamic improvement. In this article the impact of cardiac resynchronisation therapy in patients with permanent right ventricular pacing and advanced heart failure is assessed.

Evidence of Negative Effects Deriving from Right Ventricular Apical Pacing

Several recent studies evidenced deleterious effects deriving from chronic right ventricular apical pacing. The Canadian Trial of Physiologic Pacing (CTOPP) [10] was a multicentric randomised study that compared VVI pacing mode with AAI and DDD mode, considered as 'physiologic' pacing. In this trial, no differences were observed in terms of mortality and hospitalisations for patients with heart failure, but right ventricular pacing seemed to provoke a detrimental effect on left ventricular systolic function.

The Danish Study [11], conducted by Nielsen, compared AAI to DDD pacing in patients with sick sinus syndrome and confirmed these results. The investigators found an increase in the size of the atrium and a reduced ejection fraction in patients with dual-chamber pacing with a high percentage of stimulation. These negative effects were more evident in patients with systolic dysfunction and/or with a previous episode of congestive heart failure.

The MOST trial [12], which attempted to identify the best pacing mode in patients with sick sinus syndrome, compared AAI to DDD pacing. No benefits regarding mortality and cerebral ischaemic accidents were found, but in the group with ventricular pacing there was a worsening of quality of life associated with an increased risk of hospitalisation for heart failure. Sweeney [13] analysed a subgroup of patients with a narrow QRS at baseline and found a close correlation between percentage of right ventricular pacing and haemodynamic and arrhythmic events. Patients with a cumulative right ventricular pacing > 40% had an increased risk of hospitalisation for heart failure associated with an increased recurrence of atrial fibrillation.

Similar results were observed in the DAVID study [14], in which patients with a dual-chamber ICD with continuous right ventricular pacing had increased mortality (10.1% vs 6.5%) and more hospitalisations (22,6% vs 13,3%) than those with a single-chamber ICD. The MADIT II trial [15], which assessed primary prevention of ICD in patients with previous myocardial infarction and severe left ventricular dysfunction, also showed that frequency of hospitalisation for heart failure was higher in patients with ICD-DDD with constant right ventricular pacing.

All these studies underline that right ventricular pacing is not a 'physiologic' stimulation and it may have negative effects on cardiac performance due to the development of abnormal motion in the septal, apical, and inferior walls as well as of cardiac dyssynchrony deriving from LBBB [16]. Impairments of left ventricular systolic and diastolic function have been demonstrated echocardiographically also in young patients after long-term right ventricular pacing.

Clinical and Haemodynamic Effects of Upgrading from Right Ventricular Apical Pacing to Biventricular Pacing

Very few reports have investigated the potential benefits of upgrading from right ventricular apical pacing to biventricular pacing. Such studies have been limited to patients who were treated with right ventricular pacing in the setting of chronic atrial fibrillation and previous AV junction ablation. Leon et al. [17] assessed the impact of biventricular pacing in 20 consecutive patients with severe left ventricular dysfunction, advanced heart failure symptoms, chronic atrial fibrillation, and permanent pacing because of prior AV node ablation. They demonstrated significant improvements in NYHA functional class, increased left ventricular ejection fraction, and decreased end-systolic diameters associated with a reduction of hospitalisations. In a randomised single-blind study, Leclercq [18] evaluated patients with advanced heart failure and atrial fibrillation with a slow ventricular rate. Patients underwent either biventricular pacing programmed in crossover with a period of right ventricular pacing mode or biventricular pacing. Patients programmed to biventricular pacing showed a significant improvement in exercise tolerance; a reduction in the number of hospitalisations was also observed. Recently, another study [19] assessed in a long-term follow up (20 ± 19 months) the effects of upgrading on 16 consecutive patients with chronic atrial fibrillation, prior AV node ablation, and permanent right ventricular apical pacing. The 14 patients surviving after 6 months evidenced an amelioration of NYHA class, a reduction of cardiothoracic ratio and mitral regurgitation, and an increased ejection fraction. Our experience on upgrading patients with right apical ventricular pacing and heart failure (NYHA III–IV; ejection fraction < 35%), consists of 28 patients, 43% paced for sick sinus syndrome and 57% for atrio-ventricular conduction disturbances. Before and after upgrading, the patients underwent clinical and echocardiographic examinations. The results after a 26 ± 9-month follow-up period demonstrated important clinical improvement in functional class (NYHA = 1.8 vs 3.2) and a reduction in the number of hospitalisations (0.4 vs 2.4). Similarly, haemodynamic benefits were evidenced with respect to end-diastolic volume and mitral regurgitation area reduction and enhanced ejection fraction. The same results were obtained in a comparison of the upgraded patients with a similar group of patients recommended for cardiac resynchronisation therapy. The implanting procedure was simplified by the presence of stable previously inserted leads. In the major of our patients, we cannulate the coronary sinus directly with the lead until the lateral or posterolateral vein, without the use of contrasting iodine agents, and with a very short procedure time.

Discussion

Cardiac resynchronisation therapy improves heart failure symptoms in patients with LBBB and severe reduction of left ventricular systolic function [8, 9]. While the effects of upgrading from right ventricular to biventricular pacing in patients with congestive heart failure have been analysed in only a few studies, the initial results are highly encouraging. Thus, this procedure seems to be safe and feasible; procedural success is estimated to be 90–92%, with a low percentage of complications [20]. Many studies have found that chronic right ventricular pacing induces desynchronisation, which could worsen ventricular function and accelerate the progression of heart disease [21, 22]. Why do some patients develop cardiac heart failure after 'ablate and pace' procedure? In patients with heart failure, in whom symptoms persist in spite of ventricular rate control, one explanation could be that correcting the tachycardia and irregular cardiac cycles is insufficient to reverse the evolution of the underlying heart disease, and that the benefits deriving from AV node ablation are counterbalanced by the deleterious effects of right ventricular apical pacing [23]. In patients treated with AV junction ablation, it is often observed that initial well-being is followed by a re-appearance or recurrence of heart failure symptoms [24]. This implies that the natural evolution of the underlying heart disease is accelerated by the detrimental effect of long-term right ventricular pacing – a consequence that is maximised in patients with reduced ventricular performance. In our study we also observed detrimental effects of right ventricular apical pacing on systolic function. Before pacemaker implantation, 80% of the patients presented with moderate left ventricular dysfunction (ejection fraction = 0.42 ± 0.08) and NYHA I-II. After 24 months of right ventricular pacing, almost 50% of the patients showed a worsening of congestive heart failure symptoms associated with severe left ventricular dysfunction. In three patients, the procedure of upgrading to biventricular pacing became necessary very early (after 3 months). This occurrence led the suggestion that right ventricular apical pacing associated with initial left ventricular dysfunction seems to worsen ventricular performance, accelerating progression of heart disease.

Conclusions

Patients with right ventricular pacing and heart failure may be candidates for resynchronisation therapy with the upgrading to biventricular pacing.

The procedure has been shown to be simple and safe. In addition, the results of the above-mentioned studies are encouraging and show that upgraded patients may profit from a better quality of life. However, the life expectancy of these patients remains to be investigated.

References

1. Shamin W, Francis DP, Yousuffuddin M et al (1999) Intraventricular conduction delay: a prognostic marker in chronic heart failure. Int J Cardiol 70:171–178
2. Sivet H, Amin J, Padmanabban S et al (1999) Increased QRS duration reduces survival in patients with left ventricular dysfunction: results from a cohort of 2263 patients. J Am Coll Cardiol 33:145A (abs)
3. Abraham WT, Fisher WG, Smith AL et al (2002) Cardiac resynchronization in chronic heart failure. N Engl J Med 346:1845–1853
4. Sogaard P, Egeblad H, Kim WY et al (2002)Tissue Doppler imaging predicts improved systolic performance and reverse left ventricular remodelling during long-term cardiac resynchronization therapy. J Am Coll Cardiol 40:723–730
5. Yu CM, Chau E, Sanderson JE et al (2002) Tissue Doppler echocardiographic evidence of reverse remodelling and improved synchronicity by simultaneously delaying regional contraction after biventricular pacing theraphy in heart failure. Circulation 105:438–445
6. Cazeau S, Leclercq C, Lavergne T et al (2001) For the Multisite Stimulation in Cardiomyopathies (MUSTIC) Study Investigators. Effects of multisite biventricular pacing in patients with heart failure and intraventricular conduction delay. N Engl J Med 344:873–880
7. Auricchio A, Stellbrink C, Sack S et al for the pacing therapies in congestive heart failure (PATH-chf) Study Group (2002) Long term clinical effects of upgrading to biventricular pacing in patients with heart failure and ventricular conduction delay. J Am Coll Cardiol 39:2026–2033
8. Bradley DJ, Bradkey EA, Calkins H et al (2003) Cardiac resynchronization and death from progressive heart failure: a meta-analysis of randomized controlled trials. JAMA 289:730–740
9. Bristow MR, Saxon LA, Boehmer J et al For the COMPANION investigators (2004) Cardiac resynchronization therapy with or without an implantable defibrillator in advanced chronic heart failure. N Engl J Med 350:2140–2150
10. Connolly SJ, Kerr CR, Gent M et al (2000) Effect of Physiologic pacing versus ventricular pacing on the risk of stroke and death due to cardiovascular causes. N Engl J Med 342:1385–1391
11. Nielsen JC, Kristensen L, Andersen HR et al (2003) A randomized comparison of atrial and dual-chamber pacing in 177 consecutive patients with sick sinus syndrome. Echocardiographic and clinical outcome. J Am Coll Cardiol 42:614–623
12. Lamas GA, Lee KL, Sweeney MO et al (2002) Ventricular pacing or dual pacing for sinus node dysfunction. N Engl J Med 346:1854–1862

13. Sweeney MO, HellKamp AS, Kenneth A et al (2003) Adverse effect of ventricular pacing on heart failure and atrial fibrillation among patients with normal baseline QRS duration in a clinical trial of pacemaker therapy for sinus node dysfunction. Circulation 107:2932–2937
14. Wilkoff BL, Cook JR, Epstein AE et al (2002) Dual-chamber pacing or ventricula backup pacing in patients with an implantable defibrillator: the Dual Chamber and VVI Implantable Defibrillator (DAVID) trial. JAMA 288:3115–3123
15. Moss AJ, Zareba W, Hall WJ et al (2002) Prophylactic implantation of a defibrillator in patients with myocardial infarction and reduced ejection fraction. N Engl J Med 346:877–883
16. Rosenqvist M, Bergfeldt L, Haga Y et al (1996) The effect of ventricular activation on myocardial performance during pacing. Pacing Clin Electrophysiol 19:1279–1286
17. Leon AR, Greenberg JM, Kanuru N et al (2002) Cardiac resynchronization in patients with congestive heart failure and chronic atrial fibrillation. J Am Coll Cardiol 39:1258–1263
18. Leclercq C, Walker S, Linde C et al (2002) Comparative effects of permanent biventricular and right-univentricular pacing in heart failure patients with chronic atrial fibrillation. Eur Heart J 23:1780–1787
19. Valls-Bertault V, Fatemi M, Gilard M et al (2004) Assessment of upgrading to biventricular pacing in patients with right ventricular pacing and congestive heart failure after atrioventricular junctional ablation for chronic atrial fibrillation. Europace 6:438–443
20. Baker CM, Christopher TJ, Smith PF et al (2002) Addition of a left ventricular lead to conventional pacing systems in patients with congestive heart failure: feasibility, safety and early results in 60 consecutive patients. PACE 25:1166–1171
21. Lee MA, Dae MW, Langberg JJ et al (1994) Effects of long term right ventricular apical pacing on left ventricular perfusion, innervation, function and histology. J Am Coll Cardiol 24:225–232
22. Saxon LA, Stevenson WG, Middlekauff HR et al (1993) Increased risk of progressive hemodynamic deterioration in advanced heart failure patients requiring permanent pacemakers. Am Heart J 125:1306–1310
23. Mera F, De Lurgio DB, Patterson RE et al (1999) A comparison of ventricular function during high right ventricular septal and apical pacing after His-bundle ablation for refractory atrial fibrillation. Pacing Clin Electrophysiol 22:1234–1239
24. Vanderheyden M, Goethals M, Anguera I et al (1997) Hemodynamic deterioration following radiofrequency ablation of the atrioventricular pacing system. Pacing Clin Electrophysiol 20:2422–2428

Cardiac Resynchronisation Therapy: How to Identify Patients Who Will not Respond to Therapy

M.M. Gulizia, A. Ragusa, G.M. Francese

Congestive heart failure (CHF) is the major cause of mortality, morbidity, and hospitalisation in patients aged ≥ 60 years in Europe and the USA, with a prevalence in this latter from 0.4% up to 2% [1]. In addition to the clinical symptoms such as left ventricular dysfunction, reduced exercise tolerance, and impaired quality of life, these patients often have a markedly shortened life expectancy, with a further worsening in those with heart conduction defects [2–5]. Despite major advances in medical therapy [6-16], mortality and morbidity remain still high [17].

Cardiac resynchronisation therapy (CRT) was introduced in the early 1990s [18]. It was approved by the FDA in 2001 and was classified in the American College of Cardiology/American Heart Association/North American Society of Pacing and Electrophysiology/Heart Rhythm Society 2002 guideline update for the implantation of pacemaker and anti-arrhythmic devices with evidence level IIA [19] for patients with idiopathic or ischaemic cardiomyopathy and severe heart failure (NYHA functional class III or IV) despite optimised medical therapy, with left ventricular ejection fraction < 35%, QRS duration > 120 ms, and left ventricular end-diastolic diameter > 55 mm. These guidelines were based on two controlled trials: Multisite Stimulation in Cardiomyopathy (MUSTIC) [20] with a crossover design and Multicenter InSync Randomised Clinical Evaluation (MIRACLE) [21] a parallel placebo trial.

The results of MUSTIC [20], PATH-CHF (Pacing Therapies for Congestive Heart Failure study) [22, 23], and the preliminary data from the Italian InSync Registry (InSIR) [24, 25] demonstrated the enhancing effect of car-

Cardiology Department, S. Luigi – S. Currò Hospital, Catania, Italy

diac resynchronisation therapy (CRT) on heart haemodynamic performance, working ability, and quality of life in a large number of patients with CHF and uncoordinated contraction, but while the majority of patients 'feel better' with CRT and the benefit has an On-Off effect (COMPANION study) [26–31], still 20–30% of patients did not respond to CRT, emphasising the need for additional selection criteria to identify potential responders [32].

Table 1 shows the proposed patient selection of the major studies on CRT. All the studies reported in this table demonstrated a statistical ($P < 0.001$) improvement in mean NYHA class in the biventricular paced population, as well as an increase ($P < 0.001$) in the mean distance walked in 6 min (with the exception, for this latter, of the Contak ICD Trial). All these studies also showed an improvement in the quality of life of the patients by a reduction of more than 30% of the Minnesota Living with Heart Failure test score, but no definite indication has been given towards finding any clinical routine-practice predictors that would identify patients who will or will not respond to CRT.

Table 1. Proposed patient selection of the major studies on CRT

Study (number randomised)[a]	NYHA class	QRS	Sinus	ICD	Status
MUSTIC AF (43)	III	> 200b	AF	No	Published
PACMAN (328)	III	≥ 150	Normal	No	Enrolled
MUSTIC SR (58)	III	> 150	Normal	No	Published
VecToR (420)	II,IV	≥ 140	Normal	No	Published
MIRACLE (453)	III,IV	≥ 130	Normal	No	Published
MIRACLE ICD (369)	III,IV	≥ 130	Normal	Yes	Published
MIRACLE ICD II (186)	II	≥ 130	Normal	Yes	Published
CARE HF (800)c	III,IV	≥ 120	Normal	Y/N	Published
COMPANION (>1600)	III, IV	≥ 120	Normal	Y/N	Published
CONTAK CD (227)	III,IV	≥ 120	Normal	Yes	Published
PATH-CHF (41)	III,IV	≥ 120	Normal	No	Published
PATH-CHF II (89)	III,IV	≥ 120	Normal	No	Published

[a]EF ≤ 35% for all

[b]RV paced QRS

[c]Echo-based criteria for < 150 ms

QRS QRS duration at standard electrocardiogram, Sinus patients in sinus rhythm (normal) or atrial fibrillation (AF), *ICD* biventricular ICD device implantation

At present, although no definite guideline has been given about the selection of patients who will or will not respond to CRT, recent data from many authors' studies may provide indications and clinical routine-practice predictors that can identify patients who will respond to CRT.

Leclerq et al. [33] identified a clinical predictive parameter in the LVEF ($P < 0.036$) and an acute predictive one when an increase was recorded in cardiac output and a decrease in PCWP by more than 10% during DDD BiV pacing compared to baseline AAI mode.

In another study, Kass et al. [34] demonstrated the positive correlation existing between the baseline QRS duration and the dP/dt_{max} during left ventricle and BiV pacing. However, because of some discrepancies in the response to BiV pacing observed in some patients with wide QRS, authors postulate that finding the optimal pacing site can play a major role in CRT.

The same results were found by Auricchio et al. [35], who underlined the importance of a baseline QRS duration > 150 ms, which was able to identify most of the responders to BiV pacing.

To determine whether some factors could predict the long-term clinical effectiveness of CRT, Alonso et al. [36] studied 26 patients with drug-refractory heart failure and wide QRS implanted with a BiV pacemaker. NYHA class, exercise tolerance, and LVEF were recorded at baseline and after pacemaker implantation. Patients were divided into two groups: group I, responders; group II, non-responders. QRS duration and axis at baseline and during BiV pacing, interventricular conduction time, and left and right ventricular lead positions were compared between the two groups. Only QRS duration during BiV pacing differed between the two groups, with a significantly shorter value in group I than in group II (154 ± 17 ms vs 177 ± 26 ms; $P = 0.016$).

In a study on the sensitivity and specificity of QRS duration in predicting the acute benefit in CHF patients (PATH-CHF I and II) treated with CRT, Kadhiresan et al. [37] demonstrated that at smaller QRS duration thresholds the specificity tends to be lower, while accuracy was highest (80%) at a QRS duration of 155 ms, with positive and negative predictive values of 77% and 92% respectively.

Performing cardiac catheterisation in 22 CHF patients with a dual-sensor micromanometer to measure LV and aortic pressure during sinus rhythm and LV free wall pacing, Nelson et al. [38] demonstrated that, although mechanical dyssynchrony is a key predictor for pacing efficacy in CHF patients with conduction delay, combining information about QRS and basal dP/dt_{max} provides an excellent tool by which to identify maximal responders.

Other authors [39], speculating on the idea that pacing two sites with the longest conduction delay will result in the largest improvement in cardiac function in CHF, demonstrated that applying CRT in these sites does not necessarily produce better haemodynamic improvement in CHF patients.

Some authors [40] have hypothesised that the percentage increase in QRS duration at short atrioventricular delays during BiV pacing can distinguish responder from non-responder sites, while others [41] have demonstrated, in a group of 18 CHF patients in atrial fibrillation treated with BiV pacing compared to a group of 56 in sinus rhythm, that CRT improved both patient groups, suggesting that inter- and intraventricular resynchronisation had a more important effect than atrioventricular delay optimisation.

In partial contrast with these just-mentioned results, in the analysis of 54/316 patients enrolled in the InSIR [42], LVEDD was the only significant predictor of clinical outcome. The authors postulate that this could be due to the poor contractility reserve of a very dilated left ventricle, as shown by the LVEF percentage increasing only in the responders group.

The recent studies have suggested the role of assessing systolic asynchrony to predict improvement of systolic function or LV reverse remodelling [43–49] [defined as a reduction of left ventricle end systolic volume (LVESV)] > 15% 3 months after CRT, while the non-responders are defined by a reduction of LVESV ≤ 15%). Mechanical dyssynchrony is not necessarily related to electrical dyssynchrony, and the presence of substantial left ventricular dyssynchrony is a major predictor of response to CRT. Indeed, the absence or lesser extent of ventricular dyssynchrony can identify non-responders to CRT. Moreover, many patients with a wide QRS complex do not exhibit LV dyssynchrony, whereas many patients with a narrow QRS complex may demonstrate LV dyssynchrony. These considerations suggest that electrocardiography is not an accurate marker of electromechanical delay, as electrical delay may not occur in patients with left bundle branch block, whereas significant mechanical asynchrony is absent in nearly 30% of patients with prolonged QRS duration [50]. Thus, many investigators are looking for any features that will predict the clinical response in the individual patient who is the optimal candidate for CRT but did not respond to CRT.

NYHA functional class IV, marked dilatation of the left ventricle (DTD > 60 mm), severe mitral regurgitation, an unstable haemodynamic status, and a VTI of aortic flow ≤ 12 cm are considered to be associated to a negative response to CRT [51]. Furthermore, many authors have suggested that the likelihood of responding to CRT is lower in patients with ischaemic heart disease, sustained ventricular tachycardia, and severe mitral regurgitation [52], whereas others have demonstrated that the percentages of responders to CRT were comparable in the group of patients with ischaemic disease and in those with idiopathic cardiomyopathy, underlining that the aetiology of heart failure was not related to the response to CRT [53].

Given the limitations of surface ECG, the authors in the CARE-HF study proposed some echocardiographic parameters to investigate the presence of ventricular dyssynchrony [54, 55]. Thus, in patients with a QRS duration of 120–150 ms it is possible to evaluate the presence of ventricular dyssynchrony by the presence of the following echocardiographic parameters: (1) a prolonged aortic pre-ejection delay (> 140 ms), (2) an increased mechanical interventricular delay (> 40 ms), and (3) a left ventricular segmental post-systolic contraction (LVPSC).

The first echocardiographic parameter is derived from the measurement between the onset of the QRS complex and the beginning of the aortic flow on pulsed-wave Doppler imaging. The second echocardiographic parameter can be evaluated by assessing the extent of interventricular mechanical delay, defined as the time difference between the onset of the pulmonary and the aortic flow (left and right ventricular pre-ejection intervals = IVMD) during pulsed-wave Doppler imaging. An IVMD ≥ 40 ms is considered indicative of interventricular dyssynchrony, and in the MIRACLE trial this index was reduced by 19% after CRT. Finally, LVPSC is defined as the maximal local wall inward movement occurring later than the start of the trans-mitral Doppler flow signal.

The prolongation of the delay of the first two parameters just cited results in a decrease in left ventricular contraction duration and a decrease in regional ejection fraction. Moreover, Yu et al. [55] using tissue Doppler imaging (TDI) found a large mechanical delay between the free right ventricular wall and the lateral wall of the left ventricle, which was completely reversed after CRT. So, as described by other authors [56], a simple rule can be represented by: the longer the aortic pre-ejection delay, and the shorter the left ventricular filling duration, the more advanced the ventricular dyssynchrony. However, besides the interventricular dyssynchrony, which is defined as an asynchronous right–left ventricular contraction and relaxation occurring in left bundle branch block patients that produces abnormal septal motion with a reduced interventricular septal contribution to global left ventricular performance, there are other forms of asynchrony that may contribute to ventricular dyssynchrony [57].

Briefly, the atrioventricular dyssynchrony is an abnormal conduction of the AV node which results in: a delay between atrial and ventricular contraction; mitral valve incompetence with occurrence of late diastolic regurgitation; shortened ventricular filling time, limiting diastolic stroke volume; and, often, immediate occurrence of atrial systole with early passive filling, hence reducing left ventricular filling. In this case left ventricular performance can be improved by adequate atrioventricular timing. It has been proposed that the optimal atrioventricular delay should provide the longest left ventricular filling time without premature truncation of the A-wave by mitral valve closure. This approach is widely accepted as a simple method by which to optimise atrioventricular delay, although it is not clear whether atrioventricular timing optimisation is needed or whether an atrioventricular delay of 100 or 120 ms would be appropriate for all patients.

At present attention is focused on the intraventricular dyssynchrony as data revealing that a lower degree of intraventricular dyssynchrony results in a lower benefit from CRT. It occurs when a portion of the left ventricle is prematurely activated and generates regions of both early and delayed contraction that will contribute to altered LV performance [51]. Using M-mode echocardiography, Pitzalis et al. [43] demonstrated that a septal-to-posterior wall motion delay (SPWMD) ≥ 130 ms was a marker of intraventricular dyssynchrony. However, the SPWMD cannot be obtained, either because the septum is akinetic after extensive anterior infarction or because the maximal posterior motion is not defined. In addition, it is often not possible to obtain a perpendicular M-mode section of the proximal left ventricle. TDI can provide accurate information about intraventricular dyssynchrony by assessing peak systolic velocity at different regions of the myocardium and the timing of peak systolic velocity. Bax et al. [46] measured intraventricular dyssynchrony by placing two sample volumes on the basal parts of the septum and lateral wall, and a delay ≥ 60 ms, referred as septal-to-lateral delay, was an indicator of substantial intraventricular dyssynchrony. Yu et al. [50] used TDI to assess intraventricular dyssynchrony into 12 myocardial segments. For each segment the time from onset of QRS complex to peak systolic velocity was measured and two parameters were obtained: the maximal difference between peak systolic velocities of any 2 of the 12 segments (intraventricular dyssynchrony defined as difference > 100 ms) and the SD of all 12 time intervals measuring time to peak systolic velocity (dyssynchrony index SD > 33 ms) Only patients with an index > 33 ms demonstrated reverse remodelling after CRT. More recently, Yu et al. [49] utilised tissue synchronisation imaging (TSI), a parametric imaging derived from 2D TDI which automatically calculates and colour-codes the time to peak tissue velocity in every position in the image with reference to QRS signal, using the six basal mid-segmental model. The cut-off of the SD of the peak systolic velocities of the LV segments was 34.4 ms. The commonest site of most severe delay was the inferior wall (45%), followed by the lateral wall (30%), posterior wall (25%), septal wall (16%), and anteroseptal wall (5%). However, only the presence of lateral wall delay at baseline was associated with a reverse remodelling response (sensitivity 47%, specificity 89%) [49, 57]. Therefore a simple algorithm could be used to identify responders or non-responders to CRT in which the combination of these two parameters, lateral wall delay and SD > 34.4 ms, gave a specificity of 87% and a sensitivity of 82% (Fig. 1). Ansalone et al. [45] have also shown that the most delayed wall was the lateral one (35%), while the inferior wall and the septum infrequently show the latest mechanical activity; furthermore, these authors demonstrated that biven-

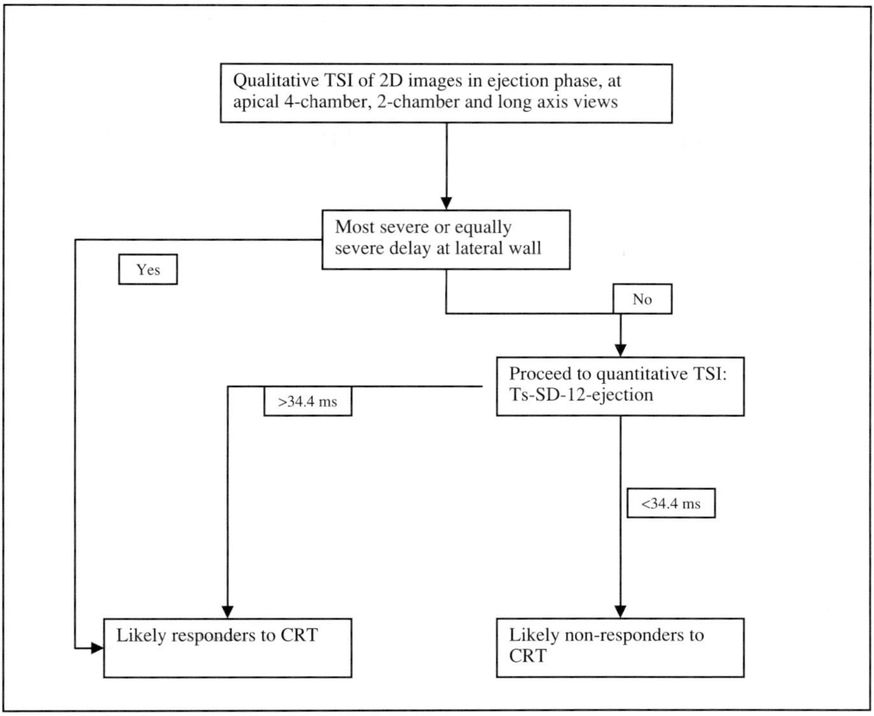

Fig. 1. Suggested algorithm for assessing systolic asynchrony by tissue synchronisation imaging (TSI) to identify responders and non-responders to cardiac resynchronisation therapy and predict reverse remodelling (modified from [49]). *2D* two dimensional, *SD* standard deviation

tricular pacing provided additional benefit when applied at the most delayed site. A limitation of TDI with velocity imaging is its inability to determine whether the motion represents contraction or is merely passive. Strain and strain rate allows direct assessment of the degree of myocardial deformation during systole; strain is expressed as the percentage of segmental shortening or lengthening in relation to the original length, while strain rate measures the rate of local deformation. Compared with TDI, strain rate differentiates better between active systolic contraction and passive displacement, which is of particular importance in ischaemic patients with scar tissue [58]. Tissue tracking and strain rate imaging have also proved useful in assessing longitudinal resynchronisation. The latter is interpreted as a decrease in percentage of the extent of LV basal segments displaying delayed longitudinal contraction (an active contraction after closure of the aortic valve), and CRT reduced the extent of this form of diastolic contraction. Sogaard et al. [47] focused on late or postsystolic longitudinal contraction at the base of the left ventricle, and delayed longitudinal contraction is considered a superior predictor of CRT (less extensive mechanical asynchrony, less response to CRT).

In conclusion, cardiac resynchronisation therapy (CRT) is now considered an established therapy for patients with heart failure, with good clinical results, although 20–30% do not respond. Many investigators are looking for reliable predictors of patient response to CRT. Although no definite guideline has been given as of today about the selection of patients who will or will not respond to CRT, recent data from many authors' studies may provide indications and clinical routine-practice predictors that can identify patients.

At present, several echocardiographic methods to assess dyssynchrony have been proposed, varying from conventional to advanced approaches, primarily involving TDI, trans thoracic (TT), TSI, strain, and strain rate. It currently unclear which of these parameters provides optimal information on dyssynchrony and which parameters may actually allow prospective identification of responders and non-responders to CRT. However, based on the assessment of AV, interventricular, and intraventricular dyssynchrony, accurate prediction of response to CRT will be feasible. In particular TDI may allow precise assessment of intra-and interventricular dyssynchrony and could be included in the selection of candidates for CRT. Moreover, based on the assessment of the site of latest activation in LV, echocardiography can guide LV lead positioning and may be used to optimise AV delay and V-V delay.

References

1. Brown AM, Cleland JG (1998) Influence of concomitant disease on pattern of hospitalization in patients with heart failure discharged from Scottish hospitals in 1995. Eur Heart J 19:1063–1069
2. Cohn JN, Johnson G, Ziesche S et al (1991) A comparison of enalapril with hydralazine-isosorbide dinitrate in the treatment of chronic congestive heart failure. N Engl J Med 325:303–310
3. Anonymous (1983) A placebo-controlled trial of captopril in refractory chronic congestive heart failure. Captopril Multicenter Research Group. J Am Coll Cardiol 2:755–763
4. Stevenson WG, Stevenson LW, Middlekauff HR et al (1996) Improving survival for patients with atrial fibrillation and advanced heart failure. J Am Coll Cardiol 28:1458–1463
5. Aaronson KD, Schwartz S, Chen T-M et al (1997) Development and prospective validation of a clinical index to predict survival in ambulatory patients referred for cardiac transplant evaluation. Circulation 95:2660–2667
6. Opie LH (1995) Fundamental role of angiotensin-converting enzyme inhibitors in the management of congestive heart failure. Am J Cardiol 75:3F–6F
7. Packer AC, Gheorghiade M, Young J et al (1993) Withdrawal of digoxin from patients with chronic heart failure treated with angiotensin-converting-enzyme

inhibitors. N Engl J Med 329:1–7
8. Anonymous (1993) Effect of ramipril on mortality and morbidity of survivors of acute myocardial infarction with clinical evidence of heart failure. The Acute Infarction Ramipril Efficacy (AIRE) Study Investigators. Lancet 342:821–828
9. Cohn JN, Tognoni G for the Valsartan Heart Failure Trial Investigators (2001) A randomized trial of the angiotensin-receptor blocker valsartan in chronic heart failure. N Engl J Med 345:16667–16675
10. Packer M (1998) Do beta-blockers prolong survival in chronic heart failure? A review of the experimental and clinical evidence. Eur Heart J 19:B40–B46
11. Packer M, Bristow MR, Cohn JN et al (1996) The effect of carvedilol on morbidity and mortality in patients with chronic heart failure. N Engl J Med 334:1349–1355
12. Packer M, Coats AJS, Fowler MB et al for the Carvedilol Prospective Randomized Cumulative Survival Study Group (2001) Effect of carvedilol on survival in severe chronic heart failure. N Engl J Med 344:1651–1658
13. Dargie HJ (2001). Effect of carvedilol on outcome after myocardial infarction in patients with left-ventricular dysfunction: the CAPRICORN randomised trial. Lancet 357:1385–1390
14. Anonymous (2000) Effects of metoprolol CR in patients with ischemic and dilated cardiomyopathy. The Randomized Evaluation of Strategies for Left Ventricular Dysfunction Pilot Study. Circulation 101: 378–384
15. Goldstein S, Fagerberg B, Hjalmarson A et al; MERIT-HF Study Group (2001) Metoprolol controlled release/extended release in patients with severe heart failure: analysis of the experience in the MERIT-HF study. J Am Coll Cardiol 38:932–938
16. The Beta-Blocker Evaluation of Survival Trial Investigators (2001) Trial of the beta-blocker bucindolol in patients with advanced chronic heart failure. N Engl J Med 344:1659–1667
17. Zannad F, Briancon S, Juilliere T et al (1999) Incidence, clinical and etiologic features and outcomes of advanced chronic heart failure: the EPICAL study. J Am Coll Cardiol 33:734–742
18. Abraham WT, Hayes DL (2003) Cardiac resynchronization therapy for heart failure. Circulation 108:2596–2603
19. Gregoratos G, Abrams J, Epstein AE et al (2002) ACC/AHA/NASPE 2002 guidelines update for implantation of cardiac pacemakers and antiarrhythmia device. J Am Coll Cardiol 40:1703–1719
20. Cazean S, Leclercq C, Lavergne T et al (2001) Effects of multisite biventricular pacing in patients with heart failure and interventricular conduction delay. N Engl J Med 344:873–880
21. Abraham WT, Fisher WG, Smith AL et al (2002) Cardiac resynchronization in chronic heart failure. N Engl J Med 346:1845–1853
22. Huth C, Friedl A, Klein H, Auricchio A (2001) Pacing therapies for congestive heart failure considering the results of the PATH-CHF study. Z Kardiol 90(Suppl 1):10–15
23. Auricchio A, Stellbrink C et al (1999) Pacing therapies for congestive heart failure. (PATH-CHF study.) Rationale, design and endpoints of a prospective, randomized, multicentric study. Am J Cardiol 83:130–135
24. Padeletti L, Porciani MC, Santini M et al (2001) InSync Italian Registry: long term clinical results of cardiac resynchronization. Europace Suppl 2:B58:787
25. Gulizia M, Ricci R, Lunati M et al (2001) InSync Italian Registry: does biventricular pacing impact on patients hospitalizations? Europace Suppl 2:B59:816
26. Cazeau S, Ritter P et al (1994) Four chamber pacing in dilated cardiomyopathy. Pacing Clin Electrophysiol 17:1974–1979

27. Saxon L, Boehemer J, Hummel J (1999) Biventricular pacing in patients with CHF: two prospective randomized trials (Vigor CHF). Am J Cardiol 83:120D–123D
28. Gras D, Mabo P, Tang T et al (1998) Multisite pacing as a supplemental treatment of CHF: preliminary results of the Medtronic InSync study (NASPE abstr). Pacing Clin Electrophysiol 21:2249–2255
29. Abraham WT (2001) Late breaking clinical trial session at ACC 2001. Am Coll Cardiol 38:604–605
30. Bristow MR, Feldman AM, Saxon LA (2000) Heart failure management using implantable device for ventricular resynchronization: comparison of medical therapy pacing, and defibrillation in chronic heart failure (COMPANION) trial. COMPANION Steering Committee and COMPANION Clinical Investigators. J Card Fail 6:276–285
31. Medtronic InSync ICD cardiac resynchronization system. www.fda.gov
32. Leclerq C, Kass DA (2002) Retiming the failing heart: principles and current clinical status of cardiac resynchronization. J Am Coll Cardiol 39:194–201
33. Leclercq C, Cazeau S, Le Breton H et al (1998) Acute hemodynamic effects of biventricular DDD pacing in patients with end-stage heart failure. J Am Coll Cardiol 32:1825–1831
34. Kass DA, Chen CH, Curry C et al (1999) Improved ventricular mechanics from acute VDD pacing in patients with dilated cardiomyopathy and ventricular conduction delay. Circulation 30:1567–1573
35. Auricchio A, Stellbrink C, Block M et al (1999) Effect of pacing chamber and atrioventricular delay on acute systolic function of paced patients with congestive heart failure: the Pacing Therapies for Congestive Heart Failure Study Group: the Guidant Congestive Heart Failure Research Group. Circulation 99:2993–3001
36. Alonso C, Leclercq C, Victor F et al (1999) Electrocardiographic predictive factors of long-term clinical improvement with multisite biventricular pacing in advanced heart failure. Am J Cardiol 84:1417–1421
37. Kadhiresan V, Vogt J, Auricchio A et al (2000) Sensitivity and specificity of QRS duration to predict acute benefit in heart failure patients with cardiac resynchronization. NASPE 2000, part II, p 555[AQ7]
38. Nelson G, Curry CW, Wyman BT et al (2000) Predictors of systolic augmentation from left ventricular preexcitation in patients with dilated cardiomyopathy and intraventricular conduction delay. Circulation 101:2703–2709
38. Nelson G, Curry CW, Wyman BT et al (2000) Predictors of systolic augmentation from left ventricular preexcitation in patients with dilated cardiomyopathy and intraventricular conduction delay. Circulation 101:2703–2709
39. Butter C, Auricchio A, Stellbrink C et al (2001) Longer LV-RV delay may not yield better iVRT outcome in HF. Europace Suppl 2 B11:649
40. Yu Y, Auricchio A, Butter C et al (2001) Assess effectiveness of BiVRT using surface RS duration. Europace Suppl 2 B11:770
41. Achilli A, Bocchiardo M, Sassara M et al (2001) Biventricular stimulation: comparison of results of sinus rhythm and chronic atrial fibrillation patients. Europace Suppl 2 B11:612
42. Montenero AS, Santini M, Lunati M et al (2001) InSync Italian Registry: baseline predictive factors of the clinical outcome. Europace Suppl 2 B49:613
43. Pitzalis MV, Iacovello M, Romito R et al (2002) Cardiac resynchronization therapy tailored by echocardiographic evaluation of ventricular asynchrony. J Am Coll Cardiol 40:1615–1622
44. Yu CM, Fung WH, Lin H et al (2003) Predictors of left ventricular reverse remodel-

ling after cardiac resynchronization therapy for heart failure secondary to idiopathic dilated or ischemic cardiomyopathy. Am J Cardiol 91:684–688
45. Ansalone G, Giannatoni P, Ricci R et al (2001) Doppler myocardial imaging in patients with heart failure receving biventricular pacing treatment. Am Heart J 142:881–896
46. Bax JJ, Marwich TH, Molhoek SG et al (2003) Left ventricular dyssynchrony predicts benefit of cardiac resynchronization therapy in patients with end-stage heart failure before pacemaker implantation. Am J Cardiol 92:1238–1240
47. Sogaard P, Egeblad H, Kim WY et al (2002) Tissue Doppler imaging predicts improved systolic performance and reverse left ventricular remodeling during long term cardiac resynchronization therapy. J Am Coll Cardiol 40:723–730
48. Yu CM, Fung JW, Zhang Q et al (2004) Tissue Doppler imaging is superior to strain rate imaging and postsystolic shortening on the prediction of reverse remodelling in both ischemic and nonischemic heart failure after cardiac resynchronization therapy. Circulation 110:66–73
49. Yu CM, Zhang Q, Fung JW et al (2005) A novel tool to assess systolic asynchrony and identify responders of cardiac resynchronization therapy by tissue synchronization imaging. J Am Coll Cardiol 45:677–684
50. Yu CM, Lin H, Zhang Q et al (2003) High prevalence of ventricular systolic and diastolic asynchrony in patient with congestive heart failure and normal QRS duration. Heart 89:54–60
51. Achilli A, Patruno N, Pontillo D et al (2004) La terapia di resincronizzazione cardiaca per il trattamento dello scompenso cardiaco. Ital Heart J Suppl 5:445–456
52. Diaz-Infante E, Berruezo A, Mont L et al (2004) Predictors of lack of clinical improvement at mid-term follow-up with cardiac resynchronization therapy. Rev Esp Cardiol 57:279–282
53. Molhoek SG, Bax JJ, van Erven L et al (2004) Comparison of benefit from cardiac resynchronization therapy in patients with ischemic cardiomyopathy versus idiopathic dilated cardiomyopathy. Am J Cardiol 93:860–863
54. Cleland JGF, Daubert JC, Erdmann E et al; CARE-HF study steering committee and investigators (2001) The CARE-HF study (Cardiac Resynchronisation in Heart Failure study): rationale, design and end-points. Eur J Heart Fail 3:481–489
55. Yu CM, Chau E, Sanderson JE et al (2002) Tissue Doppler echocardiographic evidence of reverse remodeling and improved synchronicity by simultaneously delaying regional contraction after biventricular pacing therapy in heart failure. Circulation105:438–445
56. Gras D, Cebron JP, Brunel P et al (2003) Selection of patients for cardiac resynchronization therapy. In: Gulizia M (ed) Mediterranean Cardiology Meeting 2003: new advances in heart failure and atrial fibrillation. Springer, Milan, pp 237–241
57. Bax JJ, Ansalone G, Breithardt OA et al (2004) Echocardiographic evaluation of cardiac resynchronization therapy: ready for routine clinical use? J Am Coll Cardiol 44:1–9
58. Ascione L, Accadia M, Iengo R et al (2005) How to detect dyssynchrony and how to correct it. In: Gulizia M (ed) Mediterranean Cardiology Meeting 2003: new advances in heart failure and atrial fibrillation. Springer, Milan, 165–173

Controversial and Emerging Indication for CRT: Atrial Fibrillation

M. Brignole[1], P. Jaïs[2]

Introduction

Randomised trials have shown that in patients affected by atrial fibrillation (AF) the 'rhythm control strategy,' which uses medication to maintain sinus rhythm, increases the rate of hospitalisation, with no improvement in mortality and no or little symptomatic benefit, as compared with the 'rate control strategy.' However, both pharmacological strategies give, respectively, largely incomplete rhythm or rate control. Indeed, maintaining sinus rhythm with the use of anti-arrhythmic drugs is challenging, owing to the limited efficacy and potentially deleterious effects of the drugs [1–4]. However, the control of heart rate achievable with pharmacologic therapy is also imperfect and, in many patients, difficult to achieve. Moreover, acute studies have shown that during AF irregular RR intervals are associated with a negative haemodynamic effect, which is independent of heart rate [5], and that this effect is reversed by regularisation of the rhythm [6].

Curative catheter ablation has been established as an effective therapeutic option for treating atrial fibrillation that is resistant to pharmacologic rhythm control, with successful long-term maintenance of sinus rhythm without the need for anti-arrhythmic drugs [7, 8]. AV junction ablation and pacing therapy offer theoretically perfect control of heart rate; consequently, the expected results are superior to those observed with drug therapy [9, 10]. Catheter ablation is easier for rate control than for rhythm control. Creating heart block and implanting a permanent pacemaker provide regularisation of the ventricular rate, and the use of biventricular pacemakers

[1]Centro Aritmologico, Dipartimento di Cardiologia, Ospedali del Tigullio, Lavagna (Genua), Italy; [2] Hôpital Cardiologique du Haut-Lévêque and Université Victor Segalen, Bordeaux II, Bordeaux-Pessac, France

may prevent the adverse effect of right ventricular pacing on left ventricular function [11].

Thus, both non-pharmacological strategies seem to be able to provide better (potentially optimal) rate and rhythm control than pharmacological therapies. Two recently published studies, one using AV junction ablation [10] and the other using curative left atrial catheter ablation [8] have shown a great improvement in quality of life, exercise capacity, and cardiac performance compared with the pre-ablation evaluation.

The present study compares the effect of optimal rate control (RATE) obtained with AV junction ablation and bi-ventricular pacing with optimal rhythm control (RHYTHM) obtained with catheter ablation using the populations of the above studies [8, 10].

Methods

The results of two recently published studies, one using AV junction ablation (RATE) [10] and the other using curative left atrial catheter ablation (RHYTHM) [8] have been compared. There were 56 and 58 patients, respectively, with persistent or permanent AF (with the exception of 9% of patients of the RHYTHM study who had a paroxysmal form), which was severely symptomatic and refractory to pharmacological therapy. The two populations had similar baseline characteristics except that the RATE patients were older (70 ± 8 vs 56 ± 10 years) and 50% of them had left-bundle-branch block (LBBB) (Table 1); minor differences were also present regarding gender, NYHA functional class, and left ventricular end diastolic diameter. There were also some differences in pharmacological therapy at enrolment (Table 2). The RATE study was a prospective randomised, single-blind, 3-month cross-over comparison between right ventricular (RV) and left ventricular (LV) pacing (months 0–6) and between RV and biventricular (BiV) pacing (months 7–12); total follow-up lasted 12 months. RYHTHM was a case-control parallel study. For the purpose of the present comparison, only the 58 patients belonging to the congestive heart failure arm were considered; total follow-up lasted 12 ± 7 months. For a comprehensive description of the study protocol, inclusion and exclusion criteria, and outcome measures, refer to the original publications [8, 10].

Procedural success rate and complications as well as clinical events that occurred during the study period were compared between the two studies. Symptoms, quality of life, exercise capacity, and echocardiographic LV function measures were compared between the 41 patients of the RATE group who completed the BiV pacing phase (i.e. at month 9 or 12) and the 34 patients of the RHYTHM group who were seen at 1-year follow-up. Symptom

Table 1. Patients' characteristics at enrolment. *LV* left ventricle, *NYHA* New York Heart Association classification, *LVEDD* left ventricular end diastolic diameter, *LVESD* left ventricular end systolic diameter

	Rate control group	Rhythm control group	*P* value
Number of patients	56	58	
Age, years	70 ± 8	56 ± 10	0.001
Gender, males	34 (61%)	51 (88%)	0.001
Duration of atrial fibrillation, years	6.6±4.2	6.7±3.7	0.9
Persistent/permanent AF	56 (100%)	53 (91%)	0.03
Bundle-branch block	28 (50%)	0 (0%)	0.001
Holter monitoring:		*(on 53 patients)*	
Mean heart rate, bpm	88 ± 20	89 ± 11	0.7
Maximum heart rate, bpm	142 ± 41	154 ± 30	0.1
Inadequate heart rate[a]	34 (61%)	29 (50%)	0.2
Associated structural heart disease			
Coronary artery disease	17 (30%)	12 (21%)	0.2
Others	39 (70%)	46 (79%)	0.2
NYHA functional class	2.5 ± 0.5	2.3 ± 0.5	0.04
Standard echocardiogram:			
LV ejection fraction, %	38 ± 14	35 ± 7	0.2
LV ejection fraction < 40%	33 (59%)	38 (66%)	0.3
LVEDD, mm	56 ± 9	60 ± 8	0.01
LVESD, mm	44 ± 10	46 ± 9	0.3

[a]Inadequate ventricular rate control was defined as a mean ventricular rate < 80 bpm without exercise during Holter monitoring before the procedures

Table 2. Concomitant pharmacological therapy at enrolment

Drug	Rate control group n = 56	Rhythm control group n = 58	*P* value
Digoxin	40 (71%)	17 (29%)	0.001
Diuretics	44 (79%)	32 (55%)	0.01
Nitrates	12 (21%)	NA	
Ace-inhibitors/AT-II blockers	40 (71%)	42 (72%)	0.4
Beta-blockers	29 (52%)	56 (97%)	0.001
Calcium-antagonists	11 (20%)	16 (28%)	0.2
Aspirin	4 (7%)	10 (17%)	0.09
Warfarin	47 (85%)	58 (100%)	0.001
Amiodarone	7 (12%)	41 (71%)	0.001

and the Specific Symptom Scale in the RATE study and the 36-item Short Form of the Medical Outcome Study and the Symptom Checklist questionnaires in the RHYTHM study were used to measure symptoms and quality of life. Exercise capacity was evaluated by the 6-min walked distance in the RATE study and by exercise time and capacity in the RHYTHM study.

The comparison between the two study populations was made by unpaired t test for continuous variables and by Fisher's exact test for proportions. To make the measures of the two studies comparable, the intrapatient comparison that had been performed in the original study between enrolment and follow-up was reported as percentage of change. The respective percentages were then compared between the two study populations.

Results

A stable rate or rhythm control was achieved in 98% of RATE patients and in 78% of RHYTHM patients ($P = 0.001$). At least one procedure was necessary in 11% and 50% of patients, respectively ($P = 0.001$) (Table 3). Two RHYTHM patients who had heart failure symptoms after failed ablation received successful AV junction ablation and AV pacing. Severe peri-procedural complications occurred in 0% and 3% of patients (difference not significant). During a follow-up of 12 months (Table 4), compared with pre-ablation measures, NYHA class improved by 30% in RATE patients and by 39% in RHYTHM patients (difference not significant). In the RATE study, the Minnesota Living with Heart Failure Questionnaire score improved by 49%, the Specific Symptom Scale total score by 53%, and the Karolinska score by 54%. In the RHYTHM study, the Physical and the Mental summary scores of the 36-item Short Form of the Medical Outcome Study questionnaire increased by 53% and 40%, respectively, and the frequency and severity scores of the Symptom Checklist questionnaire increased by 45% and 57%, respectively (all differences not significant compared with RATE quality of life measures). In the RATE study, the 6-min walked distance increased by 19%; in the RHYTHM study, exercise time increased by 9.4% and exercise capacity by 17% (difference not significant). Congestive heart failure recurred during the follow-up in 11% of RATE and in 5% of RHYTHM patients (difference not significant). The RHYTHM patients had significantly greater improvement in LV function (+60% vs +10%, $P = 0.001$), reduction of LV diastolic diameters (-10% vs +2%, $P = 0.001$), and LV systolic diameters (-17% vs -5%, $P = 0.001$). There were six deaths in the RATE study and one in the RHYTHM study ($P = 0.05$). The mean age of the six patients who died in the RATE study was 75±4 years; five of those patients (83%) had LBBB.

Table 3. Procedures and outcome. CS coronary sinus

	Rate control group	*P* value	Rhythm control group	
Undergoing initial procedure	56		58	Performing initial procedure
Failures: no CS pacing (2), no stable AV block (3), threshold increase (1):	6 (11%)	0.001	29 (50%)	Failure: AF persistence
Stable rate control after correction	55 (98%)	0.001	45 (78%)	Stable sinus rhythm after repeated ablation (5 with drugs
Severe complications	0 (0%)	0.3	2 (3%)	Severe complications: tamponade (1), stroke (1)
Length of follow-up, months	12		12 ± 7	Length of follow-up, months
Clinical events during follow-up				Clinical events during follow-up
Death (sudden 3, heart failure 3)*	6 (11%)	0.05	1 (1%)	Death
Congestive heart failure	6 (11%)	0.2	3 (5%)	Congestive heart failure

Discussion

This is the first attempt to compare two recent, non-pharmacological, innovative therapies that are not yet fully established. Although the methodological limitations of this kind of comparison are obvious, nevertheless to our knowledge no prospective randomised trial has yet been designed for this purpose, and many years of follow-up will probably be necessary before such a study can be concluded. Therefore, our results provide the background to perform a proper randomised controlled trial.

Nonetheless, the results should be interpreted with caution, taking in account the following considerations:

1. Non-pharmacological rate and rhythm control strategies are very effective in improving quality of life and exercise capacity during 1 year of follow-up. While NYHA class was used in both studies, quality of life and exercise capacity were evaluated by different outcome measures. Thus,

Table 4. Improvement of quality of life, exercise capacity and left ventricular function during the follow-up compared with baseline evaluation. *NYHA* New York Hear Associaton classification, *LHFQ* Minnesota Living with Heart Failure questionnaire, *SSS* Specific Symptom Scale, *SF 36* 36-item Short Form of the Medical Outcome Study questionnaire, *SCL* Symptom Checklist

	Rate control group (BIV pacing) ($n = 41$ patients)			Rhythm control group ($n = 34$ patients)			
Outcome measure[a]	Absolute improvement vs baseline	Improvement vs baseline (%)	*P* value*	Outcome measure	Absolute improvement vs baseline	Improvement vs baseline (%)	*P* value*
NYHA	-0.7 ± 0.6 points out of 4	30	0.02	NYHA	-0.9 ± 0.5 points out of 4	39	0.001
Minnesota LHFQ	-23 ± 16 points out of 105	49	0.001	SF 36 (physical)	+24 ± 21 points out of 100	53	0.001
Karolinska questionnaire	-4.3 ± 2.6 points out of 16	54	0.001	SF 36 (mental)	+21 ± 19 points out of 100	40	0.001
SSS total	-12 ± 11 points out of 60	53	0.001	SCL (frequency)	-13 ± 9 points out of 64	45	0.001
				SCL (severity)	-10 ± 8 points out of 64	57	0.001
6-minute walked distance	From 293 ± 108 to 350 ± 116 m (+57 m)	19	0.001	Exercise time	from 11 ± 4 to 14 ± 5 min	9.4	0.001
				Maximal exercise capacity	from 123 ± 44 to 144 ± 55 Watts	17	0.001
LV ejection fraction	+4 ± 9 points	10	0.004	LV ejection fraction	+21 ± 13 points	60	0.001
LVEDD	+1 ± 6 mm	-2	0.2	LVEDD	-6 ± 6 mm	10	0.03
LVESD	-2 ± 6 mm	5	0.02	LVESD	-8 ± 7 mm	17	0.001

*Intrapatient comparison with baseline valves

NYHA, $P = 1.0$; LHFQ vs SF36 physical: $P = 0.9$; LHFQ vs SF36 mental: $P = 0.6$; Karolinska vs SF36physical: $P = 0.9$; Karolinska vs SF36mental: $P = 0.3$; SSS vs SCL frequency: $P = 0.6$; SSS vs SCL severity: $P = 0.9$; 6-min walked distance vs exercise time: $P = 0.4$, 6-min walked distance vs exercise capacity: $P = 0.9$; EF, $P = 0.001$; LVEDD, $P = 0.001$; LVESD, $P = 0.001$

the results could be compared only indirectly, by comparing the percent variations from baseline to the end of the follow-up. However, they were very similar in terms of improvement in quality of life and exercise capacity. It is likely that the greater improvement of cardiac performance obtained with the rhythm control therapy was counterbalanced by the lower procedural success rate of this therapy and by the potentially deleterious effects of antiarrhythmic drugs, which were continued in some patients.

2. Advanced age and the presence of LBBB are independently associated with poorer survival in population-based studies of patients with heart failure [12, 13]. In one study [12], patients ≥ 75 years the age of those who died in the RATE study had an odds ratio of 4.2 (CI 3.5–5.1) to die after 1 year compared to the odds ratio of 1.6 (CI 1.3–1.9) of patients age 50–64 years as which affected five of the six patients who died in the RATE study had a odds ratio of1.9 (CI 1.4–2.3) to die after 1 year compared to those without LBBB. Thus, it seems that the great difference in age and the presence of LBBB can explain sufficiently the observed difference in mortality between the two studies. The 1-year mortality rate of our population was 11%, which is very similar to that of the large series of patients affected by AF and mild-to-moderate heart failure enrolled in the V-HeFT II study [14]. In some population-based studies, mortality at 1 year was higher, ranging from 8% up to 60% [12, 13, 15]. The large disparity between patient-fatality rates observed in the RHYTHM study and the rates reported in population-based studies is due clearly to some selection criteria of the patients, making mortality rates difficult to compare.

Perspectives

What scenario is likely in the next few years? Both strategies will probably become established in clinical practice, and many patients with drug-refractory symptomatic AF will benefit from one or the other therapy. The advantage of a curative approach that maintains sinus rhythm should be weighed against the lower success rate, the need to perform a second procedure in many patients, and the potential for severe complications. The choice of one or the other therapy may well depend on the individual characteristics of the patients. For example, younger patients with narrow QRS and absence of LV dyssynchrony could first undergo an attempt of curative left atrial catheter ablation. Conversely, older patients with wide QRS and LV dyssynchrony will probably benefit more from resynchronisation therapy. Since the risk of arrhythmic sudden death remains a major issue, an ICD back-up should be considered in those patients with severely depressed systolic function.

References

1. The AFFIRM First Antiarrhythmic Drug Substudy Investigators (2003) Maintenance of sinus rhythm in patients with atrial fibrillation: an AFFIRM substudy of the first antiarrhythmic drug. J Am Coll Cardiol 42:20–29
2. The Atrial Fibrillation Follow-up Investigation of Rhythm Management (AFFIRM) Investigators (2002) A comparison of rate control and rhythm control in patients with atrial fibrillation. N Engl J Med 347:1825–1833
3. Van Gelder IC, Hagens VE, Bosker HA et al (2002) A comparison of rate control and rhythm control in patients with recurrent persistent atrial fibrillation. N Engl J Med 347:1834–1840
4. Hohnloser SH, Kuck KH, Lilienthal J (2000) Rhythm or rate control in atrial fibrillation–Pharmacological Intervention in Atrial Fibrillation (PIAF): a randomized trial. Lancet 356:1789–1794
5. Clark D, Plumb V, Epstein An et al (1997) Hemodynamic effects of irregular sequences of ventricular cycle lenghts during atrial fibrillation. J Am Coll Cardiol 30:1039–1045
6. Daoud EG, Weiss R, Bahu M et al (1996) Effect of irregular ventricular rhythm on cardiac output. Am J Cardiol 78:1433–1436
7. Haïssaguerre M, Jaïs P, Shah DC et al (1998) Spontaneous initiation of atrial fibrillation by ectopic beats originating in the pulmonary veins. N Engl J Med 339:659–666
8. Hsu LF, Jaïs P, Sanders P et al (2004) Catheter ablation for atrial fibrillation in congestive heart failure. N Engl J Med 351:2373–2383
9. Brignole M, Menozzi C, Gianfranchi L et al (1998) Assessment of atrioventricular junction ablation and VVIR pacemaker versus pharmacological treatment in patients with heart failure and chronic atrial fibrillation. A randomized controlled study. Circulation 98:953–960
10. Brignole M, Gammage M, Puggioni E et al (2005) Comparative assessment of right, left and bi-ventricular pacing in patients with permanent atrial fibrillation. Eur Heart J 26:712–722
11. Stevenson WG, Stevenson LW (2004) Atrial fibrillation and heart failure - five more years. N Engl J Med 351:2437–2438
12. Jong P, Vowinckel E, Liu PP et al (2002) Prognosis and determinants of survival in patients newly hospitalized for heart failure: a population-based study. Arch Intern Med 162:1689–1694
13. Baldasseroni S, De Biase L, Fresco C et al (2002) Cumulative effect of complete left bundle-branch block and chronic atrial fibrillation on 1-year mortality and hospitalization in patients with congestive heart failure. A report from the Italian network on congestive heart failure (in-CHF database). Eur Heart J 23:1692–1698
14. Carson P, Johnson G, Dunkman B, et al (1993) The influence of atrial fibrillation on prognosis in mild to moderate heart failure. The V-HeFT studies. Circulation 87 (suppl VI):102–110
15. Blackledge HM, Tomlinson J, Squire IB (2003) Prognosis for patients newly admitted to hospital with heart failure: survival trends in 12 220 index admissions in Leicestershire 1993–2001. Heart 89:615–620

Cardiac Resynchronisation Therapy in Patients with NYHA Class I-II

C. Linde

Background

Chronic heart failure (HF) due to systolic dysfunction is a major health problem, and there is an increasing prevalence as a result of better survival after acute myocardial infarction, improved diagnostic methods, and aging of the population. In the USA, there are approximately five million HF patients in a total population of nearly 294 million [1], while in Europe there are 10 million in a total of 666 million people. Asymptomatic left ventricular dysfunction (ALVD) is estimated to have a similar prevalence [2, 3]. The prognosis of HF is poor if the underlying cause cannot be treated. Recent advances in drug treatment, particular those that modify neurohormones, have been shown to reduce HF-related morbidity and mortality [4–6].

Overt HF symptoms generally follow ALVD, which is linked to increased morbidity and mortality [5–7]. In the Framingham trial, a mortality rate of 40% over a 5-year follow-up was found in patients with a marginally reduced left ventricular ejection fraction (LVEF) (< 50%) [6]. In the SOLVD prevention study, the development of HF was studied in patients with ALVD defined by a LVEF of < 35%. Over 8.3 months, 30% in the placebo group, compared to 21% in the enalapril group, developed overt HF. If electrical dyssynchrony accompanies left ventricular (LV) dysfunction, the prognosis is worse [8–10]. Health-care expenditures on HF typically account for 1–2% of total health budgets, of which hospitalisations account for 60–70% of costs [11–13]. Thus, in addition to optimal HF medication, interventions that would halt disease progression and thereby reduce hospitalisation will reduce health-care expenditure in these patients.

Department of Cardiology, Karolinska University Hospital, Stockholm, Sweden

Cardiac resynchronisation therapy (CRT) has recently emerged as new and additional form of treatment for patients with chronic HF and evidence of ventricular dyssynchrony. The clinical efficacy of CRT is now established in patients with moderate to severe (NYHA class III–IV) HF [14, 15]. Reverse ventricular remodelling has consistently been demonstrated with CRT [16–18]. It reflects prevention of disease progression and is possibly associated with better outcome. Recent data [19] suggest that reverse LV remodelling by CRT can also be observed in less symptomatic HF patients (NYHA class II) patients. The purpose of this chapter is to elucidate the rationale for CRT in patients with ALVD with prior HF symptoms or with mild systolic HF (NYHA class II) and to discuss ongoing studies in these patients.

The Effects of CRT in Patients with Classical Indications for CRT

In studies including 3- to 6-months of follow-up, CRT, either alone or combined with an implantable cardioverter-defibrillator (ICD), has been shown to improve symptoms, exercise tolerance, and quality of life [14, 15, 20] and to reverse LV remodelling [16–18] in patients with moderate to severe HF and wide QRS. Two studies have focused on morbidity and mortality with longer follow-up periods in similar patients. One of these demonstrated reduced HF-related deaths and hospitalisations by CRT whereas reduced overall mortality was only demonstrated in combination with ICD therapy [21]. Recently, however, total mortality and HF-related hospitalisations were found to be reduced by CRT compared to control treatment in the CARE-HF trial [22]. Thus, there is a clear evidence for improvements in total and HF-related mortality by CRT per se, which justifies the choice of a CRT device without a defibrillator in many HF patients, especially in the elderly.

Present Knowledge Regarding the Effects of CRT in NYHA II Patients

Whether CRT has similar benefits in patients with less severe HF remains controversial [23]. One recent study focused on patients with NYHA class-II HF and a classical indication for an ICD [19]. This was a relatively small, randomised, double-blind, parallel-controlled 6-month study on optimal medical therapy of HF patients. All of the patients had NYHA class-II symptoms, an LVEF ≤ 35%, and a left ventricular end-diastolic diameter (LVEDD) ≥ 55 mm. In this study, 101 patients were randomised to CRT OFF and 85 to CRT ON. Based on the clinical composite endpoint developed by Packer [24] to assess HF patients, significant improvement of CRT compared to control treatment was shown (Fig. 1).

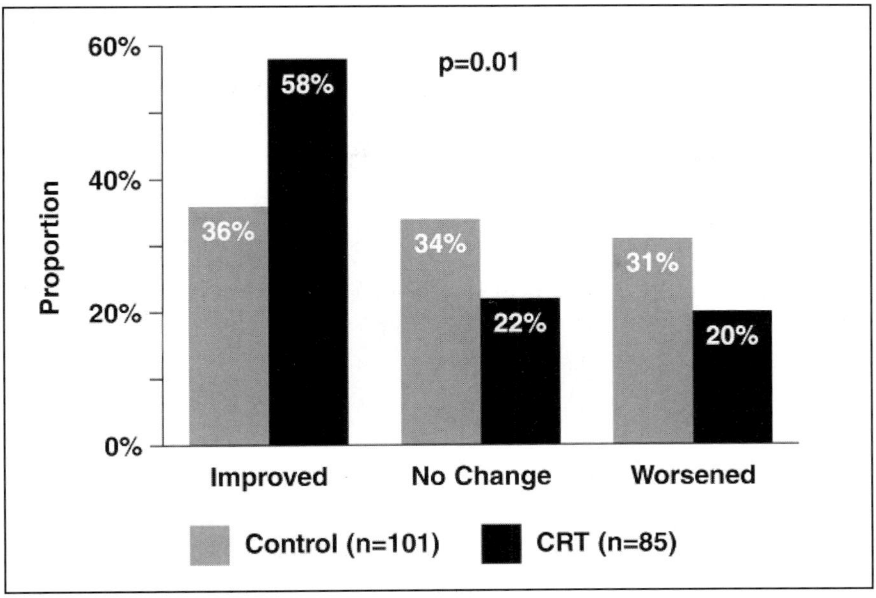

Fig. 1. The clinical composite endpoint in the treatment and control groups at 6 months in the Miracle ICD II trial. From [19], with permission

Reverse Remodelling

Although patients with pathological LV remodelling experience progressive worsening of HF, slowing or reversing of remodelling has only recently been recognised as a goal of treatment [25]. Reverse remodelling by inhibitors of angiotensin converting enzyme (ACEIs), in particular β-blockers [26, 27], has been linked to reduced morbidity and mortality in all classes of systolic HF. Furthermore, these observations have been substantiated by large trials [28–30]. A consistent finding in the CRT trials designed with 3- to 6-months follow-up is an 8–15% reduction in LVEDD and an increase in LVEF of 4–6% [15–17, 23, 31], expressed in units of absolute value. In the CONTAK-CD trial, significant reverse remodelling could also be demonstrated in the subgroup of NYHA class I–II patients after 6 months of CRT, even though benefits were less pronounced than in the much larger group of NYHA III–IV patients [23]. In the MIRACLE ICD II study, significant reverse remodelling by CRT was seen in NYHA class-II patients (Fig. 2) [19]. These preliminary observations suggest that CRT might favourably impact outcomes in patients with less severe symptoms of HF, LV systolic dysfunction, and ventricular dyssynchrony.

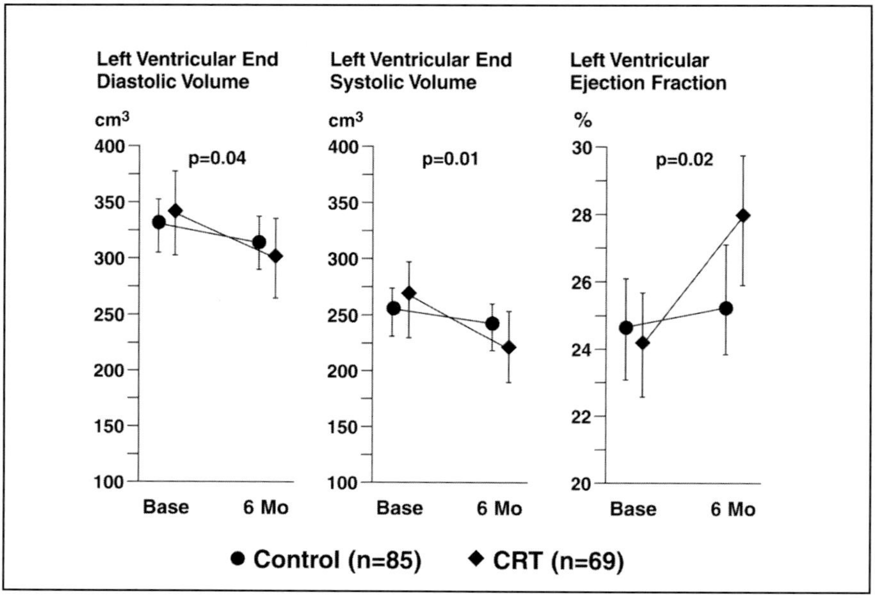

Fig. 2. The change in left ventricular (LV) volumes and LV ejection fraction after 6 months of either cardiac resynchronisation therapy or no pacing

Ongoing and Future Trials To Assess the Effects of CRT in NYHA Class I–II Patients

To test the hypothesis that CRT might favourably impact outcomes in patients with less severe symptoms of HF, LV systolic dysfunction, and ventricular dyssynchrony, the REsynchronization [reVErses Remodeling in Systolic left vEntricular dysfunction (REVERSE)] study has been initiated. This study aims at assessing the safety and efficacy of CRT in addition to optimal medical therapy in patients with ALVD (NYHA I ACC/AHA stage C) or mild HF (NYHA II) [32].

The REVERSE study is a prospective, multi-centre, randomised, double-blind, parallel-controlled clinical trial designed to establish whether CRT combined with optimal medical treatment can attenuate HF disease progression over at least 12 months compared to optimal medical treatment alone, in patients with mild HF. Inclusion criteria are: NYHA I ACC/AHA stage C or II HF, QRS duration ≥ 120 ms, LV ejection fraction ≤ 40%, LVEDD ≥ 55 mm, and an optimised pharmacological regimen [33].

After successful implantation of an atrio-biventricular device (CRT pacemaker or CRT defibrillator, according to the patients' needs) approximately 500 patients from 100 centres in the USA, Canada, and Europe will be randomised to CRT versus no CRT, and followed for at least 12 months (24 months in Europe). The primary endpoint is the HF clinical composite response, and LV end-systolic volume index is the first-order secondary endpoint. Enrolment started in September 2004 and is expected to be completed in 2006.

The MADIT CRT aims at investigating whether prophylactic CRT inhibits or slows symptomatic HF. Patients with previous myocardial infarction and NYHA I–II, or patients with non-ischaemic cardiomyopathy in NYHA II will be randomised to either the CRT or control group if they have an EF < 30%, sinus rhythm, and QRS> 130 ms. The primary endpoint is time to mortality (considering all causes) or HF event. This study will include 1820 subjects with an estimated follow-up time of 24 months.

Conclusions

Cardiac resynchronisation therapy improves HF symptoms and reduces HF-related hospitalisations and total mortality in patients with moderate to severe HF and ventricular dyssynchrony. In smaller studies, CRT has also been shown be beneficial in patients with less symptomatic HF. The effects of CRT on HF outcomes is therefore currently being studied in patients with NYHA II heart failure or ALVD.

References

1. Anonymous (2003) Heart disease and stroke statistics - 2004 update. American Heart Association. In: http://www.americanheart.org/downloadable/heart/1079736729696HDSStats2004UpdateREV3-19-04.pdf
2. Mosterd A, Hoes AW, de Bruyne MC et al (1999) Prevalence of heart failure and left ventricular dysfunction in the general population; The Rotterdam Study. Eur Heart J 20:447–455
3. McDonagh TA, Robb SD, Murdoch DR et al (1998) Biochemical detection of left-ventricular systolic dysfunction. Lancet 351:9–13
4. Konstam MA, Kronenberg MW, Rousseau MF et al (1993) Effects of the angiotensin converting enzyme inhibitor enalapril on the long-term progression of left ventricular dilatation in patients with asymptomatic systolic dysfunction. SOLVD (Studies of Left Ventricular Dysfunction) Investigators. Circulation 88:2277–2283
5. The SOLVD Investigators (1992) Effect of enalapril on mortality and the development of heart failure in asymptomatic patients with reduced left ventricular ejection fractions. N Engl J Med 327:685–691
6. Wang TJ, Evans JC, Benjamin EJ et al (2003) Natural history of asymptomatic left ventricular systolic dysfunction in the community. Circulation 108:977–982
7. Levy D, Kenchaiah S, Larson MG et al (2002) Long-term trends in the incidence of and survival with heart failure. N Engl J Med 347:1397–1402
8. Venkateshawar K, Gottipaty K, Krelis P (1999) The resting electrocardiogram pro-

vides a sensitive and inexpensive marker of prognosis in patients with chronic congestive heart failure. J Am Coll Cardiol 33:145A (abs)
9. Baldasseroni S, Opasich C, Gorini M et al (2002) Left bundle-branch block is associated with increased 1-year sudden and total mortality rate in 5517 outpatients with congestive heart failure: a report from the Italian network on congestive heart failure. Am Heart J 143:398–405
10. Silvet H, Amit J, Padmanabhan S (1999) Increased QRS-duration reduces survival in patients with left ventricular dysfunction: results form a cohort of 2263 patients. J Am Coll Cardiol 33:145A (abs)
11. McMurray J, McDonagh T, Morrison CE et al (1993) Trends in hospitalization for heart failure in Scotland 1980–1990. Eur Heart J 14:1158–1162
12. Berry C, Murdoch DR, McMurray JJ (2001) Economics of chronic heart failure. Eur J Heart Fail 3:283–291
13. Ryden-Bergsten T, Andersson F (1999) The health care costs of heart failure in Sweden. J Intern Med 246:275–284
14. Cazeau S, Leclercq C, Lavergne T et al (2001) Effects of multisite biventricular pacing in patients with heart failure and intraventricular conduction delay. N Engl J Med 344:873–880
15. Abraham WT, Fisher WG, Smith AL et al (2002) Cardiac resynchronization in chronic heart failure. N Engl J Med 346:1845–1853
16. Stellbrink C, Breithardt OA, Franke A et al (2001) Impact of cardiac resynchronization therapy using hemodynamically optimised pacing on left ventricular remodeling in patients with congestive heart failure and ventricular conduction disturbances. J Am Coll Cardiol 38:1957–1965
17. Linde C, Leclercq C, Rex S et al (2002) Long-term benefits of biventricular pacing in congestive heart failure: results from the MUltisite STimulation in cardiomyopathy (MUSTIC) study. J Am Coll Cardiol 40:111–118
18. St John Sutton MG, Plappert T, Abraham WT et al (2003) Effect of cardiac resynchronization therapy on left ventricular size and function in chronic heart failure. Circulation 107:1985–1990
19. Abraham WT, Young JB, Smith AL et al (2004) Combined cardiac resynchronization and implantable cardioversion defibrillation in advanced chronic heart failure: the MIRACLE ICD Trial. Circulation 110:2864–2868
20. Young JB, Abraham WT, Smith AL et al (2003) Combined cardiac resynchronization and implantable cardioversion defibrillation in advanced chronic heart failure: the MIRACLE ICD Trial. JAMA 289:2685–2694
21. Bristow MR, Saxon LA, Boehmer J et al (2004) Cardiac resynchronization therapy with or without an implantable defibrillator in advanced chronic heart failure. N Engl J Med 350:2140–2150
22. Cleland JGF, Daubert JC, Erdmann E et al (2001) on behalf of the CARE-HF Steering Committee and Investigators. The CARE-HF study (Cardiac Resynchronisation in Heart Failure study) rationale, design and end-points. Eur Heart Failure 3:481–489
23. Higgins SL, Hummel JD, Niazi IK et al (2003) Cardiac resynchronization therapy for the treatment of heart failure in patients with intraventricular conduction delay and malignant ventricular tachyarrhythmias. J Am Coll Cardiol 42:1454–1459.
24. Packer M (2001) Proposal for a new clinical end point to evaluate the efficacy of drugs and devices in the treatment of chronic heart failure. J Card Fail 7:176–182
25. Cohn JN, Ferrari R, Sharpe N (2000) Cardiac remodeling – concepts and clinical implications: a consensus paper from an international forum on cardiac remode-

ling. Behalf of an International Forum on Cardiac Remodeling. J Am Coll Cardiol 35:569–582

26. Bristow MR, Gilbert EM, Abraham WT et al (1996) Carvedilol produces dose-related improvements in left ventricular function and survival in subjects with chronic heart failure. MOCHA Investigators. Circulation 94:2807–2816
27. Kawai K, Takaoka H, Hata K et al (1999) Prevalence, predictors, and prognosis of reversal of maladaptive remodeling with intensive medical therapy in idiopathic dilated cardiomyopathy. Am J Cardiol 84:671–676
28. The Cardiac Insufficiency Bisoprolol Study II (CIBIS-II)(1999): a randomised trial. Lancet 353:9–13
29. Packer M, Coats AJ, Fowler MB et al (2001) Effect of carvedilol on survival in severe chronic heart failure. N Engl J Med 344:1651–1658
30. Effect of metoprolol CR/XL in chronic heart failure: Metoprolol CR/XL (1999) Randomised Intervention Trial in Congestive Heart Failure (MERIT-HF). Lancet 353:2001–2007
31. Lau CP, Yu CM, Chau E et al (2000) Reversal of left ventricular remodeling by synchronous biventricular pacing in heart failure. Pacing Clin Electrophysiol 23:1722–1725.
32. Hunt SA, Baker DW, Chin MH et al (2002) ACC/AHA guidelines for the evaluation and management of chronic heart failure in the adult: executive summary. J Heart Lung Transplant 21:189–203
33. Linde C, Gold M, Abraham WT, Daubert JC (2005) for the REVERSE study group. Rationale and design of a randomised controlled clinical study to assess if cardiac resynchronisation therapy can slow disease progression in mild to moderate heart failure – The Resynchronisation reVerses Remodelling in aSymptomatic left vEntricular dysfunction (REVERSE) study. Am Heart J (in press)

Cardiac Resynchronisation Therapy: Is It Antiarrhythmic or Proarrhythmic?

G. Turitto, N. El-Sherif

Introduction

Cardiac resynchronisation therapy (CRT) was defined in an American Heart Association Science Advisory as 'a relatively new therapy for patients with symptomatic heart failure resulting from systolic dysfunction' [1]. In addition to improving a variety of indices of functional status, CRT may decrease morbidity and mortality. A recent meta-analysis concluded that CRT reduces mortality from progressive heart failure and suggested a trend toward longer survival in patients treated with this approach [2]. Total mortality was also reduced in two recent trials, one of which included CRT in combination with defibrillation therapy [3, 4].

Although a delayed or halted progression of cardiac dysfunction may be sufficient to prevent malignant ventricular tachyarrhythmias, there is still lingering uncertainty regarding the presence and magnitude of antiarrhythmic effects of CRT per se. Furthermore, there is experimental and anecdotal clinical evidence that left ventricular pacing may have proarrhythmic potential, thus mandating the presence of a back-up defibrillation function in CRT devices. This review aims at reviewing evidence in favour or against an antiarrhythmic effect of CRT.

Evidence for a Proarrhythmic Effect of Left Ventricular Pacing

Basic Studies

Medina-Ravell et al. were the first to point out that the common design for

Cardiac Electrophysiology, New York Methodist Hospital and State University of New York – Downstate Medical Center, Brooklyn, NY, USA

CRT, i.e. simultaneous pacing of the right ventricular endocardium and left ventricular epicardium, is associated with a nonphysiological ventricular activation sequence. This may augment transmural heterogeneity of repolarisation intrinsic to ventricular myocardium and, as a consequence, prolong the QT and JT intervals on ECG [5]. Their study tested this hypothesis by assessing the effects of biventricular pacing (BiVP), left ventricular epicardial pacing (LVEpiP), and right ventricular endocardial pacing (RVEndoP) on ventricular repolarisation, specifically on QT and JT interval and transmural dispersion of repolarisation (TDR), and their roles in arrhythmogenesis in patients who received CRT. The cellular mechanisms underlying the pacing-site-dependent alterations in ventricular repolarisation were studied in an experimental model consisting of an arterially perfused rabbit LV wedge preparation in which transmembrane action potentials from endocardium and epicardium could be simultaneously recorded together with a transmural ECG. In the experimental preparation, TDR was defined as the difference between the longest and shortest repolarisation times across the LV wall. The authors showed that switching from endocardial to epicardial pacing resulted in a change of activation sequence between epicardium and endocardium, which was associated with an increase in QT interval and TDR without a parallel increase in endocardial and epicardial transmembrane action potential duration (APD). An increase in TDR manifested as a more positive and broader T wave on the transmural ECG. In six preparations, switching from endocardial to epicardial pacing produced a net increase in QT and TDR by 17 ± 5 and 22 ± 5 ms, respectively, at a basic cycle length of 1000 ms ($P < 0.05$). A more recent study examined the cellular basis for QT prolongation after reversal of the direction of activation of the LV wall [6]. Based on previous investigations documenting the contribution of M cells to TDR, this study postulated that delayed activation and repolarisation of M cells, coupled with earlier activation and repolarisation of epicardial cells, may result in QT prolongation, development of transmural heterogeneity, and torsade de pointes after a shift from endocardial to epicardial activation of the LV wall in the absence or presence of rapidly activating delayed rectifier potassium current (I_{Kr}) blockade. This hypothesis was tested in a 1-dimensional mathematical model of transmural conduction and in the coronary-perfused canine LV wedge preparation. The results of the mathematical simulation and the experimental data confirmed that intrinsic electrical heterogeneity exists within the ventricular myocardium and is amplified when the normal direction of activation of the ventricular wall is reversed. Epicardial activation augments TDR because the epicardial action potential activates and repolarises earlier while the M cells with the longest APD, located in the deep subendocardium, activate and repolarise later compared with endocardial activation of the ventricular wall. The additional conduction delay encountered between epicardial and M regions during epicardial stimulation contributes to the amplification of TDR. M cells play a crucial role in QT prolongation, amplification of TDR, and induction of torsade de pointes that develop after a shift from endocardial to epicardial activation of the LV myocardium. The delayed activation and repolarisation of M cells, when coupled with earlier activation of repolarisation of epicardial cells, create the substrate for the development of reentry.

In another study, the roles of voltage output, interventricular delay, and pacing sites in the development of ventricular arrhythmias were investigated during BiVP or LV pacing [7]. Voltage-sensitive dye was used in eight ischaemic Langerdorff-perfused guinea-pig hearts to measure ventricular activation times and to examine conduction patterns during multisite pacing from three RV and four LV sites. Isochronal maps of RV and LV activation were plotted. Ischaemia was produced by gradually halving the perfusion output over 5 min. Pacing the RV apex and the base of the LV anterior wall was associated with the most homogeneous and rapid activation pattern (28 ± 9 ms vs 41 ± 12 ms with the other configurations, $P < 0.01$), and no inducible arrhythmia. In six hearts, ventricular tachycardia could be induced when pacing from the right and left free walls with 20 ms of interventricular delay, at six-fold the pacing threshold output. In four hearts, simultaneous RV and LV pacing at high-voltage output induced ventricular fibrillation with complex three-dimensional propagation patterns, independently of the pacing sites. During BiVP with ischaemia, pacing at high-voltage output with a long interventricular delay is likely to induce ventricular arrhythmias, particularly when left and right pacing results in a conduction pattern orthogonal to the orientation of the ventricular myocardial fibres.

Clinical Studies

In a study by Medina-Ravell et al., the QT interval, JT interval, and TDR were measured in 29 patients with heart failure during RVEndoP, BiVP, and LVEpiP [5]. The data were collected perioperatively ($n = 29$), 24 h after the operation ($n = 19$), and during the first follow-up period, ranging from 1 to 2 weeks after the procedure ($n = 12$). LVEpiP and BiVP led to significant QT and JT prolongation. LVEpiP also enhanced TDR, defined as the interval between the peak and the end of the T wave ($T_{peak\text{-}end}$). Frequent R-on-T extrasystoles generated by BiVP and LVEpiP but completely inhibited by RVEndoP occurred in four patients, of whom one developed multiple episodes of nonsustained polymorphic ventricular tachycardia and another suffered incessant torsade de pointes. These data suggest that, in a subpopulation of patients with prolonged QT intervals, secondary to heart failure, electrolyte abnormalities, or exposure to agents with class III antiarrhythmic actions, a BiVP- or LVEpiP-dependent increase in QT interval and TDR may be a potential risk for the development of torsade de pointes. Similar occurrences of ventricular tachyarrhythmias developing or worsening immediately after CRT were the subject of two case reports [8, 9].

Evidence for an Antiarrhythmic Effect of Left Ventricular Pacing

Basic Studies

It is possible that changes described in experimental models of LV epicardial pacing may apply only to the first few hours of LV pacing in human subjects. Previous studies have shown that changes in the transmural activation sequence can lead to enduring changes in cardiac repolarisation (i.e. 'remodeling') [10, 11]. Further studies are needed to establish whether potentially proarrhythmic abnormalities that may be associated with the initiation of CRT are mitigated during long-term follow-up. At the present time, no data are available on the presence and degree of electrical remodeling after initiation of CRT.

Clinical Studies

There is evidence that beneficial structural and contractile LV remodeling after CRT has a favourable effect on the frequency of spontaneous and inducible ventricular tachyarrhythmias. The Ventak CHF Investigators reviewed the frequency of device therapy in patients, serving as their own controls, who were enrolled in this CRT study [12]. Of 54 patients enrolled in the Ventak CHF trial, 32 could be analysed. Each of them completed three blinded months programmed to BiV pacing and a second randomly assigned 3-month period of no pacing. Of the 32 patients, 13 (41%) received appropriate therapy for a ventricular tachyarrhythmia at least once in the 6-month monitoring period following implantation. Five patients (16%) had at least one tachyarrhythmic episode while programmed to BiV pacing, whereas 11 (34%) had at least one episode while programmed to no pacing. Three patients (9%) received therapy in both pacing periods, two with BiV pacing only. The decrease in necessary therapy for tachycardia during the BiV pacing period was statistically significant ($P = 0.035$). The authors concluded that, although CRT does not obviate the need for an ICD, it might diminish the need for appropriate tachyarrhythmia therapy. Other studies have shown that BiVP is associated with a decrease in the inducibility of ventricular tachycardia [13, 14]. Finally, there is anecdotal evidence that electrical storms may also be suppressed by CRT [15, 16].

Several markers of ventricular electrical vulnerability may be ameliorated by CRT, which may provide indirect evidence for the antiarrhythmic effect of this therapy. Heart rate variability (HRV) was evaluated during periods of pacing and no pacing in recipients of CRT [17, 18]. In a study by Adamson et al., HRV was examined in 50 patients implanted with a BiVP system who were randomised to therapy-on ($n = 25$) or therapy-off ($n = 25$) [17]. HRV was computed as the standard deviation of the atrial cycle length sensed from the system over 2 months of continuous monitoring. A comparison of HRV between CRT-on and CRT-off groups showed that HRV was higher in CRT-on than in CRT-off patients (148 ± 47 ms for CRT-on vs 118 ± 45 ms for CRT-off; $P = 0.02$), despite the lack of difference in mean atrial cycle length (844 ± 129 ms for CRT-on vs 851 ± 110 ms for CRT-off; $P = 0.82$). These authors concluded that CRT shifts cardiac autonomic balance toward a more favourable profile that is less dependent on sympathetic activation. An increase in HRV during CRT was also reported by groups who used conventional Holter recordings to analyse HRV parameters [18].

Microvolt T-wave alternans (TWA) has been proposed as a strong independent predictor of malignant ventricular tachyarrhythmias and sudden cardiac death. We recently investigated the prevalence of TWA during different pacing modalities in a group of patients who received CRT [19]. TWA was recorded with commercially available equipment in 16 such patients during atrial pacing (AAI) at a rate of 110/min, as well as during DDD-RV pacing and DDD-BiV pacing at the same rate and with short atrioventricular delay, in order to obtain ventricular capture. Criteria for positive TWA were: alternans > 1 min with Valt (square root of alternans power) > 1.9 μv and alternans ratio (ratio of alternans to standard deviation of background noise) > 3 in ≥ 1 orthogonal lead or ≥ 2 precordial leads. In this study, AAI and RV pacing resulted in a high prevalence of tachycardia-induced TWA, while BiV pacing was associated with amelioration of all TWA indices (Figs. 1, 2).

Conclusions

Available evidence supports the hypothesis that CRT results in favourable structural and electrical remodeling. Whether this effect would obviate the need for back-up defibrillation capability in CRT devices is unclear and should be the focus of further studies.

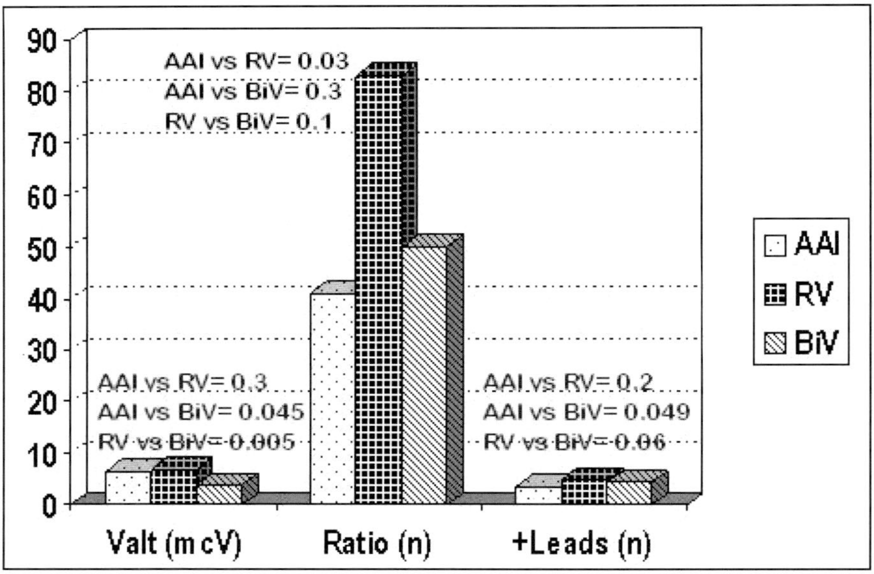

Fig. 1. T-wave alternans parameters obtained in 16 patients with CRT devices during atrial pacing (*AAI*), right ventricular pacing (*RV*), and biventricular pacing (*BiV*) at a rate of 110/min. BiV pacing resulted in a significant improvement in T-wave alternans parameters compared to AAI or RV pacing

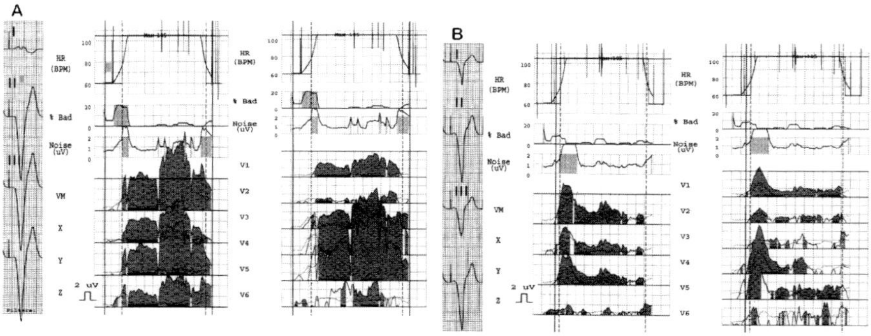

Fig. 2. **A** T-wave alternans (TWA) during RV pacing; **B**: TWA during BiV pacing. Abnormal TWA values were ameliorated when switching from RV to BiV pacing

References

1. Strickberger SA, Conti J, Daoud EG et al (2005) Patient selection for cardiac resynchronization therapy. Circulation 111:2146–2150
2. Bradley DJ, Bradley EA, Baughman KL et al (2003) Cardiac resynchronization and death from progressive heart failure. A meta-analysis of randomized controlled trials. JAMA 289:730–740
3. Bristow MR, Saxon LA, Boehmer J et al (2004) Cardiac-resynchronization therapy with or without an implantable defibrillator in advanced chronic heart failure. N Engl J Med 350:2140–2150
4. Cleland JGF, Daubert J-C, Erdmann E et al (2005) The effect of cardiac resynchronization therapy on morbidity and mortality in heart failure. N Engl J Med 352:1539–1549
5. Medina-Ravell VA, Lankipalli RS, Yan GX et al (2003) Effect of epicardial or biventricular pacing to prolong QT interval and increase transmural dispersion of repolarization. Does resynchronization therapy pose a risk for patients predisposed to long QT or torsade de pointes? Circulation 107:740–746
6. Fish JM, Di Diego JM, Nesterenko V et al (2004) Epicardial activation of the left ventricular wall prolongs QT interval and transmural dispersion of repolarization. Implications for biventricular pacing. Circulation 109:2136–2142
7. Garrigue S, Reuter S, Efimov IR et al (2003) Optical mapping technique applied to biventricular pacing: potential mechanisms of ventricular arrhythmias occurrence. Pacing Clin Electrophysiol 26(1 Pt 2):197–205
8. Guerra JM, Wu J, Miller JM et al (2003) Increase in ventricular tachycardia frequency after biventricular implantable cardioverter defibrillator upgrade. J Cardiovasc Electrophysiol 14:1245–1247
9. Cori AD, Bongiorni MG, Arena G et al (2005) New-onset ventricular tachycardia after cardiac resynchronization therapy. J Interv Card Electrophysiol 12:231–135
10. Geller JC, Rosen MR (1993) Persistent T-wave changes after alteration of the ventricular activation sequence: new insights into cellular mechanisms of cardiac memory. Circulation 88:1811–1819
11. Libbus I, Rosenbaum DS (2003) Transmural action potential changes underlying ventricular electrical remodeling. J Cardiovasc Electrophysiol 14: 394–402
12. Higgins SL, Yong P, Sheck D et al (2000) Biventricular pacing diminishes the need for implantable cardioverter defibrillator therapy: Ventak CHF Investigators. J Am Coll Cardiol 36: 824–827
13. Zagrodzky JD, Ramaswamy K, Page RL et al (2001) Biventricular pacing decreases the inducibility of ventricular tachycardia in patients with ischemic cardiomyopathy. Am J Cardiol 87:1208–1210
14. Kowal RC, Wasmund SL, Smith ML et al (2004) Biventricular pacing reduces the induction of monomorphic ventricular tachycardia: a potential mechanism for arrhythmia suppression. Heart Rhythm 1:295–300
15. Garrigue S, Barold SS, Hocini M et al (2000) Treatment of drug refractory ventricular tachycardia by biventricular pacing. Pacing Clin Electrophysiol 23:1700–1702
16. Tanabe Y, Chinushi M, Washizuka T et al (2003) Suppression of electrical storm by biventricular pacing in a patient with idiopathic dilated cardiomyopathy and ventricular tachycardia. Pacing Clin Electrophysiol 26(Pt 1):101–102
17. Adamson PB, Kleckner KJ, VanHout WL et al (2003) Cardiac resynchronization therapy improves heart rate variability in patients with symptomatic heart failure. Circulation 108:266–269

18. Livanis EG, Flevari P, Theodorakis GN et al (2003) Effect of biventricular pacing on heart rate variability in patients with chronic heart failure. Eur J Heart Fail 5:175–178
19. Turitto G, Houy S, Gupta R et al (2004) Right ventricular but not biventricular pacing increases markers of ventricular electrical instability. J Am Coll Cardiol 43 (Suppl A):149A

Impact of CRT on Mortality: What Are the Preliminary Results from the CARE-HF Trial?

M. Lunati, G. Magenta

CARE-HF Study Design and Study Results

The Cardiac Resynchronization-Heart Failure (CARE-HF) trial [1] was a multicentre, international randomised trial whose aims were:

1. To assess the effect on morbidity and mortality of adding CRT to optimised pharmacological therapy in patients with moderate and severe heart failure (HF) due to left ventricular systolic dysfunction (LVSD) complicated by cardiac dyssynchrony (CD)
2. To investigate the mechanisms underlying the observed effect and to identify markers predicting success or failure of CRT.

The main inclusion criteria were: chronic HF, NYHA class III/IV, with a high standard of pharmacological therapy, LVSD and dilation (EF $\leq$ 35% ; LVEDD $\geq$ 30 mm/heights in meters), cardiac dyssynchrony (QRS $\geq$ 150 ms or QRS $\geq$ 120 ms and two of the following echo criteria: aortic preejection delay $\geq$ 140 ms, interventricular mechanical delay $\geq$ 40 ms, delayed activation of the posterolateral LV wall).

Between January 2001 and March 2003, 813 patients were enrolled at 82 European centres. Patient randomised to CRT (404) received a Medtronic Insync or Insync III device that provided atrial-biventricular stimulation (without backup ICD); the implant success rate was 96%.

The primary endpoint was a composite of death from any cause or an unplanned hospitalisation for a major cardiovascular event. The principal secondary outcome was death from any cause, classified according to mode. At completion of the study (September 30, 2004) the rate of cross-over before primary endpoint was < 5%, survival status was ascertained on all patients,

SC Elettrofisiologia, Dipartimento Cardiologico 'A. De Gasperis', Azienda Ospedaliera Niguarda Cà Granda, Milan, Italy

mean follow-up from randomisation was 29.4 months.

Baseline characteristics were similar in the two groups (males 73%, mean age 66 years, mean ejection fraction 25%, mean QRS duration 160 ms, mean use of a beta-blocker 74%).

By the end of the study, the primary endpoint had been reached in 159 patients in the CRT group vs 224 patients in the control group (39% vs 55%; HR 0.63, 95% confidence interval 0.51–0.77, $P < 0.001$).

In the CRT group, 82 patients died as compared with 120 patients assigned to medical therapy alone (20% vs 30%; HR 0.64, 95% confidence interval 0.48–0.85, $P < 0.002$). The mode of death was sudden in 35% of the patients in the CRT group and in 32 % of the patients assigned to medical therapy; the cause of death was attributed to worsening HF in 40% of the patients in the CRT group and in 47% of the patients assigned to medical therapy.

Compared with medical therapy alone, CRT reduced interventricular mechanical delay, end-systolic volume index, area of mitral regurgitation jet. CRT increased EF and improved symptoms and quality of life ($P < 0.01$). The benefits were similar among patients with ischaemic heart disease and in those without, and were in addition to those afforded by pharmacological therapy.

In summary, the study demonstrated that in patients with advanced HF and cardiac dyssynchrony CRT improves symptoms and quality of life and reduces complications and risk of death (37% risk reduction of death or unplanned hospitalisation, 36% risk reduction of death from any cause) and should be routinely considered in such patients.

Impact of CRT on Mortality and Update on Guidelines

Approximately 20–25% of patients with advanced HF have electrocardiographic or echocardiographic evidence of inter or intraventricular dyssynchrony. CRT with the simultaneous stimulation of both ventricles improves coordination of ventricular contraction and, in a series of trials lasting up to 6 months, decreased symptoms and improved exercise capacity and ventricular function [2, 3].

In the COMPANION trial [4], the primary endpoint, composite outcome of mortality and hospitalisation for any reason, was reduced by 20% in the CRT arm and in the CRT+ICD arm during a mean follow-up of 16 months. Mortality, the secondary endpoint, was reduced by 24% relative (4% absolute), $P < 0.06$, by CRT and 36% relative (7% absolute), $P < 0.003$, by CRT + ICD. There was no difference in mortality when CRT and CRT+ICD were compared.

Meta-analyses have left some uncertainty about the effects of CRT on mortality [5, 6].

The CARE-HF trial [1] demonstrated a 37% relative (16% absolute), $P < 0.001$, reduction in the composite of death or hospitalisation for major events and a 36% relative (10% absolute), $P < 0.001$, reduction in all-cause death.

Thus, there is now clear-cut evidence that CRT, without ICD, significantly reduces the risk of death in patients with advanced HF and ventricular dyssynchrony. An ICD might further reduce the risk of sudden death, but if all cause mortality curves of COMPANION and CARE-HF are compared, it seems that HF patients died for arrhythmic events in the first 5–6 months after CRT, and after that period they died of HF progression; in other words, it seems that reverse remodelling influences electrical remodelling. Retarding the progression of cardiac dysfunction to prevent malignant arrhythmias and sudden death may be a better strategy than treating arrhythmias with an ICD once they occur, but obviously this issue needs further evaluation.

Owing to the striking evidence of the CARE-HF trial, in the recently published new guidelines (update 2005) for the diagnosis and treatment of chronic HF of the European Society of Cardiology [7], CRT can be considered in the treatment of patients with reduced EF and ventricular dyssynchrony (QRS duration [NYHA III–IV] despite optimal medical therapy:

- To improve symptoms (class of recommendation I, level of evidence A)
- To reduce hospitalisations (class of recommendation I, level of evidence A)
- To decrease mortality (class of recommendation I, level of evidence B).

CRT in combination with an ICD can be considered in patients with severe HF (NYHA III–IV), reduced EF, and ventricular dyssynchrony (QRS duration $\geq$ 120 ms):

- To improve morbidity and mortality (class of recommendation IIa, level of evidence B)

References

1. Cleland JG, Daubert JC, Erdmann E et al (2005) The effect of cardiac resynchronization on morbidity and mortality in heart failure. N Engl J Med 352:1539–1549
2. Cazeau S, Leclerq C, Lavergne T et al (2001) Effects of multisite biventricular pacing in patients with heart failure and intraventricular conduction delay. N Engl J Med 344:873–880
3. Abraham WT, Fisher WG, Smith AL et al (2002) Cardiac resynchronization in chronic heart failure. N Engl J Med 346:1845–1853
4. Bristow MR, Saxon LA, Boehmer J et al (2004) Cardiac resynchronization therapy with or without an implantable defibrillator in advanced chronic heart failure. N Engl J Med 350:2140–2150
5. Mc Alister FA, Ezekowitz JA, Wiebe N et al (2004) Systematic review: cardiac resyn-

chronization in patients with symptomatic heart failure. Ann Intern Med 141:381–390

6. Calvert M, Freemantle N, Cleland JG et al (2005) Cardiac resynchronization therapy in heart failure. Ann Intern Med 142:305–307
7. Anonymous (2005) Guidelines for the diagnosis and treatment of chronic heart failure: full text (update 2005). The Task Force for the diagnosis and treatment of CHF in the European Society of Cardiology. Eur Heart J 26:1115–1140

Loss of Resynchronisation by Biventricular Pacemakers: Mechanisms, Diagnosis and Therapy

S.S. BAROLD, B. HERWEG, A.B. CURTIS

Introduction

Ventricular resynchronisation with biventricular pacing has increased the complexity of device follow-up by virtue of additional timing cycles and new electrocardiographic manifestations [1–6]. Ventricular resynchronisation devices that memorise episodes of ventricular sensing together with preceding events have facilitated the diagnosis of loss of resynchronisation [1, 2]. The long-term stored data in resynchronisation devices are diagnostically far superior than conventional 24-h Holter recordings. Although the term 'ventricular resynchronisation' describes the mechanical effect of biventricular pacing, in this discussion the term is used simply to describe biventricular pacing (not equated with physiologic electrical resynchronisation). The term 'desynchronisation' describes the opposite electrical phenomenon, i.e. loss of biventricular pacing.

The 12-Lead Electrocardiogram

Paced QRS Complex and Status of Mechanical Ventricular Resynchronisation

The paced QRS during biventricular pacing (utilising the coronary venous system) is often narrower than the pattern registered during monochamber ventricular pacing [1, 4]. Barring ventricular fusion beats (with the conducted QRS complex), a narrower QRS implies depolarisation by both the right ventricular (RV) and left ventricular (LV) channels. Thus, measurement of

Division of Cardiology, University of South Florida College of Medicine and Tampa General Hospital, Tampa, FL, USA

QRS duration during follow-up is helpful in the analysis of appropriate biventricular capture and fusion with the spontaneous QRS complex [1, 4]. If the biventricular ECG is virtually similar to that recorded with RV or LV pacing alone and no cause is found, the conclusion that one of the leads does not contribute to biventricular depolarisation should not be automatically made without a detailed evaluation of the pacing system.

RV Lead at the Apex, and LV Lead in the Coronary Venous System

The frontal plane QRS axis is usually in the right superior quadrant. The frontal plane axis may occasionally reside in the left rather than the right superior quadrant. The QRS is often positive in lead V1 during biventricular pacing.

A negative QRS complex in lead V1 during uncomplicated biventricular pacing probably reflects differential activation of a heterogeneous biventricular substrate (ischaemia, scar, His-Purkinje participation in view of the varying patterns of LV activation in spontaneous left bundle-branch block, etc.), and may not necessarily indicate a poor (electrical or mechanical) contribution from LV stimulation. However, such a pattern in lead V1 requires exclusion of incorrect placement of lead V1 (too high on the chest), ventricular fusion (with the spontaneous QRS complex), lack of LV capture, LV lead displacement, presence of pacing via the middle cardiac vein or even unintended placement of two leads in the RV [1]. In this situation, it is also imperative to rule out marked latency (exit block or delay from the LV stimulation site), an important but poorly studied phenomenon that may generate the pattern of RV depolarisation during biventricular pacing and can be compensated by V–V timing that alters the timing between LV and RV pacing [1].

RV Lead in the Outflow Tract, and LV Lead in the Coronary Venous System

In our limited experience, we have found that during biventricular pacing with the RV lead in the outflow tract the paced QRS in lead V1 is often negative and the frontal plane paced QRS axis is often directed to the right inferior quadrant (right axis deviation) [1]. Further studies are required to confirm these preliminary findings and then determine the significance of these ECG patterns of biventricular pacing according to the RV pacing site.

Ventricular Fusion Beats with Native Conduction

In patients with sinus rhythm and a relatively short PR interval, ventricular fusion with competing native conduction during biventricular pacing may cause misinterpretation of the ECG, a common pitfall in device follow-up

[1]. Elimination of ventricular fusion may produce substantial clinical improvement. Marked QRS shortening mandates exclusion of ventricular fusion with the spontaneous QRS complex, especially in the setting of a relatively short PR interval. The presence of ventricular fusion should be ruled out by observing the paced QRS morphology during progressive shortening of the AS–VP interval in the VDD mode or the AP-VP interval in the DDD mode, if necessary. The AS–VP interval should be then programmed (with rate-adaptive function) to ensure pure biventricular pacing under circumstances that might shorten the PR interval such as increased circulating catecholamines.

Upper Rate Response of Biventricular Pacemakers

The upper rate response of biventricular pacemakers differs from those of conventional antibradycardia pacemakers because many patients with congestive heart failure (CHF) have normal sinus node function and AV conduction. In this situation, the upper rate response can assume one of two forms according to the location of the P wave in the pacemaker cycle: (1) Atrial-sensed upper rate response or a pre-empted Wenckebach upper rate response with AS–VS sequences (AS = atrial sensed event, VS = ventricular sensed event) and the P wave falling beyond the postventricular atrial refractory period (PVARP). (2) Atrial-refractory upper rate response (AR–VS) sequences (AR = atrial event detected in the PVARP) with the P wave 'unsensed' (not tracked) within the PVARP (Table 1) [2].

Table 1. Comparison of the two types of upper rate response of biventricular pacemakers in patients with normal sinus node and AV conduction (from [2])

	Wenckebach block	Atrial refractory block
VS–VS interval	< URI	< URI and < TARP
P wave sensing	All P waves are sensed beyond the PVARP	All P waves are unsensed (not tracked) in the PVARP where they cannot initiate a programmed AV delay.
PR interval	AS–VS > programmed AS–VP	AR–VS > programmed AS–VP
Ventricular pacing during established response	No	No
Entry	1. Gradual prolongation of AV delay (AS–VP) to the duration of the spontaneous PR interval (AS–VS).	1. Occurs when URI = TARP (W = 0) without intervening Wenckebach block. 2. Occurs following

continue →

Table 1 *continue*

	2. During the above, ventricular pacing contributes progressively less to ventricular fusion with the spontaneous QRS complex until ventricular pacing is inhibited by VS–VS sequences < URI.	Wenckebach block when the P–P interval < TARP. Will not occur if TARP is short (W long).
Progression with increase in atrial rate	1. No change will occur if W interval is long. AS–VS sequences continue and zone of refractory block will not be reached. 2. Wenckebach sequence may change into refractory block if W interval is short and atrial rate > TARP or P–P interval < TARP.	Remains unchanged but if the PR is long, AR may eventually move into the PVAB whereupon no AR marker will be registered.
Markers	AS–VS, AS–VS, AS–VS All P waves are followed by a spontaneous (conducted) QRS complex	AR–VS, AR–VS, AR–VS All P waves are followed by a spontaneous (conducted) QRS complex
Exit	During exit at the URI, ventricular pacing occurs with progressively more contribution to fusion with the spontaneous QRS complex until pure ventricular pacing supervenes. AS–VP sequences occur just below the programmed upper rate.	AS–VP sequences do not return when the P–P interval drops just below the programmed TARP [(AS–VP) + PVARP]. AS–VP sequences return when the P–P interval drops below the longer prevailing TARP [(AR–VP) + PVARP] because AR–VS > AS–VP.
Transient ventricular pacing	Briefly during entry and briefly during exit from established sequence	No

P–P interval Interval between two sinus P waves, *AS* atrial sensed event, *AP* atrial paced event, *AR* atrial event sensed in the atrial refractory period, *VS* ventricular sensed event, *VP* ventricular paced event, *PVARP* postventricular atrial refractory period, *PVAB* postventricular atrial blanking period, *TARP* total atrial refractory period. *URI* upper rate interval, *W* Wenckebach interval (*URI–TARP*, which is the maximal extension of the AV delay during a Wenckebach upper rate response (*maximal AV delay* programmed AV delay + W)

Pre-empted Wenckebach Upper Rate Response

In patients with normal or near normal sinus node function and AV conduction and a pacemaker with a relatively short PVARP, the Wenckebach upper rate response takes the form of a repetitive pre-empted process which consists of an attempted Wenckebach upper rate response with each cycle, associated with continual partial or incomplete extension of the programmed AV interval initiated by atrial sensing [1, 7]. The conducted spontaneous QRS complex occurs continually before completion of the upper rate interval. It is therefore sensed by the pacemaker, and pre-empts ventricular pacing (Fig. 1). In other words, the pacemaker cannot time out the upper rate interval and thus cannot emit a ventricular stimulus at its completion. This form of upper rate response tends to occur in patients with relatively normal AV conduction, a short programmed AV delay, a short PVARP (and short total atrial refractory period, TARP), but a relatively slow programmed (atrial-driven) upper rate. The occurrence of a pre-empted Wenckebach response in CHF patients may be puzzling because there are no pacemaker stimuli.

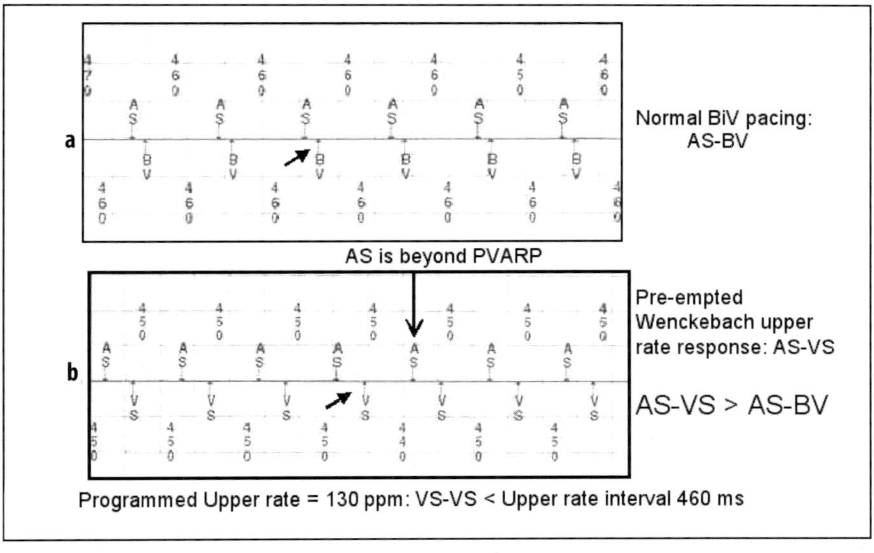

Fig. 1a, b. Stored markers from a Medtronic InSync II Marquis biventricular ICD showing the development of a pre-empted Wenckebach upper rate response during biventricular pacing. Upper rate interval (URI) = 460 ms. A There is 1:1 atrial tracking and biventricular (BV) pacing with the programmed AS–VP delay. B When the spontaneous ventricular rate exceeds the programmed upper rate (VS–VS < URI), a pre-empted Wenckebach upper rate response supervenes. AS conducts to VS so that AS–VS becomes longer than the programmed AS–VP interval. Note that the sinus P wave is sensed beyond the PVARP and that there is absence of pacemaker stimuli or pauses typical of a traditional Wenckebach upper rate response. *AS* Atrial sensed event, *VS* ventricular sensed event, *PVARP* postventricular atrial refractory period. The displayed interval durations by the programmer are approximate. (Reproduced with permission from [2])

Upper Rate Limitation with P Wave in the PVARP: Atrial Refractory Block

In a conventional antibradycardia pacemaker, a so-called fixed-ratio upper rate response follows a traditional Wenckebach upper rate response when the sinus or P–P interval ≤ TARP < upper rate interval or URI (or when P–P interval ≤ URI = TARP), and often takes the form of 2:1 block where every alternate P wave is unsensed in the PVARP. When P–P interval < TARP during biventricular pacing (in the setting of relatively normal sinus node function and AV conduction), a 2:1 block response does not occur in CHF patients because every spontaneous P wave falls in the PVARP (depicted as a AR marker) where they cannot be tracked. The conducted QRS complex (VS) linked to the P wave (AR, in the PVARP) generates a PVARP into which the next P wave will fall thereby ensuring the perpetuation of functional atrial undersensing [1, 2] (Fig. 2). Thus, no P wave can be tracked (Table 1). In this situation, the AV delay or AR-VS > programmed AS–VP. This upper rate response is probably best called a 1:1 atrial refractory upper rate response, or simply refractory a block because all the P waves are locked in the PVARP. There are no pauses and no pacemaker stimuli as in the pre-empted Wenckebach upper rate response.

Exit from Upper Rate Response and Onset of P Wave Tracking

When the upper rate response pushes the P wave into the PVARP, a device may not resume 1:1 atrial tracking when the sinus rate drops immediately below the programmed upper rate [1–3]. The P wave can remain in the

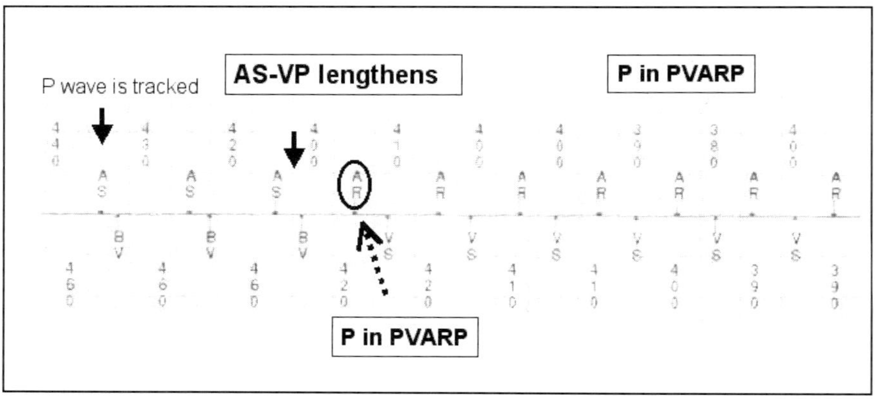

Fig. 2. Upper rate response in stored markers recorded from a Medtronic InSync II Marquis biventricular ICD. There is a typical Wenckebach upper rate response (with progressive prolongation of the AS–VP interval) which terminates with a sequence of atrial refractory block consisting of AR–VS combinations where the sinus P wave is in the PVARP and is not being tracked. The P wave conducts to the ventricle. Note the absence of pacemaker stimuli or pauses typical of traditional Wenckebach, and 'fixed-ratio' upper rate responses. (Reproduced with permission from [2])

PVARP even when the P–P interval > programmed TARP (or the atrial rate drops below the upper rate dictated by the TARP which is the sum of the programmed AS-VP + PVARP). The reason lies in the fact that AR-VS (spontaneous AV conduction) > programmed AS–VP interval (Fig. 3). Therefore, the TARP during AR–VS operation, (AR–VS) interval + PVARP must be longer than the programmed TARP, which is the sum of (AS–VP) interval + PVARP. The pacemaker will continue to operate with AR–VS cycles below the upper rate (dictated by the programmed TARP) until the P–P or sinus interval > the sum of (AR–VS) interval + PVARP, thereby allowing escape of the sinus P wave out of the PVARP (Fig. 3). Thus, restoration of resynchronisation will occur at a rate slower than the programmed upper rate (dictated by the TARP). These considerations are important in CHF patients, who may occasionally develop substantial increases in sinus

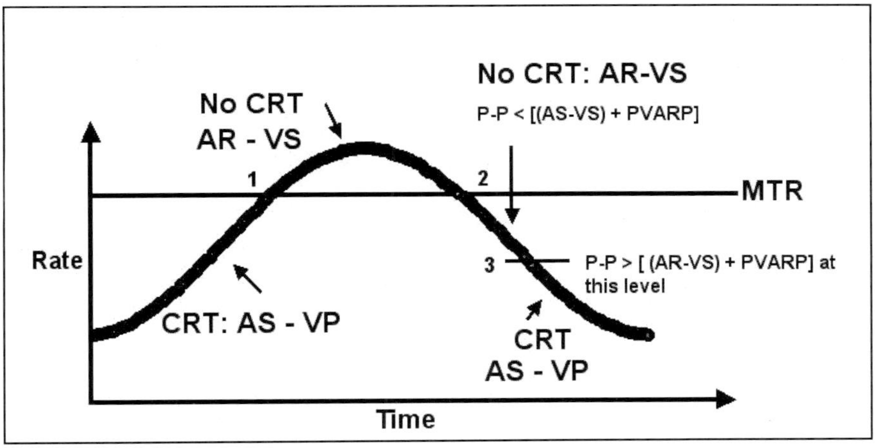

Fig. 3. Upper rate response with the P wave falling within the postventricular atrial refractory period (*PVARP*) in the setting of normal AV conduction. Ventricular resynchronisation occurs with AS–VP sequences (as programmed) when the sinus rate is below the maximum tracking rate (*MTR*). When the atrial rate exceeds the MTR at point 1, the P wave falls within the PVARP (sensed in the atrial refractory period and depicted by the AR marker) and ventricular resynchronisation is lost. The spontaneous rhythm takes over with AR–VS sequences and AR conducting to the ventricle (depicted by VS). When the sinus rate falls below the MTR at point 2, ventricular resynchronisation does not occur because the timing cycles of the device force the continuation of AR–VS sequences. Failure of ventricular resynchronisation at this stage results from the longer prevailing total atrial refractory period (TARP) which is equal to [(AR–VS) + PVARP] which is longer than the programmed TARP = [(AS–VP) + PVARP] simply because AR–VS >AS–VP. Ventricular resynchronisation with AS–VP sequences is restored at point 3 when the sinus or atrial interval (P–P) > [(AR–VS) + PVARP], at a sinus rate substantially lower than the MTR. AS atrial sensed event, VS ventricular sensed event, VP biventricular paced event, AR atrial event sensed in the atrial refractory period of the pacemaker where tracking cannot occur. (Reproduced with permission from [1])

rates despite beta-blocker therapy. The postponed restoration of atrial tracking upon emergence from the upper rate is worse in patients with first-generation devices because of double counting where 1:1 atrial tracking (AS–VP pacing) will return only when the sinus interval becomes longer than the [AR–VS] interval + PVARP + ICD (ICD = interventricular conduction delay or the interval between the RV and LV electrograms both sensed by the common sensing channel of these devices) [3, 5, 8].

Programming the Upper Rate

Inappropriately low upper rates in patients with normal sinus and AV nodal function is an important cause of ventricular desynchronisation that can deny patients the benefit of resynchronisation at high atrial rates, which are not uncommon in this patient population during exercise or situations associated with increased circulating catecholamines (especially during decompensation despite beta-blocker therapy). Relatively low upper rates must be avoided even in patients with symptomatic angina because loss of resynchronisation can itself precipitate cardiac ischaemia by increasing $MV0_2$. Loss of ventricular resynchronisation at high sinus rates can be reduced or prevented by programming a relatively high pacemaker upper rate because the risk of tracking rapid atrial rates by the implanted device (as with antibradycardia pacemakers) is not an important issue in the presence of normal AV conduction. However, the programmable values of the upper rate may be restricted in biventricular ICDs by the programmed maximum ventricular tachycardia interval to be detected.

Programming a fast upper rate may be difficult in some patients with retrograde ventriculoatrial conduction where more 'squeezing' of the AV delay to shorten the TARP may cause unfavourable haemodynamics. Alternatively, the maximum spontaneous rate could be attenuated by larger doses of beta-blockers (often better tolerated with device therapy [9]) or other drugs that depress sinus node function. In difficult or refractory cases, ablation of the AV junction should be considered to ensure continual ventricular depolarisation by the implanted device.

Loss of Resynchronisation Below the Programmed Upper Rate: Locking of P Waves in the PVARP

AR–VS, AR–VS sequences containing locked P waves within the PVARP can also occur outside of situations where a fast atrial rate (> the programmed upper rate) gradually drops below the upper rate [1–3]. There are many causes of desynchronisation that occur at rates slower than the upper rate (Table 2). For example, during sinus rhythm and synchronised biventricular pacing (below the upper rate), a ventricular premature complex (or T wave oversensing which produces the same effect) (Figs. 4, 5), by initiating a regular

PVARP, shifts pacemaker timing so that the succeeding undisturbed sinus P wave now falls in the PVARP. This P wave within the PVARP conducts to the ventricle, producing a spontaneous QRS complex sensed by the device. The sinus P waves will remain trapped in the PVARP as long as the P–P interval < [(AR–VS) + PVARP]. These forms of ventricular desynchronisation may be symptomatic, not uncommon, and can be precipitated by a variety of mechanisms (Table 2) [2]. The development of ventricular desynchronisation is favoured by a relatively fast sinus rate (but below the programmed upper rate), first-degree AV block, and a relatively long PVARP (Figs. 4, 5). 'Locking' of the P wave can often be prevented (barring reprogramming the device to eliminate the initiating mechanism, e.g. T wave oversensing) with a shorter PVARP and slowing the sinus rate with drugs. Persistent desynchronisation with 'locked' P waves is amenable to automatic disruption by special algorithms based on temporary PVARP abbreviation (Fig. 6). Refractory conditions (usually associated with marked first-degree AV block) can be treated by AV junctional ablation.

Table 2. Loss of cardiac resynchronisation during DDD or DDDR pacing in the presence of preserved RV and LV pacing

Intrinsic	1. Atrial undersensing from low amplitude atrial potentials 2. T wave oversensing and other types of ventricular oversensing such as diaphragmatic potentials 3. Long PR interval 4. Circumstances that push the P wave into the PVARP such as a junctional rhythm 5. New arrhythmia such as atrial fibrillation with a fast ventricular rate 6. Short runs of unsustained, often relatively slow, ventricular tachycardia 7. First-generation devices with a common sensing channel: ventricular double counting and sensing of far-field atrial activity
Extrinsic	1. Inappropriate programming of the AV delay or any function that prolongs the AV delay such as rate smoothing, AV search hysteresis, etc 2. Low maximum tracking rate 3. Slowing of the atrial rate upon exit from upper rate behavior 4. Functional atrial undersensing below the programmed upper rate A. precipitated by an atrial premature beat or ventricular premature beat. B. Long PVARP including post VPC automatic PVARP extension and single beat PVARP extension related to algorithms for automatic termination of endless loop tachycardia 5. Inappropriately slow programmed lower rate permitting junctional escape (cycle length < lower rate interval) in patients with periodic sinus arrest) 6. Intraatrial conduction delay where sensing of AS is delayed in the right atrial appendage. A short AS–VP interval may not be able to achieve biventricular pacing

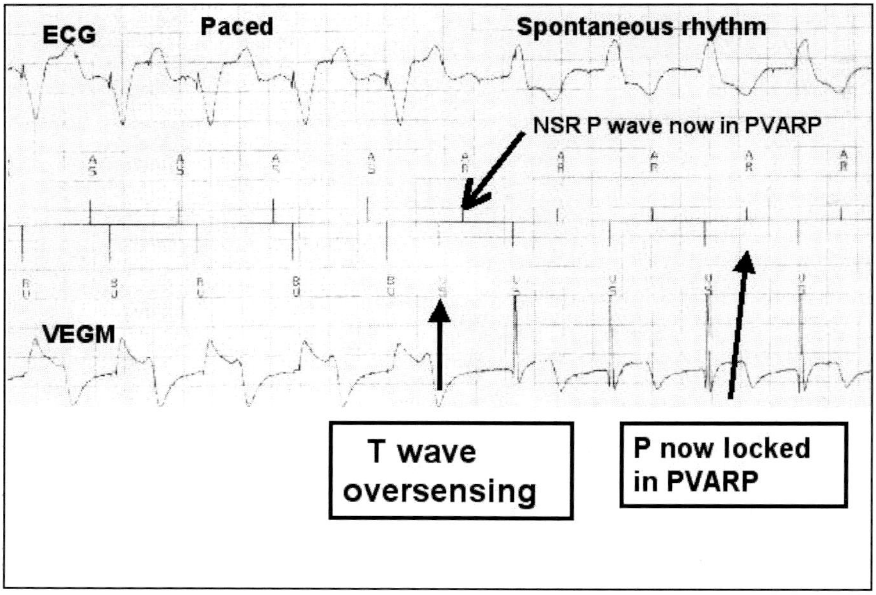

Fig. 4. Ventricular desynchronisation induced by T wave oversensing (*VS, arrow*) in a patient with marked first-degree AV block, left bundle-branch block and a Medtronic InSync II Marquis biventricular ICD. Lead II ECG is on top, markers in the middle, and the ventricular electrogram from the right ventricular apex at the bottom. The sinus rhythm remains undisturbed. VS (related to T wave oversensing) initiates a new PVARP into which the succeeding P wave is detected as AR (in the atrial refractory period) but not tracked. AR conducts to the ventricle as VS with a long PR interval thereby perpetuating the desynchronisation process with the sinus P waves (locked in the PVARP) continually conducting to the ventricle. (Reproduced with permission from [2])

Automatic Unlocking of P Waves From the PVARP. Algorithms to Restore Atrial Tracking

Special algorithms (which must be programmed) based on beat-to-beat PVARP shortening upon sensing a P wave in the PVARP are now available in the latest devices. This function promotes 1:1 atrial tracking whenever the 'effective TARP' [(AR–VS) + PVARP] prevents atrial tracking at rates below the programmed upper rate [10]. A device can detect AR–VS, AR–VS sequences suggestive of ventricular desynchronisation whereupon temporary PVARP abbreviation permits the device to sense the sinus P wave beyond the PVARP and restore atrial tracking and ventricular resynchronisation (Figs. 6, 7). In other words, the algorithm shortens the prevailing effective TARP. A P wave falling in the postventricular atrial blanking period (for pacing) cannot activate the special algorithm.

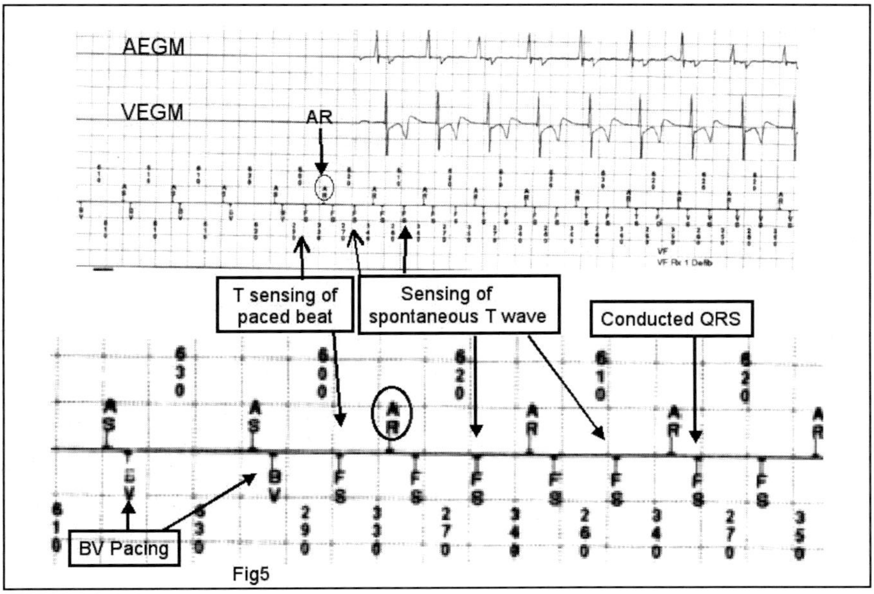

Fig. 5. Stored electrograms showing ventricular desynchronisation induced by T wave oversensing of a biventricular paced beat in a patient with a Medtronic InSync II Marquis biventricular ICD. A magnified portion at the bottom shows initiation of desynchronisation in greater detail. Note that the sinus rate is relatively fast (P–P interval = 610–630 ms, which is below the upper rate). The sequence starts with T wave oversensing of a paced beat (*first arrow on to FS*) which then initiates ventricular desynchronisation causing locking of the P wave in the PVARP (AR) which permits the emergence of the conducted spontaneous QRS complex. T wave oversensing also follows the spontaneous QRS complex. The device interpreted continual detection of both spontaneous QRS and T wave as ventricular fibrillation and subsequently delivered an inappropriate shock. T wave sensing of paced and spontaneous beats was subsequently reproduced at the time of follow-up. *AS* Atrial sensed event, *AR* atrial event detected in the atrial refractory period, *BV* biventricular pacing event, *AEGM* atrial electrogram, *VEGM* ventricular electrogram, *TS* tachycardia sense, *FS* ventricular fibrillation sense

Ventricular Triggered Mode

The ventricular triggered mode in some resynchronisation devices automatically attempts to provide resynchronisation in the presence of ventricular sensing. A ventricular sensed event initiates an immediate emission of a ventricular or usually a biventricular output (according to the programmed settings) in conformity with the programmed upper rate interval. For example, Medtronic devices offer this function in the VVIR mode, but in dual chamber devices triggering occurs upon sensing only in the programmed AV delay. The ventricular output will be ineffectual in the chamber where sens-

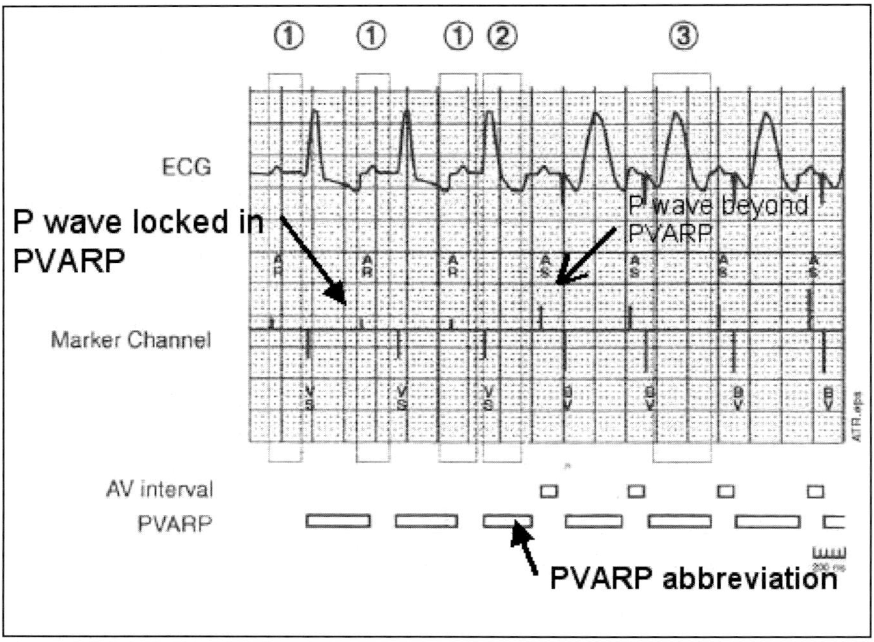

Fig. 6. Atrial tracking recovery algorithm (Medtronic) during biventricular pacing. Abbreviation of the PVARP promotes recovery of atrial tracking, and resynchronisation. The algorithm recognises VS–AR sequences only when the VS–VS interval is longer than the programmed upper rate interval. Atrial events must occur during the PVARP. After eight AR–VS cycles, the device intervenes by shortening the PVARP. The sinus P wave now resides outside the PVARP and is sensed and tracked as AS. This restores resynchronisation with AS–VP sequences. If the attempt fails, the process continues until AS–VP intervals are restored at their programmed value. *1* Atrial events in PVARP, *2* after 8 cycles the PVARP is shortened, *3* proper AS–VP sequences are restored at the programmed value

ing was initiated because the myocardium is physiologically refractory. The stimulus to the other ventricle thus attempts to provide a measure of resynchronisation. Ventricular triggering may be helpful in some patients but its true benefit is difficult to assess as the ventricles may be activated in an order that may not be haemodynamically favourable.

Atrial Fibrillation

In atrial fibrillation, the ventricular triggered mode may provide some degree of ventricular resynchronisation. Alternatively, some devices have programmable algorithms that increase the percentage of ventricular pacing and promote rate regularisation (without an overall increase in the ventricu-

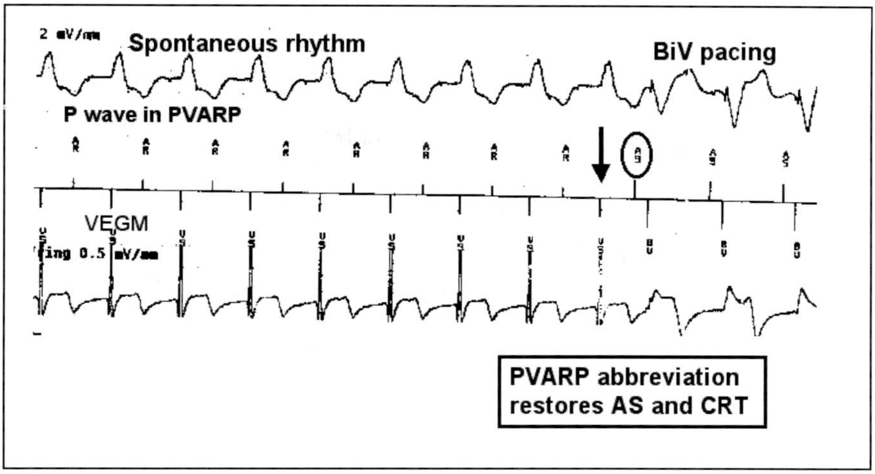

Fig. 7. Same patient and format as in Fig 4. On the left, the pattern of ventricular desynchronisation (AR–VS sequences) is identical to that in Fig 4. The ICD restores ventricular resynchronisation with an algorithm (see Fig. 6) that detects a specific number of AR–VS sequences (interpreted by the device as loss of resynchronisation) and then temporarily abbreviates the PVARP (*arrow*). The shorter PVARP permits P wave tracking and restores resynchronisation (AS–VP sequences at the programmed value) on the *right* of the recording. (Reproduced with permission from [2])

lar rate) by dynamic matching with the patient's own ventricular responses (up to the programmed maximum tracking rate). Activation of this algorithm or relying on the triggered response for resynchronisation does not result in control of the ventricular rate, and should not be a substitute for ablation of the AV junction in patients with drug-refractory rapid ventricular rates.

Cardiac resynchronisation by virtue of reverse remodelling may promote the return of sinus rhythm in some patients, but no firm data are yet available [11]. Furthermore, patients with permanent atrial fibrillation may have a greater likelihood of staying in sinus rhythm after cardioversion when it is performed after several months of device therapy and aggressive antiarrhythmic therapy [12]. This raises the question as to whether an atrial lead should be implanted during the initial procedure (with or without intraoperative cardioversion) in patients with permanent atrial fibrillation in whom cardioversion might be contemplated in the future.

Intra- and Interatrial Conduction Delay

Some patients have intraatrial conduction delay so that the atrial channel senses the atrial electrogram from the atrial appendage late and during the isoelectric portion of the PR interval [13]. The AS–VS interval (as seen by the pacemaker) during spontaneous AV conduction becomes quite short and can measure only 50–60 ms. Such patients may not tolerate an AS–VP interval of 40 ms or less to produce biventricular pacing, which in all likelihood might be associated with some degree of fusion with the spontaneous conducted QRS complex. This situation calls for one of two options: (1) using the ventricular triggered mode upon sensing the QRS complex after the sensed P wave – a trial of the triggered mode might produce the desired clinical improvement; (2) ablation of the AV junction with subsequent optimisation of the AV delay.

Conclusions

The physician must ensure that biventricular pacing takes place 100% of the time. The percentage of biventricular pacing and ventricular sensing must be carefully checked in the stored memorised data retrieved from the device. Devices must be programmed carefully to prevent desynchronisation (Table 3).

Table 3. Optimal programming of cardiac resynchronisation devices (modified from [1])

Parameters	Management
AV delay	1. A long AV delay should not be used. 2. Optimise the AS–VP delay and avoid ventricular fusion with the spontaneous conducted QRS complex 3. Program rate-adaptive (dynamic) AV delay off during temporary pacing for testing (with VDD mode slower than sinus rate to sense atrial activity) 4. Program rate-adaptive AV delay for long-term pacing
Atrial sensing and PVARP	1. Short PVARP (aim for 250 ms); may have to use algorithms for the automatic termination of endless loop tachycardia 2. Program off the post-VPC PVARP extension and the pacemaker-mediated tachycardia termination algorithm based on one cycle of PVARP extension 3. Automatic mode switching off in devices using a relatively long PVARP mandated by the mode switching algorithm
Upper rate	Relatively fast upper rate so the patient does not have 'break-through' ventricular sensing within their exercise zone. Initial upper rate of 140/min is often appropriate in the absence of myocardial ischaemia during pacing at this rate
AV conduction	1. Use drugs that impair AV conduction to avoid ventricular fusion or double counting in devices with a common sensing channel 2. Consider ablation of the AV junction in patients with a long PR interval or intraatrial conduction delay difficult to manage as well as refractory double counting (common sensing channel)

Troubleshooting loss of resynchronisation may be difficult and requires a thorough knowledge of biventricular pacemaker function, timing cycles, and complex algorithms. Partial (as in fusion beats), intermittent, or complete desynchronisation should always be ruled out in patients presenting with decompensated CHF, bearing in mind that the optimal or effective AV delay and other indices may change with time [14].

References

1. Barold SS, Herweg B, Giudici M (2005) Electrocardiographic follow-up of biventricular pacemakers.Ann Noninvasiv Electrocardiol (in press)
2. Barold SS, Herweg B (2005) Upper rate response of biventricular pacemakers. J Interv Card Electrophysiol12:129–136
3. Kay GN (2004) Troubleshooting and programming of cardiac resynchronization therapy. In: Ellenbogen KA, Kay GN, Wilkoff BL (Eds) Device Therapy for Congestive Heart Failure. Saunders, Philadelphia, pp 232–293
4. Steinberg JS, Maniar PB, Higgins SL et al (2004) Noninvasive assessment of the biventricular pacing System. Ann Noninvasive Electrocardiol 9:58–70
5. Barold SS, Garrigue S, Israel CW et al (2004) Arrhythmias of biventricular pacemakers and implantable cardioverter-defibrillators. In: Barold SS, Mugica J (Eds) The Fifth decade of Cardiac Pacing. Blackwell-Futura, Elmford, pp 101–117
6. Lau CP, Barold SS, Tse HF et al (2003) Advances in devices for cardiac resynchronization in heart failure. J Interv Card Electrophysiol 9:167–181
7. Barold SS, Sayad D, Gallardo I (2002) Upper rate response of pacemakers implanted for nontraditional indications: the other side of the coin. Pacing Clin Electrophysiol 25:1283–1284
8. Barold SS, Herweg B, Gallardo I (2003) Double counting of the ventricular electrograin biventricular pacemakers and ICDs. Pacing Clin Electrophysiol 26:1645–1648
9. Aranda JM Jr, Woo GW, Conti JB, Schofield RS, Conti CR, Hill JA. Use of cardiac resynchronization therapy to optimize beta-blocker therapy in patients with heart failure and prolonged QRS duration. Am J Cardiol. 2005;95:889–891
10. Medtronic InSync II Marquis 7289 reference Manual, Minneapolis, MN 2003:165–230
11. Malinowski K (2003) Spontaneous conversion of permanent atrial fibrillation into stable sinus rhythm after 17 months of biventricular pacing. Pacing Clin Electrophysiol 26:1554–1555
12. Butter C, Winbeck G, Schlegl M et al (2004) Management of atrial fibrillation in cardiac resynchronization therapy. Eur Heart J Suppl 6D:106–111
13. Daubert JC, Pavin D, Jauvert G, Mabo P (2004) Intra- and interatrial conduction delay: implications for cardiac pacing. Pacing Clin Electrophysiol 27:507–525
14. O'Donnell D, Nadurata V, Hamer A et al (2005) Long-term variations in optimal programming of cardiac resynchronization therapy devices. Pacing Clin Electrophysiol 28 Suppl 1:S24–S26

CARDIAC PACING:
TECHNICAL AND CLINICAL ASPECTS

Right Ventricular Pacing: Is It Really That Bad?

A. Curnis[1], G. Sgarito[2], G. Mascioli[1], L. Bontempi[1], T. Bordonali[1], G. Ciaramitaro[2], E. De Maria[1], S. Novo[2], L. Dei Cas[1]

Introduction

The era of the pacemaker began with the work of the Swedish surgeon Senning in 1958. Subsequently, endocardial right ventricular apex (RVA) became the most extensively used site for cardiac pacing because it was easily accessible, even by infrequent implanters, and, with its short fluoroscopy time and few peri/post-operative complications, provided stable and reliable chronic pacing parameters.

However, animal data and recent findings in humans have led to questions regarding the safety of pacing the heart from the RVA. In fact, even though this kind of stimulation was effective, it was suboptimal from a physiologic point of view. Many studies now support the conclusion that RVA pacing contributes to left ventricular dysfunction in patients with normal cardiac function and in those whose cardiac function is impaired.. Moreover, impairment of the normal heart in patients undergoing RVA pacing seems to be only a matter of time.

Although RVA pacing maintains heart rate and atrioventricular synchrony (providing that a dual-chamber device is implanted), it is associated with increased morbidity and mortality when compared with patients with normal atrioventricular conduction. The result is an increase in end-systolic volume and wall stress, energetic inefficiency, and reduced systolic and diastolic function and cardiac output; this may also lead to asymmetric septal hypertrophy, myofibrillar disarray, increased myocardial catecholamine concentration, and perfusion and metabolic abnormalities.

[1] Divisione e Cattedra di Cardiologia, Facoltà di Medicina e Spedali Civili di Brescia;
[2] Divisione e Cattedra di Cardiologia, Facoltà di Medicina, Policlinico 'Paolo Giaccone', Palermo, Italy

Effects of Right Ventricular Apical Pacing

About 80 years ago, Wiggers pointed out that RVA pacing in animals caused a prolonged initial rise of intraventricular pressure and an increase of the isometric contraction phase, resulting in a prolonged ventricular systole. Other studies in animal models observed that RVA stimulation is responsible for anomalous contraction patterns, leading to a negative inotropic effect because of a detrimental consequence on maximal oxygen consumption.

The potential deleterious effects of RVA pacing in humans have been lately highlighted in several reports in which an increased incidence of symptomatic congestive heart failure was found in patients paced at the RVA.

Recently, Nielsen et al. published the first randomised trial that compared the echocardiographic changes in left atrium (LA) size and left ventricular (LV) size and function (primary end-point) during rate-adaptive AAI and DDD in patients with sick sinus syndrome (SSS) and relatively normal atrioventricular (AV) conduction [1]. In their study, 177 consecutive patients were randomised to treatment with one of three rate-adaptive pacemakers: AAIR, DDDR with a short atrioventricular delay (110–150 ms) (DDDR-s), or DDDR with a fixed long atrioventricular delay (≥ 250 ms) (DDDR-l).

During a mean follow-up of 3 R pacing caused increased LA diameter, and DDDR-s also caused decreased LVFS. These results clearly demonstrate how a high proportion of RV pacing (90% in DDDR-s arm vs 17% in DDDR-l arm) may provoke a decrease in LV function. Atrial fibrillation was also more common in the DDDR group, indicating that ventricular desynchronisation promotes atrial fibrillation, probably through LA dilation. These data underline, as demonstrated elsewhere, that what is achieved via improved rate-responsive and atrioventricular synchrony is countered by the more frequent delivery of single-site ventricular stimulation [2, 3].

Harmful consequences of RVA pacing were also evident in the DAVID trial that provided important insight into negative effect of RVA pacing on LV performance behind some of the current thinking [4].

In this randomised clinical trial, the efficacy of dual-chamber rate-responsive pacing at 70/min (DDDR-70) was compared with back-up ventricular pacing at 40/min (VVI-40) in patients with standard indication for ICD implantation but without indication for antibrady pacing. All enrolled patients (506) had an ejection fraction ≤ 40% and were on optimal medical therapy for LV dysfunction. At the end of the study, there was a strong trend toward higher mortality and hospitalisation for new or worsened congestive heart failure in the DDDR-70 arm. In this group, the AV delay was not optimised in order to preserve intrinsic AV contraction, so nearly 60% of all ventricular beats were paced compared with 1% in the VVI-40 group.

The results of the DAVID trial were consistent with those of the recent

MOST study, which demonstrated an association between the percentage of RVA pacing (while maintaining AV synchrony) and heart failure and atrial fibrillation in patients affected with sick sinus syndrome and non-enlarged QRS [5, 6].

In the Multicenter Automatic Defibrillator Implantation II trial (MADIT II), the incidence of new or worsened heart failure was 14.9% in the control group vs 19.9% in those implanted with a device ($P = 0.09$) [7].

In retrospective, post-hoc analysis of the MADIT-II database, approximately 40% of the ICD-treated patients had dual-chamber devices (mostly set at DDD 60–70 beats/min) and 60% had single-chamber ones (mostly set at VVI 60 beats/min). Patients with dual-chamber ICD paced the ventricle about 85% of the time, whereas those with single-chamber units paced the ventricle only 15% of the time. The slightly increased occurrence of heart failure was clearly associated with dual-chamber ICD units having a higher frequency of ventricular pacing.

Pathophysiology of Right Ventricular Pacing

After RV pacing, in the early stimulated territory, there is initial shortening at low chamber stress (small pressure load) because this motion is principally converted to pre-stretch of the opposite region, i.e. the still-inactive muscle. As systole progresses, the late-activated region must develop higher load, re-lengthening the early-activated muscle. The net result of this mechanism is a decline in ejection and depression of systolic chamber function. Furthermore, higher end-systolic volumes cause a right shift of the pressure–volume loop, with reduced width (stroke volume) and area, and of the end-systolic pressure/volume relation [8]. This phenomenon was first demonstrated in animals in 1985 by Park et al. [9] and, subsequently, by Pak et al. [10] in a study on humans.

There are also important regional and global metabolic/energetic consequences that arise from dyssynchrony; in fact, the prematurely activated myocardium develops less overall work, consuming less energy, while the late-activated free wall operates under a higher load, with larger metabolic demand, with the net consequence of a compromise of systolic function and reduced energetic efficiency.

Recently, Prinzen et al. [11] used magnetic resonance tagging methods to asses circumferential strain, regional external work, and regional total work in normal canine hearts under sinus rhythm and RV apex vs LV basal pre-excitation. Reciprocal increases and decreases in strain and work were observed, with reduced values in the early-activated myocardium and higher values in the late-activated regions.

Moreover, van Oosterhout et al. demonstrated that dyssynchronous contraction due to RVA pacing generated myocardial hypertrophy in the territory remote to the pacing site. Regional dyssynchrony also rapidly generated regional blood-flow gradients, with higher flow in the late-activated higher-stress region; later, however, the flow became more homogeneous, with the development of hypertrophy and adaptive changes [12]. Inhomogeneous contraction is also a mechanism for delaying muscle relaxation and likely contributes to diastolic dysfunction. Furthermore, papillary muscle discoordination following the altered ventricular activation sequence leads to mitral valve dysfunction with mitral regurgitation [13–15].

These functional abnormalities of ventricular pacing appear to have potentially deleterious effects over time, leading to ventricular remodelling. Experimental studies have demonstrated that long-term RV apical pacing induces anomalous histologic changes (myofibrillar disarray) and molecular abnormalities not observed in 'normal' heart failure, such as marked reduction in protein expression for gap junction connexin, excitation–contraction coupling proteins, and increased stress kinase expression/activation in the late-activated lateral endocardium [16–18].

Selective Site Pacing

Current data indicating that even patients with underlying ventricular dysfunction but minimal symptoms can be adversely affected by discoordinated ventricular activity due to RVA pacing have led electrophysiologists to focus on an alternative pacing site, especially in sites close to the native conduction system (such as the RV outflow tract and His bundle).

There is a great deal of interest in RV septal pacing despite some very confusing results. In 16 patients with chronic atrial tachyarrythmia and complete AV-block, Victor et al. evaluated the long-term functional and haemodynamic effects of right ventricular outflow tract (RVOT) vs RVA pacing. After 3 months of RVOT pacing, no symptomatic improvement or haemodynamic benefit was observed, also in those patients with an ejection fraction $< 40\%$ [19].

Similar results were obtained in the Right Ventricular Outflow Versus Apical Pacing (ROVA) trial, which enrolled patients with chronic AF, heart failure, and LV systolic dysfunction. There was no consistent incremental benefit associated with long-term RV outflow tract or dual-site RV pacing either in patients following AV nodal ablation or in those receiving pharmacologic heart rate control [20].

Opposite results were obtained by others authors. De Cock et al. compared nine studies (217 patients) with regarding the haemodynamic effect of

RVOT pacing. The data from this meta-analysis suggested that RVOT pacing may offer a modest but significant benefit over RVA [21].

As for His bundle pacing, only studies with a small number of patients have been published. Desmuckh demonstrated the feasibility and safety of this approach in a group of 14 patients with chronic heart failure and chronic AF who were candidates for the ablate-and-pace strategy. Direct His bundle pacing led to a decrease in left ventricular end-diastolic diameter (LVEDD) and left ventricular end-sistolic diameter (LVESD) and in New York Heart Association (NYHA) class and to an increase in LV ejection fraction [22]. Perhaps the major problem, accounting for the inconsistent findings, is that these trials have not used the same pacing site.

Conclusions

As discussed above, the more frequently the RV apex is paced, the more likely cardiac performance will be compromised. This explains why, although maintenance of AV synchrony afforded by conventional DDDR is intuitively superior to VVIR, this has been surprisingly difficult to prove. Large randomised clinical trials have reached a consensus that there is no survival benefit in patients conventionally DDDR paced; furthermore, DDDR pacing may be associated with an increased risk of death among ICD patients.

These trials have highlighted the importance of developing sophisticated pacemakers and ICDs capable of minimising, in patients without AV block, RV pacing, thus preserving normal ventricular activation while providing physiologic pacing support.

A reliable alternative to RV pacing may well be biventricular pacing, which seems to be a valid option to preserve LV function in patients who present with LV dysfunction and heart failure symptoms. In addition, there is the option to use CRT for 'primary prevention' in selected patients who require ventricular pacing for electrical reasons.

References

1. Nielsen JC, Kristensen L, Andersen HR et al (2003) A randomized comparison of atrial and dual-chamber pacing in 177 consecutive patients with sick sinus syndrome: echocardiographic and clinical outcome. J Am Coll Cardiol 42(4):614–623
2. Connolly SJ, Kerr CR, Gent M et al (2000) Effects of physiologic pacing versus ventricular pacing on the risk of stroke and death due to cardiovascular causes. Canadian Trial of Physiologic Pacing Investigators. N Engl J Med 342(19):1385–1391
3. Lamas GA, Lee KL, Sweeney MO et al (2002) Ventricular pacing or dual-chamber pacing for sinus-node dysfunction. N Engl J Med 346(24):1854–1862

4. Wilkoff BL, Cook JR, Epstein AE et al (2002) Dual-chamber pacing or ventricular backup pacing in patients with an implantable defibrillator: the Dual Chamber and VVI Implantable Defibrillator (DAVID) Trial. JAMA 288(24):3115–3123
5. Sweeney MO (2002) Effect of pacing mode and cumulative percent time ventricular paced on heart failure in patients with sick sinus syndrome and baseline QRS duration ≤120 milliseconds in MOST. Pacing Clin Electrophysiol 25:561 (abs)
6. Sweeney MO, Hellkamp AS, Ellenbogen KA for MOde Selection Trial Investigators et al (2003) Adverse effect of ventricular pacing on heart failure and atrial fibrillation among patients with normal baseline QRS duration in a clinical trial of pacemaker therapy for sinus node dysfunction. Circulation 107(23):2932–2927
7. Moss AJ, Zareba W, Hall WJ et al (2002) Prophylactic implantation of a defibrillator in patients with myocardial infarction and reduced ejection fraction. N Engl J Med 346(12):877–883
8. Nelson GS, Berger RD, Fetcs BJ et al (2000) Left ventricular or biventricular pacing improves cardiac function at diminished energy cost in patients with dilated cardiomyopathy and left bundle branck block. Circulation 102:3053–3059
9. Park RC, Little WC, O'Rourke RA (1985) Effect of alteration of left ventricular activation sequence on the left ventricular end-systolic pressure-volume relation in closed-chest dogs. Circ Res 57(5):706–717
10. Pak PH, Maughan WL, Baughman KL et al (1998) Mechanism of acute mechanical benefit from VDD pacing in hypertrophied heart: similarity of responses in hypertrophic cardiomyopathy and hypertensive heart disease. Circulation 98(3):242–248
11. Prinzen FW, Hunter WC, Wyman BT et al (1999) Mapping of regional myocardial strain and work during ventricular pacing: experimental study using magnetic resonance imaging tagging. J Am Coll Cardiol 33(6):1735–1742
12. van Oosterhout MF, Arts T, Bassingthwaighte JB et al (2002) Relation between local myocardial growth and blood flow during chronic ventricular pacing. Cardiovasc Res 53(4):831–840
13. Mark JB, Chetham PM (1991) Ventricular pacing can induce hemodynamically significant mitral valve regurgitation. Anesthesiology 74:375–377
14. Sassone B, De Simone N, Parlangeli R et al (2001) Pacemaker-induced mitral regurgitation: prominent role of abnormal ventricular activation sequence versus altered atrioventricular synchrony. Ital Heart J 2(6):441–448
15. Tse HF, Yu C, Wong KK et al (2002) Functional abnormalities in patients with permanent right ventricular pacing: the effect of sites of electrical stimulation. J Am Coll Cardiol 40:1451–1458
16. Vernooy K, Verbeek XA, Peschar M et al (2003) Relation between abnormal ventricular impulse conduction and heart failure. J Interv Cardiol 16(6):557–562
17. Karpawich PP, Justice CD, Cavitt DL et al (1990) Developmental sequelae of fixed-rate ventricular pacing in the immature canine heart: an electrophysiologic, hemodynamic, and histopathologic evaluation. Am Heart J 119(5):1077–1083
18. Adomian GE, Beazell J (1986) Myofibrillar disarray produced in normal hearts by chronic electrical pacing. Am Heart J 112(1):79–83
19. Victor F, Leclercq C, Mabo P et al (1999) Optimal right ventricular pacing site in chronically implanted patients: a prospective randomized crossover comparison of apical and outflow tract pacing. J Am Coll Cardiol 33(2):311–316
20. Stambler BS, Ellenbogen K, Zhang X et al (2003) Right ventricular outflow versus apical pacing in pacemaker patients with congestive heart failure and atrial fibrillation. J Cardiovasc Electrophysiol 14(11):1180–1186

21. de Cock CC, Giudici MC, Twisk JW (2003) Comparison of the haemodynamic effects of right ventricular outflow-tract pacing with right ventricular apex pacing: a quantitative review. Europace 5(3):275–278
22. Deshmukh P, Casavant DA, Romanyshyn M et al (2000) Permanent, direct His-bundle pacing: a novel approach to cardiac pacing in patients with normal His-Purkinje activation. Circulation 101(8):869–877

The Importance of Minimising Right Ventricular Pacing in Patients with Sick Sinus Syndrome: Why and How?

A.B. Curtis, S.S. Barold, B. Herweg

Introduction

It is now generally accepted that the avoidance of left ventricular (LV) dyssynchrony explains the remarkable long-term haemodynamic benefit of AAI compared with VVI pacing in patients with sick sinus syndrome. This finding was documented in two Danish studies carried out in 1997 and 1998 [1, 2]. Compared to the AAI group (with normal LV depolarisation), the VVI group (with LV dyssynchrony) exhibited a higher incidence of congestive heart failure (CHF), a significant reduction in LV fractional shortening, a larger left atrial (LA) diameter, and a higher cardiovascular mortality. A number of more recent studies (reviewed in this chapter) have now firmly established that long-term right ventricular (RV) pacing (mostly apical) can cause LV dysfunction and CHF on the basis of mechanical LV dyssynchrony [3–13]. Consequently, minimising potentially harmful RV pacing has become an important goal in treating patients with sick sinus syndrome, since they generally have less cumulative need for pacing over time than patients with AV block.

The Dual-Chamber and VVI Implantable Defibrillator (DAVID) Trial

The DAVID trial compared the clinical effectiveness of dual-chamber implantable cardioverter defibrillators (ICDs) programmed to the DDDR pacing mode at 70 ppm vs the VVI mode at 40 ppm in patients with LV ejection fraction (LVEF) ≤ 40% [4, 5]. The atrioventricular (AV) delay was programmed according to the clinical judgment of the investigators and was

University of South Florida College of Medicine and Tampa General Hospital, Tampa, FL, USA commonly set at 180 ms, thereby favouring ventricular pacing in the majority of patients. The patients had no indication for antibradycardia pacing and no persistent atrial arrhythmias. Twelve percent of the patients were in NYHA classes III and IV. One-year survival free of the primary combined endpoint of hospitalisation for CHF or death was lower in patients paced in the dual-chamber mode (73.3%) than in patients randomised to ventricular backup pacing (83.9%) (hazard ratio 1.61, 95% confidence intervals 1.06–2.44). Ventricular backup pacing produced up to 3.5% ventricular and no atrial pacing, while dual-chamber pacing (DDDR-70) produced approximately 60% atrial- and ventricular-paced heart beats. The poor outcome in the dual-chamber paced group correlated with the percentage of ventricular pacing and suggested that RV pacing caused LV dyssynchrony. The DAVID study concluded that unnecessary RV apical pacing delivered as part of the DDDR arm produced LV ventricular desynchronisation with impaired LV haemodynamic performance that was ultimately harmful. The depression of LV function by RV apical pacing (mean LVEF = 27% in the DAVID trial) may be more important in ICD patients that start with poor LV function and a common prior history of CHF.

The Mode Selection Trial (MOST)

MOST was a randomised trial of DDDR vs VVIR pacing in 2010 patients with sick sinus syndrome who were followed for 6 years. The study demonstrated an association between the percentage of RV pacing in the DDDR mode (with maintenance of AV synchrony) and CHF in patients with sick sinus syndrome and QRS < 120 ms [6]. The harmful consequences of RV pacing in MOST appeared related to nonphysiologic LV contraction. A cumulative percent of ventricular pacing index (Cum%VP) < 10% was associated with lower rates of CHF-related hospitalisations, while an index > 90% was associated with higher rates.

For DDDR pacing, the risk of CHF hospitalisation increased linearly until the Cum%VP reached 40% and then it was level from 40 to 100%. A related analysis showed that ventricular pacing > 40% in the DDDR mode was associated with a 2.6-fold increased risk of hospitalisation due to heart failure compared with pacing < 40% of the time. For VVIR pacing, the risk of CHF hospitalisation was level from 0 to 80% and increased with increased Cum%VP from 80 to 100%. In a related analysis, ventricular pacing > 80% of the time in the VVIR mode was associated with a 2.5-fold increased risk of CHF-related hospitalisation compared with pacing < 80% of the time.

The MOST study also found a correlation between the Cum%VP index and the development of atrial fibrillation presumably induced by LV dysfunction. The incidence of atrial fibrillation increased linearly in the DDDR and VVIR modes up to a Cum%VP of 80–85%. The risk of atrial fibrillation in the DDDR group was increased by 1% for each 1% increase in Cum%VP up to 85%. In the VVIR group the risk was increased by 0.7% for each 1% increase in Cum%VP up to 80%.

Multicenter Automatic Defibrillator Trial II (MADIT II)

A subanalysis by Steinberg et al. [7, 8] of the MADIT II data involving 567 ICD patients (54% with a single-chamber device and 46% with a dual-chamber device programmed with an AV delay of 190 ± 43 ms) indicated that the harmful effects of RV pacing were correlated with the percentage of ventricular pacing, confirming the findings of MOST [4]. Steinberg et al. divided the MADIT II ICD patients into two groups since the vast majority of them had Cum%VP under 10% or over 90% (bimodal distribution): (1) Cum%VP ≤ 50% group 1 ($N = 369$) consisted of patients with very little pacing (median Cum%VP = 0.2%), and (2) Cum%VP > 50% group 2 ($N = 198$) consisted of patients being paced most of the time (Cum%VP = 95.6%). Group 2 patients (30%) had a significantly higher probability of new or worsened CHF (CHF hospitalisation) at 2 years vs only 17% in group 1 ($P < 0.001$). A similar pattern emerged with the combined endpoint of CHF hospitalisation or death ($P < 0.001$). Group 2 patients were also more likely to undergo ICD therapy for ventricular tachycardia/fibrillation ($P < 0.005$), raising the possibility that RV pacing is proarrhythmic. It is highly unlikely that the results can be explained solely in terms of sicker patients requiring more pacing.

The Danish AAIR vs DDDR Trial

Andersen et al. [3] reported the results of the first randomised trial comparing the AAIR and DDDR modes of pacing in 117 consecutive patients who received a first pacemaker for sick sinus syndrome [1]. The patients were followed for 2.9 ± 1.1 years and had normal AV conduction (according to previously used arbitrary criteria by these investigators), and no bundle-branch block. The primary endpoints were changes from baseline to last follow-up in LA size and LV function, as determined by M-mode echocardiography. The patients were randomised to three arms: AAIR, DDDR-s (short rate-adaptive AV delay, 110–150 ms), and DDDR-l (fixed long AV delay, ≥ 250 ms) modes. The AV delay was not optimised because the study was designed to evaluate the effect of cumulative RV pacing. The AAIR group exhibited no significant change in LA and LV diameters and LV fractional shortening.

However, the LA diameter increased significantly in both DDDR groups (more marked in the DDDR-s group), while LV fractional shortening decreased significantly in the DDDR-s group but not in the DDDR-l group.

The AAIR vs DDDR trial clearly documented the detrimental effects of LV dyssynchrony produced by long-term nonphysiologic RV pacing in patients with sick sinus syndrome [3]. The DDDR-s group with 90% RV pacing developed LA dilatation and decreased LV fractional shortening, but the DDDR-l group with 17% RV pacing developed LA dilatation but no change in LV fractional shortening. Atrial fibrillation (diagnosed on the basis of a 12-lead ECG at planned follow-up visits) was more common in the DDDR group, indicating that LV desynchronisation promotes atrial fibrillation, probably by causing LA dilatation.

The results of the AAIR vs DDDR study are in accordance with the data from the DAVID and MOST studies and the subanalysis of the MADIT II study (in which sequential LV function was not evaluated) with hospitalisation for CHF as the endpoints [4, 5, 8].

The New Jersey Study of Pacemakers and Heart Failure (MIDAS 9)

This study enrolled a cohort of patients with no history of CHF who underwent initial pacemaker implantation ($n = 11{,}426$). These patients were compared with a cohort of randomly selected patients without pacemakers or a CHF diagnosis ($n = 11656$) [10]. The pacemakers consisted of 73% dual-chamber and 27% single-chamber devices, the latter group probably containing < 1% single-chamber atrial pacemakers. No programming or Cum%VP data were available. The median length of follow-up was about 33 months, ranging from ≥ 2 years to 5 years.

During the study period, 20% of the paced group were hospitalised for CHF hospitalisation compared with 12.5% of the control group ($P < 0.0001$). Deaths from CHF were also more frequent in the paced group than in the control group ($P < 0.035$). In addition, the pacemaker group had a higher rate of the combined endpoint of first CHF hospitalisation or death from CHF than the control group ($P < 0.0001$); these events began early after implantation and persisted throughout the analysis. The difference from the control group was more marked with single-chamber pacemakers (hazard ratio = 1.59) than with dual-chamber devices (hazard ratio = 1.36). There was a 32% increase in the adjusted risk for fatal or nonfatal CHF in the single-chamber pacemaker group compared with the dual-chamber pacemaker group [10]. Although the paced group was more likely to have heart disease than the control group, the data point in the same direction as the results from the aforementioned trials.

Importance of Monitoring Left Ventricular Function in Pacemaker Patients

The advent of cardiac resynchronisation therapy has underscored the importance of monitoring LV function in patients attending a routine pacemaker follow-up service [14]. In this respect, O'Keefe et al. [9] evaluated the change in the nuclear-determined LVEF over a period of approximately 18 months (baseline 25–40%) in 207 patients with a variety of conditions. The analysis was limited to patients with an increase of LVEF $\geq$ 10% (148 patients) and to those with a decrease of LVEF $\geq$ 7% (59 patients). Twenty-two patients had pacemakers (mostly DDDR): six showed an increase in LVEF, and 11 a decrease. The strongest independent predictor of LVEF decrease was the presence of a permanent right ventricular pacemaker (odds ratio 6.6, P = 0.002). Although the numbers were small, and the presence of a pacemaker (no programming or Cum%VP data were provided) probably identified a sicker group of patients at the beginning of the study, the results do highlight the importance of careful follow-up of LV function in pacemaker patients with the view to consider upgrading to a biventricular system for primary prevention of CHF in selected patients.

Pacing Methodology

The results of the DAVID, MOST, MADIT II, Danish AAIR vs DDDR, and Post AV Nodal Ablation Evaluation (PAVE) studies should be considered a wake-up call to avoid or minimise RV pacing if possible [3–8, 15–17]. Table 1 outlines how RV pacing can be minimised in patients with sick sinus syndrome using present pacemaker technology.

Algorithms involving the automatic search for AV conduction (such as AV search hysteresis promoting functional AAIR pacing) have been refined so that correctly programmed devices can probably reduce RV pacing by 50% or more in suitable patients; but data are sparse [30–31]. Large trials are needed to determine the efficacy of 'AV conduction search' algorithms [33–34]. New pacing modes with automatic mode switching from DDDR to AAIR and back to AAIR according to the status of AV conduction are now available (Figs. 1–3). These systems virtually eliminate RV pacing in ICD patients who do not have a clear indication for pacing [27, 35]. During antibradycardia pacing in patients with sick sinus syndrome or paroxysmal AV block, this new pacing mode can also reduce RV pacing but to a lesser degree [36–38]. In this respect, a multicentre randomised single-blind crossover evaluation was conducted in 13 European and five Canadian centres involving patients (N = 65 with 55% sick sinus syndrome) who received a Medtronic EnRhythm Model P1501 DR pace-

Table 1. Methodology of pacing in sinus syndrome

Method	Comments
Do not pace if it is not necessary	1. Use the DDD(R) or DDI(R) mode with a long AV delay and slow lower rate according to the behaviour of the spontaneous rhythm. 2. When the stable PR interval is ≥ 0.28 ms, seek the optimal paced AV delay by echocardiography to avoid more unfavourable haemodynamics related to a very long spontaneous PR interval compared to a shorter PR interval with RV pacing and LV dyssynchrony [19].
Alternative single-site RV pacing	Pooled data from many studies suggest that RV outflow (or septal) pacing provides somewhat better acute haemodynamic performance than RV apical pacing [20]. An acute improvement does not necessarily translate into long-term improvement in LV function. At present, long-term studies involving RV pacing sites other than the apex are difficult to interpret and have yielded mixed results in terms of LV function [21].
Bifocal RV pacing (2 RV sites)	Limited experience with mixed results [22–25].
AAI and AAIR modes	Small risk of AV block in carefully selected patients (1–2% per year). Rarely used in the USA for fear of litigation. In Europe, AAI and AAIR modes are considered viable and acceptable in carefully screened patients without bundle-branch block and delayed AV conduction.
His bundle pacing	Evolving technique in its infancy; technically demanding [26].
Programming manoeuvres	Functional AAIR pacing: 1. Using the DDDR (or DDIR) mode with a fixed long AV delay (250–300 ms) in patients with normal AV conduction is of limited value in preventing RV pacing [3, 27, 28]. During AV block, pacing occurs with the programmed long AV delay. Complications: A. Long atrial refractory period may cause atrial undersensing and limits the programmable upper rate. B. Long AV delay favours endless loop tachycardia. C. Long AV delay may cause AV desynchronisation arrhythmia (repetitive nonreentrant VA synchrony) [29] with functional loss of atrial capture. D. Interlocks with ICDs because of

	long AV delay. E. In the DDIR mode, functional VVIR pacing occurs during AV block if the sinus rate is faster than the lower rate or sensor-driven rate. 2. AV search hysteresis (autointrinsic conduction search, Search AV+) in the DDDR mode [30–31]). These algorithms allow the functional AV delay to be longer than the programmed AV delay as long as AV nodal conduction is intact. During AV block, the AV delay is more appropriate than the above situation in part 1 using a fixed long AV delay. Modest benefit in reducing Cum%VP even in patients without AV block but substantial data are not available.
Biventricular pacing	Consider biventricular pacing in patients with LVEF ≤ 35%, especially when mitral regurgitation is present and Cum%VP is expected to be high.
New pacing modes in which the algorithm maintains AAI or AAIR pacing. Automatic mode switching DDDR → AAIR → DDDR. Return to AAIR from DDDR is achieved by periodic AV conduction checks by the device monitoring for conducted VS. First- and second-degree AV block are tolerated in the AAIR mode up to a predetermined programmable limit. Supraventricular tachyarrhythmias activate automatic mode switching to the DDIR mode (AAIR → DDIR or DDDR →DDIR)	Pacemakers with automatic mode switching DDDR → AAIR → DDDR according to AV conduction are effective in minimising RV pacing but clinical benefit and long-term results (including impact on atrial fibrillation) are unknown at this time. The algorithms allow occasional cycles of second-degree AV block for a short period but an occasional patient may become symptomatic. 1. Medtronic's Managed Ventricular Pacing (MVP) has no AV interval (ending in VS) so that no ventricular pacing will occur after a long PR (AS–VS or AP–VS) interval. Sustained marked 1st-degree AV block may be haemodynamically important and symptomatic like retrograde VA conduction [27]. 2. In ELA's AAISafeR 2 pacemaker, ventricular pacing is delivered for 1st-degree AV block after a number of consecutive long PR (AS–VS: 350 ms) or (AP–VS: 450 ms) intervals. The response to 1st degree AV block can be programmed for exercise (considered when the atrial rate > 100 bpm), rest or both [32]. There is a non-sustained switch and a long-lasting switch to the DDDR mode. Both of the above systems are efficient in reducing RV pacing, especially in patients with ICDs who often do not require rate support.

AP Atrial pacing event, *AS* atrial sensed event, *AV* atrioventricular, *Cum%VP* cumulative percentage of ventricular pacing, *ICD* implantable cardioverter-defibrillator, *LV* left ventricular, *LVEF* left ventricular ejection fraction, *RV* right ventricular, *VA* ventriculoatrial, *VS* ventricular sensed event

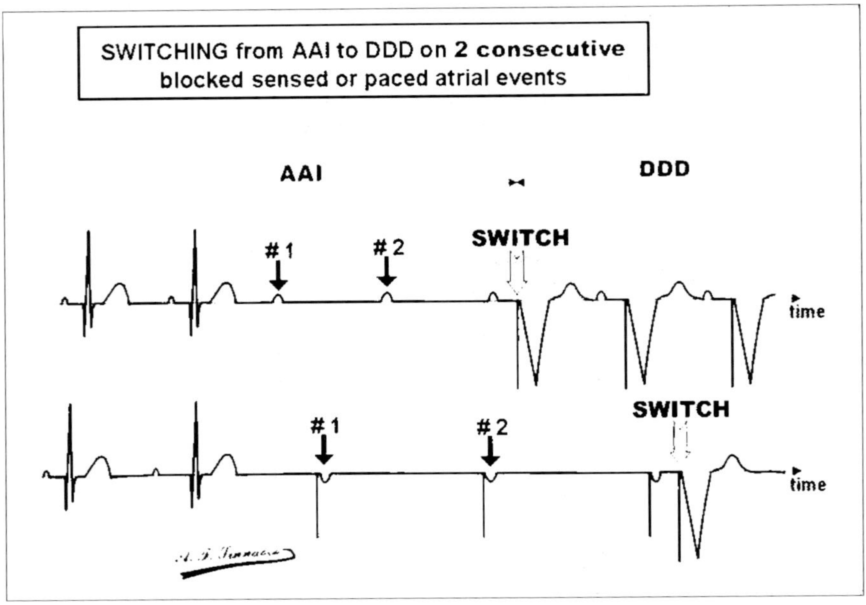

Fig. 1. Mode switching by the AAISafeR (ELA) pacemaker in response to two consecutive blocked P waves. (Courtesy of Roland X. Stroobandt, MD)

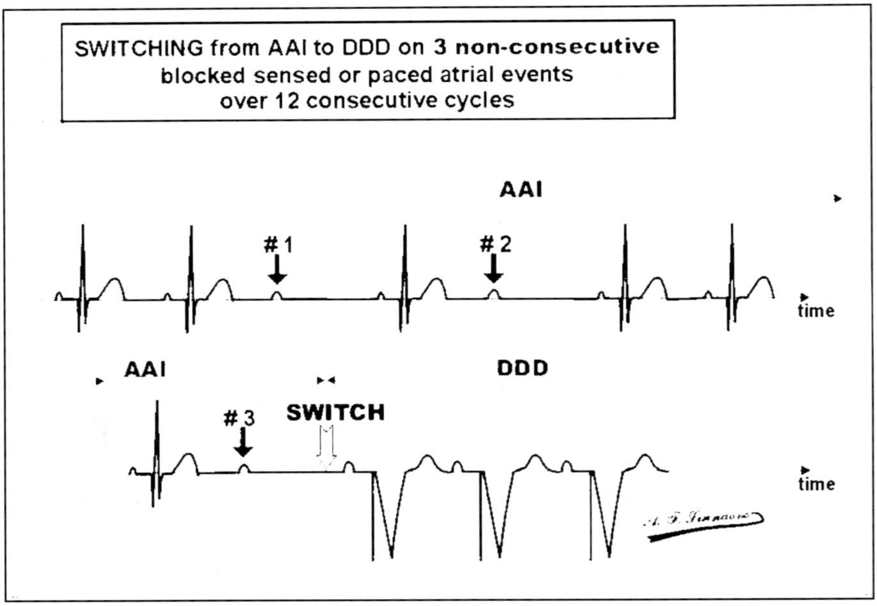

Fig. 2. Mode switching of the AAISafeR (ELA) pacemaker in response to three non-consecutive blocked P waves over 12 cycles. (Courtesy of Roland X. Stroobandt MD)

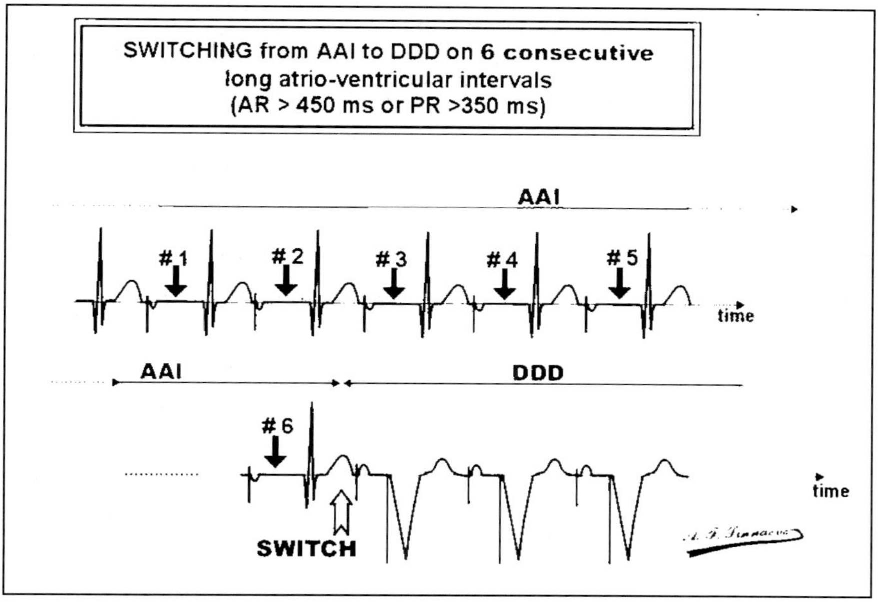

Fig. 3. Mode switching by the AAISafeR (ELA) pacemaker in response to six consecutive, critically long PR intervals. Note that a pacing algorithm that has no defined AR (AP–VS) or PR (AS–VS) interval (AV interval terminating with VS) would result in pacing in the AAIR mode irrespective of the duration of the AR or PR interval. Thus, a very long AR or PR interval could produce unfavourable haemodynamics similar to those in the pacemaker syndrome associated with retrograde ventriculoatrial conduction. *AR* Atrial paced event, *PR* atrial sensed event-ventricular sensed event. (Courtesy of Roland X. Stroobandt MD)

maker [36]. Patients were randomised to Managed Ventricular Pacing (MVP) or DDDR pacing mode for one month and switched over to the alternate mode for a second month. The MVP mode reduced RV pacing significantly in patients with sick sinus syndrome (absolute median reduction 65.6%, $P < 0.001$). It is clear that the efficacy of systems that promote functional AAIR pacing by withholding RV pacing will depend on the selection of the type of patients being investigated.

During pacemaker follow-up, the Cum%VP data stored in the pacemaker memory should be carefully evaluated to determine whether it can be reduced by altering pacemaker parameters. Unfortunately, recording of a paced event (VP) involves several mechanisms other than a pure paced beat, such as ventricular fusion and pseudofusion beats. This means that the percentage of true ventricular paced beats has been underestimated in the various trials, making conclusions about the harmful effects of RV pacing even more important. A pacemaker with an appropriate algorithm and programmability could store these paced ventricular events in its memory and display them upon retrieval by the clinician. This would allow the mechanisms of such events to be determined and subsequently prevented. In addition, the data would help in the design of pacemakers capable of withholding RV stimulation in a variety of circumstances in which pacing is not warranted.

The use of 'prophylactic' biventricular antibradycardia pacing in patients with poor LV function has not yet found its way into the standard guidelines. Nevertheless, some physicians believe that ventricular resynchronisation should be used for 'primary prevention' at the time of initial device implantation or replacement, before the development of CHF in selected patients, regardless of QRS duration, if the LVEF is ≤ 35%, especially if there is associated mitral regurgitation and when a large Cum%VP is expected. At this juncture, patients with sick sinus syndrome and LVEF ≤ 35% should probably receive a conventional RV pacemaker with appropriate algorithms to minimise RV pacing if the clinical situation suggests that RV pacing is likely to be infrequent. The question of primary prevention of LV dysfunction and CHF with biventricular pacing needs to be addressed in large trials.

References

1. Andersen HR, Nielsen JC, Thomsen PE et al (1997) Long-term follow-up of patients from a randomised trial of atrial versus ventricular pacing for sick-sinus syndrome. Lancet 350:1210–1216
2. Nielsen JC, Andersen HR, Thomsen PE et al (1998) Heart failure and echocardiographic changes during long-term follow-up of patients with sick sinus syndrome randomized to single-chamber atrial or ventricular pacing. Circulation 97:987–995
3. Andersen HR, Nielsen JC, Kristensen L et al (2003) A randomized comparison of atrial and dual chamber pacing in 177 consecutive patients with sick sinus syndrome. Echocardiographic and clinical outcome. J Am Coll Cardiol 42:614–623
4. Wilkoff BL, Cook JR, Epstein AE et al (2002) Dual-chamber pacing or ventricular backup pacing in patients with an implantable defibrillator: the Dual Chamber and VVI Implantable Defibrillator (DAVID) Trial. JAMA 288:3115–3123
5. Wilkoff BL; Dual Chamber and VVI Implantable Defibrillator trial investigators (2003) The Dual Chamber and VVI Implantable Defibrillator (DAVID) Trial: rationale, design, results, clinical implications and lessons for future trials. Card Electrophysiol Rev 7:468–472
6. Sweeney MO, Hellkamp AS, Ellenbogen KA et al for the MOST Investigators (2003) Adverse effect of ventricular pacing on heart failure and atrial fibrillation among patients with normal baseline QRS duration in a clinical trial of pacemaker therapy for sinus node dysfunction. Circulation 107:2932–2937
7. Moss AJ, Zareba W, Hall WJ et al (2002) Prophylactic implantation of a defibrillator in patients with myocardial infarction and reduced ejection fraction. N Engl J Med 346:877–883

8. Steinberg JS, Fischer A, Wang P et al (2005) The clinical implications of cumulative right ventricular pacing in the Multicenter Automatic Defibrillator Trial II. J Cardiovasc Electrophysiol 16:359–365
9. O'Keefe JH Jr, Abuissa H, Jones PG et al (2005) Effect of chronic right ventricular apical pacing on left ventricular function. Am J Cardiol 95:771–773
10. Freudenberger RS, Wilson AC, Lawrence-Nelson J et al; Myocardial Infarction Data Acquisition System Study Group (MIDAS 9) (2005) Permanent pacing is a risk factor for the development of heart failure. Am J Cardiol 95:671–674
11. Barold SS (2003) Adverse effects of ventricular desynchronization induced by long-term right ventricular pacing. J Am Coll Cardiol 42:624–626
12. Tantengo MV, Thomas RL, Karpawich PP (2001) Left ventricular dysfunction after long-term right ventricular pacing in the young. J Am Coll Cardiol 37:2093–2100
13. Thambo JB, Bordachar P, Garrigue S et al (2004) Detrimental ventricular remodeling in patients with congenital complete heart block and chronic right ventricular apical pacing. Circulation 110:3766–3772
14. Thackray SD, Witte KK, Nikitin NP et al (2003) The prevalence of heart failure and asymptomatic left ventricular systolic dysfunction in a typical regional pacemaker population. Eur Heart J 24:1143–1152
15. Post AV nodal ablation evaluation (PAVE) Trial. http://www.heartrhythmfoundation.org/research/pave/default.asp
16. PAVE Trial: Biventricular pacing superior to RV pacing in atrial fibrillation patients treated with Ablate and Pace therapy. http://www.medscape.com/viewarticle/471604
17. Daoud E, Doshi R, Fellows C et al; the Investigators of the PAVE Study (2004) Ablate and pace with cardiac resynchronization therapy for patients with reduced ejection: subanalysis of PAVE study. Heart Rhythm 1(suppl):S59
18. Barold SS, Herweg B, Sweeney MO (2005) Minimizing right ventricular pacing. Am J Cardiol 95:966–969
19. Iliev II, Yamachika S, Muta K et al (2000) Preserving normal ventricular activation versus atrioventricular delay optimization during pacing: the role of intrinsic atrioventricular conduction and pacing rate. Pacing Clin Electrophysiol 23:74–83
20. de Cock CC, Giudici MC, Twisk JW (2003) Comparison of the haemodynamic effects of right ventricular outflow-tract pacing with right ventricular apex pacing: a quantitative review. Europace 5:275–278
21. Barold SS, Herweg B (2005) Right ventricular outflow tract pacing: Not ready for prime time. J Interv Card Electrophysiol (in press)
22. Vlay SC (2003) Alternatives when coronary sinus pacing is not possible. Pacing Clin Electrophysiol 26:4–7
23. da Silva Menezes A (2004) Outcome of right ventricular bifocal pacing in patients with permanent atrial fibrillation and severe dilated cardiomyopathy due to Chagas disease: three years of follow-up. J Interv Card Electrophysiol 11:193–198
24. O'Donnell D, Nadurata V, Hamer A et al (2005) Bifocal right ventricular cardiac resynchronization therapies in patients with unsuccessful percutaneous lateral left ventricular venous access. Pacing Clin Electrophysiol 28(Suppl 1):S27-S30
25. Zamparelli L, CioffiL, Di Costanzo S et al (2003) Dual-site right ventricular pacing in heart failure patients. In: Gulizia M (Ed) Mediterranean Cardiology Meeting 2003. New Advances in Heart Failure and Atrial Fibrillation, Spriger, Milan, pp 401–404
26. Deshmukh PM, Romanyshyn M (2004) Direct His-bundle pacing: present and future. Pacing Clin Electrophysiol 27:862–870

27. Sweeney MO, Shea JB, Fox V et al (2004) Randomized pilot study of a new atrial-based minimal ventricular pacing mode in dual-chamber implantable cardioverter-defibrillators. Heart Rhythm 1:160–167
28. Nielsen JC, Pedersen AK, Mortensen PT et al (1999) Programming a fixed long atrioventricular delay is not effective in preventing ventricular pacing in patients with sick sinus syndrome. Europace 1:113–120
29. Barold SS, Levine PA (2001) Pacemaker repetitive nonreentrant ventriculoatrial synchronous rhythm. A review. J Interv Card Electrophysiol 5:45–58
30. Deering TF, Wilensky M, Tondato F et al (2003) Auto intrinsic conduction search algorithm: a prospective analysis. Pacing Clin Electrophysiol 26:1080 (abs)
31. Milasinovic G, Sperzerl J, Compton S et al; Worldwide EnPulse Investigators (2004) Search AV+: A new feature to promote intrinsic ventricular activation. Europace 6(Suppl 1):32 (abs)
32. Savoure A, Frohlig G, Galley D et al (2005) A new dual-chamber pacing mode to minimize ventricular pacing. Pacing Clin Electrophysiol 28(Suppl 1):S43-S46
33. Olshansky B, Day J, McGuire M et al (2005) Inhibition of unnecessary RV pacing with AV search hysteresis in ICDs (INTRINSIC RV): design and clinical protocol. Pacing Clin Electrophysiol 28:62–66
34. Sweeney MO, Nsah E, McGrew F et al; The SAVE PACe Investigators and Medtronic, Inc (2005) Reduction in ventricular pacing and its long-term clinical outcomes: Preliminary results of the SAVE PACe Trial. Heart Rhythm 2:S322 (abs)
35. Steinhaus D, Schöls W, Johnson WB et al; EnTrust-study investigators (2005) Managed ventricular pacing: how well does it work? Heart Rhythm 2:S34 (abs)
36. Gillis AM, Pürerfellner H, Israel C et al; Medtronic EnRhythm Clinical Study Investigators (2005) Reduction of Unnecessary Right Ventricular Pacing due to the Managed Ventricular Pacing (MVP) Mode in Patients with Symptomatic Bradycardia: Benefit for both Sinus Node Disease and AV Block Indications. Heart Rhythm 2:S34 (abs)
37. Anselme F, Defaye P, Mabo P et al (2005) First clinical results of AAIsafeR 2, a new mode to prevent ventricular pacing. Heart Rhythm 2:S246 (abs)
38. Davy JM, Victor J, Mabo P et al (2005) Determining optimal dual-chamber algorithm to favor spontaneous AV conduction: preliminary results of the SAVE R study. Heart Rhythm 2:S323 (abs)

Drug-Induced, Drug-Provoked and Drug-Associated Bradycardia

I.E. Ovsyshcher

Introduction

Bradycardia or bradyarrhythmia is present if the heart rate, i.e. ventricular rate, is less than 60 bpm in the setting of sinus rhythm, a variety of atrial rhythms, atrial fibrillation/flutter, junctional, or idioventricular rhythm [1] and advanced atrioventricular (AV) block. Drug-induced bradycardia in adults is frequently observed. This paper will discuss clinically significant and symptomatic bradycardia [1], i.e. bradycardia responsible for the development of syncope, near-syncope, and confusional state, and bradycardia which is accompanied by premature ventricular beats with short–long intervals, non-sustained ventricular tachycardia, QT prolongation, low cardiac output, and/or poor left ventricular function (these bradycardias can lead to torsades de pointes and to new onset or deterioration of previous heart failure).

Types of Bradycardia Observed in Patients Treated by Drugs Inducing Bradycardia: Definitions

Three types of bradycardia maybe observed during therapy with drugs inducing bradycardia:

1. *Drug-induced bradycardia.* In the heart with normal sinus and AV node and normal infranodal conduction, drug-induced bradycardia may be due to overdosage and toxic effect of medication, or to a synergistic 'brady effect' of several medications.

Electrophysiology, Faculty of Health Sciences, Ben Gurion University of the Negev, Beer Sheva, Israel

2. *Drug-provoked bradycardia.* In the heart with underlying latent disease of the sinus and/or AV node, and/or infranodal conduction system, bradycardia may be due to a trigger effect of even sub-therapeutic doses of drugs inducing bradycardia. This kind of 'drug-induced' bradycardia should be classified as drug-provoked bradycardia. It is important to note that generally drugs inducing bradycardia (β- and calcium channel blockers and most anti-arrhythmic drugs) have no influence on infranodal conduction.
3. *Drug-associated bradycardia.* In patients with underlying latent disease of the sinus and/or AV node, and/or infranodal conduction, significant bradycardia may be associated with drugs inducing bradycardia but not due to a brady effect of these drugs. Frequently the difference between bradycardia associated with drugs is invisible and the former may be confused with the later.
4. In patients with normal heart therapeutic doses of drugs inducing bradycardia generally cannot cause clinically significant bradycardia, especially due to AV block. This suggestion is logical extension of previous three.

   All definitions based on level of evidence C.

Drugs Inducing Bradycardia

Clinically significant bradycardia can be induced by β-blockers, non-dihydropyridine calcium channel antagonists, digitalis, and anti-arrhythmic drugs [1–7]. Other drugs include sympatholytic anti-hypertensives, tedisamil, carbamazepine, cimetidine, anti-depressants, lithium, opioid blockers, and cocaine [3, 8]. This last group has generated relatively little data in the literature.

Severe symptomatic bradycardia has been observed after the eating of honey (called mad honey) produced from the nectar of rhododendrons (of the family Ericaceae) [9]. Grayanotoxins extracted from this honey and injected to rats cause severe bradycardia.

There are case reports regarding a toxic effect of doxorubicin and anti-smoking remedy (herbs) leading to symptomatic bradycardia due to heart block [10, 11].

Bradyarrhythmia develops more commonly with amiodarone, sotalol and other β-blockers, propafenone, or flecainide than with procainamide, quinidine, or disopyramide; combined drug therapy increases the risk of significant bradycardia [7, 8, 12]. Advanced age, a history of prior myocardial infarction, decreased systolic performance, and ventricular arrhythmias (i.e. factors strongly associated with sinus node dysfunction and supra- and infranodal conduction disturbances) are independent predictors of bradyarrhythmic complications of drug therapy [3–8].

An interesting study was published recently regarding high-degree heart block in patients treated with β-blockers and non-dihydropyridine calcium channel antagonists [2]. During AV block, sinus rhythm was 79 ± 17 bpm and troly 'caused by the drugs' was uncommon, being observed in only 8%. The majority of patients presenting with second- or third-degree AV block during therapy with β- or calcium channel blockers will continue to suffer from AV block even after discontinuation of these medications. Importantly, in most of these patients heart block was infranodal, and even when the block resolved after the medication was discontinued, it usually recurred in the absence of drug therapy. In fact, this would be expected because both β- and calcium channel blockers have no effect on infranodal conduction.

Thus, it cannot be predicted whether a patient with AV block that appeared during therapy with bradycardia-inducing drugs can expect a benign course after discontinuation of the 'wrong' medication. Moreover, was been emphasised by the authors, in the vast majority of these patients the 'offending' drug cannot be blamed for AV block, but rather plays a bystander role, i.e. in these patients AV block was drug-associated, but not drug-induced, and only occasionally was drug-provoked AV block observed (i.e. the drug played a trigger role in AV block initiation). It is very possible that clinically significant and symptomatic 'drug-induced' bradycardia in other patients (without heart block) is also mostly due to underlying sinus and/or AV node disease [1, 6, 8, 12, 13]. In these cases 'drug-induced' bradycardia should be classified as drug-provoked or drug-associated bradycardia.

This is of clinical importance because in the 2002 ACC/AHA/NASPE guidelines for pacemaker implantation [14], definitions of various clinical forms of drug-induced bradycardia are missing, and pacemaker implantation is generally considered unnecessary in patients with significant drug-induced bradycardia.

Is Drug-Induced Bradycardia Evidence of Pro-arrhythmia?

Since many of the inducing bradycardia and anti-arrhythmic drugs have a depressant effect on both sinus node automaticity and AV nodal conduction, sinus bradycardia, sinus pauses, sinus arrest, and/or various degrees of supranodal AV block may occur. It is often stated in the literature that bradycardia appearing during treatment by the mentioned groups of drugs is a 'pro-arrhythmic complication' [3–6], a term connoting aggravation of treated arrhythmia or the development of a new tachyarrhythmia [4]. However, 'drug-induced bradycardia' due to either sinus node dysfunction or various degrees of both supra- and infra-nodal AV block appears more common in patients with underlying sinus or/and AV node diseases (usually latent), which frequently occur in patients with structural heart disease [1–6, 12, 13]. Furthermore, true pro-arrhythmic events commonly occur within several days from the start of drug therapy with initially relatively low doses [3–6], whereas bradycardia usually appears after prolonged drug treatment, and only sometimes during a loading process, as with amiodarone [6, 13], especially in the management of malignant ventricular arrhythmia.

Thus, characterisation of drug-induced bradycardia as a pro-arrhythmic complication is inaccurate because it represents largely a manifestation of underlying disease of the sinus and/or conduction system or drug overdosage. Of note, bradycardia itself may predispose to bradycardia-dependent pro-arrhythmic tachyarrhythmias.

Bradycardia Requiring Permanent Pacing

There are no data in the literature regarding the incidence of drug-induced bradycardia in specific cardiac conditions. According to a review of 26 published reports, the incidence of development of drug-induced bradycardia necessitating pacemaker implantation was estimated at 1–15% of patients on a variety of anti-arrhythmic agents used for different indications [1, 7]. In a recent report [13] based on a study of 8770 post-myocardial infarction patients with recent-onset atrial fibrillation, amiodarone use was associated with an increased risk of pacemaker insertion (odds ratio, OR: 2.14, 95% confidence interval, CI). Digoxin was the only other medication associated with an increased risk of pacemaker insertion (OR: 1.78, 95% CI). A strong association between prior sinus node dysfunction or conduction disturbances and the need for a permanent pacemaker was also demonstrated. (OR: 3.32, 95% CI). In another report [12] on amiodarone treatment of patients with atrial fibrillation, bradycardia requiring permanent pacing occurred in 1.4% of patients.

In a study of patients with atrial fibrillation treated only with sotalol, bradycardia requiring permanent pacing was observed in 2.5% and dose reduction in about 14% of patients [15]. Among 78 patients with a DDDR system implanted for symptomatic bradycardia and paroxysmal or persistent atrial fibrillation, the bradycardia was drug-induced (mostly by amiodarone and sotalol) in 33% [7]. Before pacemaker implantation, the drug dosage had to be reduced or the agent discontinued in these patients, owing to bradycardia despite unsatisfactory rhythm and rate control. After pacemaker implantation, the drug could be used again and was more effective at either the same or an increased dosage [7].

Zeltser et al. [2] recently published a study regarding drug-induced AV block. They concluded that AV block is commonly 'related to drugs' but is rarely 'caused by drugs' (see above).

The incidence of pacemaker implantation for 'drug-induced' bradycardia varies considerably [1, 7]. This variability depends on several factors: drug type, drug combination, and diversity of patient cohorts (patients with normal heart versus patients with sinus and/or AV node dysfunction and conduction disturbances). In addition, the need for pacemaker implantation was decided on the basis of individual clinical judgement rather than published guidelines.

Clinical Implications and Conclusions

'Drug-induced bradycardia' is a multifarious and an important but poorly defined clinical problem. Its characterisation as a pro-arrhythmia is unwarranted. 'Drug-induced bradycardia' is common and frequently represents a manifestation of underlying sinus and/or AV node dysfunction and conduction disturbances, i.e. drug-*provoked* and drug-*associated* bradycardia. True drug-*induced* bradycardia is caused by drug overdosage and/or drug toxicity or combination of 'drugs-inducing bradycardia' in inappropriate doses due to their synergistic effect. In patients with symptomatic or clinically significant true drug-induced bradycardia, one must decide whether to stop or reduce the drug therapy or to continue it if there is no acceptable alternative, in which case pacing therapy should be considered. In patients with drug-provoked bradycardia a similar approach should be suggested. In patients with drug-associated bradycardia, especially due to high-degree AV block, pacing implantation should be considered [2]. Frequently, clinical differences between drug-induced, drug-provoked, and drug-associated bradycardias maybe invisible and they may be poorly differentiated.

Little is known about when bradycardia discovered in patients treated with 'offending' drugs merely unmasks the presence of clinically important underlying sinus or conduction system disease or both. Little also is known about the natural history and prognosis of patients with drug-induced bradycardia.

References

1. Ovsyshcher IE, Barold SS (2004) Drug-induced bradycardia: to pace or not to pace? Pacing Clin Electrophysiol 27:1144–1147
2. Zeltser D, Justo D, Halkin A et al (2004) Drug-induced atrioventricular block: prognosis after discontinuation of the culprit drug. J Am Coll Cardiol 44:105–108
3. Podrid PJ (1995) Aggravation of arrhythmia by antiarrhythmic drugs. In: Podrid PJ, Kowey PR (eds) Cardiac arrhythmia. Mechanisms, diagnosis and management.

Williams & Wilkins, Baltimore, pp 507–522
4. Friedman PL, Stevenson WG (1998) Proarrhythmia. Am J Cardiol 82:50N-58N
5. Zipes DP (1987) Proarrhythmic effect of antiarrhythmic drugs. Am J Cardiol 59:26E-31E
6. Hofman R, Leisch F (1995) Symptomatic bradycardia with amiodarone in patients with pre-existing conduction disorders. Wien Klin Wochenschr 107:640–644
7. Israel CW, Ehrlich JR, Barold SS et al (2002) Treatment of tachyarrhythmias with pacing and antiarrhythmic drugs. In: Israel CW, Barold SS (eds) Advances in the treatment of atrial tachyarrhythmias: pacing, cardioversion, and defibrillation. Futura, Armonk, NY, pp 305–323
8. Yusuf S, Camm AJ (2003) Sinus tachyarrhythmias and the specific bradycardia agents: a marriage made in heaven? J Cardiovasc Pharmacol Ther 8:89–105
9. Onat F, Yegen BC, Lawrence R et al (1991) Site of action of grayanotoxins in mad honey in rats. J Appl Toxicol 11(3):199–201
10. Kilickap S, Akgul E, Aksoy S et al (2005) Doxorubicin-induced second degree and complete atrioventricular block. Europace 7:227–230
11. Kolettis TM, Oikonomou G, Novas I et al (2005) Transient complete atrioventricular block associated with herb intake. Europace 7:225–226
12. Hauser TH, Pinto DS, Josephson ME et al (2003) Safety and feasibility of a clinical pathway for the outpatient initiation of antiarrhythmic medications in patients with atrial fibrillation or atrial flutter. Am J Cardiol 91:1437–1441
13. Essebag V, Hadjis T, Platt RW et al (2003) Amiodarone and the risk of bradyarrhythmia requiring permanent pacemaker in elderly patients with atrial fibrillation and prior myocardial infarction. J Am Coll Cardiol 15:249–254
14. Gregoratos G, Abrams J, Epstein AE et al (2002) ACC/AHA/NASPE 2002 guideline update for implantation of cardiac pacemakers and antiarrhythmia devices: summary article. A report of the American College of Cardiology/American Heart Association Task Force on Practice Guidelines (ACC/AHA/NASPE Committee to Update the 1998 Pacemaker Guidelines). Circulation 106:2145–2161
15. Chung MK, Schweikert RA, Wilkoff BL et al (1998) Is hospital admission for initiation of antiarrhythmic therapy with sotalol for atrial fibrillation required? J Am Coll Cardiol 32:169–176

The Sleep Apnoea Syndrome: CPAP or Cardiac Pacing?

P.E. Vardas, E. Simantirakis, S.E. Schiza

Sleep apnoea syndrome is a serious health problem that according to the National Institute of Health afflicts 18 million Americans. Its incidence is estimated to be 4% in men and 2% in women in a population of middle-aged adults considered to be healthy [1]. Sleep apnoea is divided into two types, obstructive and central. Obstructive sleep apnoea syndrome is defined as repeated episodes of upper airway occlusion during sleep with consequent excessive daytime sleepiness, impaired quality of life, and abnormal cardiopulmonary function. The central type of the syndrome is characterised by simultaneous absence of inspiratory airflow and respiratory movements due to dysfunction of the central respiratory control mechanisms. Patients with sleep apnoea display increased morbidity and mortality, mainly because the syndrome is linked to an increased risk of cardiopulmonary diseases [2], and also have an increased risk of being involved in traffic accidents [3], as well as a decline in their family, social, and professional lives [4].

Sleep Apnoea Syndrome Therapy

Central Sleep Apnoea

The central type of apnoea is often seen in patients with congestive heart failure (CHF). Its appearance has known to be dependent on the cause and degree of seriousness of CHF, and SAS has been recorded in 40–60% of patients with CHF [5, 6]. Its presence is related to the patients' prognosis [7] and the progress of CHF, as it is associated with increased sympathetic nerve activity, higher urinary and plasma norepinephrine concentration, and, possibly, elevated endothelin.

Cardiology Department, University Hospital of Crete, Heraklion, Greece

The haemodynamic improvement of patients with CHF is often associated with a significant reduction of central sleep apnoea. However, in cases where despite therapy of CHF, the patients continue to suffer from central sleep apnoea, more drastic therapy is required. Treatment with theophylline or the nocturnal administration of oxygen has been used, but evaluations show that, although the seriousness of the symptoms may be reduced, the long-term improvement of the patients' prognosis remains an unknown quotient. Continuous positive airway pressure (CPAP) therapy has been found to increase ejection fraction and the transplant-free survival rate [7, 8], but a number of studies have shown that patients with CHF often do not tolerate CPAP therapy, quite apart from the fact that the ventilation device is cumbersome and constraining for the patient [9, 10]. The efficacy of CPAP in CHF patients with central sleep apnoea may be related to a decrease in the obstructive component accompanying central sleep apnoea or may be due to some direct haemodynamic effects of CPAP.

Recently, cardiac pacing has been investigated as an alternative method of therapy for sleep apnoea. In one well-designed study by Garrigue et al. [11] in patients with mildly reduced function of the left ventricle who were being paced for conventional indications, atrial pacing at a rate 15 bpm higher than the average nocturnal heart rates significantly reduced episodes of central type sleep apnoea. Certainly, further studies are needed to confirm the findings and to evaluate whether the beneficial result continues over the long-term and whether there is an improvement in the quality of life and prognosis of such patients.

In addition, recently the role of cardiac resynchronisation therapy (CRT) as a therapy for central sleep apnoea and Cheyne–Stokes breathing in patients with CHF was investigated. In these patients it is known that CRT improves the haemodynamic and functional status and reduces mortality. Concerning central sleep apnoea, it was found that CRT led to a significant decrease in Apnoea Hypopnoea Index (AHI) (19.2 ± 10.3 to 4.6 ± 4.4, $P < 0.001$) and Pittsburg Sleep Quality Index (PSQI) (10.4 ± 1.6 to 3.9 ± 2.4, $P < 0.001$) without Cheyne–Stokes respiration and to a significant increase in Sao_2 min ($84 \pm 5\%$ to $89 \pm 2\%$, $P < 0.001$) [12]. So, CRT led to a clear reduction of central sleep apnoea and to an increased quality of sleep in patients with heart failure and sleep-related breathing disorders. However, further studies are necessary to evaluate the prognostic implications of breathing patterns and their therapy in patients with CHF.

Obstructive Sleep Apnoea

Obstructive apnoea has been associated with numerous cardiopulmonary diseases, particularly arterial hypertension, stroke, cardiac arrhythmias, and pulmonary hypertension. Our understanding of the nature and pathophysiology of the disorder is very limited. Anatomical narrowing of the airway, inversed collapsibility of the airway tissues, disturbance in reflexes that affect upper airway calibre, and pharyngeal muscle function all contribute to upper airway occlusion during sleep [13]. However, there is much data to suggest that obstructive sleep apnoea is a systematic illness rather than a local abnormality, a manifestation of a metabolic syndrome [14]. To date, a variety of types of therapy have been used, including upper airway surgery, weight loss, oral appliances, and nasal CPAP. From 1981, the latter has been considered the therapy of choice and has proved to be highly effective in alleviating symptoms, reducing morbidity and mortality, and improving quality of life [15–17]. However, patient compliance with CPAP is a problem and has been found to range from 65–80% , mainly because of problems with the nasal mask interface, acceptance of treatment, and poor educational programmes before CPAP titration [18, 19]. Thus new therapeutic methods remain the aim of ongoing research. Recently, it was found that increasing and stabilising the cardiac rhythm during sleep by atrial pacing can be helpful in patients with sleep apnoea [11]. This followed the observation that some patients who had received a pacemaker with atrial overdrive pacing to reduce the incidence of atrial tachyarrhythmias reported a reduction in breathing disorder after the implantation of the pacemaker. In this study, atrial pacing at a rate of 15 bpm higher than the average nocturnal rate led to a reduction not only in episodes of central type apnoea, but also in episodes of obstructive sleep apnoea [11].

Similar results were reported in an earlier small study by Kato et al. [20], which found that after physiological cardiac pacing in three patients with a mixed type of the syndrome, AHI was reduced with the increase in the average heart rate. In such patients, it seems that cardiac pacing, by improving cardiac function and avoiding periodic breathing that may play a role in the pathophysiology of some cases of obstructive sleep apnoea syndrome, could reduce the number of secondary obstructive events. It should be noted, however, that in a more recent study, Pepin et al. [21] stated that they were unable to find beneficial effects of pacing in another, more representative population with moderate to severe, predominantly obstructive sleep apnoea and mean left ventricular ejection fraction of 64 ± 13% who had been paced for conventional indications.

Furthermore, Luthje et al. [22] found in another study that in patients with normal or impaired left ventricular function, atrial pacing had no effect on the AHI and oxygen desaturation. In another study by our department with a crossover design, we evaluated prospectively the effects of atrial pacing after 24 h and 1 month in patients with pure obstructive sleep apnoea syndrome and compared it with the established CPAP therapy [23]. We found that although CPAP therapy was highly effective, atrial pacing had no effect on the treatment of such patients. From the findings of these studies, it becomes obvious that correctly programmed cardiac pacing may have some place in the therapy of patients with obstructive apnoeic episodes, but further study is necessary to estimate which subgroups of patients stand to benefit.

In conclusion, CPAP therapy, despite the limited compliance, remains the first-line therapy for patients with sleep apnoea syndrome. The role of cardiac pacing in the treatment of such patients still remains obscure and more studies are needed to evaluate whether it could benefit some subgroup or subgroups of patients.

References

1. Young T, Palta J, Dempsey J et al (1993) The occurrence of sleep disordered breathing among middle-aged adults. N Engl J Med 328:1230–1235
2. Leung RST, Bradley TD (2001) Sleep apnea and cardiovascular disease. Am J Respir Crit Care Med 164:2147–2165
3. Teran-Santos J, Jimenez-Gomez A, Cordero-Guevara J (1999) The association between sleep apnea and the risk of traffic accidents. Cooperative Group Burgos–Santander. N Engl J Med 18:847–851
4. Yamamoto H, Akashiba T, Kosaka N et al (2000) Long-term effects of nasal continuous positive airway pressure on daytime sleepiness, mood and traffic accidents in patients with obstructive sleep apnoea. Respir Med 94:87–90
5. Javaheri S, Parker TJ, Limining JD et al (1998) Sleep apnea in 81 ambulatory male patients with stable heart failure: types and their prevalences, consequences and presentations. Circulation 97:2154–2159
6. Lanfranchi PA, Braghiroli A, Bosimini E et al (1999) Prognostic value of nocturnal Cheyne–Stokes respiration in chronic heart failure. Circulation 99:1435–1440
7. Malone S, Liu PP, Holloway R et al (1991) Obstructive sleep apnoea in patients with dilated cardiomyopathy: Effects of continuous positive airway pressure. Lancet 338:1480–1484
8. Kaneko Y, floras JS, Usui K et al (2003) Cardiovascular effects of continuous positive airway pressure in patients with heart failure and obstructive sleep apnoea. N Engl J Med 348:1233–1241
9. Calverley PM (1996) Nasal CPAP in cardiac failure: Case not proven. Sleep 19(Suppl 10):S236-S239
10. Buckle P, Millar T, Kryger M (1992) The effect of short-term nasal CPAP on Cheyne-Stokes respiration in congestive heart failure. Chest 102:31–35
11. Garrigue S, Bordier P, Jais P et al (2002) Benefit of atrial pacing in sleep apnoea syndrome. N Engl J Med 346:404–412
12. Sinha AM, Skobel EC, Breithardt OA et al (2004) Cardiac resynchronization therapy improves central sleep apnea and Cheyne–Stokes respiration in patients with chronic heart failure. J Am Coll Cardiol 44:68–71
13. Hudgel DW (1992) Mechanisms of obstructive sleep apnea. Chest 101:541–549

14. Vgontzas AN, Bixler ED Chrousos GP (2003) Metabolic disturbances in obesity versus sleep apnea: The importance of visceral obesity and insulin resistance. J Intern Med 254:32–44
15. Sullivan CE, Issa FG, Berthon-Jones M, Eves L (1981) Reversal of OSAHS by continuous positive airway pressure applied through the nose. Lancet 1:862–865
16. Anonymous (1994) American Thoracic Society indications and standards for use of nasal continuous positive airway pressure (n-CPAP) in sleep apnea syndromes. Am J Respir Crit Care Med 150:1738–1745
17. Redline S, Adams N, Strauss ME et al (1998) Improvement of mild sleep-disordered breathing with n-CPAP compared with conservative therapy. Am J Respir Crit Care Med 157[3 Pt 1]:858–865
18. Rolte I, Olson LG, Saunder NA (1991) Long-term acceptance of continuous positive airway pressure in obstructive sleep apnea. Am Rev Respir Dis 144:130–133
19. Pepin JL, Krieger J, Rodenstein D et al (1999) Effective compliance during the first 3 months of continuous positive airway pressure. A European prospective study of 121 patients. Am J Respir Crit Care Med 160:1124–1129
20. Kato I, Shiomi T, Sasanabe R et al (2001) Effects of physiological cardiac pacing on sleep-disordered breathing in patients with chronic bradydysrhythmias. Psychiatry Clin Neurosci 55:257–258
21. Pepin JL, Defaye P, Garrigue S et al (2005) Overdrive atrial pacing does not improve obstructive sleep apnoea syndrome. Eur Respir J 25:343–347
22. Luthje L, Unterberg-Buchwald C, Dajani D et al (2005) Atrial overdrive pacing in sleep apnea patients with implanted pacemaker. Am J Respir Crit Care Med 172(1):118–122
23. Simantirakis EN, Schiza SE, Chrysostomakes SI et al (2005) Assessment of atrial overdrive pacing as a treatment for obstructive sleep apnoea hypopnoea syndrome. A prospective, randomised, crossover study (abstract). Heart Rhythm 2005, 26th Annual Scientific Sessions, New Orleans, LA, 4–7 May 2005

Rate-Responsive Pacing Controlled by the TVI Sensor in the Treatment of Sick Sinus Syndrome

F. Dorticós[1], M.A. Quiñones[1], F. Tornes[1], Y. Fayad[1], R. Zayas[1], J. Castro[1], A. Barbetta[2], F. Di Gregorio[2]

Introduction

Cardiac rate adaptation to changes in metabolic demand for blood supply is essential for the optimisation of exercise capacity and general well-being, especially for people inclined to an active life-style. Since patients affected by sick sinus syndrome often present with different forms of chronotropic incompetence [1], dual-chamber rate-responsive pacing is usually indicated in the electrical treatment of this disease. Sensors of various kind are currently applied to regulate the pacing rate, but the ideal goal to precisely meet the physiological needs by an artificial control system has not yet been fully achieved [2]. Indeed, activity sensors, which are generally based on an accelerometer, are highly sensitive and quickly reactive during dynamic exercise, but they cannot detect conditions of isometric exercise, post-exercise recovery, or mental stress, which would normally entail cardiovascular compensation. In addition, the accelerometer indications are not specific, since the sensor can induce a rate increase even in response to passive movements. Sensors designed to record changes in physiological parameters indicating exercise or fatigue, such as minute ventilation, are more specific, but usually slow and less sensitive. Sensors of different manifestations of adrenergic tone, e.g. Q–T interval, pre-ejection interval, unipolar ventricular impedance, and peak endocardial acceleration (PEA), generally provide a good approximation of the expected rate regulation [3–6], but may require complex hardware [7], can be affected by positive feedback from the pacing rate itself [8], or may be unreliable under particular conditions [9].

[1]Department of Arrhythmias and Cardiac Pacing, Institute of Cardiology and Cardiovascular Surgery, La Havana, Cuba; [2]Medico Clinical Research, Rubano (Padua), Italy

A new and interesting advancement in sensor technology is the application of trans-valvular impedance (TVI) in the assessment of cardiac haemodynamics. TVI is the impedance recorded between the right atrium and ventricle with standard pacing electrodes that can be either in contact with the myocardium or floating in the blood [10, 11]. It is well-known that cardiac impedance changes in-phase with the cardiac cycle, in a fashion suggesting an inverse correlation with the ventricular volume. This relationship can be applied to infer relative modifications in end-diastolic volume (EDV), end-systolic volume (ESV), stroke volume (SV), and ejection fraction (EF) from absolute impedance measurements [12, 13]. Simultaneous monitoring of SV and preload can account for the influence of intrinsic heart regulation on myocardial contraction, as predicted by Starling's law. The fraction of SV changes that is not ascribed to the preload effect represents the adrenergic component of inotropic regulation [14–16], which can be correlated with the sinus rate in patients endowed with physiological chronotropic competence [17, 18]. Impedance measurement in trans-valvular configuration is especially suitable for the practical implementation of this haemodynamic model, since the TVI signal is quite stable and allows reliable DC recording. The theoretical expectation has been confirmed by previous experience demonstrating that end-diastolic TVI decreases under conditions of increased preload and increases when preload is reduced, while end-systolic TVI and signal peak-to-peak amplitude are increased by adrenergic stimulation [15, 17–19].

In addition to the development of advanced novel sensors, the current strategy for rate-responsive pacing improvement is oriented toward matching different sensors together, thus extending the sensitivity to a variety of different conditions and increasing the reliability of the system, thanks to sensor cross-checking [20, 21]. This principle has been applied in the design of a new dual-chamber rate-responsive pacemaker (Sophòs 100 by Medico) that is equipped with the TVI sensor integrated by an accelerometer. Pilot implantations of this device have been done in our center, with the aim of testing the effectiveness of rate adaptation in patients affected by sinus node disease.

Materials and Methods

The study was approved by the local Ethical Committee and the enrolled patients provided written informed consent. Seven patients presenting with sick sinus syndrome, marked bradycardia at rest, and depressed chronotropic response were implanted with the DDD-R pacemaker Sophòs 100 along with the atrial lead model 366 and the ventricular lead model 340 (Medico, Padua, Italy), positioned in the right atrial appendage and the right ventricular apex, respectively. Both leads are tined bipolar and bear porous Ti electrodes coated with Pt.

The TVI measurement is obtained by the application of subthreshold square-current pulses of 125-µs duration and amplitude automatically adapted to the detected impedance, up to a maximum of 45 µA. With a dual-lead system, TVI can either be derived between the ring atrial electrode and the tip ventricular electrode (Ar-Vt configuration) or between the ring atrial electrode and the ring ventricular electrode (Ar-Vr configuration). The most appropriate recording configuration is chosen in each patient after evaluation of the TVI waveform transmitted by telemetry, selecting the signal with the most physiological timing (minimum TVI in telediastole and maximum peak at the end of the T wave) and the best signal-to-noise ratio are chosen. The minimum and maximum TVI in each cardiac cycle are processed to get the current values and the reference resting values. The comparison of resting and current parameters provides information on myocardial contractility changes, which are expressed by the TVI inotropic index. Pacing rate changes above the basic rate are proportional to the inotropic index, with a slope specified by the individual rate-gain.

The rate-response profile of the accelerometric sensor corresponds to a dual-slope linear increase in pacing rate as a function of the acceleration detected in excess of a programmable threshold. The first slope is specified by the difference between the pacing rate associated with moderate activity (snap rate) and the basic rate, while the second slope results from the difference between the sensor upper rate and the snap rate. In the Sophòs 100 rate-responsive system, the accelerometer and the TVI sensor are closely interdependent and sensor cross-checking is applied since at the early stages of the processing procedure, to cut down the risk of false-positive reactions. In addition, the indications provided by each of the two sensors can be blended in programmable proportion to obtain the final pacemaker rate.

The present study was designed to assess the effectiveness and reliability of the pacemaker sensors in daily living and during different types of physical activity, including walking, biking, and stair climbing. The latest follow-up check was performed at 6, 4, and 2 months from the implantation in four, one, and two patients, respectively, and comprised technical tests of the pacemaker, physical stress tests under controlled conditions, and 24-h Holter monitoring. Data are presented as mean ± SD; the statistical significance of differences was evaluated by two-tailed paired Student *t* test.

Results

Regular pacemaker operation was confirmed throughout the observation period, although the entire patient group could be checked only at 2-months follow-up, due to the different implantation times. Pacing function was tested in unipolar mode, while sensing was assessed in bipolar mode. Atrial and ventricular pacing threshold at 2 months averaged 2.0 ± 0.7 and 1.7 ± 0.8 V, respectively. Atrial and ventricular sensing threshold averaged 1.9 ± 1.3 and 5.3 ± 2.4 mV, respectively. Neither pacing nor sensing threshold was affected by turning on the pacemaker sensors.

The sensitivity of the accelerometric sensor was tested in standard configuration during a short (3-min) fast walk. The maximal rate indicated by the accelerometer under exercise conditions ranged from 88 to 138 bpm (mean 109 ± 17), with the average time-course shown in Fig. 1. With standard kinetic regulation, the time taken to reach the maximal rate indicated by the accelerometer after exercise start and to return to the basic rate after exercise end was in the order of 90 s.

The response of the haemodynamic sensor was assessed by fast walking for 6–15 min, which entailed a clear-cut increase in end-systolic TVI and peak-to-peak amplitude of the TVI signal (Fig. 2). As a result, the TVI-derived inotropic index was significantly increased with respect to resting conditions (Fig. 3). The time-course of pacing rate adaptation in a representative patient is shown in Fig. 4. In this case, the TVI sensor was in Ar-Vt configuration, with TVI rate gain set at 0.375 and standard kinetic regulation. Little changes in rate were induced by the transition from supine to standing up position, while the start of exercise triggered a quick rise in the TVI-indicated rate, which was completed in less than 2 min. This fast reac-

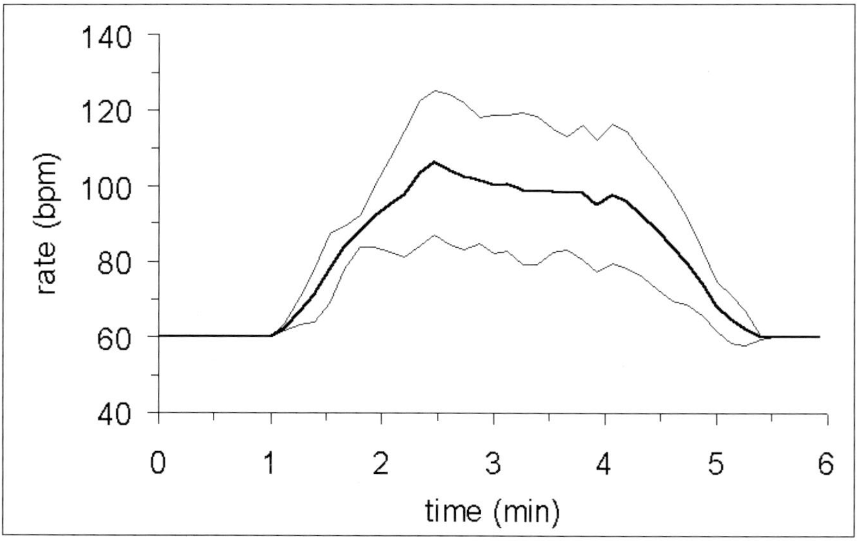

Fig. 1. Average accelerometer indicated rate (*thick line*) ± 1 standard deviation (*thinner lines*) in the entire patient group during fast walk. The activity started at 1 min and lasted for 3 min

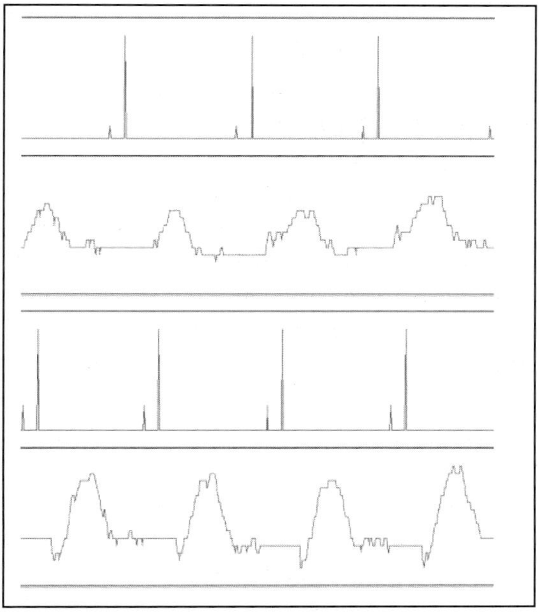

Fig. 2. Pacemaker event markers and TVI waveform transmitted to the programmer by telemetry. *Upper panel* DDD pacing with the patient standing up at rest; l*ower panel* atrium-driven pacing with the patient standing up still after walking for 15 min. Note the increase in maximum TVI and signal peak-to-peak amplitude induced by physical stress

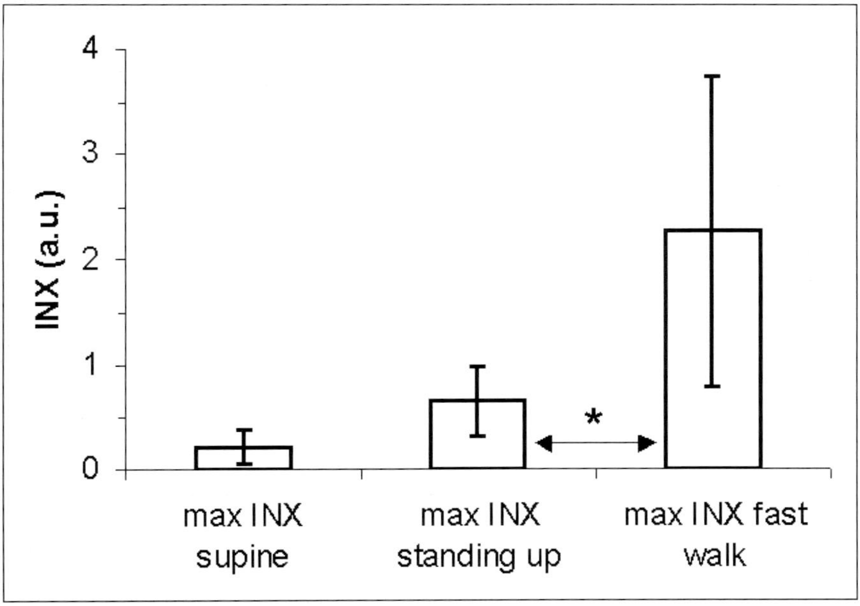

Fig. 3. Group mean ± 1 standard deviation of the maximum inotropic index (*Inx*) recorded in the supine position, standing up at rest, and standing up at the end of a 6- to 15-min fast walk. The exercise induced increase in Inx is statistically significant (**P* < 0.05)

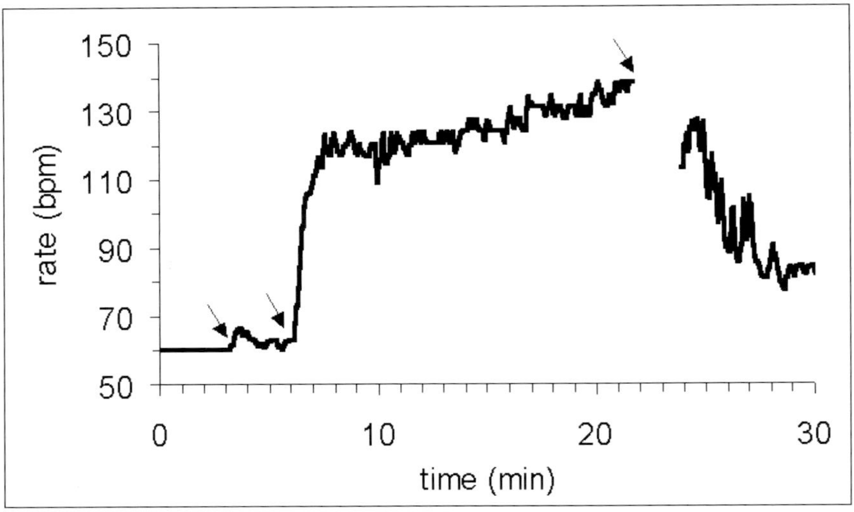

Fig. 4. Time-course of TVI-indicated rate in a patient undergoing a fast-walk test (same case as in Fig. 2). The patient was lying in supine position in the first 3 min, during which he was paced at the basic rate. In the next 3 min (interval between the first two arrows), the patient was standing upright without moving. Thereafter, he walked at his maximum speed for 15 min: the third arrow marks the exercise end. In the following recovery stage, the patient was standing up again with no motion. At the end of the stress, the acquisition was broken for few minutes to allow TVI waveform recording (Fig. 2, lower panel). See text for details and comments

tion was followed by a slower rate increase as a function of exercise duration. When the patient stopped exercising, the TVI-indicated rate remained elevated in the early recovery phase and progressively decreased thereafter, so that 50% of the maximal rate increase was removed in about 4 min.

All patients also underwent a stair-climbing test (three storeys, repeated twice), which increased the inotropic index from 0.14 ± 0.10 (maximal value recorded at rest) to 0.85 ± 0.52 ($P < 0.05$). In some cases, an incremental stress test with the ergometric bicycle was also performed, increasing the exercise power in 25-W steps every 3 min. Under such conditions, the TVI inotropic index progressively increased as a function of time, with a response proportional to the exercise energy cost (Fig. 5).

The TVI- and accelerometer-indicated rate trends were recorded in each patient in 24 h of daily living. The indications of the two sensors were generally consistent and allowed a clear discrimination of periods of rest and activity (Fig. 6). Sensor blending and cross-check further improved the specificity of the rate-responsive system (Fig. 7). Simultaneous Holter monitoring did not show any evidence of tachycardia due to inappropriate pacing, thus both sensors were left permanently enabled with standard settings in all patients.

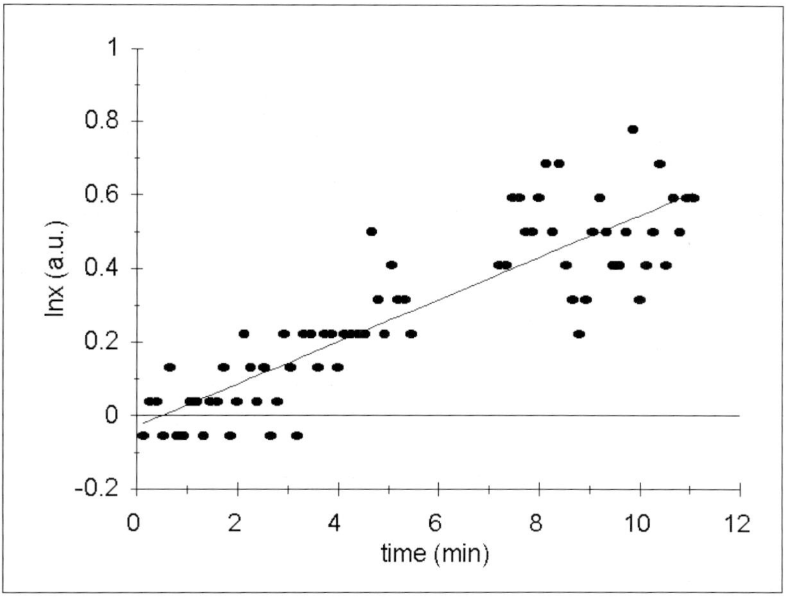

Fig. 5. Inotropic index (Inx) as a function of time, during incremental stress test with the ergometric bicycle. The power was increased in 25-W steps every 3 min. The Inx trend is described by the regression line: *Inx = 0.057*min – 0.028,* with $r^2 = 0.76$ and standard error of the slope = 0.004

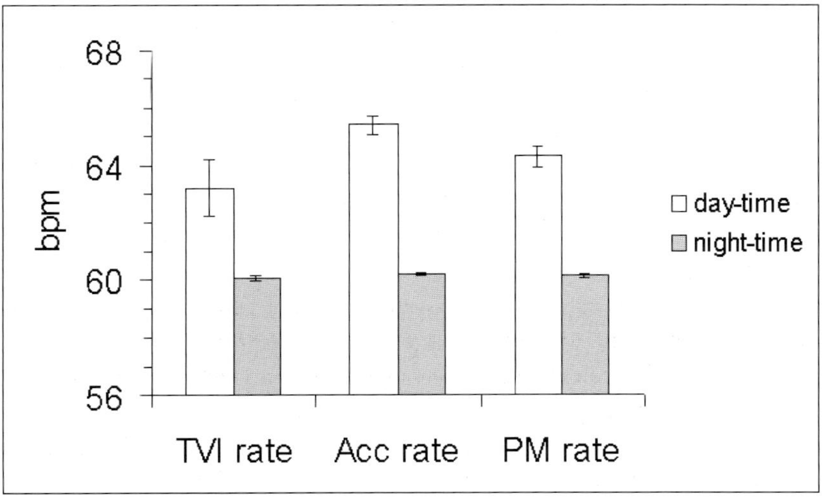

Fig. 6. Whole group mean ± standard deviation of the rate indicated by the TVI sensor, by the accelerometer sensor, and applied by the pacemaker (PM) after 50–50 sensor blending, in day-time (*white bars*) and night-time (*grey bars*). All differences between day-time and night-time rates are statistically significant ($P < 0.01$)

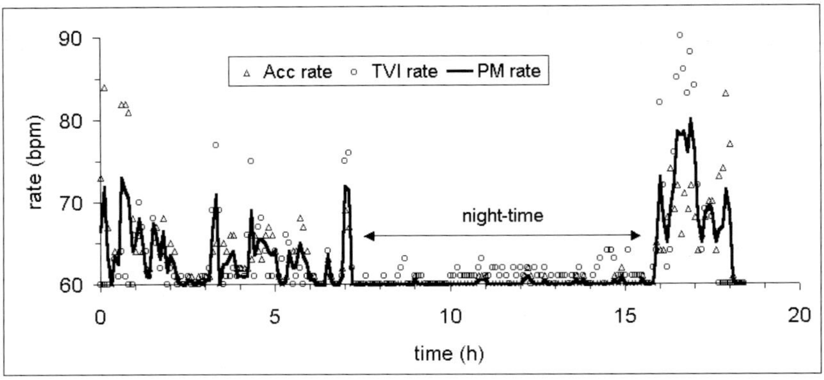

Fig. 7. Trends of the rate indicated by the accelerometer (*open triangles*) and the TVI sensor (*open circles*) in a 24-h observation of a representative patient. The rate actually applied by the pacemaker (PM) after sensor cross-checking and 50–50 blending is indicated by the marked curve

Discussion

Rate-responsive systems relying on haemodynamic sensors adapt the pacing rate following changes in inotropic tone, with the aim of restoring the correlation between cardiac rate and myocardial contractility, which is ensured by the extrinsic regulation of the heart under physiological conditions. Usually, haemodynamic sensors can detect different manifestations of the ventricular contraction strength, like the right ventricular d*P*/d*t*, the pre-ejection interval, the peak endocardial acceleration, and the unipolar ventricular impedance waveform [3, 22–25]. It is well-known, however, that contraction strength is not a univocal reflection of contractility modulation, since it is also heavily affected by ventricular preload, which can change independently of the autonomic nervous system input [14, 16]. TVI is the first sensor that takes into account the influence of cardiac intrinsic regulation on haemodynamic performance, by monitoring SV and preload at the same time [17–19]. This feature improves the specificity of the rate-responsive system, preventing undue pacing-rate modifications induced by postural changes [9]. Integration with the accelerometer makes the dual-sensor system even more sensitive and selective, as suggested for other haemodynamic sensors [26].

Our experience confirms that TVI sensor shows a physiological response to physical activity and is characterised by quick rate adaptation at exercise onset and additional modulation reflecting increasing fatigue. After the stress, the TVI-indicated rate decreases slowly, supporting the patient in the recovery phase [27]. In daily life, the pacemaker rate-responsive system effectively discriminates periods of rest and activity, avoiding at the same time high rate pacing. The activation of the TVI sensor, which implies the application of sub-threshold current pulses to allow impedance sampling, does not influence the basic pacemaker functions of pacing and sensing. As a result, the implanted device proved effective and reliable throughout the follow-up.

Haemodynamic monitoring may have several applications in permanent cardiac pacing besides rate regulation, including confirmation of ventricular activity, optimisation of pacemaker configuration, and assessment of the patient's clinical condition and response to the therapy [19, 28]. These additional features will be available in forthcoming devices of the Sophòs family, which promise to be a breakthrough in pacing technology and advanced new tools in the medical care of pacemaker patients.

References

1. Rosenqvist M (1990) Atrial pacing for sick sinus syndrome. Clin Cardiol 13:43–47
2. Santini M, Ricci R, Pignalberi C et al (2004) Effect of autonomic stressors on rate control in pacemakers using ventricular impedance signal. Pacing Clin Electrophysiol 27:24–32
3. Ruiter JH, Heemels JP, Kee D et al (1992) Adaptive rate pacing controlled by the right ventricular preejection interval: clinical experience with a physiological pacing system. Pacing Clin Electrophysiol 15:886–894
4. Clementy J, Kobeissi A, Garrigue S et al (2001) Validation by serial standardized testing of a new rate-responsive pacemaker sensor based on variations in myocardial contractility. Europace 3:124–131
5. Greco EM, Ferrario M, Romano S (2003) Clinical evaluation of peak endocardial acceleration as a sensor for rate responsive pacing. Pacing Clin Electrophysiol 26[Pt I]:812–818
6. Griesbach L, Gestrich B, Wojciechowski D et al (2003) Clinical performance of automatic closed-loop stimulation systems. Pacing Clin Electrophysiol 26[Pt I]:1432–1437
7. Rickards AF, Bombardini T, Corbucci G et al (1996) An implantable intracardiac accelerometer for monitoring myocardial contractility. Pacing Clin Electrophysiol 19:2066–2071
8. Fananapazir L, Bennett DH, Faragher EB (1983) Contribution of heart rate to QT interval shortening during exercise. Eur Heart J 4:265–271
9. Cron TA, Hilti P, Schächinger H et al (2003) Rate response of a closed-loop stimulation pacing system to changing preload and afterload conditions. Pacing Clin Electrophysiol 26[Pt I]:1504–1510
10. Di Gregorio F, Morra A, Finesso M et al (1996) Transvalvular impedance (TVI) recording under electrical and pharmacological cardiac stimulation. Pacing Clin Electrophysiol 19[Pt II]:1689–1693
11. Morra A, Panarotto D, Santini P et al (1997) Transvalvular impedance (TVI) sensing: a new way toward the hemodynamic control of cardiac pacing. In: Vardas PE (ed) Europace '97. Monduzzi Editore, Bologna, pp 529–533
12. Chirife R (1991) Acquisition of hemodynamic data and sensor signals for rate con-

trol from standard pacing electrodes. Pacing Clin Electrophysiol 14:1563–1565
13. Chirife R, Ortega DF, Salazar A (1993) Feasibility of measuring relative right ventricular volumes and ejection fraction with implantable rhythm control devices. Pacing Clin Electrophysiol 16:1673–1683
14. Chirife R, Tentori MC, Mazzetti H et al (2001) Hemodynamic sensors: are they all the same? In: Raviele A (ed) Cardiac Arrhythmias 2001. Springer, Milan, pp 566–575
15. Di Gregorio F, Curnis A, Pettini A et al (2002) Trans-valvular impedance (TVI) in the hemodynamic regulation of cardiac pacing. In: Mitro P, Pella D, Rybár R, Valočik G (eds) Cardiovascular Diseases 2002. Monduzzi Editore, Bologna, pp 53–57
16. Chirife R (2003) Hemodynamic assessment with implantable pacemakers. How feasible and reliable is it? In: Raviele A (ed) Cardiac Arrhythmias 2003. Springer, Milan, pp 705–712
17. Gasparini G, Curnis A, Gulizia M et al (2003) Can hemodynamic sensors ensure physiological rate control? In: Raviele A (ed) Cardiac Arrhythmias 2003. Springer, Milan, pp 725–731
18. Gasparini G, Curnis A, Gulizia M et al (2005) Rate-responsive pacing regulated by cardiac haemodynamics. Europace 7:234–241
19. Bongiorni MG, Soldati E, Arena G et al (2005) Haemodynamic assessment by transvalvular impedance recording. In: Gulizia MM (ed) Emerging pathologies in cardiology. Springer, Milan, pp 323–330
20. Leung SK, Lau CP, Tang MO et al (1996) New integrated sensor pacemaker: comparison of rate responses between an integrated minute ventilation and activity sensor and single sensor modes during exercise and daily activities and nonphysiological interference. Pacing Clin Electrophysiol 19[Pt II]:1664–1671
21. Barold SS, Clémenty J (1997) The promise of improved exercise performance by dual sensor rate adaptive pacemakers. Pacing Clin Electrophysiol 20[Pt I]:607–609
22. Bennett T, Sharma A, Sutton R et al (1992) Development of a rate adaptive pacemaker based on the maximum rate-of-rise of right ventricular pressure (RV dP/dt_{max}). Pacing Clin Electrophysiol 15:219–234
23. Pichlmaier AM, Braile D, Ebner E et al (1992) Autonomic nervous system controlled closed loop cardiac pacing. Pacing Clin Electrophysiol 15:1787–1791
24. Osswald S, Cron T, Gradel C et al (2000) Closed-loop stimulation using intracardiac impedance as a sensor principle: correlation of right ventricular dP/dt_{max} and intracardiac impedance during dobutamine stress test. Pacing Clin Electrophysiol 23:1502–1508
25. Plicchi G, Marcelli E, Parlapiano M et al (2002) PEA I and PEA II based implantable haemodynamic monitor: pre clinical studies in sheep. Europace 4:49–54
26. Erol-Yilmaz A, Tukkie R, De Boo J et al (2004) Direct comparison of a contractility and activity pacemaker sensor during treadmill exercise testing. Pacing Clin Electrophysiol 27:1493–1499
27. Dorticós F, Quiñones MA, Tornes F et al (2005) Transvalvular impedance in the autoregulation of a cardiac pacemaker. In: Gulizia MM (ed) Emerging pathologies in cardiology. Springer, Milan, pp 347–354
28. Occhetta E, Magnani A, Bortnik M et al (2003) Hemodynamic sensors: their impact in clinical practice. In: Raviele A (ed) Cardiac Arrhythmias 2003. Springer, Milan, pp 713–718

Preliminary Test of a New Haemodynamic Pacemaker: Evaluation of Sensor Safety

N. Galizio[1], J. Gonzalez[1], H. Fraguas[1], J. Barra[1], S. Graf[1], E. De Forteza[1], R. Chirife[2], F. Di Gregorio[3]

Introduction

The autonomic nervous system stimulation of the heart affects simultaneously chronotropism, dromotropism, and inotropism. Intracardiac haemodynamic sensors detect changes in the performance of the heart, which depends on the inotropic regulation of myocardial fibres. These sensors, designed to monitor changes in ventricular volumes at every beat, look promising since they could have an important function in haemodynamic monitoring for physiological rate adaptation, for beat-to-beat capture confirmation, in patients with neurocardiogenic syncope, for the follow-up of patients with heart failure, to indicate the best interventricular delay in cardiac resynchronisation therapy and to identify arrhythmias and their haemodynamic impact in automatic implantable defibrillators [1–13].

Intracardiac haemodynamic sensors include:

- Intraventricular pressure
- Peak endocardial acceleration
- Ventricular impedance
- Transvalvular impedance

Transvalvular impedance (TVI) is a measure of blood impedance between right atrium and ventricle. The low-amplitude constant current is driven from the source to the atrial ring and ventricular ring or tip of conventional electrodes. TVI is inversely related to right ventricular volume: TVI increases during ventricular systole, throughout the QT period, and decreases during passive and active ventricular filling. The minimum TVI is

[1] Institute of Cardiology and Cardiovascular Surgery. Favaloro Foundation, Rene G. Favaloro University Foundation, Buenos Aires; [2] Hospital Fernández, Buenos Aires, Argentina; [3] Medico Clinical Research, Rubano (Padua), Italy

sensitive to all conditions known to modify the preload. The maximum TVI corresponds to end-systolic volume (ESV), which is sensitive to changes in cardiac contractility [8, 9, 13] (Fig. 1).

TVI data have been processed to get an index of cardiac contractility corrected for the intrinsic regulation effects on systolic volume, which correlated well with corresponding changes in sinus rate under adrenergic challenge [14]. The TVI-derived inotropic index has been successfully used to control the rate-responsive function of an experimental external pacemaker. In June 2004, the first DDD rate-responsive implantable pacemaker featuring TVI recording (Shopós 100 Medico, Padua, Italy) was developed.

Study Objective

Since measurement of TVI requires the injection of a low-voltage pulsed carrier signal between the pacing electrodes [7, 15, 16], the aim of the study was to evaluate whether TVI sensor operation could interfere with the conventional pacing and sensing functions of the pacemaker, testing at the same time the overall reliability of the pacer and the sensitivity to changes in the inotropic cardiac state.

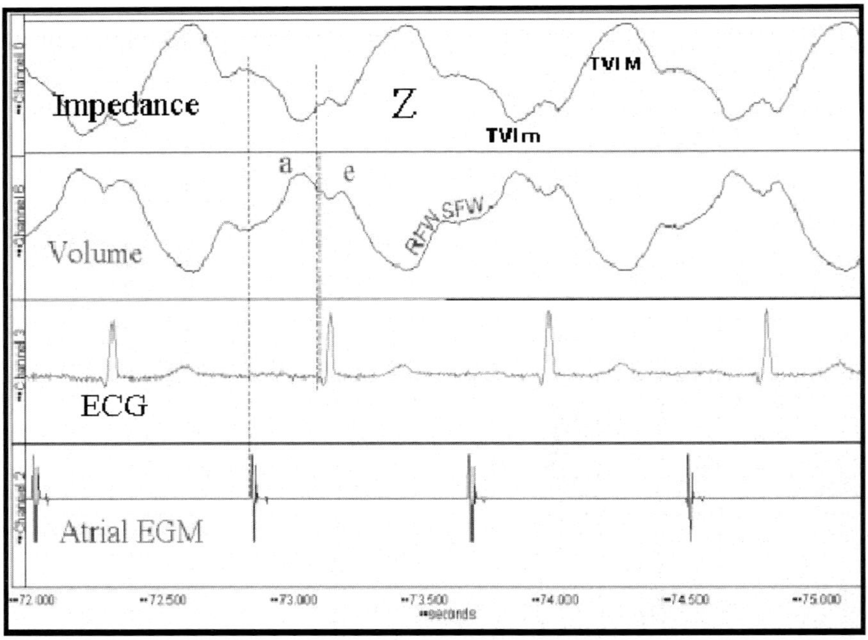

Fig. 1. TVI and volume waveforms, ECG, and atrial electrogram

Methods

Animals

The experimental study was performed in three castrated adults, male, Corrediale-Romey-Marsh sheep, aged 2.5 years, body weight 56–62 kg. The animals had been treated for internal and external parasites (cypermethrin 5% topically; nitroxynil, 10 mg/kg s.c., Dovenix, Merial). On arrival at the animal house the sheep were vaccinated against clostridial diseases (Miloxan, Merial). After a quarantine period of 15 days the animals were entered into the study protocol.

Experimental Protocol Consent

The experimental protocol was approved by the Institutional Animal Care and Use Committee of Favaloro University and the study was conducted according to the 1996 Guide to the Care and Use of Laboratory Animals published by the United States National Research Council [17].

Surgical Procedures

Implantation of Subcutaneous Electrodes for Holter Recordings

Before surgery, three pairs of subcutaneous electrodes were implanted for Holter recording. Cables were tunnelled subcutaneously to emerge at the interscapular space and connected to the Holter recorder, which was fastened at the back of the sheep (Fig. 2).

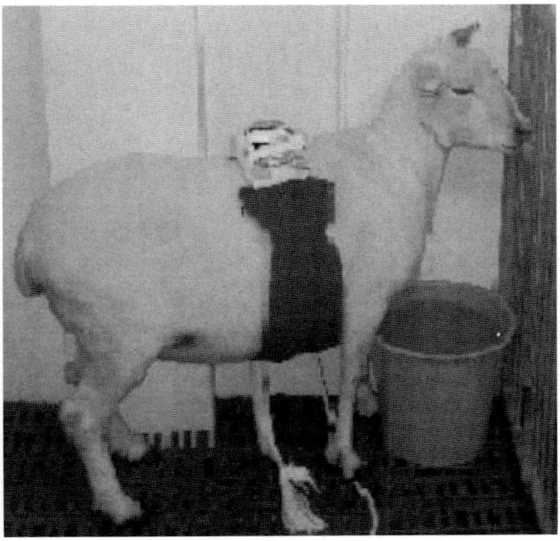

Fig. 2. Holter recorder fastened on the back of the sheep

Anaesthesia and Intraoperative Monitoring

After 24 h starvation, general anaesthesia was induced with sodium thiopental and maintained with 1.5–2% halothane, carried in pure oxygen (2.5 l/min) under assisted ventilation. Surface ECG and PCO_2 were continuously displayed in a monitor. Heart rate and blood oxygen saturation was measured by pulse oximetry.

Data Acquisition

Blood pressure was measured using a pressure transducer (Gould 6600 series transducer). Aortic pressure and ECG signals were registered on a six-channel-signal conditioner (Gould 5900) and simultaneously on a chart recorder which allowed signals to be displayed on the screen of a PC monitor.

Instantaneous pressure and ECG signals were sampled and analysed offline on a computer equipped with a multichannel 12-bit analogue-to-digital converter. Signals were digitised every 4 ms and stored as ASCII text files.

Surgery

With the animals in right lateral decubitus, a screw-in pacing lead (Oscor HT 52 PSBV) and a tined ventricular lead (Medico 340) were inserted via the jugular vein and implanted in the right atrium and right ventricular apex, respectively, guided by fluoroscopy by means of a C-arm angiographic apparatus.

TVI was measured either between atrial ring and ventricular ring (Ar–Vr) or atrial ring and ventricular tip (Ar–Vt) electrodes, whichever configuration resulted in the best signal resolution. After that, atrial and ventricular pacing and sensing thresholds were measured with TVI ON and OFF. The pacemaker was then placed subcutaneously in the lateral surface of the neck.

Finally, recording of arterial pressure and ECG was performed during baseline conditions and during intravenous infusion of isoproterenol (2 μg/ml).

Pacemaker Operation and Program

The TVI sensor was designed to work synergistically with an accelerometric sensor.

The indications provided by the two sensors can be integrated by a blending process, with relative weighting of each sensor programmable from 0 to 100%.

Even when the pacing rate results from the blending of the two sensors, the pacemaker diagnostic functions allow separate storage of the TVI-indicated rate and the accelerometer-indicated rate. In the Sophós pacemaker, TVI is sampled at 16-ms intervals. The digital data are processed at the end of each cardiac cycle to work out the minimum diastolic impedance and the maximum systolic impedance, which are the basis for calculating the inotropic index and the TVI-indicated rate.

The pacemaker was programmed in bipolar mode for atrial and ventricular sensing and pacing. The lower rate was set at 80 beats per minute (bpm), the upper rate at 160 bpm and the A-V interval at 40 ms in order to obtain appropriate ventricular pacing.

Holter Monitoring

Holter recording was performed after 2 weeks and 4 weeks of implantation, looking for pacemaker malfunctions (undersensing or oversensing).

Results

The TVI recording configuration was Ar–Vr in two sheep and Ar–Vt in one sheep. The pacemaker automatically sets the intensity of the current pulses to be applied for TVI measurement to ensure the best signal resolution. TVI pulse amplitude was 10 μA in the Ar–Vt and 18 μA and 21 μA in Ar–Vr configurations.

Ventricular capture thresholds showed a small increase after 2 weeks of implantation, as usual, but there was no difference between measures with TVI ON or OFF, neither was there any difference in ventricular sensing thresholds (Fig. 3). The same result was obtained between measures in atrial capture and sensing thresholds with TVI ON or OFF (Fig. 4).

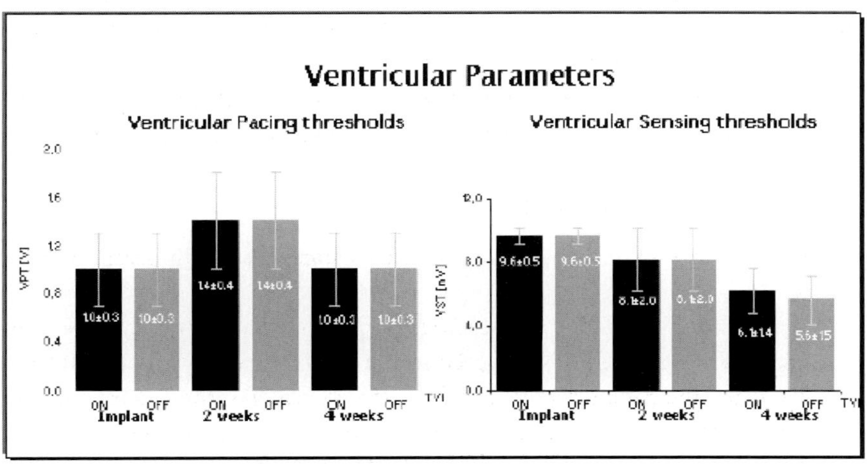

Fig. 3. Ventricular capture and sensing threshold at implantation and 2 and 4 weeks after implantation

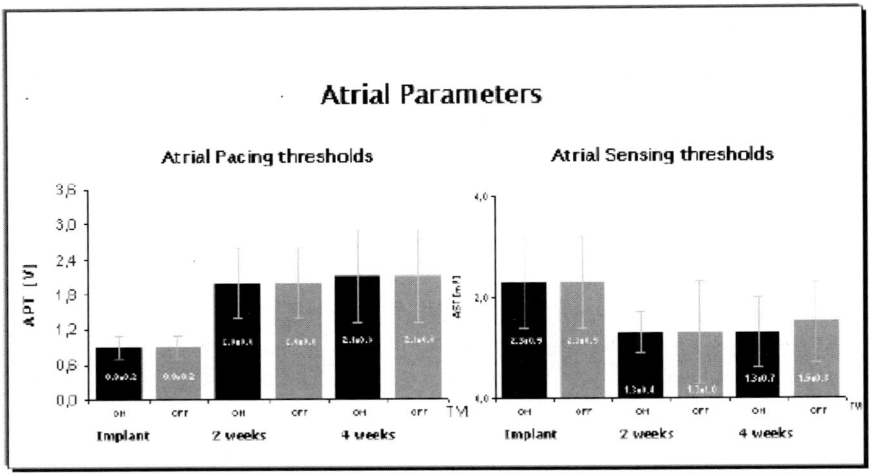

Fig. 4. Atrial capture and sensing threshold at implantation and 2 and 4 weeks after implantation

Figure 5 shows normal sinus rhythm before pacemaker implantation (Fig. 5a) and normal pacemaker function after implantation (Fig. 5b). Sporadic atrial undersensing was found after 2 weeks (Fig. 5c). This was corrected by reprogramming the atrial sensitivity.

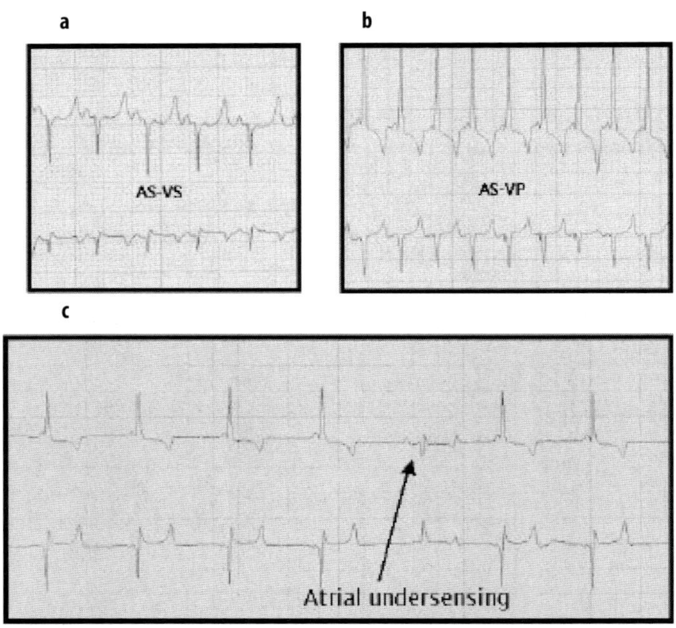

Fig. 5. a Normal sinus rhythm; **b** normal pacemaker function after implantation; **c** sporadic atrial undersensing

Conclusions

In the present animal model study, the pacemaker Sophós 100 proved fully reliable in a 1 month follow-up period. TVI sensor operation did not interfere with conventional pacemaker functions, opening the way to its implantation in human beings.

References

1. Bennett T, Sharma A, Sutton R et al (1992) Development of a rate adaptive pacemaker based on the maximum rate-of-rise of right ventricular pressure (RV dP/dtmax). Pacing Clin Electrophysiol 15:219–234
2. Pichlmaier AM, Braile D, Ebner E et al (1992) Autonomic nervous system controlled closed loop cardiac pacing. Pacing Clin Electrophysiol 15:1787–1791
3. Rickards AF, Bombardini T, Corbucci G et al (1996) An implantable intracardiac accelerometer for monitoring myocardial contractility. Pacing Clin Electrophysiol 19:2066–2071
4. Clementy J, Kobeissi A, Garrigue S et al (2000) Validation by serial standardized testing of a new rate-responsive pacemaker sensor based on variations in myocardial contractility. Europace 3:124–131
5. Griesbach L, Gestrich B, Wojciechowski D et al (2003) Clinical performance of automatic closed-loop stimulation systems. Pacing Clin Electrophysiol 26[Pt I]: 1432–1437
6. Gasparini G, Curnis A, Gulizia M et al (2003) Can hemodynamic sensors ensure physiological rate control? In: Raviele A (ed) Cardiac arrhythmias 2003. Springer, Milan, pp 725–731
7. Schaldach M (1990) Automatic adjustment of pacing parameters based on intracardiac impedance measurements. Pacing Clin Electrophysiol 13:1702–1710
8. Di Gregorio F, Morra A, Finesso M, Bongiorni MG (1996) Transvalvular impedance (TVI) recording under electrical and pharmacological cardiac stimulation. Pacing Clin Electrophysiol 19[Pt II]:1689–1693
9. Bongiorni MG, Soldati E, Arena G et al (1997) Trans valvular impedance as a marker of cardiac activity. In: Vardas PE (ed) Europace '97. Monduzzi, Bologna, pp 525–528
10. Occhetta E, Magnani A, Bortnik M et al (2003) Hemodynamic sensors: their impact in clinical practice. In: Raviele A (ed) Cardiac arrhythmias 2003. Springer, Milan, pp 713–718
11. Bongiorni MG, Soldati E, Arena G et al (2003) Transvalvular impedance: does it allow automatic capture detection? In: Raviele A (ed) Cardiac arrhythmias 2003. Springer, Milan, pp 733–739
12. Chirife R, Tentori MC, Mazzetti H et al (2001) Hemodynamic sensors: are they all the same? In: Raviele A (ed) Cardiac arrhythmias 2001. Springer, Milan, pp 566–575
13. Chirife R (2003) Hemodynamic assessment with implantable pacemakers. How feasible and reliable is it? In: Raviele A (ed) Cardiac arrhythmias 2003. Springer, Milan, pp 705–712
14. Di Gregorio F, Curnis A, Pettini A et al (2002) Trans-valvular impedance (TVI) in the hemodynamic regulation of cardiac pacing. In: Mitro P, Pella D, Rybár R, Valočik G (eds) Cardiovascular diseases 2002. Monduzzi, Bologna, pp 53

15. Chirife R, Ortega DF, Salazar A (1993) Feasibility of measuring relative right ventricular volumes and ejection fraction with implantable rhythm control devices. Pacing Clin Electrophysiol 16:1673–1683
16. Arthur W, Kaye GC (2001) Clinical use of intracardiac impedance: current applications and future perspectives. Pacing Clin Electrophysiol 24[Pt I]:500–506
17. Galizio N, Gonzalez J, Chirife R, et al (2005) Initial experience of implanted pacemakers with intracardiac haemodynamic sensor. In: Gulizia M (ed) Emerging pathologies in cardiology. Springer, Milan, pp 339–345

From Analog to Digital Technology: What Are the Clinical Benefits?

R. MANTOVAN[1], G. CORBUCCI[2]

Introduction

In 1995, Nicholas Negroponte, theorist and researcher at MIT (Massachusetts Institute of Technology), published 'Being Digital,' in which he examined new technological developments and their impact on the world [1]. The title of his book has now become a catch-phrase to describe a technological revolution that has substantially modified our social, economic, and intercultural conditions.

This evolving scenario is founded on the process that transforms analogic signals into digital signals. Digitalisation consists of translating data into a numerical sequence of 0s and 1s (binary system). Thus encoded, differing signals (static or moving images, sounds, written texts) become homogeneous and can be handled simultaneously in a rapid and flexible manner, while maintaining their quality and stability.

The digital 'breakthrough' has brought ever greater interaction-integration to sectors that for a long time developed separately. Information technology, telecommunications, media, electronics, and mathematics are now converging to create a set of products and services that are radically changing our way of living and working [2]. Mobile telephones, CDs, Internet, electronic diaries, DVDs, MP3 players, video cameras, digital cameras, and satellite and cable TV are just a few of the numerous applications of this 'synthetic' technology.

The concept of synthesis accurately reflects the nature of these new instruments, which are both integrated and interactive, flexible and dynam-

[1]Cardiovascular Department, Ospedale Regionale 'S. Maria dei Battuti', Treviso; [2]Vitatron Medical Italia S.r.l., Bologna, Italy

ic. Likewise, it embodies increased speed in handling and transmitting data, as seen in faster means of communication (sms, e-mail) and the greater quantity of information exchanged as a result of data compression (by means of specific algorithms).

The Internet is one of the greatest manifestations of the digital era. Connecting through the web annuls distance, bringing together remote locations in business (e-commerce, on-line shopping, on-line conferences) and in services for the citizen (outsourcing, tele-medicine, home banking).

In digital format, data are easy to handle and can be compressed without undergoing any alteration in their contents. Bits enable a vast wealth of information to be contained in small space, as in the case of digital libraries (on-line or stored in memory devices such as CD-ROMs). High resolution, as evidenced by the ability to record or reproduce the finest details, is achieved in both music and images. Indeed, CD-ROMs offer clearer and more subtly nuanced sound reproduction than the old vinyl records; similarly, digital images achieve greater definition than traditional photography. Another particular feature of digital applications is that of stability over time; CD-ROMs, for instance, conserve their performance quality longer than vinyl records do.

The History of Digital Technology

The digital revolution is rooted in the distant past. In the 18th century [3], French artisans were experts in weaving elaborately decorated cloth. The looms used in this process were 'programmed' by means of a method that was perfected by Joseph Jacquard at the beginning of the 19th century. Jacquard used punched cards, in which the holes served to position the threads according to a precise design. Each hole allowed a hook with a thread attached to it to be inserted into the design. Where there was no hole in the card, the hook could not pass through, and the corresponding coloured thread could not therefore be inserted into the weave. A punched card was provided for each single operation, and the whole set of cards constituted the complete programme of the weaving process.

Jacquard's punched cards were taken up by the manufacturers of calculating machines. In 1890, the census taken in the United States was carried out with the aid of calculating machines designed by Hermann Hollerith, who had adapted the system of punched cards to meet the specific needs of the census. Hollerith added an electrical device to detect the presence of perforations in the cards. The data collected in the census were analysed in a tenth of the time that the previously used method would have taken. This success prompted Hollerith to seek other applications for this technology; he founded a company for the production of accounting machines, which subsequently became the International Business Machine (IBM) Corporation.

After 1937, punch-card technology, together with the electrical mechanisms designed by Hollerith, proved to be so efficient that many engineers suggested combining it with the more recent model of calculating machine that was being designed by Howard Aiken, a professor of applied mathematics at the University of Harvard. Aiken drew up a plan to develop mechanical calculators that could work on mathematical problems in a sequential manner. Subsequently, with the support of the International Business Machine Corporation and the University of Harvard, and with the help of four co-workers from IBM, he built the first modern computer. Named *Automatic Sequence Controlled Calculator* (also known as the *Harvard Mark I computer*), this machine was unveiled at Harvard in August 1944. Instructions and data were fed into the computer by means of a punched paper tape. The digital logical components were constructed on the basis of electrical, electronic, and mechanical principles, while the operations were controlled by means of switches and relays. The Mark I was capable of performing 200 additions per minute, and could work out sines and cosines in about one minute. Compared with modern computers, this machine was huge and somewhat limited in terms of speed and flexibility. Nevertheless, it was the first machine that truly possessed all the characteristics of a modern computer.

The first electronic computer suitable for generic use was built in 1946 by Eckert and Mauchly of the University of Pennsylvania. The rapid-response electronic components used in their *ENIAC* (*Electronic Numerical Integrator and Computer*) enabled two 10-digit numbers to be multiplied in 30 ms – a hundred times faster than the Mark I. The ENIAC was made up of 18 000 valves and 6000 switches so that it could perform 5000 additions per second. It was a huge machine, occupying the entire perimeter of a 9 x 15 m room, weighing 30 tons and requiring 80 fans to prevent its components from overheating.

Technological progress in electronics continued to gather speed. In the 1960s and 1970s, when computers became capable of high-powered calculation, digital signal processing (DSP) began to open new doors in the world of science.

In many cases, the signals that are of clinical and scientific interest are produced by sensors that detect seismic vibrations, images, sound waves, etc. DSP is a fusion of mathematics, algorithms, and the techniques used to analyse these signals once they have been converted into digital form. This analysis may have various objectives, such as image enhancement, speech recognition and generation, or data compression for transmission and storage.

The sectors in which DSP technology now find application are many and various, as are the objectives for which it is used:

- Space sector: enhancement of images from space, data compression, analyses of data from space probes using 'smart' sensors.
- Commercial sector: compression of sounds and images for multi-media presentation, special effects for films, video conferences.
- Telephone sector: compression of voice and other data, echo reduction, signal multiplexing, filtering.
- Military sector: radar, sonar, encrypted communication.
- Industrial sector: oil and mineral prospecting, process control and monitoring, non-destructive testing, CAD and design instruments.
- Scientific sector: seismic recording and analysis, acquisition of various types of signal, frequency analysis, modelling and simulation.
- Medical sector: diagnostic imaging (computerised tomography, nuclear magnetic resonance, ultrasonography), image storage and retrieval, electrocardiographic and encephalographic analyses [47].

The Analog and the Fully Digital Pacemaker

The Analog Pacemaker

Standard stimulators are only concerned with establishing whether or not the endocavitary potential is present; no attempt is made to evaluate it qualitatively. The signal that the pacemaker receives from the lead is an analog electrical signal; that is to say, it is a signal which varies over time. The analog signal can assume any of the infinite values encompassed within a certain interval. Proper functioning of the pacemaker and the delivery of appropriate stimulation therapy depend exclusively on the exact detection of the intrinsic cardiac signals – when they are present, of course.

In order to achieve good sensing, the hardware of the pacemaker is equipped with filters that screen out useless signals, while the software provides a range of parameters, such as refractory period, blanking period, sensitivity and polarity of sensing, in order to mask or avoid the detection of undesired signals. The refractory periods and the blanking periods do not eliminate the problem of the disturbance which is added to the useful signal; they simply prevent the device from 'seeing' it, which, in itself, is incorrect. In reality, the device should always be able to 'see' and to interpret the cardiac rhythm in real time. In spite of the filters and careful programming of the pacemaker, the difficulty of correctly detecting the signals remains the weak point of the system and reveals the limits of the technology currently in use in cardiac stimulators, which handles the signals analogically.

Pacemakers utilise very little of the information contained in the intracardiac signal. Indeed, illustration of how the input signal into the pacemaker is processed in an analog system reveals that this is the only information utilised.

The signal passes through an analog amplifier, which increases its amplitude. The amplified signal passes through an analog filter that screens out the undesired components and lets the useful ones through. Thus amplified and filtered, the signal reaches the sensing circuit, where a comparator compares it with a threshold value determined by the sensitivity programmed. The sensing circuit is of paramount importance, in that all decisions regarding the pacemaker's stimulation therapy are based on the output from this unit. The device decides whether to deliver the impulse, to switch the mode of stimulation, or to activate one or more of the many functions available, solely on the basis of sensing. Without the sensing circuit, the pacemaker would simply be a generator of electrical impulses.

Once sensing has been carried out, the rest of the information contained in the signal is lost, that is to say, it is not utilised, except for periodic measurements of the amplitude of the atrial or ventricular signal. The signal provides information only when it exceeds the sensing threshold (programmed sensitivity), thereby allowing the pacemaker's microprocessor to calculate the cardiac cycle and to establish which pacing therapy to activate. Of the morphology of the signal, nothing remains. Some pacemakers memorise intracardiac signals (EGM) only for diagnostic purposes. This memorisation is 'passive,' in that the device does not utilise the signal to 'decide' which therapy to deliver.

Pacemakers based on analog technology do not have the necessary equipment to 'read' the morphology of the signal; they cannot therefore discriminate between a sinus P wave and a retrograde P wave, a tachyarrhythmia or a ventricular far-field wave. With analog technology, cardiac events are classified solely on the basis of the time lag between consecutive sensing events.

The Fully Digital Pacemaker

The term 'digital' must not be confused with 'electronic.' The pacemakers in current use receive analog signals, which are detected analogically.

DSP technology, as applied to cardiac stimulators, may be regarded as the digital processing of intracardiac signals [8-10]. And this is the great innovation: the input signals entering the pacemaker are converted into digital form before any decision is taken as to the appropriate therapy to be delivered!

A digital signal is one that assumes a quantifiable number of values in a certain interval (meaning that the values can be counted). Unlike the analog signal, which is continuous, the digital signal is discrete.

In order to convert an analog signal into a digital one, its value needs to be measured at regular time intervals (sampling). The result of this sampling is a sequence of numerical values – graphically, a sequence of equidistant points along the time axis. The profile of the original signal is reconstructed by ideally joining up the points obtained. The number of points, and therefore the degree of resolution, depends on the sampling frequency, i.e. on the number of measurements taken during a given unit of time.

Once the intracardiac signal has been converted into digital format, the pacemaker has to be equipped with the capability to 'read' the information it contains, just as a cardiologist is able to interpret the cardiac events recorded on an ECG. The task of enabling the pacemaker to read and put together the information yielded by the morphology, amplitude, and duration of the digital signal is left to the software designers.

The first stage is a standard amplifier that serves to increase the amplitude of the signal in order to make it compatible with the digital conversion system: from this stage on, every analysis of the signal is based on software algorithms. The signal is converted into digital form by means of an analog-digital converter, which samples the input signal. The quality of the sampled signal depends on the sampling frequency, that is to say, on the number of samples taken per second. A high sampling frequency means high resolution, high quality of the reconstructed signal, and therefore reliability.

With DSP technology, all data are in numerical format and can be used by a high-speed microprocessor in the pacemaker to process and bring together information of clinical and technical interest. The results obtained have a direct bearing on the optimisation of the follow-up in terms of quality, time, and reliability, in that the stimulator can provide more reliable diagnostic and therapeutic suggestions [11].

Clinical Benefits

With the increasing number of applications for devices for bradycardia, tachycardia, and non-conventional applications, the complex arrhythmias and signal morphologies present a challenge to analog-based systems. It become evident that digitising of these signals opens a new word of opportunities. Inappropriate classification of cardiac signals by a device leads DSP may offer reliable recognition of local versus remote signals. In ICD therapy, electrogram morphology discrimination offers an additional approach to improve discrimination of supraventricular tachyarrhythmias from ventricular tachycardia.

Further automation of many pacemaker functions can be realised. This is especially true for automation of programmable parameters related to technical functioning of the device, relieving physicians from time-consuming procedures.

Conclusions

The advent of digital technology in implantable cardiac stimulators will open up new frontiers for the automatic analysis and diagnosis of endocardial signals. This will dramatically increase the reliability of the therapies delivered and the amount of information that can be processed and stored for clinical and scientific purposes. In the next few years, we can expect specific algorithms to be developed for morphological discrimination of the far-field R-wave in the atrium and the retrograde P-wave. The use of blanking periods will gradually be phased out, since the system will instantly classify what it receives from the implanted electrodes, without needing to mask undesired signals. Such devices will really and continuously monitor every cardiac event.

References

1. Negroponte N (1995) Being digital. Knopf, New York, pp 133–225
2. Cimino JJ, Bakken S (2005) Personal digital educators. N Engl J Med 352(9):860–862
3. Smith RJ, Dorf RC (1992). Circuits, devices and systems. Wiley, New York, pp 428–429
4. Tompkins WJ (1993) Biomedical digital signal processing. Prentice Hall, Englewood Cliffs, pp 1–4
5. Zareba W (2002) New era for digital ECG: FDA requires digital ECG submission for tested drugs. Ann Noninvasive Electrocardiol 7(1):1–3
6. Warner RA, Hill NE (1999) Using digital versus analog ECG data in clinical trials. J Electrocardiol 32(Suppl 1):103–107
7. Batchvarov V, Hnatkova K, Malik M (2002) Assessment of noise in digital electrocardiograms. PACE 25(Pt 1):499–503
8. Van Hemel NM, Wohlgemuth P, Engbers JG et al (2004) Form analysis using digital signal processing reliably discriminates far-field R waves from P waves. PACE 27:1615–1624
9. Padeletti L, Barold SS (2005) Digital technology for cardiac pacing. Am J Cardiol 95:479–482
10. Love CJ (2004) The Digital Pacemaker. PACE 27(Pt I):707–708
11. Scipione P, Capestro F, Cecchetti P et al (2005) The innovative fully digital pacemakers: may they improve our patients management? Europace (in press) (abs)

What Are the Benefits of Morphological Signal Analysis Using Digital Technology?

R. TUKKIE

Digital technology is all around us. However only since the late 1970s has digital technology been incorporated into cardiac pacemakers. Memory, circuits, and counters became larger, faster, and more accurate. Improvements in sensor-driven pacing, dual-chamber pacing, and specific algorithms such as mode switching and overdrive pacing were made possible because of the advances in digital technology. The first microprocessors in cardiac pacing were introduced in the DGP-1 platform made by Vitatron b.v. (Arnhem, The Netherlands), the same company who recently introduced digital signal processing (DSP).

Standard pacemakers will amplify the intracardiac signal, then filter the signal using high- and low-pass filters, after which the signal is sensed by the pacemaker if it exceeds a certain programmable threshold. However, the true morphology of the signal is no longer present after this process and a certain amount of information is lost. Classification of intracardiac events and events of extracardiac origin based on timing and morphology is not possible in these analogue devices. Filters and blanking periods are a suboptimal solution to this problem. This may result in serious adverse events for the pacemaker patients such as undersensing of atrial arrhythmias.

In the new digital pacemakers, DSP will process the analogue electrical signals coming from the heart (atrium or ventricle) into a digital format. After digitising the intracardiac signal, the pacemaker will use specially designed algorithms to make certain decisions or discriminate between signals from different origins. To sample a signal reliably, a very high sampling rate has to be achieved. The current DSP platform samples at a rate of 800

Kennemer Gasthuis, Haarlem, The Netherlands

samples per second, allowing reliable description of the signal in which all relevant information is contained. After the signal is digitised by the analogue-to-digital converter, flexible filters are used to yield the components of the intracardiac signal, which are of clinical interest. The main engineering challenge consisted of designing a DSP circuit without increasing the power consumption. This has been achieved in the currently available commercial digital pacemakers.

Now that we have DSP, numerous opportunities arise which will make pacing more physiological and reliable. The first application, which is currently being evaluated, is discriminating far-field R waves (FFRW) from true atrial signals. FFRW are usually managed by extending the post-ventricular atrial blanking period. However, by doing so, we increase the risk of 2:1 sensing and tracking of atrial tachyarrhythmias. In addition, FFRW sensing may result in false detection of atrial tachyarrhythmias, leading to unnecessary mode switches with loss of atrioventricular synchrony and incorrect diagnostic counters for atrial tachycardias and atrial fibrillation. A recent study by Van Hemel et al. demonstrated that a novel DSP algorithm reliably separated FFRW from P waves [1]. Data from 100 bipolar and unipolar intracardiac atrial recordings from 31 patients were collected during pacemaker replacement and analysed off line. Sensitivity and specificity of FFRW detection were 99.3% and 100%. Moreover, no P waves were falsely classified. The DSP algorithm is therefore capable of preventing false mode switches. Further studies are on their way using data collected from implanted pacemakers during 24-h external Holter recordings and bicycle exercise. These results will provide further information on the accuracy of this specific DSP algorithm, and ultimately this algorithm will be incorporated in future devices.

Looking to the future, it seems that the future is digital. Numerous opportunities arise from digital signal processing, not only in pacemakers but also in implantable cardioverter–defibrillators (ICDs). New applications of digital morphology discrimination could be the discrimination of fusion beats, especially in auto-capture devices. Improved sensing of supraventricular tachycardias in ICDs could reduce the incidence of inappropriate therapies, thereby greatly improving patient quality of life and the acceptance of ICDs. In the coming years many of these new applications will find their way into clinical practice.

Reference

1. Van Hemel NM, Wohlgemuth P, Engbers J et al (2004) Form analysis using digital signal processing reliably discriminates far-field R waves from P waves. Pacing Clin Electrophysiol 27:1615–1624

How Can New Technologies Help Make Follow-Up Easier?

V. LEONHARDT, C. VAN GROENINGEN

Introduction

In the Western world, health care budgets are increasingly under pressure. With an increasingly older population, more people require more medical care. In addition, medical standards have become higher and people are remaining active longer and thus expecting better care. At the same time, the relative number of people working is decreasing.

In the USA, the number of implantations of cardiac device has increased by 7% per year, from 294 000 in 2001 to 401 000 in 2005 (pacemaker, ICD, and CRT devices combined) and the number of follow-ups (FUs) doubled in the same period. This rise in FUs translates into an increasing burden on individual clinics and especially on specialised centres. For example, in our clinic the number of implantations rose dramatically, from only 46 in 1999 to 385 in 2004, and we have now 6500–7500 FUs per year. The ever-growing demand on medical care therefore calls for new technologies to be developed.

Increasing Follow-Up Burden

A pacemaker implantation and more specific dual chamber systems seem to be cost-effective treatments. The reimbursement of an implantation renders a profit when cost for staff and materials are deducted. However, clinicians' reimbursement for FUs does not counter-balance the costs of an average 5 years of FU. This is a growing financial problem for the clinic.

Facharzt für Innere Medizin, Berlin, Germany

One of the reasons that FUs are a problem is that, over the years, pacemakers have become increasingly complex. In the late 1970s, pacemaker memories were small and only a few parameters were stored. With increasing memory size, counters were added to basically store sensed and paced events; as sensing circuits remained analog and pacing therapies remained simple, there was no extra information to store anyway. Pacemaker FUs thus consisted of simply checking the functionality of the pacemaker device.

The introduction of microprocessors (DPG-1, Vitatron Medical), in 1981, created the possibility to make intelligent decisions based on rate and rhythm information. Simultaneously, more data could be stored, and Holters and histograms were added that stored more clinically relevant data over longer periods of time. This meant that during FU this clinical data had to be analysed and interpreted in order to optimise pacemaker therapy.

Over the years, memory size has continued to increase (more counters, Holters, and histograms) and information about relevant arrhythmic episodes can be stored as markers or, currently, as digitally stored IEGMs. All these developments have led to an increase in time and effort needed to carry out proper follow-up.

Digital vs Analogue Technology

In 2003, Vitatron introduced the world's first fully digital pacemaker. In conventional pacemakers, the analogue input is digitised in an analog/digital (AD) converter to store the IEGM, but for event sensing only the analogue signal is used. In fully digital devices, the analogue input out of the heart is amplified and then digitised. All subsequent steps, filtering, event detection, IEGM storage, and signal analysis, are performed on this digital signal (Fig. 1). Digitisation allows digital signal processing (DSP) in pacemakers, a technology that has been used in many types of electronic equipment available for the consumer for more than 15 years and which includes CDs, mobile telephones, and handheld cameras to mention a few. This is equipment that requires many times more energy than is available in pacemakers. A mobile phone has a battery capacity of 0.72 mA that lasts about 1 week with the typical current consumption of 4.2 Ah. A pacemaker battery has nearly double the capacity (1.36 mA), but it is of course unacceptable to change pacemakers every 2 weeks. It therefore was an impressive engineering feature to make DSP possible while maintaining an acceptable life span for the pacemaker. For a life span of 9 years, the power consumption had to be reduced to 0.03 Ah.

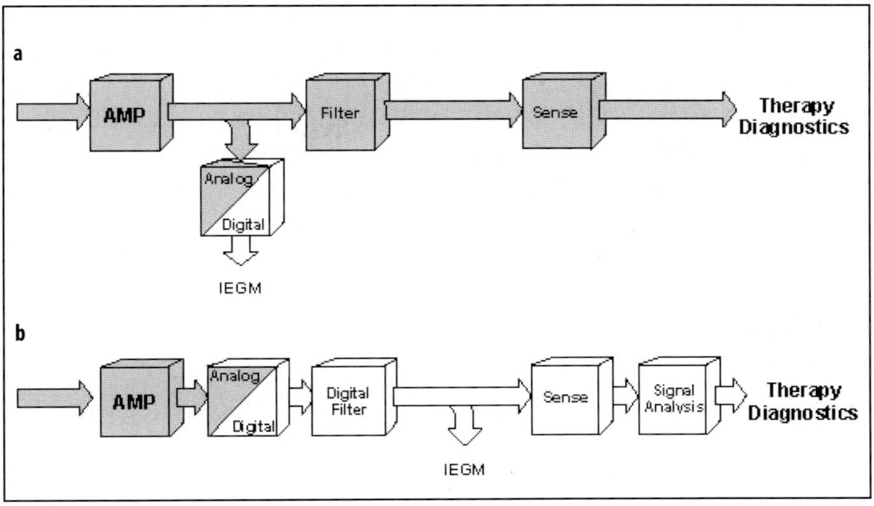

Fig. 1. a Design of conventional pacemakers. The entire signal processing is done on the analog signal. Only the IEGM is digital. **b** Design of digital pacemakers. The signal is converted as soon as possible and all signal processing is done digitally

New Technologies Making Follow-Up Easier

The resulting digital pacemaker is able to analyse the cardiac signals based on the morphology of the signal. Morphology analysis can be used to distinguish between PACs, retrograde, and physiologic atrial events, and to reduce the detection thresholds without fear of noise, far fields, or muscle potentials [1]. In the future, morphology will be used to reveal pathologies, for instance, ischaemia.

The increased storage capabilities have added more data that must be analysed at each FU. It could be considered that in this aspect digital pacemaker technology has brought the healthcare system from bad to worse.

Automaticities

To reduce FU duration, a number of basic pacemaker settings have been made automatic or semi-automatic. Auto-sensing and auto-capture features make cumbersome threshold testing at each FU redundant, thus freeing-up FU time.

Long-Distance Follow-Up

Another development is long-distance FU. Pacemaker patients can check their pacemakers at home, and in case disturbing diagnostics are detected an alarm is sent to specialised centres or the physician in attendance. In theory, this reduces the FU burden because patients only come to the clinic for FU when required. However, in practice, it is yet not totally clear which problems require the attention of a physician, and patients are often referred to the clinic 'just in case', thereby increasing the FU burden. Of course, it is expected that in-home analysis will improve as the systems performing the analysis mature over time. An example of an expert system having this potential is the Therapy Advisor – although currently it is only available for use in the clinic.

Therapy Advisor

In light of clinicians' limited time available for FUs, it is annoying to realise that a lot of FU time is spent on interrogating and adapting pacemaker settings that are important for the proper functioning of the device itself and its collection of clinically relevant data. This is a problem especially with the devices of atrial fibrillation patients. FUs should be about patient management and diagnostics about their treatment.

To handle the problem of the complicated and time-consuming interpretation of the large amount of pacemaker data, Vitatron developed the Therapy Advisor, which is an expert system that, in the time needed to interrogate the collected diagnostic data from the pacemaker, analyses the data for clinically relevant information. It identifies clinical issues, guides the physician to the specific diagnostics for evaluation if desired, and provides programming recommendations. By guiding the physician through these complicated issues, he or she can focus on important clinical questions and take care of them during the limited FU time.

Evaluation of the Therapy Advisor

Currently, two studies are in progress to evaluate the performance of the Therapy Advisor and physicians' satisfaction with its use: the C-STAR and the T-STAR registries. Both registries are international, multi-centre, prospective Post Marketing Studies aimed at gathering data related to the usefulness and appropriateness of the Therapy Advisor.

C-STAR was the first study and it focuses on the general diagnostics; the focus of T-STAR is atrial tachycardia.

C-STAR [2]

Methods

In the C-STAR registry, all patients with a class I or class II pacing indication and a Vitatron C-series pacemaker are included. Physicians follow each patient per normal practice. Each of the patients receives the standard of medical care that is typically provided by the investigator with respect to device FU, management of co-morbidities, etc. The registry does not require specified FU visits. However, in order to have the patient's data contribute to the study objectives, the data of at least two follow-ups within a different time frame in the first 12 months following discharge are required.

In the first interim analysis, data use was limited to the enrolment/implant, 2-month FU, and 6-month FU, and the data passed all validation levels. Patients were only included in this interim analysis if both the CRF data and diskette data were available for a FU. This resulted in 96 patients with a 2-month FU being analysed and 33 of these with an additional 6-month FU.

The interim analysis focuses on the opinion of the clinician regarding the helpfulness of the Therapy Advisor in assessing the patient's condition, making an efficient FU, and optimising pacemaker programming and drug regimen.

Results

The most common diagnostic observations generated by the Therapy Advisor are listed in Table 1. The total number of messages was 169, with 131 messages for the 2-month FU ($n = 96$) and 39 messages for the 6-month FU ($n = 33$). Since it is possible for the Therapy Advisor to generate more than one message per patient, this resulted in a percentage for both the 2-month FU and the 6-month FU of more than 100%.

The investigators' opinions about the helpfulness of the Therapy Advisor in assessing the patient's condition were positive to neutral; only 11.6% were negative. Within the group of patients with both a 2- and a 6-month FU, the percentage of positive-minded investigators increased from 36.4% at the 2-month FU to 72.7% at the 6-month FU.

Table 1. The five most common Therapy Advisor (TA) messages

Message	Frequency of follow-up		
	All FUs ($n = 129$)	2-months ($n = 96$)	6-months ($n = 33$)
TA has nothing significant to report	68	48 (50%)	20 (61%)
Fast V rhythm detected	31	25 (26%)	6 (18%)
High sensed atrial rates	21	18 (19%)	3 (9%)
Retrograde conduction detected	14	8 (8%)	6 (18%)
P-wave sensing problem suspected	12	10 (10%)	2 (6%)

With regard to whether the Therapy Advisor helps to optimise programming, the pacemaker investigators were mostly neutral (48.1%). Between the 2- and 6-month FU, the negative responses decreased, from 18.2% to 3.0% in favour of positive responses, which increased from 18.2 to 42.4%.

About optimising the drug regimen, most investigators were neutral (56.6%). Negative scores decreased from 27.3% to 18.2% when 2- and 6-month FUs are compared.

Finally, regarding FU efficiency, physicians were again positive to neutral (50% and 31%, respectively.) The number of positive answers increased from 36% at the 2-month FU to 67% at the 6-month FU.

In a large number of cases (50–60%), the Therapy Advisor had nothing significant to report, and the opinion of physicians about the Therapy Advisor in assessing the patient and FU efficiency in these cases was also analysed. For patient assessment, more than 30% of physicians were negative after the 2-month FU, with not a single one positive. At 6 months, there were no negative opinions and almost 80% were positive. The same holds for FU efficiency: the almost 25% negative answers at 2 months disappeared at the 6-month FU whereas the positive answers increased from 25% to almost 60% (Fig. 2).

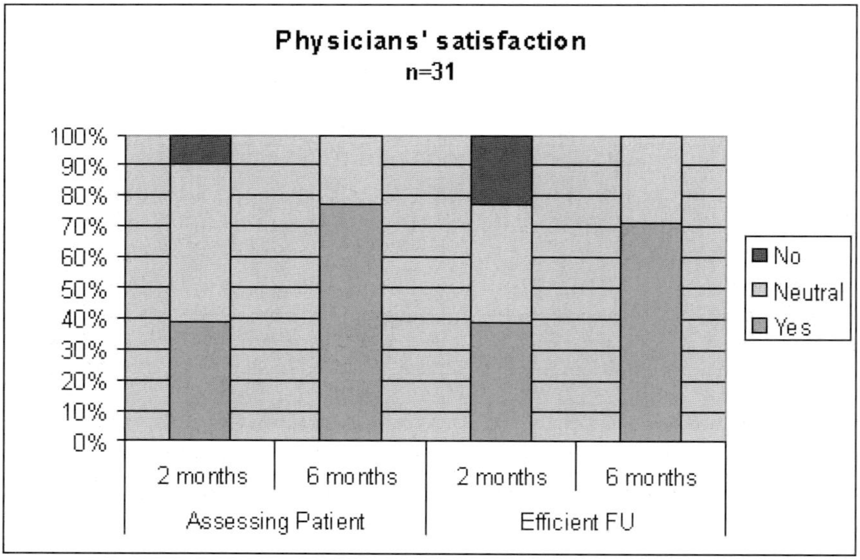

Fig. 2. Physicians satisfaction: compared at 2- and 6-months FU physicians are clearly more satisfied about the helpfulness of the Therapy Advisor in assessing the patient and improving FU efficiency

Discussion

The majority of investigators rated the contribution of the Therapy Advisor in assessing the patient and making the FU more efficient neutral to positive. Over time, trust in the Therapy Advisor increased, as indicated by the increase in investigator satisfaction between the 2- and 6-month FU. This increase was particularly observed for assessment of the patient's condition and making the FU more efficient. Increased trust is also indicated by the higher satisfaction with the message 'Nothing significant to report' during the 6-month FU than at the 2-month FU. Apparently, the investigators did not trust the message in the beginning and felt that it was necessary to collect all diagnostic information. After doing this a couple of times, the physicians learned that the message was useful and reliable.

This, it appears that, as investigators use Therapy Advisor over time, they become acquainted with its features and increasingly appreciate its usefulness.

Conclusions

Pacemaker follow-ups are a burden for health budgets in general and for the clinic in particular. A reason for this is that during the last several years pacemakers have become increasingly complicated and able to store greater amounts of data. Programming the pacemaker properly and analysing the collected data for clinically relevant details have likewise become more complicated. Consequently, a new field of relevant diagnostics was needed to cope with the increased demands of digital pacemakers on clinicians' time during patient FU.

New technologies can bring solutions. In the case of pacemakers, automaticities are taking increasing care of checking and re-programming basic functions, such as sensing and pacing thresholds. Long-distance FU have made it possible to spare patients coming to the clinic on schedule 'just in case,' so that they now are able to come only when required. This is a promising technique although it still requires adjustment. The Therapy Advisor is a next step. It analyses all the data collected by the pacemaker, directing the physician to the clinically relevant issues. Again, this is a field under development but the interim results of the C-STAR registry show a high degree of satisfaction among physicians and a growing acceptance and trust in this new technology. New technologies such as the Therapy Advisor thus allow the physician to forget the technique behind the pacemaker and focus on the clinical aspects of the pacemaker patient.

References

1. van Hemel NA, Wohlgemuth P, Egbers JG et al (2004) Form analysis using digital signal processing reliably discriminates far-field R waves from P waves. PACE 27:1615-1624
2. Schuchert A (2004) C-STARegistry. In: Proceedings of the 11th international symposium on progress in clinical pacing. Centro Scientifico Editore Rome p 5
3. Love CJ (2004) The digital pacemaker. PACE 27:707–708

Interference of Cellular Phones and Metal Detectors With Pacemakers and ICDs: Still a Problem?

E. Occhetta, L. Plebani, M. Bortnik, P. Marino

Electromagnetic interference (EMI) may affect the behaviour of some medical electrical equipment, including cardiac pacemakers and implanted cardioverter-defibrillators (ICDs) [1]. EMI occurs when an electronic device is subjected to any electromagnetic field with an amplitude higher than the interference threshold. The effects on the device depend on the energy of the electromagnetic signal interfering with the normal function of the electronic circuit, with the following possibilities:

- A temporary malfunction
- An alteration of the device during exposure to interference
- A permanent alteration of the circuit due to the interference

Electromagnetic fields may be of various natures, and their ability to interfere with the electronic device depends mainly upon two factors:

- The frequency range of the electromagnetic field – either the carrier or its modulation – which may fall within the operative range of the device
- The power of the electromagnetic wave, which, when relevant, can modify the behaviour of the active device

Nowadays there are multiple sources of environmental EMI signals, e.g. metal detector gates (airports, supermarkets, jewellers, banks, etc.), which may generate dangerous electromagnetic fields; however, while some authors [2, 3] have reported no interference with pacemaker functioning, other studies [4–7] have found interference, sometimes significant.

In the Spiced Teas study [7] interactions between acoustomagnetic electronic article surveillance gates and pacemakers have been reported for vir-

Divisione Clinicizzata di Cardiologia, Facoltà di Medicina e Chirurgia, Università degli Studi del Piemonte Orientale 'A. Avogadro', Novara, Italy

tually all the pacemakers tested (50 patients, 6 different types of pacemakers). Interactions included asynchronous pacing, atrial and ventricular oversensing, and even paced beats resulting from the direct induction of current in the pacemaker. Other modern applications have also been investigated, such as automatic toll payment radiofrequency systems: in this case no interference effect on pacemakers was found [8].

Although the effects of electromagnetic interference on cardiac pacemakers have been widely studied, there are still many perplexities about the consequences on more sophisticated devices such as ICDs. Fetter et al. [9] evaluated the electromagnetic interference generated in a working environment by large welding machines and motors on patients with implanted ICDs; they did not observe any interference with normal ICD functional operation.

The Spiced Teas study [7] has reported the absence of interference between electronic article surveillance devices and correct functioning of ICDs. The authors suppose that this immunity to electromagnetic interference is due to complex detection algorithms and programmable rate cut-off parameters, which of course are not present in pacemaker sensing systems.

Mathew et al. [10] and McIvor [11], on the other hand, have reported inappropriate discharge of ICDs as a result of exposure to electromagnetic interference from electronic article surveillance devices, perhaps because of complex interference between arrhythmia detection and automatic gain control.

In 1989, Karson et al. [12] reported a case of inadvertent ICD activation by a magnet located in the loudspeaker of a stereo system. Other anecdotal reports have been published of inappropriate ICD shocks caused by EMI from a magnetic bingo wand [13], remote controls of toys [14], slot machines [15], and an electric razor [16]; in this last case, EMI was caused by defective insulation of the electrode and could not be evoked with an intact electrode. Most of the previous reports of EMI in ICDs involved earlier, less sophisticated devices with epicardial screw-in sensing leads. Theoretically, endocardial leads should be better protected from EMI, because of both the spatial orientation of the endocardial bipole and the endocardial location itself [17].

Another common medical source of EMI is transcutaneous electric nerve stimulation (TENS), a widely used method of relieving various musculoskeletal pains. Several well-documented cases of spurious shocks triggered by TENS application in patients with a variety of lead configurations and sensing algorithms have been described [18, 19].

An ever more common source of electromagnetic waves in today's environment is cellular phones; they may be clinically relevant sources of EMI and may affect pacemaker and ICD function [20–23]. Patients with an implanted pacemaker or ICD are so alarmed at the interference phenomenon that there have been urgent calls for studies to evaluate the problem [24–29].

Currently there are no standards prescribing limits for pacemaker compatibility. The IEC standard 601-1-2 [30] is not adequate, recommending testing with an electric field of 3 V/m modulated sinusoidally with 1 KHz when digital mobile phones with 2 W output may produce up to an amplitude of 120 V/m at a 2 cm distance [20]. There is an European standard to which pacemakers designers conform, named EN 50061/A1 [31]. This norm specifies voltages as a function of frequency below which (30 MHz) pacemakers must function undisturbed. Although the standard of 30 MHz does not cover the mobile phone frequencies, Irnich [20] found that most pacemakers were resistant to 2 W digital GSM (Global System for Mobile Communication) fields, suggesting that most manufacturers have developed resistant models without having mobile phone compatibility as a design criterion.

Cellular phones may be divided in two different systems utilised in Europe and North America:

1. Analogue transmission: transmission passes through a continuous wave which has modulation variations in frequency. The carrier frequency in this system may be about 450 MHz (NMT 450) or around 900 MHz (NMT 900, European TACS, and American FDMA).
2. Digital transmission: several simultaneous conversations are allowed on the same line; to do this, a carrier frequency of around 900 MHz for the European GSM system and 800–900 MHz for the American NADC, TDMA, and CDMA systems is coded. In digital transmission systems the signal is coded and modulated at a frequency which on the GSM system is around 217 Hz. The system also has an energy saving mechanism, called DTX, which is activated when the user is in the listening mode, with an additional modulation of 2 Hz and 8 Hz.

All these systems operate on a power of 0.6–1 W in the USA and from 20 mW to 2 W in Europe, with a mean value of 0.8 W. It is, therefore, theoretically possible that a mobile phone operating near enough to a pacemaker may cause interference in its working condition. Numerous studies have been carried out on this matter both in vitro [25, 32] and in vivo [27, 28, 33–36], which discuss the question of the significance and nature of the interference: briefly, it was shown that interference was around 20–30%, always with the telephone in close proximity, within 20 cm. In the majority of cases the interference was considered insignificant, with brief inhibition, conversion to asynchronous mode, and synchronisation of atrial-triggered stimulation; in each case interference took place when the phone was placed on the pacemaker itself, the sensitivity of the pacemaker was at its maximum, the device used GSM digital technology, and interference occurred almost exclusively when the phone was in the calling or receiving mode.

Less clear is the question of interference by cellular telephones in the operation of more sophisticated devices such as the ICDs [23, 24, 26, 29]. An electromagnetic field interfering with an ICD may alter its working mechanisms in the following ways:

- By not allowing for correct recognition of an arrhythmia (undersensing), resulting in failure to deliver cardioversion or defibrillation therapy
- By generating false recognition of an arrhythmia (oversensing), which may induce inappropriate delivery (most uncomfortable for the patient), or may even induce a serious arrhythmia such as ventricular fibrillation
- By inhibition of pacing, which of course may be very dangerous after shock delivery.

The few data presently available indicate that shielding by the body is an important element of protection from external interference [26]. Bassen et al. [37] documented an in vitro inappropriate delivery of therapy induced by digital telephone signals. In vivo studies by Chiladakis et al. (36 patients) [26], Stanton et al. (25 patients) [38], Wilke et al. (50 patients) [39], and Altamura et al. (200 patients) [40] investigated different types of telephones, analogue and digital. They found that no interference was produced when the telephone antenna was kept directly over the ICD, and there was no interference effect on recognition of induced ventricular fibrillation, pacing/sensing functions, or telemetry data.

Notwithstanding these findings, some ICD today are equipped with special filters which may reduce EMI from mobile telephones. Interesting results emerged when these filters were tested on pacemakers and ICDs [41]. A previous study by ourselves [29] evaluated quite a large cohort of ICD models on today's market. Using either analogue (TACS) or digital (GSM) European phone systems, patients were monitored by means of surface ECG and telemetric intracardiac electrogram with sensing markers, using an identical protocol for each group (Fig. 1):

1. Telephone in direct contact with both the ICD and the programming head of the programmer
2. Telephone in direct contact with the ICD alone (head of the programmer moved away)
3. Telephone positioned in the area of the pacing/sensing ventricular lead
4. Telephone held in patient's hands

Following manoeuvres were carried out for each position:

1. Telephone in receiving and calling mode (frequency around 900 MHz)
2. Telephone in active conversation (speaking, frequency around 900 MHz modulated at 217 Hz)
3. Telephone in passive conversation mode (listening, with activation for the digital transmission phone of the discontinuous transmission mode – DTX – frequency modulated at 2–8 Hz)

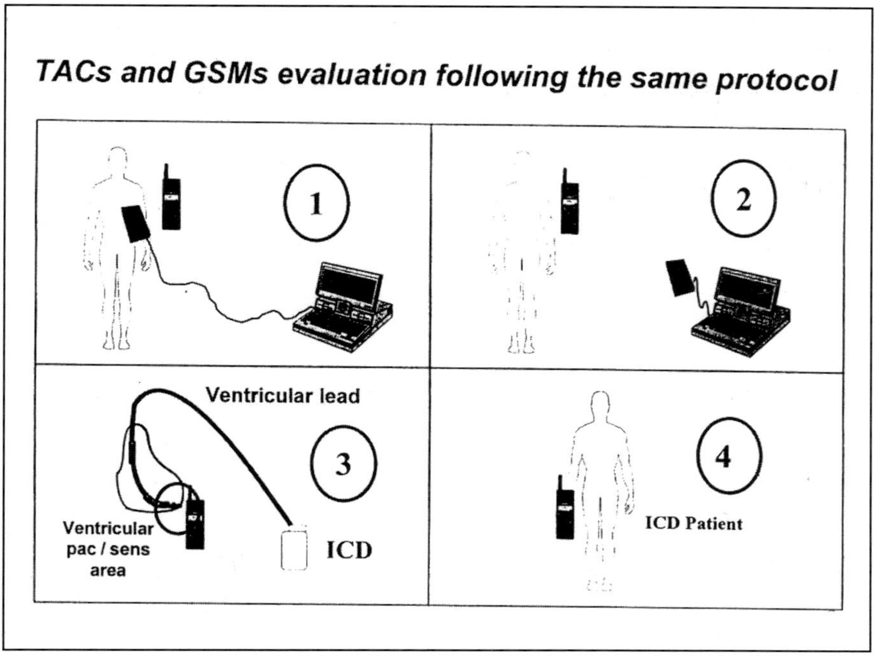

Fig. 1. Protocol of cellular phone evaluation: *1* the telephone in direct contact with both the ICD and the programming head of the programmer; *2* the telephone in direct contact with the ICD alone (head of the programmer moved away); *3* the telephone positioned in the area of pacing/sensing ventricular lead; *4* the telephone placed in the hands of the patient

In no patient there was any interference induced by the electromagnetic field from a cellular phone causing false arrhythmia recognition, even under the maximum limit condition, with the telephones placed in direct contact with the ICD. Conversely, for both the analogue and the digital system, constant interference on telemetric transmission between the programmer and the ICD was observed when the phone in receiving or calling mode was in direct contact with the telemetric head. Sometimes the interference was so great to cause loss of telemetric monitoring of the intracardiac ECG, even if there was no inappropriate reprogramming.

In a subgroup of five patients, we also evaluated the presence/absence of interference caused by cellular phones during ventricular arrhythmia induction and recognition. There was no evidence of interference with arrhythmia detection. The implanted system recognised the arrhythmia correctly and appropriately delivered a defibrillation shock. No difference was observed when we compared timing of ICD discharge with cellular phones operating versus inactive (Fig. 2).

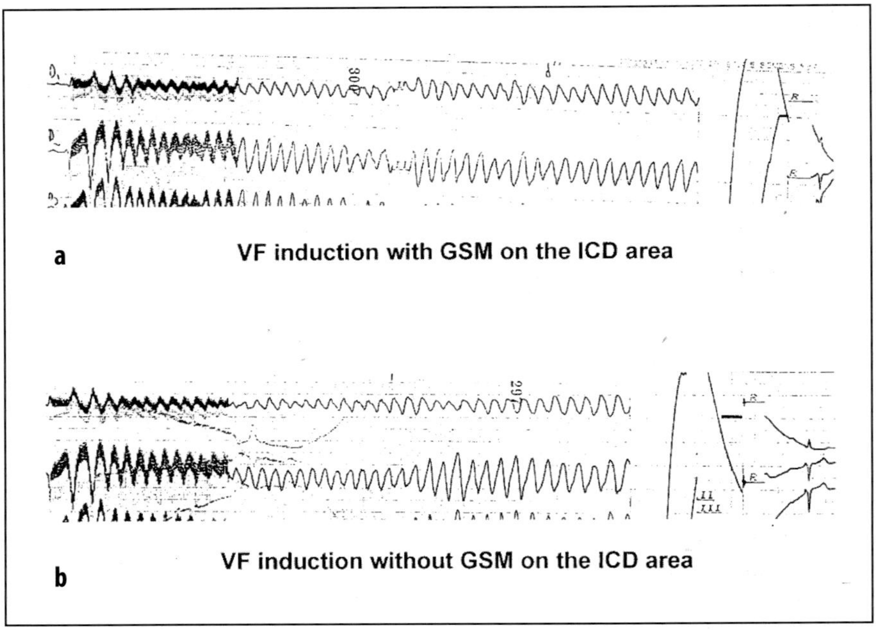

Fig. 2a, b. Test performed during Defender ICD (Ela Medical) implantation. **a** During the first ventricular fibrillation induction a GSM phone was active (ringing in receiving mode): the time before the 13 J shock was 7 s. **b** During a second ventricular fibrillation induction without GSM (phone OFF) the time before the shock was very similar (8 s)

Conclusions

1. Patients with an implanted pacemaker or ICD may safely use a cellular phone, provided they do not use it in closer range than 20 cm to the device when in receiving and conversation mode. This means: it is advisable for the patient not to keep the cellular telephone in the breast pocket of his/her jacket, on the same side as the device.
2. Use of a cellular telephone could be permitted, even in cardiac environments where programming and telemetric checking up of pacemakers and defibrillators is being carried out, if it is kept at least 1 m away from electronic devices.
3. If the patient has a cellular telephone, it would be useful to determine any possible interference effect on his/her own pacemaker/ICD in order to give psychological reassurance and allow resumption of work in industrial facilities [42].

References

1. Pinski SL, Trohman RG (2002) Interference in implanted cardiac devices. Part 1. Pacing Clin Electrophysiol 25:1367–1381
2. Copperman Y, Zarfati D, Laniado S et al (1988) The effect of metal detector gates on implanted permanent pacemakers. Pacing Clin Electrophysiol 11:1386–1387
3. Wilke A, Kruse T, Hesse H, et al (1998) Interactions between pacemakers and security systems. Pacing Clin Electrophysiol 21:1784 (abs)
4. Dodinot B, Godenir JP, Costa AB et al (1993) Electronic article surveillance: a possible danger for pacemaker patients. Pacing Clin Electrophysiol 16:46–53
5. Beaugeard D, Kacet S, Bricout M et al (1992) Interferences entre les stimulateurs cardiaques et les détecteurs de vol dans les magasins. Arch Mal Coeur 85:1457–1461
6. Lucas EH, Johnson D, McElroy BP (1994) The effects of electronic article surveillance systems on permanent cardiac pacemakers: an in vitro study. Pacing Clin Electrophysiol 17:2021–2026
7. McIvor ME, Reddinger J, Floden E et al (1998) Study of pacemakers and implantable cardioverter defibrillators triggering by electronic article surveillance devices (SPICED TEAS Study). Pacing Clin Electrophysiol 21:1847–1861
8. Barbaro V, Bartolini P, Donato A et al (1997) Electromagnetic interference between automatic toll payment RF systems and cardiac pacemakers (abs). Proceedings of 1st Int Congress Cardiostim Transmediterranéen. Rabat, Morocco, p 55
9. Fetter JC, Benditi DG, Stanton MS (1996) Electromagnetic interference from welding and motors on implantable cardioverter defibrillators as tested in the electrically hostile work site. J Am Coll Cardiol 28:423–427
10. Mathew P, Lewis C, Neglia J et al (1997) Interaction between electronic article surveillance systems and implantable defibrillators: insights from a fourth generation ICD. Pacing Clin Electrophysiol 20:2857–2859
11. McIvor ME (1995) Environmental electromagnetic interferences from electronic article surveillance devices: interactions with an ICD. Pacing Clin Electrophysiol 18:2229–2230
12. Karson TH, Grace K, Denes P (1989) Stereo speaker silences automatic implantable cardioverter defibrillator. N Engl J Med 320:1628–1629
13. Ferrick KJ, Johnston D, Kim SG et al (1991) Inadvertent AICD activation while playing bingo. Am Heart J 121:206–207
14. Ching Man K, Davidson T, Langberg JJ et al (1993) Interferences from a hand held radiofrequency remote control causing discharge of an implantable defibrillator. Pacing Clin Electrophysiol 16:1756–1758
15. Seifert T, Block M, Borggrefe M et al (1995) Erroneous discharge of an implantable cardioverter defibrillator caused by an electric razor. Pacing Clin Electrophysiol 18:1592–1594
16. Madrid A, Sanchez A, Bosch E et al (1997) Dysfunction of implantable defibrillators caused by slot machines. Pacing Clin Electrophysiol 20(Pt II):212–214
17. Glotzer TV, Gordon M, Sparta M et al (1998) Electromagnetic interference from a muscle stimulation device causing discharge of an implantable cardioverter defibrillator. Epicardial bipolar and endocardial bipolar sensing circuits are compared. Pacing Clin Electrophysiol 21:1996–1998

18. Crevenna R, Stix G, Pleiner J et al (2003) Electromagnetic interference by transcutaneous neuromuscular electrical stimulation in patients with bipolar sensing implantable cardioverter defibrillators: a pilot safety study. Pacing Clin Electrophysiol 26(Pt I):626–629
19. Vlay SC (1998) Electromagnetic interference and ICD discharge related to chiropractic treatment. Pacing Clin Electrophysiol 21:2009
20. Irnich W (1996) Mobile telephones and pacemakers. Pacing Clin Electrophysiol 19:1407–1409
21. Hayes DL (1996) Wireless phones and pacemaker interaction. Pacing Clin Electrophysiol 19:1405–1406
22. Roelke M, Bernestein AD (1997) Cardiac pacemakers and cellular telephones. N Engl J Med 336:1518–1519
23. Santini M (2001) Digital cellular telephones and ICDs. Eur Heart J 22:1251–1252
24. Hayes DL, Carrillo RG, Gretchen K et al (1996) State of the science: pacemaker and defibrillator interference from wireless communication devices. Pacing Clin Electrophysiol 19:1419–1430
25. Irnich W, Batz L, Muller R et al (1996) Electromagnetic interference of pacemakers by mobile phones. Pacing Clin Electrophysiol 19:1431–1446
26. Chiladakis JA, Davlouros P, Agelopoulos G et al (2001) In-vivo testing of digital cellular telephones in patients with implantable cardioverter-defibrillators. Eur Heart J 22:1337–1342
27. Hekmat K, Salemink B, Lauterbach G et al (2004) Interference by cellular phones with permanent implanted pacemakers: an update. Europace 6:363–369
28. Elshershari H, Celiker A, Ozer S et al (2002) Influence of D-Net (EUROPEAN GSM-Standard) cellular telephones on implanted pacemakers in children. Pacing Clin Electrophysiol 25:1328–1330
29. Occhetta E, Plebani L, Bortnik M et al (1999) Implantable cardioverter-defibrillators and cellular telephones: is there any interference? Pacing Clin Electrophysiol 22:983–989
30. Anonymous (1994) International Electrotechnical Commission: IEC Standard 601-1-2: Safety of medical electrical equipment – electromagnetic compatibility, requirements and tests. Bureau Central de la Commission Electrotechnique International, Geneva, Switzerland
31. European Committee for Electrotechnical Standardization: CENELEC Standard EN 50 061:1988/A1:1995: Safety of implantable cardiac pacemakers. Central Secretariat, Brussels, Belgium
32. Barbaro V, Bartolini P, Donato A et al (1995) Do European GSM mobile cellular phones pose a potential risk to pacemaker patients? Pacing Clin Electrophysiol 18:1218–1224
33. Barbaro V, Bartolini P, Donato A et al (1996) Electromagnetic interference of analog cellular telephones with pacemakers. Pacing Clin Electrophysiol 19:1410–1418
34. Hayes DL, Wang PT, Reynolds DW et al (1997) Interference with cardiac pacemakers by cellular telephones. N Engl J Med 336:1473–1479
35. Sparks PB, Mond HG, Joyner KH et al (1996) The safety of digital mobile cellular telephones with minute ventilation rate adaptive pacemakers. Pacing Clin Electrophysiol 19:1451–1455
36. Altamura G, Toscano S, Castro A et al (1996) Possibili conseguenze delle interferenze dei telefoni cellulari sui pacemakers impiantati: esperienza in 200 casi. G Ital Cardiol 26(suppl 1):129 (abs)

37. Bassen H, Moore HJ, Ruggera PS et al (1995) Cellular phone interference testing of implantable cardiac defibrillators. In-vitro. Circulation 92:I-738 (abs)
38. Stanton MS, Grice SE, Trusty J et al (1996) Safety of various cellular phone technologies with implantable cardioverter defibrillators. Pacing Clin Electrophysiol 19:II-583 (abs)
39. Wilke A, Grimm W, Funk R et al (1996) Influence of D-Net (European GSM-Standard) cellular phones on pacemaker function in 50 patients with permanent pacemakers. Pacing Clin Electrophysiol 19:1456–1458
40. Altamura G, Gentilucci G, Magris B et al (1996) I telefoni cellulari non inducono falsi 'riconoscimenti' nei pazienti portatori di defibrillatore automatico impiantabile. G Ital Cardiol 26(suppl 1):134 (abs)
41. Selznick L, Mueller H, Chavez T (1996) Cellular telephone technology and its effect on implantable cardiac pacing systems. Technology update, Pacesetter[AQ8]
42. Gurevitz O, Fogel RI, Herner ME et al (2003) Patients with an ICD can safely resume work in industrial facilities following simple screening for electromagnetic interference. Pacing Clin Electrophysiol 26:1675–1678

Can Patients With Implanted Pacemakers/ICD Undergo Magnetic Resonance Imaging?

S. Sermasi, M. Marconi, M. Mezzetti, G. Piovaccari

Introduction

Magnetic resonance imaging (MRI) is a rapidly expanding diagnostic tool used in a wide range of clinical applications, such as oncology, musculoskeletal disorders, and pathologies of the central nervous and cardiovascular systems. About 35 million MRI studies are performed yearly worldwide [1]. In addition, the use of innovative cardiac-device-based therapies, including pacemakers and ICDs, with new indications for primary prevention of sudden cardiac death and heart failure, is also rapidly increasing, resulting in an estimated 50–75% probability of a patient being indicated for an MRI over the lifetime of their device. In the USA, about 200 000 device recipients could have benefited from MRI in 2004 [2]. However, current pacemakers and ICDs and their connected leads have not been designed to be MRI safe. Moreover, there is a great difference among MRI scanners and devices, some of which may be state-of-the-art but connected to old leads when newer pacemakers or ICDs are replaced. Although the problem persists, MRI manufacturers' are working with the Food and Drug Administration (FDA) in the USA to modify the situation [3–7]. Nonetheless, current labelling for pacemakers and defibrillators systems includes a warning against MRI procedures for patients with such devices.

Background

The use of MRI in clinical practice has been gaining in popularity since the early 1980s. At that time, there was concern that any implanted metal object

Department of Cardiovascular Diseases, Operative Unit of Cardiology, Infermi Hospital, AUSL Rimini, Rimini, Italy

might be pulled out of the body or damaged by the very strong magnetic field generated by MRI. However, both pacemakers and ICDs utilise nonferrous metals, and there are no reports of devices being ripped out the body [8]. In contrast, animal studies, in vitro and in vivo, and anecdotal reports on humans have revealed several potential problems affecting the implanted system when exposed to the magnetic fields generated by MRI.

Potential Risks

Several studies have addressed the potential risks of using MRI in patients with pacemakers and ICDs. First, the magnetic field was shown to potentially induce a current in the lead, causing rapid cardiac stimulation [7]; however, since the applied currents are mostly subthreshold they are without clinical consequences [9]. Second, the reed switch in a pacemaker or ICD does not necessarily remain closed in response to strong magnetic fields (0.5, 1.5, 3.0 Tesla), and the state of the reed switch may not be predictable with certainty under clinical conditions [8, 10]. Third, magnetic fields inhibit or trigger pacemakers, resulting in patients having their ICD disabled during MRI or in false detection of tachyarrhythmias, leading to inappropriate ICD intervention [11]. Arrhythmogenic risks depend on scan parameters, patient, device position [12–14], and the design of the device, i.e. modern devices are less prone to the effects of MRI because of better built-in electromagnetic interference (EMI) protection circuitry [6, 15, 16]. Finally, MRI may produce considerable heading at the tip of the lead and changes of pacing parameters in long-term experiments [17–19].

Comments

When there is a strongly appropriate clinical justification for an MRI study in a patient with a pacemaker or an ICD, general medical opinion is that many possible risks can be avoided or managed by an expert clinical team, appropriate device programming, and close monitoring of the patient both during the scan and after the study.

While the FDA recognises that MRI is a very powerful diagnostic tool that may be safe for application in pacemaker and ICD recipients, it will not remove the warnings and contraindications for this population until there is better knowledge of the mechanisms associated with the potential risks of complications.

MRI safety for device patients is important and will become increasingly relevant with time. The majority of manufacturers are actively involved in designing devices that do not interfere with a multiplicity of EMI generators, including MRI [4–6]. The goal is the development of a truly MRI-compatible device. In the meantime, one possible solution is to replace the pacemaker's wire cable with a fibre-optic lead and to use an implantable low-power semiconductor laser for sensing and regulating heartbeat [20].

References

1. Martin ET (2005) Can cardiac pacemakers and magnetic resonance imaging systems co-exist? Eur Heart J 26:325–327
2. Kalin R, Stanton MS (2005) Current clinical issues for MRI scanning of pacemaker and defibrillator patients. PACE 28:326–328
3. Fisher JD (2005) MRI: safety in patients with pacemakers or defibrillators: is it prime time yet? PACE 28:263
4. Smith JM (2005) Industry viewpoint: Guidant: pacemakers, ICDs. PACE 28:264
5. Stanton MS (2005) Industry viewpoint: Medtronic: pacemakers, ICDs and MRI. PACE 28:265
6. Levine PA (2005) Industry viewpoint: St. Jude Medical: pacemakers, ICDs and MRI. PACE 28:266–267
7. Hayes DL, Holmes DR, Gra JE (1987) Effect of 1.5 Tesla nuclear magnetic resonance imaging scanner on implanted permanent pacemakers. J Am Coll Cardiol 10:782–786
8. Garcia-Bolao I, Albaladejo V, Benito A et al (1998) Magnetic resonance imaging in patient with a dual chamber pacemaker. Acta Cardiol 53:33–35
9. Lauck G, Von Smekal A, Wolke S et al (1995) Effects of nuclear magnetic resonance imaging on cardiac pacemakers. PACE 18:1549–1555
10. Luechinger R, Zeijlemaker VA, Scheidegger MB et al (2002) Pacemaker reed switch behavior in 0.5, 1.5, and 3.0 Tesla magnetic resonance imaging units: are reed switches always closed in strong magnetic fields? PACE 25:1419–1423
11. Gimbel JR, Kanal E, Schwartz KM et al (2005) Outcome of magnetic resonance imaging (MRI) in selected patients with implantable cardioverter defibrillators (ICDs). PACE 28:270–273
12. Rozner MA, Burton AW, Kumar A (2005) Pacemaker complications during magnetic resonance imaging. J Am Coll Cardiol 45:161–162
13. Gimbel JR, Wilkoff B (2003) Artifact mimicking tachycardia during magnetic resonance imaging in a patient with implantable loop recorder. Heart 89:e10
14. Faris OP, Shein MJ (2005) Government viewpoint: U.S. Food & Drug Administration: pacemakers, ICDs, and MRI. PACE 28:268–269
15. Loewy J, Loewy A, Kendall EJ (2004) Reconsideration of pacemakers and MR imaging. Radiographics 24:1257–1267
16. Del Ojo JL, Moya F, Villalba J et al (2005) Is magnetic resonance imaging safe in cardiac pacemaker recipients? Pacing Clin Electrophysiol 28(4):274–278
17. Sommer T, Vahlhaus C, Lauck G et al (2000) MR imaging anf cardiac pacemakers: in vitro evaluation and in vivo studies in 51 patients at 0.5 T. Radiology 215:869–879

18. Martin ET, Coman JA, Shellock FG et al (2004) Magnetic resonance imaging and cardiac pacemaker safety at 1.5 Tesla. J Am Coll Cardiol 43:1315–1324
19. Luechinger R, Zeijlemaker VA, Pedersen EM et al (2005) In vivo heating of pacemaker leads during magnetic resonance imaging. Eur Heart J 26:376–383
20. High Tech Rochester. Inventor of MRI to work with pacemaker inventor on MRI-compatible pacemaker. Available at http://www.htr.org

SYNCOPE:
EVALUATION AND THERAPIES

Syncope in Children and Adolescents: What Are the Peculiar Features?

W. Wieling[1], N. van Dijk[1], K.S. Ganzeboom[1], J. P. Saul[2]

Epidemiology

Syncope can be defined as a temporary loss of consciousness and postural tone secondary to lack of adequate cerebral blood perfusion. The incidence of syncope coming to medical attention is increased in two age groups, the old and the young (Fig. 1). An incidence peak occurs around the age of 15 years, with the incidence in females being more than twice that in males [1, 2]. A lower peak occurs in older infants and toddlers, most commonly referred to as 'breath-holding spells' [3].

The incidence of syncope in young subjects coming to medical attention varies between approximately 0.5 and 3 cases per 1000 (0.05–0.3%) [2]. Syncopal events which do not reach medical attention occur much more frequently. In a survey of students averaging 20 years of age, 20% of male and 50% of female students report having experienced at least one syncopal episode [4]. By comparison, the prevalence of seizures in a similar age group is about 5 per 1000 (0.5%) [5]. Cardiac syncope is even less common. The most common cause of syncope in young subjects is reflex syncope and in particular a vasovagal faint [2–4], which is diagnosed in about 80% of the paediatric patients presenting with syncope [6].

Clinical Characteristics of Reflex Syncope

The term 'reflex syncope' is used to label a heterogeneous group of disorders characterised by episodic vasodilation and/or bradycardia resulting in a transient

[1]Academic Medical Center, University of Amsterdam, Amsterdam, The Netherlands;
[2]Medical University of South Carolina, Charlston, SC, USA

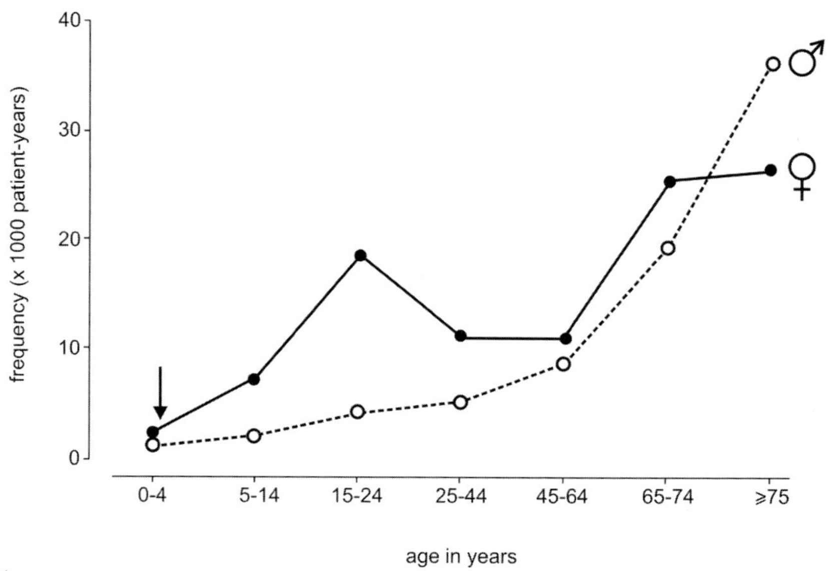

Fig. 1. Frequency of fainting as a reason for encounter in general practice in the Netherlands. Data obtained from the general practitioners' transition project in an analysis of 93 297 patient-years. *Arrow* indicates that a small peak occurs between 6 and 18 months of age (breath-holding spells)

failure of blood pressure (BP) control [7]. The circumstances surrounding reflex syncopal events often include a change in posture, but may be associated with a wide variety of common situations (Table 1) and physical factors. The more common forms of reflex syncope seen in young subjects are described below [1].

Table 1. Typical reflex syncope triggers

Prolonged standing, especially in combination with warm temperature, confined spaces, or crowding ('church syncope')
Emotional circumstances, pain (e.g. venipuncture, sight of blood)
Fasting, lack of sleep, fatigue, menstruation, illness with fever
Micturition
Directly after intense exercise
Hyperventilation and straining (self-induced syncope)
Stretching, coughing
Standing quickly, arising from squat
Rapid weight loss
Certain medications, alcohol, and illegal drugs (must be distinguished from intoxication)

Vasovagal Syncope

A combination of peripheral arterial and venous vasodilation followed closely by relative bradycardia is the most common physiological scenario observed during syncope in young subjects [7]. Two clinical scenarios in particular are known to provoke vasovagal faints in the young. First are situations that increase pooling of venous blood, such as standing motionless. The second are situations of intense emotion or pain.

The clinical presentation of vasovagal syncope varies widely both within and among young patients. They often, but not always, experience prodromal symptoms (Table 2). Episodes may occur without an identifiable trigger, even in patients who are sitting or going about normal daily exercise. Events that occur in these patients while supine in the absence of an emotional stimulus are unlikely to be vasovagal [1].

Table 2. Typical premonitory symptoms of reflex syncope

Lightheadedness, dizziness
Palpitations
Weakness
Dimming or blurred vision
Nausea, epigastric distress
Feeling warm or cold
Facial pallor
Sweating, dilated pupils

Initial Orthostatic Hypotension

(Pre)syncope upon standing is observed much more commonly in the young than in adults. Almost all teenagers and adolescents are familiar with feelings of lightheadedness within a few seconds of standing up quickly, which typically resolves spontaneously within 30 s [8]. The transient fall in pressure is caused by vasodilatation in active muscles during standing up, and is not seen upon a passive head-up tilt (Fig. 2). Patients with severe complaints tend to be tall with an asthenic habitus and poorly developed musculature. The mechanism underlying the excessive fall in pressure in these patients remains to be established.

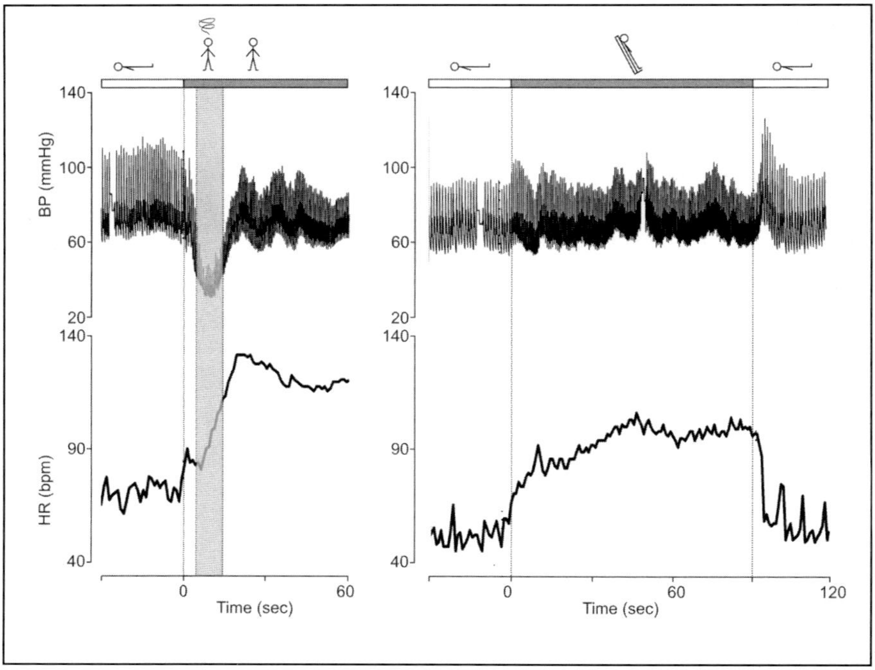

Fig. 2. Changes in HR and BP in a patient with a history of 10 years of almost daily near-syncope and occasional syncope upon standing up. Note the marked initial fall in finger BP with lightheadedness on standing and right panel after head-up tilt, but not with passive head-up tilt

Postural Orthostatic Tachycardia Syndrome

Postural orthostatic tachycardia syndrome (POTS) is defined by symptoms of cerebral and retinal hypoperfusion and an excessive increase in heart rate (HR) in the upright posture with a low normal arterial BP [9]. Reduced cerebral blood perfusion has been documented. In the average adolescent, an increase in HR of more than 35 bpm or a rise to more than 120 bpm after 2 min of standing can be considered excessive [10].

POTS is more common in females, with a ratio of about 4:1. Actual loss of consciousness occurs in a minority of the subjects. The prevalence of POTS in the general population is probably low.

Fainting 'Larks'

Hyperventilation decreases CO_2, causing cerebral vasoconstriction and pre-syncope. Straining impedes venous return and also decreases cerebral blood-flow. These adjunctive influences, in combination with orthostatic stress, have been applied by young subjects for self-induced fainting as entertainment or for avoiding an undesirable task, such as a school examination ('fainting lark') [1].

Autonomic Failure

Primary global autonomic neuropathy as a cause of syncope is extremely rare in young subjects. It has been reported in association with a variety of syndromes [11] and may also occur in the setting of chronic diseases, or in patients using vasoactive medications.

Breath-Holding Spells

Syncope may occur in toddlers during crying [2, 3, 7]. The spells have been described in two varieties: pallid, which seems to be the result of sudden transient asystole, typically after a short cry, and cyanotic after a more prolonged cry, which mechanism most likely is similar to the fainting lark, as the hyperventilation of crying is combined with the straining of a prolonged silent cry. The onset is typically between 6 months and 2 years of age, and the spells are generally self-resolving by the age of 3–4 years. Though frightening, these spells have not been associated with serious outcomes such as sudden infant death.

Associated Syndromes

Psychogenic (Pseudo-syncope)

A conversion reaction is a rare cause of transient loss of consciousness, but may occur in adolescents, especially females. The diagnosis should be considered when the number of events is high (up to several times a day) and there is no associated physical injury. The duration of the unconsciousness is often prolonged (10–30 min) despite a supine posture. During an episode, the eyes may be tightly closed with a lid flutter, while during true syncope or epilepsy the eyes are often open and deviated. An unusual posture may be assumed. Passive lifting and dropping of an extremity rarely demonstrates limpness or unawareness of pain [12]. When BP is monitored, it is normal or elevated. Typically, patients use the events to (un)consciously avoid an unpleasant emotional situation. Illicit substance abuse, in particular alcohol and cocaine, are also associated with unexplained episodes of syncope.

Migraine

When related to the basilar artery, migraines can be a cause of syncope [12]. Although specific cerebral flow deficits have not been documented, prodromal symptoms can suggest brainstem or cerebellar ischaemia. Attacks may start with bilateral visual symptoms, dysarthria, vertigo, diplopia, nystagmus, and/or ataxia, may progress to syncope, and may be followed by a more typical migraine headache (not always present). Arterial pressure is typically normal or mildly elevated. A (family) history of migraines is common both in patients with syncope and in those with basilar migraine.

Diagnostic Evaluation

Basic Assessment

Reflex syncopal disorders have an excellent prognosis, but may have a dramatic impact on quality of life. Diagnosing these disorders, therefore, is of great importance. A detailed patient and family history is the most crucial part of the initial work-up. In young patients without known heart disease, a typical history (Tables 1-3) combined with a normal physical examination and ECG can be used to diagnose reflex syncope and to determine whether the episode might be due to a non-syncopal condition or has a potentially malignant aetiology. Physical exam should focus on the heart and BP. HR and BP should be assessed with the patient in supine position and again after 3 minutes standing.

Extended Assessment

History and physical examination should be used to guide the subsequent diagnostic work-up. Otherwise, most tests are unlikely to produce diagnostic results [13]. Ambulatory (loop) ECG recorders should be used in patients with palpitations associated with syncope. Echocardiography should be obtained when a heart murmur is present. When syncope occurs during physical exertion, echocardiography and an exercise test should be performed. Syncope occurring in the cool-down phase after exercise is likely to be neurally mediated, but should also be treated with suspicion. Electroencephalography may be indicated for patients showing prolonged loss of consciousness, seizure activity, or a significant post-ictal phase of lethargy and confusion. Electrophysiological study has a minor role in paediatric patients with syncope, but may be warranted if there is a high suspicion of a tachyarrhythmia.

Tilt Testing

In patients with recurrent 'atypical' vasovagal or unexplained syncope, tilt table testing can be helpful. Drawbacks of head-up tilt testing are the high false positive and false negative rates. Tilt testing is therefore not the most appropriate tool for diagnosing patients with vasovagal syncope, but may be reassuring and instructive to the patient. In patients with conversion reactions, loss of consciousness may occur with no significant decreases in HR, BP, or cerebral blood flow.

Distinguishing Syncope from Epilepsy

Myoclonic jerks mimicking a seizure may occur during syncope [14]. Typically, prolonged asystole of about 10 s is needed in adults before myoclonic jerks occur. In young persons the anoxic threshold is reported to be lower, and it is lowest in early childhood. Clinical features by which seizure may be distinguished from syncope are summarised in Table 3.

Table 3. Features distinguishing syncope from seizures

Syncope	Seizure
Jerks begin after falling	Jerks begin while standing
Typically pale	May be cyanotic
LOC usually < 1–2 min	LOC often > 5 min
Incontinence less common	Incontinence more common
No tongue biting	Tongue biting in about 25% of cases
Post-syncopal confusion typically mild or absent, but prolonged fatigue is common	Post-ictal confusion universal and often prolonged
Difficult in standing until recovery is complete	Standing often possible early in recovery

Therapy of Reflex Syncope
The treatment of reflex syncope is subject of ongoing research [15, 1]

Aborting the Acute Episode

For acute management of an episode, recognition of pre-syncopal symptoms and applying physical manoeuvres, such as lying down, is usually sufficient to avoid loss of consciousness. More subtle manoeuvres have also demonstrated effectiveness without drawing as much attention to the patient – an important point for many adolescents. Leg crossing and muscle tensing are easily taught and highly effective in young patients. Squatting is even more effective, and can be used as an emergency measure when symptoms develop more rapidly.

Preventing (Pre-)syncopal Events

The most important therapy is education and reassurance. Patients should be informed that the risk of sudden death is virtually non-existent, but that physical injury is of some concern. Initial advice should include early recognition of warning symptoms and avoidance of triggering events.

Non-Pharmacological. A low-salt diet should be avoided and hydration status optimised. Manoeuvres can be used as a preventive measure. In highly motivated patients with recurrent symptoms, 'tilt training' may reduce recurrences. Patient compliance may, however, limit its use in young subjects. In patients with blood phobia, psychological deconditioning is the first choice of therapy.

Pharmacological. Pharmacological therapy should be reserved for patients whose symptoms recur despite non-pharmacological treatment, since undesirable side effects often outweigh any positive effects. β-Blockers are commonly prescribed, but have been demonstrated in most trials to be ineffective and frequently have side effects. The mineralocorticoid fludrocortisone is used in combination with high salt and fluid intake to increase blood volume. Mild fluid retention and occasional hypertension are generally the only significant side effects, making it the best tolerated agent in paediatric patients. Of other medications, including β-agonists, the side effects are often intolerable. An unresolved issue is how long prophylactic therapy should be advised.

Pacing. Even in the instance of cardioinhibitory syncope with prolonged asystoles, pacemaker therapy should be avoided whenever possible. Conventional therapy is almost always possible and clearly preferable in young patients.

Breath-holding spells. Most patients can be dealt with through reassurance and instructions to maintain the child in a supine position rather than upright during a spell. When asystole is documented, the muscarinic blocker glycopyrollate may be helpful. Only in rare cases is pacing required.

Acknowledgements
This article has been revised from ref. [1], with permission from the BMJ Publishing Group.

References

1. Wieling W, Ganzeboom KS, Saul JP (2004) Reflex syncope in children and adolescents. Heart 90:1094–1100
2. Driscoll DJ, Jacobsen SJ, Porter CJ et al (1997) Syncope in children and adolescents. J Am Coll Cardiol 29:1039–1045

3. Lombroso CT, Lerman P (1967) Breathholding spells (cyanotic and pallid infantile syncope). Pediatrics 39:563–581
4. Ganzeboom KS, Colman N, Reitsma JB et al (2003) Prevalence and triggers of syncope in medical students. Am J Cardiol 91:1006–1008
5. Wallace H, Shorvon S, Tallis R (1998) Age-specific incidence and prevalence rates of treated epilepsy in an unselected population of 2 052 922 and age-specific fertility rates of women with epilepsy. Lancet 352:1970–1973
6. Massin MM, Bourguignont A, Coremans C et al (2004) Syncope in pediatric patients presenting to an emergency department. J Pediatr 145:223–228
7. Saul JP (1999) Syncope: etiology, management, and when to refer. J S C Med Assoc 95:385–387
8. Dambrink JH, Imholz BP, Karemaker JM et al (1991) Postural dizziness and transient hypotension in two healthy teenagers. Clin Auton Res 1:281–287
9. Low PA, Sandroni P, Singer W et al (2002) Postural tachycardia syndrome – an update. Clin Auton Res 12:107–109
10. Wieling W, Karemaker JM (1999) Non-invasive continuous recording of heart rate and blood pressure in the evaluation of neurovascular control. In: Mathias CJ, Bannister R (eds) Autonomic failure: a textbook of clinical disorders of the autonomic nervous system. Oxford University Press, Oxford
11. Axelrod F (2002) Genetic autonomic disorders. Clin Auton Res 12(suppl 1):1–47
12. van Dijk JG (2003) Conditions which mimic syncope. In: Benditt DG, Blanc JJ, Brignole M, Sutton R (eds) The evaluation and treatment of syncope: a handbook for clinical practice. Blackwell/Futura, New York
13. Steinberg LA, Knilans TK (2005) Syncope in children: diagnostic tests have a high cost and low yield. J Pediatr 146:355–358
14. Hoefnagels WA, Padberg GW, Overweg J et al (1991) Transient loss of consciousness: the value of the history for distinguishing seizure from syncope. J Neurol 238:39–43
15. Brignole M, Alboni P, Benditt DG et al (2004) Guidelines on management (diagnosis and treatment) of syncope – update 2004. Europace 6:467–537

Syncope in Patients with Autonomic Nervous System Disturbances: Which Diagnosis and Treatment?

C.J. Mathias

Introduction

Syncope is a condition in which there is transient loss of consciousness due to reduction in cerebral blood flow. The term syncope is often used synonymously with fainting, blackouts, passing out, and swooning. It is a common condition with both neurological (autonomic and non-autonomic) and cardiac causes. Psychologic and psychiatric conditions resulting in pseudosyncope are difficult to separate from true syncope [1].

There is increasing recognition that disturbances of the autonomic nervous system account for a large proportion of syncope cases. This was emphasised in a study of 641 patients with recurrent syncope and presyncope, in whom major neurological (non-autonomic) and cardiac causes had been previously excluded [2]. Following autonomic and allied investigations, half of the patients had an autonomic cause (Fig. 1). This highlighted the role that the autonomic nervous system plays–in part through the baroreceptor reflex, with efferents to the heart and sympathetic efferents to blood vessels in the heart – in the maintenance of blood pressure and thus in the causation of syncope.

This review provides a classification of disturbances of the autonomic nervous system that result in syncope. An outline of treatment options follows.

Neurovascular Medicine Unit, Faculty of Medicine; Imperial College London at St Mary's Hospital, Autonomic Unit, National Hospital for Neurology & Neurosurgery, Queen Square; Institute of Neurology, University College London, London, United Kingdom

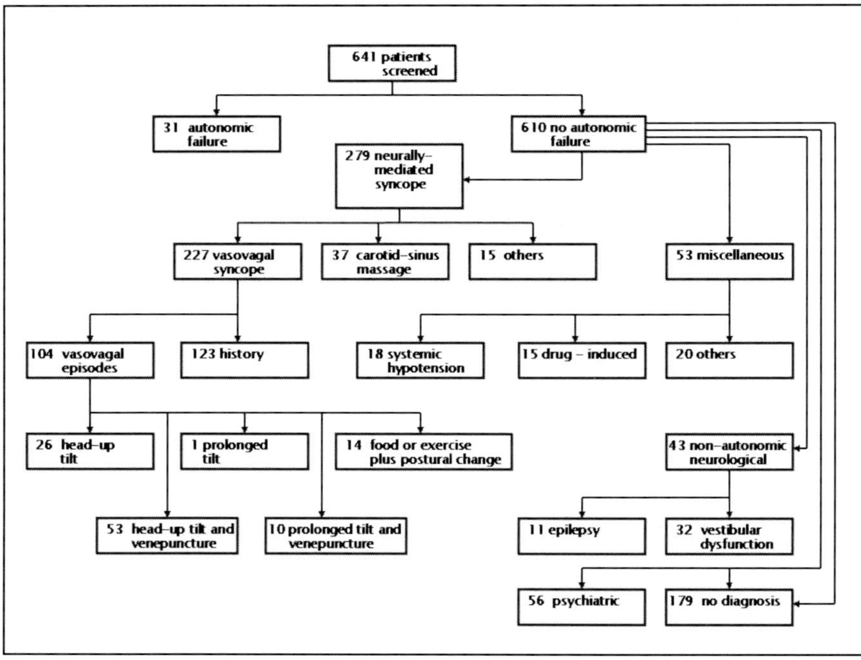

Fig. 1. Flow diagram showing investigations and diagnosis in 641 patients with recurrent syncope and presyncope. (Adapted from [2])

Diagnosis and Evaluation

Autonomic disturbances resulting in syncope may be intermittent (neurally mediated syncope and the postural tachycardia syndrome) (Table 1), due to drugs (Table 2), or the result of damage to the autonomic nervous system as a result of primary or secondary autonomic failure [3, 4] (Table 3). Diagnosis is dependent on a precise history, detailed clinical examination, and appropriate tests [5, 6] (Table 4).

Table 1. Intermittent disturbances of the autonomic nervous system that cause syncope

Neurally mediated syncope
Vasovagal syncope
Carotid sinus hypersensitivity
Miscellaneous causes (situational syncope)
Postural tachycardia syndrome (PoTS)

Table 2. Mechanisms by which drugs, chemicals, poisons, and toxins may cause syncope. (adapted from [3])

By decreasing sympathetic activity
Centrally acting
    Clonidine, reserpine, anaesthetics

Peripherally acting via
    Sympathetic nerve endings (guanethidine, bethanidine)
        α-Adrenoceptor blockade (phenoxybenzamine)
        β-Adrenoceptor blockade (propranolol)

By increasing cardiac parasympathetic activity
    Organophosphates
    Ciguatera (reef fish) poisoning

By vasodilatation
    Jellyfish and marine animal venoms

By a first-dose effect
    Prazosin, Captopril

By causing an autonomic neuropathy
    Alcohol, thiamine (vitamin B_1) deficiency
    Vincristine, perhexiline maleate

Table 3. Disorders of the autonomic nervous system that cause syncope (adapted from [4]).

Primary autonomic failure
Acute/subacute dysautonomias
    Pure pandysautonomia
    Pandysautonomia with neurological features

Chronic autonomic failure syndromes
    Pure autonomic failure
    Multiple system atrophy (Shy-Drager syndrome)
    Autonomic failure with Parkinson's disease

Secondary autonomic failure
Congenital
    Nerve growth factor deficiency

Hereditary
    Autosomal dominant trait
        Familial amyloid neuropathy

continue →

Table 3. *continue*

Autosomal recessive trait
Familial dysautonomia, Riley-Day syndrome
Dopamine beta-hydroxylase deficiency
Metabolic
Diabetes mellitus
Chronic renal failure
Chronic liver disease
Alcohol-induced
Inflammatory
Guillain-Barre syndrome
Transverse myelitis
Infections
Bacterial: Tetanus
Viral: Human immunodeficiency virus infection
Neoplasia
Brain tumours, especially of the third ventricle or posterior fossa
Paraneoplastic, including adenocarcinomas of lung and pancreas
Trauma
Cervical and high thoracic spinal-cord transection

Table 4. Outline of investigations used in the evaluation of syncope due to disturbances of the autonomic nervous system (adapted from [6])

Head-up tilt (60°)[a]; standing[a]; Valsalva manoeuvre[a]
Pressor stimuli[a] (isometric exercise, cold pressor, mental arithmetic)
Heart rate responses to: deep breathing[a], hyperventilation[a], standing[a], head-up tilt[a]
Liquid meal challenge
Modified exercise testing
Carotid sinus massage

[a]Indicates screening autonomic tests used in our London Units
Additional autonomic and allied tests, as described in [6], may need to be performed if relevant to diagnosis and management

Treatment of Syncope Caused by Autonomic Nervous System Disturbances

The key components of treatment revolve around non-pharmacological measures, drug treatment when appropriate, and the introduction of interventions such as cardiac pacemaker when relevant.

Neurally Mediated Syncope

This depends upon the cause, the most common being vasovagal syncope (Fig. 2). Reducing or preventing exposure to precipitating causes is of importance, along with educating the patient about the disorder. A combination of non-pharmacological approaches, especially if supine blood pressure is low, should include a high-salt diet; fluid repletion; exercise to strengthen lower limb muscles; measures that activate the sympathetic nervous system, such as sustained hand grip, the use of the calf muscle pump to prevent pooling; and various manoeuvres such as leg crossing [8–11]. Patients who have symptoms suggestive of an oncoming attack should sit and ideally lie head down, if needed with the legs upright. Pharmacological measures are used when non-pharmacological measures alone are not successful, especially if the supine blood pressure is low. These include low-dose fludrocortisone and

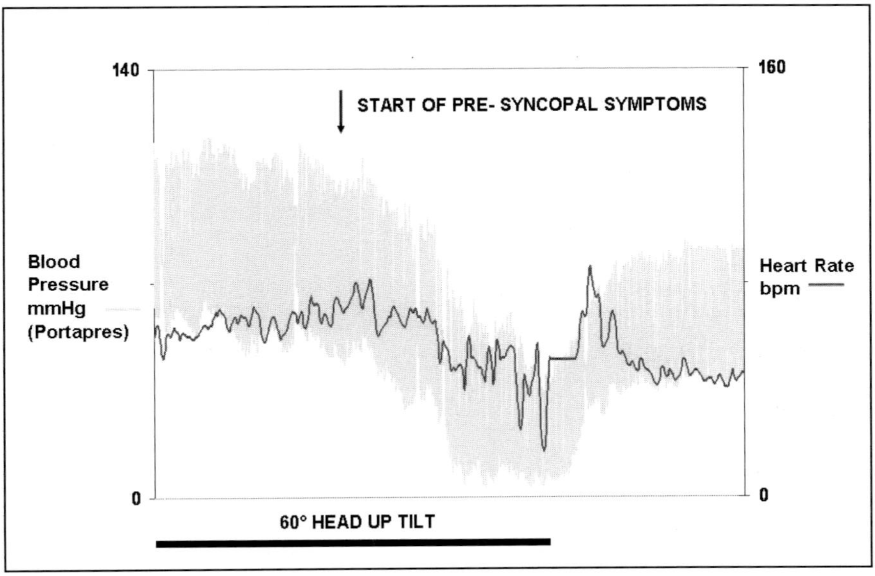

Fig. 2. Blood pressure and heart rate with continuous recordings from the Portapres II in a patient with the mixed (cardio-inhibitory and vasodepressor) form of vasovagal syncope. (Adapted from [7])

the sympathomimetics ephedrine and midodrine. 5-Hydroxytryptamine uptake release inhibitors have been used with varying success. In the cardio-inhibitory form of vasovagal syncope, a cardiac demand pacemaker is of value [12]. In some patients, especially those with phobias, cognitive behavioural psychotherapy is recommended.

In carotid sinus hypersensitivity, which is diagnosed more often in older patients, a cardiac pacemaker often is of benefit, both in the cardio-inhibitory and in the mixed forms (Fig. 3). In the vasodepressor form, non-pharmacological and drug treatment as outlined above for vasovagal syncope often is needed. In unilateral hypersensitivity, denervation of the carotid sinus nerves has been employed.

In the miscellaneous (situational) group of syncope cases, treatment is tailored to the provoking cause. Thus, in patients with high spinal cord lesions on an artificial respirator, vagal activity is not opposed by sympathetic activity and tracheal stimulation can cause bradycardia and syncope; adequate oxygenation, atropine and, in some patients, a temporary cardiac demand pacemaker is indicated [14, 15]. In micturition-induced syncope, avoidance of precipitating factors, such as alcohol, and advice to empty the urinary bladder while sitting rather than standing may be all that is required.

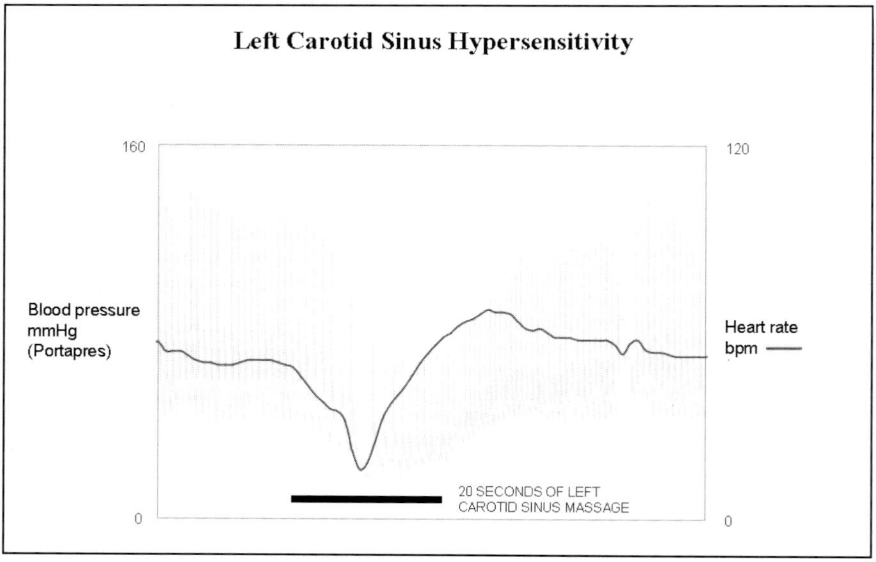

Fig. 3. Continuous blood pressure and heart rate measured non-invasively (by Portapres II) in a subject with falls of unknown cause. Left carotid sinus massage caused a fall in both heart rate and blood pressure. The findings indicate the mixed (cardioinhibitory and vasodepressor) form of carotid sinus hypersensitivity. (Adapted from [13])

Postural Tachycardia Syndrome

In this condition (Fig. 4), non-pharmacological measures are of particular importance and include avoiding hypovolaemia and contributory factors such as hyperventilation. Drugs such as fludrocortisone and midodrine are of value in some patients. Beta-adrenergic blockers, especially those that are cardioselective, reduce tachycardia. Specific approaches may be needed depending upon the cause and association; thus, in the joint hypermobility syndrome, the underlying collagen disorder (Ehlers-Danlos type III) needs to be addressed.

Drug-Induced Syncope

The pharmacological effect of drugs, their interactions with other agents, and modification of their actions in certain disease states, need to be borne in mind when syncope results from drugs. The ideal is withdrawal of drugs, but this may not always be possible, as in the treatment of parkinsonian syndromes (Table 5). Drugs such as alcohol and perhexiline maleate cause an autonomic neuropathy, and withdrawal alone may not result in recovery.

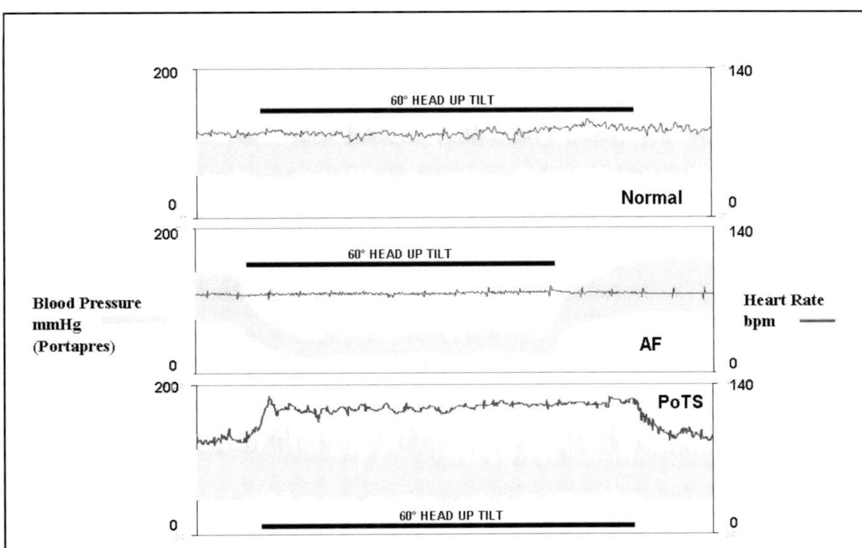

Fig. 4. Blood pressure and heart rate measured continuously before, during, and after 60° head-up tilt by Portapres II in a normal subject (*uppermost panel*) and in a subject with postural tachycardia syndrome (PoTS) (*lowermost panel*). (Adapted from [16]). The *middle panel* is from a subject with orthostatic hypotension due to autonomic failure

Table 5. The causative or contributory causes of syncope in a patient with parkinsonism (adapted from [5])

Side effects of anti-parkinsonian therapy:
L-DOPA, bromocriptine, pergolide
Combination of L-DOPA and COMT inhibitors (tolcapone)
MAO 'b' inhibitor, selegiline
Coincidental disease causing autonomic dysfunction
Diabetes mellitus
Coincidental administration of drugs for an associated condition
Antihypertensives
α-Adrenoceptor blockers (for benign prostatic hypertrophy)
Vasodilators (for ischaemic heart disease)
Diuretics (for cardiac failure)
Sildenafil (for erectile failure)
Autonomic failure
Multiple system atrophy (Shy-Drager syndrome)
Parkinson's disease with autonomic failure
Diffuse Lewy body disease

Primary and Secondary Autonomic Failure

These conditions usually require a combination of approaches. The original disorder needs to be addressed, and orthostatic hypotension (Fig. 4 middle panel), which is the usual cause of syncope, must be treated. A combination of approaches often is needed (Table 6). Drugs used for the treatment of orthostatic hypotension act in different ways and frequently can be combined in lower dosages to provide benefit while reducing side effects (Table 7).

Table 6. Non-pharmacological and major pharmacological measures used in the management of neurogenic orthostatic hypotension (adapted from [17])

Non-pharmacological measures
To be avoided
Sudden head-up postural change (especially on waking)
Prolonged recumbency
Straining during micturition and defaecation
High environmental temperature (including hot baths)
'Severe' exertion
Large meals (especially with refined carbohydrate)
Alcohol
Drugs with vasodepressor properties

continue →

Table 6. *continue*

To be introduced
Head-up tilt during sleep
Small frequent meals
High salt intake
Judicious exercise (including swimming)
Body positions and manoeuvres
To be considered
Elastic stockings
Abdominal binders
Water ingestion
Pharmacological measures
Starter drug: Fludrocortisone
Sympathomimetics: Ephedrine, midodrine
Specific targeting: Octreotide, desmopressin, erythropoietin

Table 7. Outline of the major actions by which a variety of drugs may reduce orthostatic hypotension (adapted from [17])

Reducing salt loss/plasma volume expansion
Mineralocorticoids (fludrocortisone)
Reducing nocturnal polyuria
V_2-receptor agonists (desmopressin)
Vasoconstriction: sympathetic
On resistance vessels (ephedrine, midodrine, phenylephrine, noradrenaline, clonidine, tyramine with monoamine oxidase inhibitors, yohimbine, L-dihydroxyphenylserine)
On capacitance vessels (dihydroergotamine)
Vasoconstriction: non-sympathomimetic
V_1 receptor agents – terlipressin
Ganglionic nicotinic-receptor stimulation
Anticholinesterase inhibitors: pyridostigmine
Preventing vasodilatation
Prostaglandin synthetase inhibitors (indomethacin, flurbiprofen)
Dopamine receptor blockade (metaclopramide, domperidone)
$Beta_2$-adrenoceptor blockade (propranolol)

continue →

Table 7. *continue*

Preventing postprandial hypotension
Adrenosine receptor blockade (caffeine)
Peptide release inhibitors (somatostatin analogue: octreotide)
Increasing cardiac output
Beta-blockers with intrinsic sympathomimetic activity (pindolol, xamoterol)
Dopamine agonists (ibopamine)
Increasing red cell mass
Erythropoietin

References

1. Mathias CJ, Deguchi K, Bleasdale-Barr K, Smith S (2000) Familial vasovagal syncope and pseudosyncope: observations in a case with both natural and adopted siblings. Clin Auton Res 10:43–45
2. Mathias CJ, Deguchi K, Schatz I (2001) Observations on recurrent syncope and presyncope in 641 patients. Lancet 357:348–353
3. Mathias CJ (2004) Role of autonomic evaluation in the diagnosis and management of syncope. Clin Auton Res14(Suppl 1):45–54
4. Mathias CJ (2004) Disorders of the autonomic nervous system. In: Bradley WG, Daroff RB, Fenichel GM, Jancovich J (eds) Neurology in clinical practice, 3rd edn. Butterworth-Heinemann, Boston, pp 2403–2240
5. Mathias CJ (2003)Autonomic diseases: clinical features and laboratory evaluation. J Neurol Neurosurg Psychiatry 74:iii31-iii41
6. Mathias CJ, Bannister R (2002) Investigation of autonomic disorders.In: Mathias CJ, Bannister R (eds) Autonomic failure: a textbook of clinical disorders of the autonomic nervous system, 4th edn. Oxford University Press, Oxford, pp169–195
7. Mathias CJ (2005) Orthostatic hypotension and orthostatic intolerance. In: Jameson JL, DeGroot LJ (eds) Endocrinology, 5th edn. Elsevier, Philadelphia (in press)
8. van Dijk N, Harms MP, Linzer M, Wieling W (2000) Treatment of vasovagal syncope: pacemaker or crossing legs? Clin Autonom Res 10:347–349
9. Cooper VL, Hainsworth R (2002) Effects of dietary salt on orthostatic tolerance, blood pressure and baroreceptor sensitivity in patients with syncope. Clin Auton Res 12:234–241
10. Brignole M, Croci F, Menozzi C et al (2004) Isometric arm contraction at the onset of prodromal symptoms: a new first-line treatment for vasovagal syncope.In: A Raviele (ed) Cardiac arrhythmias 2004. Springer, Milan, pp 641–650
11. Mathias CJ, Young TM (2004) Water drinking in the management of orthostatic intolerance due to orthostatic hypotension, vasovagal syncope and the postural tachycardia syndrome. Eur J Neurol 11:613–619
12. Benditt DG (1999) Cardiac pacing for prevention of vasovagal syncope. J Am Coll Cardiol 33:21–23

13. Mathias CJ (2005) Autonomic dysfunction and hypotension. In: Willerson JT, Cohn JN, WellensHJJ, Holmes DR Jr (eds) Cardiovascular medicine, 3rd edn. Elsevier, Philadelphia (in press)
14. Frankel HL, Mathias CJ, Spalding JM (1975) Mechanisms of reflex cardiac arrest in tetraplegic patients. Lancet 13:1183–1185
15. Mathias CJ (1976) Bradycardia and cardiac arrest during tracheal suction - mechanisms in tetraplegic patients. Eur J Intensive Care Med 2:147–156
16. Mathias CJ (2002) To stand on ones' own legs. Clin Med 2:237–245
17. Mathias CJ (2003) Autonomic diseases – management. J Neurol Neurosurg Psychiatry 74:42–47

Organisation of Syncope Management Units: The North American Experience

D.G. Benditt, F. Lu, K.G. Lurie, S. Sakaguchi

Introduction

European Society of Cardiology (ESC) guidelines provide a structured approach to the diagnosis and treatment of patients with syncope [1]. Among its recommendations, the ESC Syncope Task Force favoured wider use of specialised multifaceted medical units to improve the management of syncope patients. In essence, whether a physical space or a 'virtual' unit, the syncope management unit (SMU) would bring to bear appropriate multidisciplinary skills and experience more efficiently than has typically been the case [1-3].

In North America, the SMU concept has yet to be widely accepted. In part, this may be due to absence of professional organisation advocacy. The American College of Emergency Physicians has offered a 'clinical policy' covering the appropriate emergency department management of patients presenting with apparent syncope [4]. However, beyond this policy statement, there are as yet no comprehensive North American guidelines regarding the optimal evaluation and treatment of patients with transient loss of consciousness who are thought to have suffered a syncope event.

SMU Status in the US

In order to ascertain the current status of SMUs in North America, we surveyed United States and Canadian medical centres in terms of their approaches to syncope evaluation. With regard to survey target sites, since

Cardiac Arrhythmia Center, Cardiovascular Division, Department of Medicine, University of Minnesota Medical School, Minneapolis, Minnesota, USA

syncope evaluation has increasingly become the responsibility of cardiologists/electrophysiologists, we focused the survey on medical centres in which that specialty was strongly represented.

In terms of the survey itself, we were specifically interested in determining:

- Factors that impact the decision to form or not to form an SMU
- What physicians currently think about the potential utility of an SMU
- The preferred nature of the SMU, were it to be formed

In a preliminary review of study findings, only 2 of 22 reporting centres (9%) had organised an SMU. Of the two centres with an SMU, the unit was described as a 'physical space' in one case and as a 'virtual unit' (i.e., not a defined physical entity) in the other. In both cases the units were lead by a cardiologist/electrophysiologist. In one unit, only cardiology/electrophysiology participated, whereas in the second unit a variety of other specialties were also involved, including internal medicine, neurology, paediatric cardiology, and geriatrics.

Among the 20 reporting medical centres without an SMU, only 5/20 (25%) indicated that plans were being made to establish such a unit. However, 65% of respondents indicated that they would favour establishing an SMU. An approximately equal number indicated confidence that an SMU would reduce the cost of establishing an appropriate diagnosis in syncope patients. Further, in terms of the organisational make-up of the SMU, most respondents favoured a multidisciplinary unit comprising at a minimum the following medical specialties: cardiology/electrophysiology, internal medicine, and neurology. Approximately one-half of the respondents included psychiatric expertise as a necessary SMU element.

The vast majority of respondents (> 90%) indicated that they preferred cardiology/electrophysiology to be the SMU 'director' or chief organiser. However, given that the survey target sites were selected primarily from the Heart Rhythm Society (formerly North American Society of Pacing and Electrophysiology, NASPE) directory, it was inevitably heavily biased toward this specialty, and this may account for the overwhelming preference for cardiology/electrophysiology.

The survey also attempted to address the key reasons underlying the absence of an SMU at those responding institutions not having such units currently. The most common impediments were lack of leadership (55% of respondents) and an insufficient number of interested individuals (50% of respondents). However, while most respondents thought that an SMU would improve syncope management efficiency, 35% of respondents evinced ambivalence toward SMU development on the grounds that there is currently inadequate evidence of the utility of SMUs for improving diagnostic yields and reducing cost. Multi-centre studies comparing diagnostic and treatment outcomes, along with financial data, would be very helpful for promoting adoption of the SMU concept, if SMU performance proved favourable.

Economic Issues Impacting SMU Development

Improved understanding of resource requirements for evaluation and treatment of patients with cardiovascular disease is of increasing importance in the North America [5–7]. Measurements of medical care costs rely primarily on tracking International Classification of Diseases (ICD-9) codes [6, 7]. In this regard, the direct and indirect costs for treatment of arteriosclerotic diseases in the USA in 1993, estimated from Health Care Financing Administration (HCFA) national health expenditures and survey data from the National Centre for Health Statistics, were in excess of US$200 billion [7]. Clearly, even modest cost reductions in this sector would pay a substantial dividend. In contrast, the management of syncope is estimated to be approximately $1 billion annually [8]. While the syncope numbers are probably imprecise due to sampling issues and incorrect diagnoses, they nonetheless represent a relatively small proportion of the total cost of cardiovascular care. Consequently, it is not surprising that relatively little attention has been paid to issues surrounding optimisation of the management of patients who present with syncope and other forms of transient loss of consciousness.

Impact of SMU on Costs

Many factors contribute to the cost of syncope evaluation. These include the frequency with which syncope is the principal presenting medical problem to hospital emergency departments and clinics, which is probably similar in the USA to the 1% of annual emergency department visits reported from Western Europe [1, 9]. However, of perhaps greater importance is the manner in which diagnostic and treatment challenges are managed after presentation at the emergency department or clinic. A recent report detailing an Italian hospital experience quantified the extent to which low-yield, cost-ineffective tests were requested by physicians investigating presumed syncope [10]. High-yield tests were frequently overlooked. In contrast, Kenny et al. have amply demonstrated the potential cost savings associated with a well-organised SMU. Specifically, they demonstrated savings in excess of US $ 4 million in one year alone at a single hospital in Newcastle, UK, due to more efficient management of syncope and 'fall' patients [2]. The economic benefit arose in large measure from reduced readmission rates and a marked reduction of hospital in-patient days. Similar benefits may be achievable in North America, although only rarely has such an experience been published

[11]. The respondents to our survey, whether or not familiar with the Newcastle experience, appear to agree with the notion that an SMU structure offers an opportunity to reduce cost per reliable diagnosis.

Conclusions

In summary, the SMU is uncommon in North America. Furthermore, relatively few arrhythmia specialty centres are contemplating establishment of such a facility, although most survey respondents believe that an SMU would be helpful. The survey findings suggest that establishment of such a unit is impeded by lack of leadership, resource limitations within medical centres, and absence of convincing published data regarding SMU effectiveness. Thus, at least in the near term, the SMU will remain the exception rather than the rule in North American medical practice.

Acknowledgements
The authors wish to express their appreciation to the many clinicians who responded to the survey, and to Barry L.S. Detloff and Wendy Markuson, who collated survey data and assisted in preparation of the manuscript.

References

1. Brignole M, Alboni P, Benditt D et al (2004) Guidelines on management (diagnosis and treatment) of syncope. Europace 6:467–537
2. Kenny RA, O'Shea D, Walker HF (2002) Impact of a dedicated syncope and falls facility for older adults on emergency beds. Age Aging 31:272–275
3. Dey AB, Bexton RS, Tyman MM et al (1997) Impact of a dedicated 'syncope and falls' clinic on pacemaker practice in northeastern England. Pacing Clin Electrophysiol 20:815–817
4. American College of Emergency Physicians (2001) Clinical policy: critical issues in the evaluation and management of patients presenting with syncope. Ann Emerg Med 37:771–776
5. Eddy DM (1998) Performance measurement. Problems and solutions. Health Affairs 17:7–25
6. Chen J, Radford MJ, Wang Y et al (1999) Performance of the '100 Top Hospitals': what does the report card report? Health Affairs 18:53–68
7. Sun BC, Emond JA, Camargo CA (2005) Direct medical costs of syncope-related hospitalizations in the United States. Am J Cardiol 95: 668–671
8. Maisel WH (2004) Specialized syncope evaluation. Circulation 119:3621–3623
9. Blanc J-J, L'Her C, Touiza A et al (2002) Prospective evaluation and outcome of patients admitted for syncope over a 1 year period. Eur Heart J 23:815–820
10. Bartoletti A, Brignole M, Proclemer A (2004) How is syncope studied in the Italian hospitals? Ital Heart J Suppl 5:472–479
11. Shen WK, Decker WW, Smars PA et al (2004) Syncope evaluation in the emergency department study (SEEDS): a multidisciplinary approach to syncope management. Circulation 119: 3636–3645

The Syncope Unit: How To Better Organise It? The European Experience

M. Brignole

Current Syncope Management (Diagnosis and Treatment)

Syncope is a common symptom in the community and in emergency medicine. For example, in the UK, syncope and collapse (ICD code 10) are the sixth most common reason for the immediate admission of adults > 65 years to medical hospitals. Given that half of all emergency admissions involve persons over age 65, this constitutes a large volume of activity. The average length of stay for these admissions is 5–17 days, which reflects the diversity of syncope management strategies and the availability of certain tests. Hospital admission alone accounted for 74% of the cost of investigating syncope [1].

Currently, the strategies for assessing syncope vary widely among physicians as well as among hospitals and clinics. More often than not, the evaluation and treatment of syncope are haphazard and unstratified. The result is a wide variation in the diagnostic tests applied, the proportion and types of attributable diagnoses, and the proportion of syncope patients in whom the cause remains unexplained [1–5]. For example, in a prospective registry [3] enrolling patients referred to the emergency department from 28 general hospitals in Italy, carotid sinus massage was performed in 0–58% and head-up tilt tests in 0–50% of syncopal patients. Consequently the final diagnosis for neurally mediated syncope ranged from 10% to 79%. These disparate patterns of assessment can explain why pacing rates for carotid sinus syndrome vary, even within countries, from 1% to 25% of implants, depending on whether carotid sinus hypersensitivity is systematically assessed in the

Centro Aritmologico, Dipartimento di Cardiologia, Ospedali del Tigullio, Lavagna (Genua), Italy

investigation profile. Some authors have evaluated the impact of the introduction of in-hospital protocols [2, 5]. These studies showed that it is possible to improve diagnostic rates and the use of appropriate investigations. However, many inappropriate investigations and hospital admissions still occur. As a consequence, costs of investigations and costs per diagnosis have increased rather than decreased.

If the status quo for the evaluation of syncope remains unchanged, diagnostic and treatment effectiveness is unlikely to improve substantially. Furthermore, the implementation of the published syncope management guidelines will be diverse and incomplete. Thus, to maximise implementation of the guidelines it is crucial that models of care for the assessment and management of syncope are implemented and that information about the models within each organisation is adequately communicated to all parties involved with syncope patients.

It is the view of the Task Force on Syncope of the European Society of Cardiology [6, 7] that a cohesive, structured care pathway delivered either within a single syncope facility or as part of a multifaceted service is the optimal approach to quality service delivery (Table 1). Furthermore, considerable improvements in diagnostic yield and cost effectiveness (i.e., cost per reliable diagnosis) can be achieved by focusing skills and by following well-defined up-to-date diagnostic guidelines.

Table 1. Recommendations of the European Society of Cardiology for the management of the patients with syncope

A cohesive, structured care pathway–delivered either within a single syncope facility or as part of a more multifaceted service–is recommended for the global assessment of patients with syncope
Experience and training in key components of cardiology, neurology, and emergency and geriatric medicine are pertinent
Core equipment for the facility include: surface ECG recording, phasic blood-pressure monitoring, tilt-table testing equipment, external and internal (implantable) ECG loop recorder systems, 24-h ambulatory blood pressure monitoring, 24-h ambulatory ECG, and autonomic function testing
Preferential access to other tests or therapy for syncope should be guaranteed and standardised
The majority of syncope patients should be examined as out-patients or as day patients

Models Provided by Existing Syncope Management Units

The service model adopted by the Newcastle group is a multidisciplinary approach to referrals of patients with syncope or falls. All patients attend the same facility (with access to cardiovascular equipment, investigations, and trained staff) but are investigated by a geriatrician or cardiovascular physician according to the dominant symptom cited in the referral correspondence, i.e. falls or syncope. Recently, this group showed that, over a period of 1 year, the hospital at which the day-case syncope evaluation unit was based had 6116 fewer bed–days for ICD code 10 categories, comprising syncope and collapse, compared to peer teaching hospitals in the UK. This reduction translated into a significant saving in emergency hospital costs (4 million Euros). The savings were attributed to a combination of factors: reduced readmission rates, rapid access to day-case facilities for accident and emergency staff and community physicians, and reduced event rates because of effective targeted strategies for treating patients with syncope and falls [1].

The service model adopted in some Italian hospitals [8] consists of a functional unit managed by cardiologists within the Department of Cardiology, with dedicated medical and support personnel. Patients admitted to the Syncope Unit have preferential access to all other facilities and investigations within the department, including admission to cardiology wards or the intensive care unit if indicated. When appropriate, patients are jointly managed with other specialists, e.g. neurologists. The patients are referred to the Syncope Unit (SU) from the emergency department or from in-patient or out-patient clinics, but SU personnel are not usually involved in the initial evaluation of the patient. This approach substantially improved the overall management of syncope compared to peer hospitals without such a facility [8] and reduced the number of unnecessary investigations. Moreover, the appropriateness of indications and the diagnostic yield of tests increased; for example, in 66% of the patients, less than two tests were necessary for diagnosis [9].

Professional Skills Needed for the Syncope Evaluation Facility

It is probably not appropriate to be dogmatic regarding the training needs of personnel responsible for a dedicated syncope facility. These skills will depend on the pre-determined requirements of local professional bodies, the level of screening evaluation provided prior to referral, and the nature of the patient population typically encountered in a given setting. In general, experience and training in key components of cardiology, neurology, and emergency and geriatric medicine are pertinent to the assessment and diagnosis of syncope, in addition to access to other specialties, such as psychiatry, physiotherapy, occupational therapy, Ear Nose and Throat specialties, and clinical psychology.

Core medical and support personnel should be involved either full time or most of the time in management of the syncope unit, and should interact with all other stakeholders in the hospital and in the community.

Staff responsible for the clinical management of the facility should be conversant with recent guidelines on syncope management. A structured approach expedites clinical audit, patient information systems, service developments, and continuous professional training.

Equipment

Core equipment for the syncope evaluation facility includes: surface ECG recording, phased blood-pressure monitoring, tilt-table testing equipment, external and internal (implantable) ECG loop recorder systems, 24-h ambulatory blood-pressure monitoring, 24-h ambulatory ECG monitoring, and autonomic function testing. The facility should also have access to echocardiography, intracardiac electrophysiological testing, stress testing, cardiac imaging, computed tomography and magnetic resonance imaging head scans, and electroencephalography.

Patients should have preferential access to hospitalisation and to any eventual therapy for syncope, namely pacemaker and defibrillator implantation, catheter ablation of arrhythmias, etc.

Dedicated rooms for assessment and investigation are also required.

Setting

The majority of syncope patients can be investigated as out-patients or day patients. Indications for hospital admission are defined in the guidelines [6, 7].

The role of a local integrated syncope service is to set standards for the following in keeping with the objectives of the Guidelines on Syncope of the European Society of Cardiology and other appropriate guideline publications:

1. The diagnostic criteria for causes of syncope
2. The preferred approach to the diagnostic work-up in subgroups of patients with syncope
3. Risk stratification of the patient with syncope
4. Treatment to prevent the recurrence of syncope

A major objective of the syncope facility is to reduce the number of hospitalisations by offering the patient a well-defined, quick, alternative evaluation pathway.

When establishing a newly structured service, current experience suggests that careful audit of the activity of the syncope unit activity and its performance will rapidly justify the initial resource allocation and requests for additional funding, fuel further service development, and provide a legitimate magnet for increasing patient referrals.

Implementation in Clinical Practice of a Model of Structured Care Based on the Guidelines of the European Society of Cardiology

Recently, a prospective systematic evaluation of the strict adherence to the care guidelines of the European Society of Cardiology was undertaken in Italy [10]. The study consisted of consecutive patients referred for syncope to the emergency departments of 11 general hospitals. Trained core medical personnel both locally in each hospital and centrally who verified adherence to the diagnostic pathway and gave advices as needed for its correction was designated. In addition, decision-making guideline-based software was used to quantify the data. A diagnostic work-up consistent with the guidelines was completed in 465/541 patients (86%). A definite diagnosis was established in 98% (unexplained in 2%): neurally mediated syncope 66%, orthostatic hypotension 10%, primary arrhythmias 11%, structural cardiac or cardiopulmonary disease 5%, and non-syncopal attacks 6%. The initial evaluation (consisting of a history, physical examination, and standard electrocardiogram) established the diagnosis in 50% of patients. Hospitalisation for the management of syncope was appropriate in 25% and was required for other reasons in a further 13% of patients. The median in-hospital stay was 5.5 days (interquartile range 3–9). Apart from the initial evaluation, a mean 1.9 ± 1.1 appropriate tests per patient were performed in 193 patients. The mean cost per patient was € 1216 (€ 2802 for those hospitalised and € 202 for those discharged from the emergency department. In conclusion, this study showed that a structured-care approach, developed according to current guidelines of the European Society of Cardiology, can be implemented in clinical practice.

References

1. Kenny RA, O'Shea D, Walker HF (2002) Impact of a dedicated syncope and falls facility for older adults on emergency beds. Age Aging 31:272–275

2. Ammirati F, Colivicchi F, Santini M (2000) Diagnosing syncope in the clinical practice. Implementation of a simplified diagnostic algorithm in a multicentre prospective trial - the OESIL 2 study (Osservatorio Epidemiologico della Sincope nel Lazio). Eur Heart J 21:935–940
3. Disertori M, Brignole M, Menozzi C et al (2003) Management of syncope referred for emergency to general hospitals. Europace 5:283–291
4. Ammirati F, Colivicchi F, Minardi G et al (1999) Hospital management of syncope: the OESIL study G Ital Cardiol 29:533–539
5. Farwell DJ, Sulke AN (2004) Does the use of a syncope diagnostic protocol improve the investigation and management of syncope? Heart 90:52–58
6. Brignole M, Alboni P, Benditt D et al (2004) Guidelines on management (diagnosis and treatment) of syncope. Eur Heart J 25:2054–2072
7. Brignole M, Alboni P, Benditt D et al (2004) Guidelines on management (diagnosis and treatment) of syncope – Update 2004. Europace 6:467
8. Brignole M, Disertori M, Menozzi C et al (2003) The management of syncope referred for emergency to general hospitals with and without Syncope Unit facility. Europace 5:293–298
9. Croci F, Brignole M, Alboni P et al (2002) The application of a standardized strategy of evaluation in patients with syncope referred to three Syncope Units. Europace 4:351–356
10. Brignole M, Menozzi C, Bartoletti A et al (2005) The best management of syncope. Prospective systematic guideline-based evaluation of patients referred urgently to general hospitals (in press)

Water Ingestion As Prophylaxis Against Syncope: Fact or Fancy?

J. Jordan

Introduction

If you faint, it is likely that someone will offer you a glass of water – certainly, your grandmother would. Is there a scientific rational for this home remedy or is your grandmother completely off the mark? The physiological responses to acute water ingestion has been assessed in a few studies, which suggested that water drinking elicits acute changes in human physiology. These changes affect different regulatory systems, including metabolism and cardiovascular regulation, and appear to be mediated through sympathetic activation. The cardiovascular response may be exploited to attenuate symptoms in patients with orthostatic hypotension, the postural tachycardia syndrome (POTS), or neurocardiogenic (vasovagal) syncope.

Pressor Response to Water Drinking

Patients with severe orthostatic hypotension due to autonomic failure reported that they experienced fewer symptoms after they drank a glass of water. Based on these anecdotes, we decided to probe the effect of water on blood pressure in a systematic fashion. Patients with autonomic failure due to either multiple system atrophy or pure autonomic failure (Bradbury-Eggleston syndrome) were included. Drinking 480 ml tap water within 5 min elicited a profound pressor effect in these patients [1, 2]. Seated systolic blood pressure increased 33 mmHg in multiple system atrophy patients and 37 mmHg in pure autonomic failure patients [2]. The pressor effect had a

Franz-Volhard Clinical Research Center, Medical Faculty of the Charité, Max-Delbrueck-Centrum, and Helios Klinikum, Berlin, Germany

rapid onset, within 5 min after water drinking, and reached a maximum after 30–40 min. The response was sustained for more than an hour. Our findings in autonomic failure patients were reproduced by another group of investigators [3, 4]. Tetraplegic patients and cardiac transplant recipients showed a moderate pressor response to water drinking [5, 6]. Older control subjects who ingested 480 ml water exhibited a moderate increase in systolic blood pressure, which reached a maximum of 11 mmHg above baseline [1, 2]. In contrast, water drinking had no pressor effect in healthy young subjects [2, 7].

Vasoconstriction or Volume Expansion?

One study involving autonomic failure patients suggested that the pressor response to water drinking is mediated through increased systemic vascular resistance [3]. In another study, in healthy young subjects, blood pressure and systemic vascular resistance did not change after water drinking. Yet, calf vascular resistance increased significantly [7]. The paradoxical finding may be explained by compensatory dilatation in another vascular bed. Taken together, the data suggest that water drinking elicits an increase in vascular tone that contributes to the increase in blood pressure in autonomic failure patients.

Theoretical considerations and actual physiological measurements exclude volume expansion as the crucial mechanism explaining the haemodynamic response to water drinking. Solute-free water is distributed throughout extra- and intracellular spaces. If one assumes that a water load (500 ml) is absorbed but not excreted, total body water would change by 1% in a person weighing 175 lbs. Plasma volume would increase by approximately 35 ml. A substantial part of the ingested water is likely to be excreted at the time the maximal physiological response to water is observed. Indeed, plasma volume remained unchanged after water drinking [2]. In another study, water drinking had no effect on thoracic impedance [8], which correlates with thoracic blood volume [9]. Finally, it is difficult to explain increased vascular resistance through volume expansion.

Involvement of Sympathetic Mechanisms in Water-Induced Vasoconstriction?

Intuitively, one would think that the pressor response to water drinking in autonomic failure patients is not mediated by the sympathetic nervous system. Indeed, autonomic failure is tantamount to parasympathetic and sympathetic dysfunction. Initially, several vasoactive systems were implicated in the pressor response. However, neither plasma renin activity nor plasma vasopressin concentrations increased after water drinking [2]. More recent studies suggested that sympathetic efferent function is not completely lost in the majority of autonomic failure patients [10]. The incomplete loss in sympathetic efferents explains the observation that yohimbine elicits a sympathetically mediated pressor response in a large group of such patients [11–13]. Yohimbine increases sympathetic activity through blockade of alpha-2 adrenoreceptors in the central nervous system and at presynaptic sites of adrenergic neurons [13]. Paradoxically, the pressor response to yohimbine in autonomic failure patients is much greater than the response in healthy subjects. Thus, the water-induced pressor response could also be related to sympathetic activation.

We tested the effect of yohimbine and with water on separate days in autonomic failure patients. In patients with a large response to water, yohimbine profoundly raised blood pressure, whereas patients who did not respond to water exhibited a small pressor response to yohimbine or did not respond at all [2]. The observation suggests that patients who are unable to increase sympathetic activity with yohimbine do not exhibit a pressor response to water. The idea that the water pressor response is related to sympathetic activation is supported by experiments with ganglionic blockers. Interruption of ganglionic transmission with trimethaphan abolished the water-induced pressor response in two autonomic failure patients [2]. Furthermore, alpha-adrenoreceptor blockade with phentolamine attenuated the pressor effect of water drinking in animals [14]. Finally, water drinking has been shown to increase muscle sympathetic nerve traffic [7] and venous plasma norepinephrine concentrations in healthy subjects [2, 7, 15]. Thus, water drinking increases sympathetic activity.

Why is the pressor effect of water drinking enhanced in autonomic failure patients? One possible explanation is that autonomic failure patients were hypersensitive to the released norepinephrine. The hypersensitivity may be related to loss of baroreflex blood pressure buffering [16] and/or increased vascular sensitivity [17].

The sympathetic nervous system is not only involved in cardiovascular regulation, it also regulates metabolism. Thus, water-drinking-induced increases in sympathetic activity should also influence metabolism, in particular energy expenditure. We assessed the effect of drinking 500 ml water on energy expenditure and on carbohydrate and lipid oxidation rates in healthy young subjects using whole-room indirect calorimetry [18]. Water drinking caused a 30% increase in metabolic rate. In men, lipids mainly fuelled the increase in metabolic rate, while in women carbohydrates were mainly used as energy source. The total thermogenic response was about 100 kJ.

The time course of the metabolic response resembled that of the haemodynamic response. Systemic beta-adrenoreceptor blockade with metoprolol almost completely attenuated the increase in energy expenditure after water drinking [18]. Taken together, these findings suggest that water drinking increases sympathetic activity, which, in turn, drives the pressor and the thermogenic responses.

Sympathetic Activation Through a Spinal Mechanism?

Activation of the sympathetic nervous system may involve a brainstem- or spinal-reflex-like mechanism. It is less likely that water directly modulates the activity of postganglionic sympathetic neurons. In multiple system atrophy patients, the lesion to the autonomic nervous system is located in the brainstem [19]. More distal efferent sympathetic structures are, at least in part, intact [10, 20, 21]. In patients with high spinal cord injury, spinal sympathetic structures are intact but mechanically disconnected from brainstem input. In these patients, postganglionic sympathetic neurons can be activated through spinal reflexes. For example, bladder distention or muscle spasms below the spinal lesion may profoundly raise blood pressure. Water drinking increases blood pressure in multiple system atrophy patients [2] and in patients with high spinal cord injury [6]. These observations suggest that the activation of sympathetic efferents may not be explained by a brainstem mechanism. Instead, we speculate that sympathetic efferents are activated through a spinal mechanism.

What Stimulates the Sympathetic System?

The exact stimulus that triggers water-drinking-induced sympathetic activation is not known. Initially, we thought that water might elicit an 'internal cold pressor response.' However, the response to water drinking in autonomic failure patients was similar when patients ingested water at different temperatures [2]. Moreover, studies on the thermogenic effect of water drinking suggested that only 40% of the response could be explained by the energy that is required to warm the water to 37°C [18]. Drinking 37°C water also increased the metabolic rate. Clearly, water temperature is probably not the crucial stimulus of water-drinking-induced sympathetic activation.

Gastric distention increases sympathetic activity in humans [22]. The maximal response to water drinking is observed at a time when only 25% of the ingested water remain in the stomach [23]. In some autonomic failure patients, volumes of water as small as 120 ml elicit a substantial and sustained pressor response. Gastric stretch does not fully explains the sympathetic activation after water drinking. When fluids with different osmolarities were infused into the stomachs of dogs, distilled water was shown to cause a two-fold greater increase in blood pressure than normal saline [24]. In humans, infusion of hypo-osmolar solutions through a gastric tube causes a greater increase of sweat production, a sympathetic response, than infusion of isosmolar solutions [24]. Recently, we conducted similar studies in multiple system atrophy patients. In these patients, 500 ml water or isotonic saline were administered through a nasogastric tube. Water elicited a greater pressor response than saline [25].

Studies in animals have demonstrated the presence of osmoreceptive afferent nerve fibres [26]. Currently, we are exploring the possibility that water-drinking-induced sympathetic activation is related to stimulation of osmosensitive afferent nerves in the portal tract or in the liver.

Therapeutic Utility of Water Drinking in Autonomic Failure Patients

Water drinking was shown to improve standing blood pressure and orthostatic tolerance in a large subgroup of autonomic failure patients [27]. In that study, systolic blood pressure was 83 mmHg after 1 min of standing without water drinking. Upright systolic blood pressure increased to 114 mmHg 35 min after drinking 480 ml water. Water taken just before a meal prevents postprandial hypotension. In six patients, the maximal tolerated standing time increased from 5.1 min before to 11 min after water drinking. Water drinking also improved postprandial hypotension in autonomic failure patients [27]. After a meal, blood pressure decreased by 43/20 mmHg without water drinking, compared with 22/12 mmHg with drinking.

Water Drinking Attenuates Orthostatic Tachycardia

Water drinking may have therapeutic utility in postural tachycardia syndrome. Among other names, the syndrome is also referred to as POTS, idiopathic orthostatic intolerance, and chronic orthostatic intolerance. The syndrome is much more prevalent than autonomic failure, and, true to its name, it is characterised by orthostatic tachycardia rather than orthostatic hypotension [28–30]. Water drinking decreases upright heart rate in these patients by 15 beats per minute after 3 min of standing and by 10 beats per minute after 5 min of standing [27]. The effect of water drinking on orthostatic tachycardia compares favorably with established therapies, such as alpha-adrenoreceptor agonists or volume loading [29–31].

Prevention of Neurocardiogenic (Vasovagal) Syncope

So far, water drinking has not been tested in patients with spontaneous neurocardiogenic syncope. However, water drinking has been shown to delay or prevent neurocardiogenic presyncope or syncope in healthy subjects undergoing head-up tilt testing [8, 32]. In one study, subjects who tolerated standing on the head-up tilt table were subjected to incremental lower-body negative pressure while remaining in the upright position, the so-called Leeds protocol [8]. The time to presyncope or syncope was taken as a measure of orthostatic tolerance. Testing was conducted after subjects had ingested either 50 or 500 ml water. Drinking 500 ml water increased orthostatic tolerance by 5 min, which is a substantial improvement considering the supraphysiological orthostatic stress. In this study, water drinking also lowered upright heart rate, increased cardiac stroke volume, and improved cerebral blood flow regulation. In another study, healthy subjects with no history of syncope underwent head-up tilt-table testing at 60° for 45 min or until presyncope or syncope occurred. Participants were tested with or without 473 ml water drinking 5 min before tilt-table testing in a randomised and crossover fashion. During the first 30 min of tilt testing, eight of 22 subjects without water experienced presyncope compared to only one of 22 who had ingested water. On average, the time participants tolerated head-up tilt was increased 26% with water drinking. Water drinking may also be beneficial in patients with post-exercise syncope [33].

How To 'Prescribe' Water?

In patients with orthostatic hypotension, POTS, or neurocardiogenic syncope, we use water in conjunction with other nonpharmacological treatments before initiation of pharmacological therapy, or as an adjuvant to pharmacological therapy. However, more studies are required to better define the therapeutic utility of water, in particular in POTS and in neurocardiogenic syncope. There are no data on the efficacy with long-term use.

In patients with autonomic failure, we usually recommend that the daily fluid intake should be in the range of 2–3 l. However, the timing of the water intake is of major importance. Patients should drink most of the water when their orthostatic symptoms tend to be worst and before meals. In most patients, symptoms are worse in the morning and improve during the day. We tell our patients to drink a glass of water before getting up in the morning. In this setting, water may be more efficacious than commonly used pressor agents, given its more rapid onset of action [12]. Water drinking potentiates the effect of pressor drugs, such as phenylpropanolamine and pseudoephedrine [34]. The 'drug' interaction can be exploited in the treatment of orthostatic hypotension. It may also lead to dangerous elevations in blood pressure. We suggest testing the sensitivity to pressor agents with or without water in each autonomic failure patient. The approach is useful to find a reasonable initial drug dose that is large enough to provide symptomatic benefit but does not lead to excessive, potentially dangerous increases in blood pressure. We advise patients with supine hypertension not to drink water within an hour before bedtime [10, 35].

Excessive water ingestion might lead to water intoxication, in particular in autonomic failure patients. However, we have not observed this complication in clinical practice.

Conclusions

Water drinking elicits a profound pressor response in autonomic failure patients. It increases blood pressure to a lesser degree in tetraplegic patients, cardiac transplant recipients, and older healthy subjects. Blood pressure does not change in healthy young subjects. The haemodynamic response to water drinking appears to be mediated through sympathetic activation via an unknown mechanism. Water drinking improves orthostatic responses in patients with orthostatic hypotension and orthostatic tachycardia, and delays the onset of neurocardiogenic syncope in healthy subjects. Thus, water drinking may be a promising and essentially cost-free intervention for all these conditions, either as monotherapy or in conjunction with other non-pharmacological or pharmacological treatments.

References

1. Jordan J, Shannon JR, Grogan E et al (1999) A potent pressor response elicited by drinking water. Lancet 353:723
2. Jordan J, Shannon JR, Black BK et al (2000) The pressor response to water drinking in humans: a sympathetic reflex? Circulation 101:504–509
3. Cariga P, Mathias CJ (2001) Haemodynamics of the pressor effect of oral water in human sympathetic denervation due to autonomic failure. Clin Sci (Lond) 101:313–319
4. Mathias CJ (2000) A 21st century water cure. Lancet 356:1046–1048
5. Routledge HC, Chowdhary S, Coote JH et al (2002) Cardiac vagal response to water ingestion in normal human subjects. Clin Sci (Lond) 103:157–162
6. Tank J, Schroeder C, Stoffels M et al (2003) Pressor effect of water drinking in tetraplegic patients may be a spinal reflex. Hypertension 41:1234–1239
7. Scott EM, Greenwood JP, Gilbey SG et al (2001) Water ingestion increases sympathetic vasoconstrictor discharge in normal human subjects. Clin Sci Colch 100:335–342

8. Schroeder C, Bush VE, Norcliffe LJ et al (2002) Water drinking acutely improves orthostatic tolerance in healthy subjects. Circulation 106:2806–2811
9. Ebert TJ, Smith JJ, Barney JA et al (1986) The use of thoracic impedance for determining thoracic blood volume changes in man. Aviat Space Environ Med 57:49–53
10. Shannon JR, Jordan J, Diedrich A et al (2000) Sympathetically mediated hypertension in autonomic failure. Circulation 101:2710–2715
11. Biaggioni I, Robertson RM, Robertson D (1994) Manipulation of norepinephrine metabolism with yohimbine in the treatment of autonomic failure. J Clin Pharmacol 34:418–423
12. Jordan J, Shannon JR, Biaggioni I et al (1998) Contrasting actions of pressor agents in severe autonomic failure. Am J Med 105:116–124
13. Robertson D, Goldberg MR, Tung CS et al (1986) Use of alpha 2 adrenoreceptor agonists and antagonists in the functional assessment of the sympathetic nervous system. J Clin Invest 78:576–581
14. Hoffman WE, Phillips MI, Wilson E et al (1977) A pressor response associated with drinking in rats. Proc Soc Exp Biol Med 154:121–124
15. Geelen G, Greenleaf JE, Keil LC (1996) Drinking-induced plasma vasopressin and norepinephrine changes in dehydrated humans. J Clin Endocrinol Metab 81:2131–2135
16. Jordan J, Tank J, Shannon JR et al (2002) Baroreflex buffering and susceptibility to vasoactive drugs. Circulation 105:1459–1464
17. Robertson D, Hollister AS, Carey EL et al (1984) Increased vascular beta2-adrenoreceptor responsiveness in autonomic dysfunction. J Am Coll Cardiol 3:850–856
18. Boschmann M, Steiniger J, Hille U et al (2003) Water-induced thermogenesis. J Clin Endocrinol Metab 88:6015–1619
19. Benarroch EE, Schmeichel AM, Parisi JE (2000) Involvement of the ventrolateral medulla in parkinsonism with autonomic failure. Neurology 54:963–968
20. Goldstein DS, Polinsky RJ, Garty M et al (1989) Patterns of plasma levels of catechols in neurogenic orthostatic hypotension. Ann Neurol 26:558–563
21. Goldstein DS, Holmes C, Cannon RO et al (1997) Sympathetic cardioneuropathy in dysautonomias. N Engl J Med 336:696–702
22. Rossi P, Andriesse GI, Oey PL et al (1998) Stomach distension increases efferent muscle sympathetic nerve activity and blood pressure in healthy humans. J Neurol Sci 161:148–155
23. Ploutz-Snyder L, Foley J, Ploutz-Snyder R et al (1999) Gastric gas and fluid emptying assessed by magnetic resonance imaging. Eur J Appl Physiol Occup Physiol 79:212–220
24. Haberich FJ (1968) Osmoreception in the portal circulation. Fed Proc 27:1137–1141
25. Lipp A, Tank J, Franke G et al (2005) Osmosensitive mechanisms contribute to the water drinking-induced, sympathetically-mediated, pressor response in humans. Neurology (in press)
26. Adachi A (1984) Thermosensitive and osmoreceptive afferent fibers in the hepatic branch of the vagus nerve. J Auton Nerv Syst 10:269–273
27. Shannon JR, Diedrich A, Biaggioni I et al (2002) Water drinking as a treatment for orthostatic syndromes. Am J Med 355–360
28. Streeten DH, Anderson GJ, Richardson R et al (1988) Abnormal orthostatic changes in blood pressure and heart rate in subjects with intact sympathetic nervous function: evidence for excessive venous pooling. J Lab Clin Med 111:326–335
29. Jacob G, Shannon JR, Black B et al (1997) Effects of volume loading and pressor

agents in idiopathic orthostatic tachycardia. Circulation 96:575–580
30. Low PA, Schondorf R, Novak V et al (1997) Postural orthostatic tachycardia syndrome. In: Low PA (ed) Clinical Autonomic Disorders. Lippincott-Raven, Philadelphia, pp 681–697
31. Jordan J, Shannon JR, Black BK et al (1998) Raised cerebrovascular resistance in idiopathic orthostatic intolerance: evidence for sympathetic vasoconstriction. Hypertension 32:699–704
32. Lu CC, Diedrich A, Tung CS et al (2003) Water ingestion as prophylaxis against syncope. Circulation 108:2660–2665
33. Thijs RD, Reijntjes RH, van Dijk JG (2003) Water drinking as a potential treatment for idiopathic exercise-related syncope: a case report. Clin Auton Res 13:103–105
34. Jordan J, Shannon JR, Diedrich A et al (2004) Water potentiates the pressor effect of ephedra alkaloids. Circulation 109:1823–1825
35. Shannon JR, Jordan J, Costa F et al (1997) The hypertension of autonomic failure and its treatment. Hypertension 30:1062–1067

Counter-Pressure Manoeuvres to Abort Impeding Syncope: Are They Really Useful?

C. Menozzi, F. Quartieri, N. Bottoni, G. Lolli

Introduction

Vasovagal reflex syncope is the most frequent cause of transient loss of consciousness and is preceded by prodromal symptoms in about two-thirds of patients [1]. Although the long-term prognosis of reflex syncopal disorders is excellent, they may impose substantial changes in life style and cause profound psychological distress. Prodromal symptoms are present in virtually all cases of tilt-induced vasovagal syncope, which occurs, on average, 1 min after the onset of prodromal symptoms [2]. During the prodromal phase, blood pressure falls markedly; this fall usually precedes the decrease in heart rate, which may be absent at least at the beginning of this phase [2, 3]. Hypotension is caused by vasodilation in the skeletal muscles due to inhibition of sympathetic vasoconstrictive activity [2–7]. In normal and hypertensive subjects, counter-pressure manoeuvres are able to induce a significant increase in blood pressure, which is mediated largely by endogenous catecholamine release [8, 9]. Muscle sympathetic nerve discharge and vascular resistance increase during counter-pressure manoeuvres in healthy subjects [10]. A major advantage of physical counter-manoeuvres is that they may be applied at the start of hypotensive symptoms, increasing central blood volume and blood pressure, thereby giving the patient the opportunity to regain self-confidence in provocative situations.

Cardiovascular Response to Counter-Pressure Manoeuvres

Leg crossing, combined with maximum tensing of the muscles of the legs, abdomen, and buttock for the maximum tolerated time, until complete dis-

Department of Interventional Cardiology, Ospedale S. Maria Nuova, Reggio Emilia, Italy

appearance of symptoms is achieved, was the first manoeuvre proposed [11]. It has the advantage that it can be performed as a preventive measure without much effort and without drawing much attention to the patient's problem. The increase in orthostatic blood pressure is presumed to be due both to mechanical compression of the venous vascular bed in the legs and to a reflex increase in systemic vascular resistances caused by the activation of muscle mechanosensitive receptors [12, 13].

Arm tensing consists of the maximum tolerated isometric contraction of the two arms achieved by gripping one hand with the other and contemporarily abducting (pushing away) the arms for the maximum tolerated time or until complete disappearance of symptoms [14, 15]. Handgrip consists of the maximal voluntary contraction of a rubber ball (approximately of 5–6 cm diameter) taken in the dominant hand for the maximum tolerated time or until complete disappearance of symptoms [12, 14, 15].

Muscle sympathetic nerve discharge and vascular resistance increase during handgrip in healthy subjects [10]. The increase in arterial pressure can be achieved by increased peripheral resistance alone in patients who lack the capacity to increase handgrip or stroke volume because of surgical cardiac denervation following cardiac transplantation [16] or pharmacological blockade with propranolol [8]. In one study [17], there was no difference in the magnitude of cardiovascular responses between handgrip performed with one and with both hands; in another study [18], the magnitude of the increase in muscle sympathetic nerve activity was greater when the exercise was performed with two hands, but it was less than the simple sum of the responses evoked with each arm separately, suggesting that the sympathetic cardiovascular adjustments elicited by separate limbs are not simply additive, but rather exhibit an inhibitory interaction.

In 32 healthy volunteers (mean age 44 ± 12 years, 16 males), the physiological response to 2 min of isometric contraction during handgrip, arm-muscle tensing, and leg crossing (as described above) was evaluated. The tests were carried out on a tilt table at 60°; ECG tracing and noninvasive beat-to-beat arterial blood pressure (BP) were continuously recorded. Systolic BP increased from 125 ± 18mmHg to 156 ± 26mmHg during handgrip, from 123 ± 15 mmHg to 155 ± 24 mmHg during arm tensing, and from 121 ± 14 mmHg to 165 ± 26 mmHg during leg crossing (P = 0.02); diastolic BP increased from 72 ± 10mmHg to 94 ± 16mmHg during handgrip, from 73 ± 11 mmHg to 97 ± 17 mmHg during arm tensing, and from 71 ± 12 mmHg to 95±16 mmHg during leg crossing (difference not significant). Heart rate increased from 76 ± 14 bpm 84 ± 16 bpm during handgrip, from 75 ± 13 bpm to 86 ± 15 bpm during arm tensing, and from 76 ± 12 bpm to 92 ± 18 bpm during leg crossing (P = 0.04) [15].

Thus, in healthy subjects systolic BP, diastolic BP, and heart rate increased to similar extents during both handgrip and arm tensing, whereas systolic BP and heart rate increased more during leg crossing. Whether this greater increase has clinical significance is unknown.

Efficacy of Manoeuvres To Abort Vasovagal Syncope

To evaluate the efficacy of isometric arm counter-pressure manoeuvres, Brignole et al. enrolled 29 patients affected by vasovagal syncope who had: (1) a history of three syncopal episodes in the last 2 years or at least one syncopal spell in the last year and at least three episodes of presyncope in the last year; and (2) syncopal episode(s) preceded by prodromal symptoms that were recognised by the patient as symptoms of impending syncope. To confirm the vasovagal origin of the syncope and to evaluate the amount of prodromal symptoms, the patients underwent tilt testing according to the Italian Protocol [19]. The patients were trained to use arm tensing and/or handgrip in case of occurrence of symptoms of impending syncope, and were discharged with the recommendation to self-administer these manoeuvres at the maximum tolerated voluntary contraction level immediately upon the appearance of symptoms of impending syncope identical to those reported by the patients prior to treatment, and until symptoms disappeared. Thereafter, the patients were seen every 3 months in the outpatient clinic. During the follow-up of 14 ± 6 months (range 6–21), 260 episodes of impending syncope were reported by 19 patients (median 4, interquartile range 3–13). Counter-pressure manoeuvres were self-administered by these patients in 98% of cases and resulted in the abortion of syncope in 99.6% of cases. Overall, five episodes of syncope occurred in five patients (17%). In four cases, the patients were unable to start manoeuvres because of the sudden onset of syncope, and in one case the patient activated the manoeuvres but they were ineffective [14].

Krediet et al. carried out a similar study to evaluate the efficacy of leg crossing and muscle tensing in 21 patients with positive tilt test. The patients were instructed to perform manoeuvres at the onset of symptoms of fainting. Acutely prodromal symptoms disappeared in all the patients, accompanied by a significant increase in systolic and diastolic BPs. At the follow-up, 13 of 20 patients had applied manoeuvres in their everyday lives with benefit [20].

The main points of these studies is that counter-pressure manoeuvres are feasible, safe, and well-accepted by the patient and can be proposed as a new first-line treatment for those patients who are able to recognise prodromal symptoms before vasovagal reflex syncope.

While this approach seems to be very helpful in everyday life, and patients are able to implement a counter-pressure manoeuvre in the vast majority of attacks with a very high rate of success in relieving symptoms, it must nevertheless be admitted that most of these episodes would have resolved spontaneously without leading to syncope, even in the absence of counter-pressure treatment. Owing to the open design of the follow-up study, we were unable to establish the exact benefit of the treatment. The Physical Counterpressure Maneuver Trial (PC Trial) is a multi-centre, prospective, longitudinal randomised single-blind clinical trial. The main hypothesis of the study is that, in patients with definite syncope and absence of significant structural heart disease, physical counter-pressure manoeuvres decrease the total syncope burden compared to standardised intensive conventional therapy. Secondary endpoints are the time to first recurrence, pre-syncope burden, and quality of life. The study population consists of 223 patients who fulfilled the following inclusion criteria: clinical diagnosis of classical neurally mediated reflex syncope based on medical history, or a diagnosis of non-classical neurally mediated reflex syncope and a positive tilt-table test; three syncope episodes in the last 2 years or at least one syncopal spell in the last year and at least three episodes of presyncope in the last year; recognisable prodromal symptoms; age 16–70 years. The follow-up is performed quarterly and is currently ongoing. Preliminary results are expected at the end of the year.

References

1. Alboni P, Brignole M, Menozzi C et al (2001) The diagnostic value of history in patients with syncope with or without heart disease. J Am Coll Cardiol 37:1921–1928
2. Alboni P, Dinelli M, Gruppillo P et al (2002) Haemodynamic changes early in prodromal symptoms of vasovagal syncope. Europace 4:333–338
3. Brignole M, Menozzi C, Del Rosso A et al (2000) New classification of haemodynamics of vasovagal syncope: beyond the VASIS classification. Analysis of the presyncopal phase of the tilt test without and with nitroglycerin challenge. Europace 2:66–76
4. Mosqueda-Garcia R, Furlan R, Fernandez-Violante R et al (1997) Sympathetic and baroreceptor reflex function in neurally mediated syncope evoked by tilt. J Clin Invest 99:2736–2744
5. Morillo C, Eckberg D, Ellenbogen K et al (1997) Vagal and sympathetic mechanisms in patients with orthostatic vasovagal syncope. Circulation 96:2509–2513
6. Lipsitz LW, Mietus J, Moody GB et al (1990) Spectral characteristics of heart rate variability before and during postural tilt. Circulation 81:1803–1810
7. Van Lieshout JJ, Wieling W, Karemaker JM et al (1991) The vasovagal response. Clin Sci 81:575–586
8. McAllister RG (1979) Effects of adrenergic receptor blockade on the response to isometric handgrip: studies in normal and hypertensive subjects. J Cardiovasc Pharmacol 2:253–263

9. Verdecchia P, Brignole M, Delfino G et al (1983) Systolic time intervals as possible predictors of pressure response to sustained beta-adrenergic blockade in arterial hypertension. Hypertension 5:140–146
10. Seals DR (1989) Sympathetic neural discharge and vascular resistance during exercise in humans. J Appl Physiol 66:2472–2478
11. Van Lieshout JJ, ten Harkel AD, Wieling W (1992) Physical manoeuvres for combating orthostatic dizziness in autonomic failure. Lancet 11:897–898
12. Ten Harkel AD, Van Lieshout JJ, Wieling W (1994) Effects of leg muscle pumping and tensing on orthostatic arterial pressure: a study in normal subjects and patients with autonomic failure. Clin Sci 87:553–558
13. Van Dijk N, de Bruin IG, Gisolf J et al (2005) Hemodynamic effects of leg crossing and skeletal muscle tensing during free standing in patients with vasovagal syncope. J Appl Physiol 98:584–590
14. Brignole M, Croci F, Menozzi C et al (2002) Isometric arm counter-pressure maneuvers to abort impending vasovagal syncope. J Am Coll Cardiol 40:2053–2059
15. Brignole M, Croci F, Menozzi C et al (2003) Isometric arm contraction at the onset of prodromal sympotoms: a new first line treatment for vasovagal sincope? In: Raviele A (ed) Cardiac Arrhythmias 2003, Springer, Milan, pp 641–650
16. Haskell WL, Savin WM, Schroeder JS et al (1981) Cardiovascular responses to handgrip isometric exercise in patients following cardiac transplantation. Circ Res 48:I156–I161
17. Grucza R, Kahn JF, Cybulski G et al (1989) Cardiovascular and sympathoadrenal responses to static handgrip performed with one and two hands. Eur J Appl Physiol Occup Physiol 59:184–188
18. Seals DR (1989) Influence of muscle mass on sympathetic neural activation during isometric exercise. J Appl Physiol 67:1801–1806
19. Bartoletti A, Alboni P, Ammirati F et al (2000) 'The Italian Protocol': a simplified head-up tilt testing potentiated with oral nitroglycerin to assess patients with unexplained syncope. Europace 2:339–342
20. Krediet P, van Dijk N, Linzer M et al (2002) Management of vasovagal syncope: controlling or aborting faints by leg crossing and muscle tensing. Circulation 106:1684–1689

Compression Stockings to Combat Vasovagal Syncope: What Is the Rationale?

M. Madalosso, F. Giada, A. Raviele

Introduction

Syncope is defined as a sudden, transient loss of consciousness and postural tone due to cerebral hypoperfusion, followed by spontaneous recovery [1]. Syncope is a common symptom that affects up to 35–50% of the general population: it is the reason for 1–3% of emergency room visits and 1–6% of hospital admissions [2]. Syncope may have different causes: cardiovascular, non-cardiovascular and unexplained. The most frequent type of syncope is the vasovagal syncope, who accounts at least 35% of loss of consciousness.

Physiopathology of Vasovagal Syncope

The vasovagal faint is a heterogeneous condition and may be triggered by central stimuli (pain, extreme emotions, psychic stress) and peripheral stimuli (reduction in venous return to the heart, such as in prolonged standing, hot environments, hypovolaemia, or redistribution of blood volume). In daily life vasovagal syncope is common while the subject is standing [3]. On standing, the increased gravitational forces results in pooling of 500–800 ml of blood in the distensible veins below the level of the heart, i.e., the veins of the legs and the splanchnic veins, thus reducing venous return to the heart. This leads to a decrease in arterial blood pressure and cardiac output. In normal subjects there is an autonomic compensatory reflex that keeps the arterial blood pressure and the cardiac output almost normal, through vasoconstriction and tachycardia, due to sympathetic activation and parasympa-

Division of Cardiology, Cardiovascular Department, Umberto I Hospital, Mestre-Venice, Italy

thetic withdrawal, respectively. In patients who are prone to vasovagal syncope, this compensatory reflex is inadequate. Hargreaves and Muir [4] demonstrated, during orthostatic challenge, a larger increase in calf volume in patients with recurrent vasovagal syncope and a trend to greater peripheral blood pooling and reduced venous volume variability than in normal subjects. It has been postulated that, in patients with vasovagal syncope, the reduction of venous return activates an abnormal reflex, similar to the Bezold–Jarisch reflex, triggered by a vigorous contraction of an almost empty ventricular cavity. It activates intramyocardial mechanoreceptors inappropriately (the unmyelinated vagal C fibres), causing paradoxical sympathetic inhibition (peripheral vasodilation) and parasympathetic activation (bradycardia) with cerebral hypoperfusion and syncope [5]. However, the pathophysiology of vasovagal syncope is probably not so schematic, and other potential mechanisms may be responsible for this condition, such as afferent signals arising from atrial or pulmonary baroreceptors, or even from higher central nervous system centres.

Treatment of Vasovagal Syncope

In the majority of subjects vasovagal syncope is a benign condition that does not represent a threat to life and does not significantly impair quality of life. Consequently, a specific treatment is usually not indicated, and recurrence may be easily prevented by reassurance and counselling of the patient. In a minority of subjects, however, the syncopal episodes are much more frequent and often occur in the absence of predictable circumstances or warning symptoms. These episodes may be accompanied by physical injury and represent the so-called 'malignant' or 'atypical' vasovagal syncope. In these cases, as also in patients with a potential occupational hazard (pilots, truck drivers, commercial painters, roofers, and so on), a specific treatment is generally recommended.

Many forms of treatment are promoted for vasovagal syncope: non-pharmacological/physical, pharmacological, and electrical. None of them has been demonstrated to be surely effective in preventing syncopal recurrences. The substantial inefficacy of currently available therapeutic options for patients with recurrent or malignant vasovagal syncope justifies the search for alternative treatments.

Compression Elastic Stockings

One of the measures suggested in the past for the treatment of vasovagal syncope, but never tested with clinical studies, is the use of compression elastic stockings. The rationale for this therapy is the reduction in venous pooling and the increase in venous return that compression elastic stockings may induce.

Several studies have investigated the haemodynamic and clinical effects of this therapy in different clinical settings, but to the best of our knowledge no studies have been performed to evaluate the effects of compression elastic stockings in patients with vasovagal syncope. Buhs et al. [6] studied healthy subjects during daily activity that requires nearly continuous standing and walking: under those conditions, it has been shown that graduated elastic stockings had a direct anatomic effect which can be related to the transmural pressure in the veins that preserve dilation in the deep, superficial, and perforating venous system of the lower leg.

In patients with chronic venous insufficiency, compression elastic stockings have been shown to reduce the residual volume fraction, which is an indicator of improving calf muscle pump function and reflux in vein segments [7]. These favourable effects of compression elastic stockings in patients with chronic venous insufficiency seem to be a consequence of shifting blood from the superficial to the deep venous compartment of the legs [8]. This promotes venous return to the heart by means of blood milking caused by muscle contraction [9–17].

In patients with orthostatic hypotension caused by adrenergic failure, compression elastic stockings reduce the decrease in standing blood pressure by increasing total peripheral resistance and reducing venous capability [18]. In daily life this leads to a reduction of hypotension-related symptoms, such as dizziness and increased heart rhythm, and an improvement in quality of life [19].

Stic Stoc Trial

On the basis of these observations, we have planned a multi-centre, randomised, placebo-controlled study, the 'ElaSTIC STOCkings for the prevention of recurrent vasovagal syncope TRIAL' (Stic Stoc Trial).

Aim of the Study

The aim of the study is to ascertain whether, among patients suffering from recurrent vasovagal syncope, compression elastic stockings reduce the number affected by syncope recurrences, prolong the time to the first recurrence, and improve quality of life.

Study Design

Enrolled patients will be randomised to active treatment (compression elastic stockings) or placebo (non-compression stockings). The compression elastic stockings exert a pressure of 20–30 mmHg around the calves, which corresponds to class II of the European CEN classification [17]. The inactive treatment, the placebo, looks like the elastic compression stockings, but does not exert haemodynamic effects. The clinicians, nurses, and enrolled patients will be blinded to the type of stockings being worn.

Inclusion and Exclusion Criteria

To be enrolled, patients will have to meet the following criteria: vasovagal syncope and positive head-up tilt testing; at least 6 syncopal events in the patient's lifetime, the latest occurring no more than 6 months before enrolment. The following constitute exclusion criteria: non-vasovagal syncope; chronic venous and arterial insufficiency; recent (< 6 months) acute myocardial infarction; chronic severe non-cardiac diseases (terminal neoplasia, neurological disease, etc.); pregnancy.

Other Therapies

During the study period, the use of pacemakers or drugs for the prevention of vasovagal syncope, such as β-blockers, α_1-agonists, fludrocortisone, serotonin uptake inhibitors, theophylline, and scopolamine, will not be allowed.

Quality of Life

The patient's quality of life will be evaluated through a questionnaire (SF-36) filled out before treatment and again after 6 and 12 months.

Follow-Up

During follow-up, with a mean duration of 12 months, each enrolled patient will wear the stockings during the day time. Patients will be asked to keep a clinical diary, specifying the number, severity, and time of syncopal and pre-syncopal events, the circumstances in which they occur, and any associated traumas. Patients also have to report the days in which they do not wear the stockings, the reason why, and any adverse effects. Every 3 months, patients will be clinically assessed.

Primary Endpoint

The primary clinic endpoint will be syncope, since this can be easily assessed and has been successfully used in previous studies. Patients are examined within 7 days of a fainting episode. To verify the syncopal episode, patients and witnesses are asked to describe the event and the circumstances in which it occurs, stating in particular whether there was complete loss of consciousness. Patients are also examined to evaluate any severe trauma resulting from the event. The number of patients who experience syncope during follow-up, the frequency of syncope (number of times per month), and the time to first recurrence are taken as the parameters to measure the primary clinical event.

Secondary Endpoints

The secondary endpoints will be the following: (1) the number of patients with pre-syncopal recurrences, the frequency of pre-syncopal events, and time to the first pre-syncopal recurrence; (2) quality of life.

References

1. Brignole M, Alboni P, Beneditt DG et al for the Task Force on Syncope, European Society of Cardiology (2004) Guidelines on management of syncope-up date 2004. Europace 6:467–537
2. Linzer M, Pontinen M, Gold GT (1991) Impairment of physical and psychosocial function in recurrent syncope. J Clin Epidemiol 44:1037–43
3. Baron-Esquivias G, Errazquin F, Pedrote A et al (2004) Long-term outcome of patients with vasovagal syncope. Am Heart J 147:883–889
4. Hargreaves AD, Muir AL (1992) Lack of variation in venous tone potentiates vasovagal syncope. Br Heart J 67:486–490
5. Raviele A, Brignole M, Menozzi C (1997) Development of an implantable drug delivery system for the treatment of vasovagal syncope: a dream or a real prospect? In: Raviele A (ed) Cardiac Arrhythmias 1997, Springer, Milan pp 422-427
6. Buhs CL, Bedick PJ, Glover JL (1999) The effect of graded compression elastic stockings on the lower leg venous system during daily activity. J Vasc Surg 30:830–835
7. Eberhardt RT, Raggetto JD (2005) Chronic venous insufficiency. Circulation 111:2398–2409
8. Gamble J, Christ F, Gartside IB (1998) Human calf precapillary resistance decreases in response to small cumulative increases in venous congestion pressure. J Physiol 507:611–617
9. Ibelguna V, Delis KT, Nicolaides AN et al (2003) Effect of elastic compression stockings on venous hemodynamics during walking. J Vasc Surg 37:420–425

10. Agu O, Backer D, Seifalian AM (2004) Effect of graduated compression stockings on limb oxygenation and venous function during exercise in patients with venous insufficiency. Vascular 12:69–76
11. Bellard E, Fortrat JO, Dupuis JM et al (2003) Hemodynamic response to peripheral venous congestion in patients with unexplained recurrent syncope. Clin Sci 105:331–337
12. Mayberry JC, Moneta GL, De Frang RD et al (1991) The influence of elastic compression stockings on deep venous hemodynamics. J Vasc Surg 13:91–100
13. Kierkegaard A, Norgren L (1992) Compression stockings and venous function in patients with decompensated heart failure. Phlebology 7:117–120
14. Belcaro G, Laurora G, Cesarone MR et al (1992) Elastic stockings in diabetic microangiopathy. Vasa 21:193–197
15. Evers EJ, Wuppermann Th (1999) Effect of different compression therapies on the reflux in deep veins with post-thrombotic syndrome. Vasa 28:19–23
16. Gamble J, Christ F, Gartside IB (1998) Human calf precapillary resistance decreases in response to small cumulative increases in venous congestion pressure. J Physiol 507:611–617
17. Veraart JC, Pronk G, Neumann HA (1997) Pressure differences of elastic compression stockings at the ankle region. Dermatol Surg 23:935–939
18. Denq JC, Opfer-Gehrking TL, Low PA (1997) Efficacy of compression of different capacitance beds in the amelioration of orthostatic hypothension. Clin Auton Res 7:321–326
19. Gorelik O, Fishlev G, Cohen N (2004) Lower limb compression bandaging is effective in preventing signs and symptoms of seating-induced postural hypothension. Cardiology 102:177–183

β-Blockers for Prevention of Vasovagal Syncope: Who Benefits from Treatment?

R.S. Sheldon

Catecholamines and Vasovagal Syncope

Vasovagal syncope is a common problem that reduces quality of life [1–3] and may be difficult to treat. Although β-adrenergic blockers are frequently prescribed to prevent syncope, there is limited evidence for their effectiveness. However, there is considerable evidence supporting a role for catecholamine involvement in the haemodynamic response to head-up tilt, and perhaps in the vasovagal reflex itself (for review, see [4]). Both norepinephrine and epinephrine increase steadily during prolonged head-up tilt, with terminal levels of epinephrine significantly higher in patients in whom the vasovagal reflex is induced than in those resistant to prolonged tilt testing [4–6]. Older patients may release more epinephrine than younger subjects [5]. The amount of the increase in norepinephrine varies considerably from study to study. Taken together, these findings suggest that sympathetic stimulation, perhaps of β-adrenergic receptors, is important in the genesis of vasovagal syncope. Consistent with this is the ability of an isoproterenol infusion to provoke vasovagal syncope far more quickly in patients undergoing tilt tests than in those examined by simple passive prolonged head-up tilt testing [7, 8]. Whether isoproterenol simply accelerates the onset of the vasovagal reflex or identifies a subset of patients is unclear. For example, both isoproterenol and nitrates provoke syncope on tilt tests, but do so in only partly overlapping populations [9]. There is ample evidence that acute β-blockade during isoproterenol tilt tests can prevent the vasovagal reflex (for a summary, see [10]). However, they are less effective in preventing syncope during passive head-up tilt tests [6], suggesting that while stimulation of the

Libin Cardiovascular Institute of Alberta, Faculty of Medicine, University of Calgary, Alberta, Canada

β-adrenergic receptor may be important in isoproterenol tilt tests, it is significantly less important in the vasovagal reflex provoked by passive head-up tilt. Finally, Dendi and Goldstein reported a meta analysis of 19 papers and 1060 patients who received β-blockade during tilt testing. They reported that that β_1-selective adrenoreceptor blockade resulted in 68% negative tilt tests, while non-selective blockade resulted in 94% negative tilt tests. The authors concluded that non-selective β-blockers are likely to be more effective than β_1-selective blockers in preventing vasovagal syncope [10]. Unfortunately, the types of tilt tests were not reported, so it is not clear whether this was a study of the physiology of isoproterenol or a study of the physiology of vasovagal syncope. Whether the findings have therapeutic implications for patients with recurrent vasovagal syncope is also not known.

Observational Studies

Three observational studies yielded conflicting information about whether β-blockade prevents syncope. In a nonrandomised trial, Cox et al. [11] administered a variety of β-blockers to 118 syncope patients who had fainted a median three times and who had a positive tilt test. Control patients were those who either refused β-adrenergic blocker treatment or discontinued it. After 28 ± 11 months, the proportion of patients with a recurrence of syncope was 10-23% in the persistently treated patients and 42-58% in the partially or completely untreated patients. The estimated absolute effect size was about 34% with a relative reduction of 68%. We studied a cohort of 153 syncope patients who had positive tilt tests and a historical median of seven syncopal spells [12]. Syncope recurred in 17 of the 52 patients who received β-blockers and in 28 of the 101 patients who were untreated; the actuarial probability of remaining free of syncope was the same in both groups. Alegria et al. recently reported similar results in a large observational report [13]. They followed 163 patients treated with β-blockers and 75 control subjects treated with conservative, non-pharmacologic measures for 20 ± 13 months. Most (82%) patients who received a β-blocker took either atenolol or metoprolol. Patients who received β-adrenergic blockers were somewhat younger than those managed conservatively. There was a trend to a worse outcome in patients on β-blockers; 20% of control subjects and 35% of patients who received β-adrenergic blockers had at least one recurrence of syncope ($P = 0.056$). At the very least, this study provides little evidence of a beneficial effect of β-blockers.

Randomised Clinical Trials

There have been five randomised clinical trials testing the efficacy or effectiveness of β-adrenergic blockers for the prevention of syncope [14–18]. Although the results are not completely consistent, they do suggest strongly that β-blockade does not prevent vasovagal syncope. Mahanonda et al. studied 42 patients with an unspecified mix of historical presyncope and syncope, and a positive tilt test [14]. The patients then were randomised to atenolol or placebo. After 1 month, 71% of patients receiving atenolol, but only 29% of patients receiving placebo reported feeling better and had experienced fewer combined presyncopal and syncopal spells. The absolute effect size was 42% and the relative risk reduction was 61%. The frequency of presyncopal and syncopal events was 1 ± 2 vs 6 ± 9 spells per week in the atenolol vs the placebo populations, with a relative reduction of 83%.

Madrid et al. randomised 50 patients with vasovagal syncope to treatment with atenolol (50 mg daily) or placebo [15]. The subjects were selected on the basis of a clinical diagnosis provided by the investigators and all underwent passive prolonged head-up tilt testing. This modestly symptomatic study population had a median of only three lifetime syncopal spells, and were included regardless of whether the tilt test was positive or negative. Patients were followed for up to 1 year, during which there was a non-significant increase in the number of patients who had a recurrence of syncope in the group taking atenolol compared to those taking placebo. There was no significant difference in outcome in patients who had a negative or positive baseline tilt test. The authors concluded that patients with a clinical diagnosis of syncope, regardless of tilt-test outcome, did not benefit from attempted treatment with atenolol. Although this was a small study, there was not even a trend to benefit from atenolol.

Flevari et al. carried out a prospective, randomised crossover study of nadolol, propranolol, and placebo in 30 patients with recurrent vasovagal syncope and a positive tilt test [16]. Each treatment arm in this Latin Square design lasted 3 months, and the authors reported the number of presyncopal and syncopal spells for each observation period. Nadolol was selected because it is a hydrophilic non-selective β-blocker, while propranolol is a hydrophobic non-selective β-blocker. There was a remarkable 80–90% reduction in all measures of presyncope and syncope in all three treatment arms (placebo, propranolol, and nadolol), with no significant difference among the three arms. Therefore, this small study, with short observation periods, did not detect any clinical benefit from β-blockers above that seen with placebo.

Ventura et al. [17] randomised 56 patients with recurrent syncope to treatment with β-blockers or to no treatment. In a 1-year follow-up period, syncope recurred in 71% of untreated patients but in only 29% of patients who received β-blockers. In a subsequent Cox regression analysis, only β-blocker treatment predicted the absence of syncope recurrence. The strength of the conclusions of this study is compromised by its lack of placebo control and blinding.

We carried out the Prevention of Syncope Trial, whose design was previously described [18]. This randomised, placebo-controlled, double-blind trial was designed to assess the effects of metoprolol in vasovagal syncope over a 1-year treatment period. The primary hypothesis was that in patients at moderate-to-high risk for frequent recurrence of vasovagal syncope, a decision to treat with metoprolol would increase the time to the first recurrence of syncope compared to treatment with placebo. The major secondary hypotheses were that metoprolol would reduce the frequency of recurrent syncopal spells as well as the frequency, duration, and severity of presyncopal spells; and that it would improve quality of life. In addition, we hypothesised that older age or the need to use isoproterenol to induce syncope predicts a beneficial clinical response to metoprolol.

Each patient had > 2 syncopal spells and a positive tilt test. Randomisation was stratified according to ages < 42 and ≥ 42 years. Patients received either metoprolol or matching placebo at best-tolerated doses from 25 to 200 mg daily. The main outcome measure was the first recurrence of syncope. In total, there were 208 patients, mean age 42 ± 18 years who had had a median of nine syncopal spells. This was, therefore, a group of fairly symptomatic patients. Nearly 40% had at least one recurrence of syncope during the 1-year observation period, as predicted in the initial power calculations, which were based on earlier epidemiologic studies from our institution [18, 19]. The likelihood of recurrent syncope was not significantly different between groups by either intent-to-treat or on-treatment analyses. Therefore, metoprolol was no more effective than placebo in preventing vasovagal syncope in the study population as a whole. Taken together with the results of the previous four smaller studies, metoprolol, and probably β-adrenergic receptor blockade in general, appear to be ineffective in preventing vasovagal syncope in the broad patient population.

Baseline Clinical and Tilt-Test Variables

Part of the explanation for the discrepant conclusions about β-adrenergic blocker effect may relate to patient selection. There may be specific baseline variables that predict a beneficial response to β-blockers, such as age, sinus tachycardia preceding syncope during tilt, and the requirement for isoproterenol to induce syncope. We examined the effect of age on outcome of patients taking β-adrenergic blockers in a large population whose characteristics were previously reported [12, 19]. A multivariate analysis showed that age was an independent risk factor for the recurrence of syncope in patients taking β-blockers but not in untreated patients. The relative hazard of recurrent syncope for patients taking β-blockers was 3.0 at age 20, 1.0 at age 42, and 0.3 at age 70. Natale et al. reported an observational study of 112 patients who were treated with metoprolol [21]. Patients responding to metoprolol were older (55 ± 12 years vs 42 ± 15 years, $P < 0.05$). Age > 42 years was associated with a lower likelihood of syncope on metoprolol ($P < 0.02$). This was an unblinded observational study, and numerous confounding factors, such as patient selection and the placebo effect, could have biased the findings.

Accordingly the placebo-controlled Prevention of Syncope Trial contained a prespecified secondary analysis of the effects of age on patient response to metoprolol [18]. Patient randomisation was stratified at age 42, which was the age of neutral response predicted from our previous unpublished work. In a stratified analysis, we found a highly significant reduction in the likelihood of syncope in subjects ≥ 42 years old, with no detectable benefit in younger patients. Based on these studies, it seems clear that treatment with β-blockers confers no benefit on younger patients, but might be beneficial in older patients. Both studies were retrospective secondary analyses but we still lack an adequately powered study targeting older patients.

Two studies also suggested that patients who do not faint during passive drug-free tilt tests, but do so during an isoproterenol infusion are more likely to benefit from β-blockers. Natale et al. [21] used multivariate analysis to show that isoproterenol-dependent syncope gave an odds ratio of 3.6 as a predictor of response to β-blockers. Leor et al. [22] reported isoproterenol-dependent syncope predicted clinical outcome with positive and negative predictive values of 94% and 37%, respectively. As both these were observational, open-label, retrospective studies, we tested this hypothesis prospectively in the Prevention of Syncope Trial (POST) [18]. A majority of the subjects underwent a standardised tilt test consisting of a preliminary passive head-up tilt for 30 min followed, if necessary, by an infusion of isoproterenol. The effect of metoprolol on eventual clinical outcome was analysed in patients who fainted during passive head-up tilt and in those who required isoproterenol to induce a vasovagal response. The need for isoproterenol to produce a positive tilt test did not predict subsequent benefit from metoprolol. These substudy results from POST conflict with those of two previous reports [21, 22]. However, as POST was a prospective, randomised, placebo-controlled study, it seems likely that the need for isoproterenol at baseline tilt testing does not predict eventual clinical response to metoprolol.

Finally, two groups reported observational studies showing that sinus tachycardia during head-up tilt predicts an eventual response to β-blockers. Leor et al. [22] reported that during a follow-up period of 18 ± 6 months syncope recurred in only 9% of patients who had sinus tachycardia during the baseline tilt test compared to 54% who did not have sinus tachycardia ($P < 0.01$). Development of tachycardia was a better predictor of drug efficacy than an isoproterenol-induced positive tilt test. Klingenheben et al. [22] performed baseline head-up tilt, then treated patients with metoprolol and tilted them again. Syncope occurred during the second tilt test in only 17% of patients who had sinus tachycardia during the baseline tilt test compared to 80% who did not have sinus tachycardia ($P < 0.05$). These interesting preliminary results await confirmation in prospective randomised studies.

Patient Selection for β-Blocker Therapy

Clearly, β_1-selective blockers are not effective in patients under 40 years of age, and thus cannot be recommended for this group. Given the weakness of the evidence, they should not be used generally as first-line therapy. There is some evidence from non-randomised studies and from a POST subgroup analysis that β_1-selective blockers may be effective in patients older than 40 years. They might also be effective, although the data are weak, in patients who develop sinus tachycardia preceding syncope during tilt testing. It would therefore be prudent to recommend β-adrenergic blockers as therapy for the prevention of vasovagal syncope only in older patients who have already proven resistant to at least one medical attempt, or have another possible indication for β-blocker treatment. For example, one might reasonably suggest that β-blockers be used for patients with both recurrent vasovagal syncope and hypertension.

References

1. Ganzeboom KS, Colman N, Reitsma JB et al (2003) Prevalence and Triggers of Syncope in Medical Students. Am J Cardiol 91:1006–1008
2. Linzer M, Pontinen M, Gold DT et al (1991) Impairment of physical and psychosocial function in recurrent syncope. J Clin Epidemiol 44:1037–1043
3. Rose S, Koshman ML, Spreng S et al (2000) The relationship between health-related quality of life and frequency of spells in patients with syncope. J Clin Epidemiol 53:1209–1216
4. Mosqueda-Garcia R, Furlan R, Tank J et al (2000) The elusive pathophysiology of neurally mediated syncope. Circulation 102:2898–2906
5. Ermis C, Samniah N, Sakaguchi S et al (2004) Comparison of catecholamine

response during tilt-table-induced vasovagal syncope in patients, < 35 to those > 65 years of age. Am J Cardiol 93:225–227

6. Kikushima S, Kobayashi Y, Nakagawa H et al (1999) Triggering mechanism for neurally mediated syncope induced by head-up tilt test: role of catecholamines and response to propranolol. J Am Coll Cardiol 33:350–357
7. Almquist A, Goldenberg IF, Milstein S et al (1989) Provocation of bradycardia and hypotension by isoproterenol and upright posture in patients with unexplained syncope. N Engl J Med 320:346–351
8. Sheldon R, Killam S (1992) Methodology of isoproterenol-tilt table testing in patients with syncope. J Am Coll Cardiol 19:773–779
9. Delepine S, Prunier F, Leftheriotis G et al (2002) Comparison between isoproterenol and nitroglycerin sensitized head-upright tilt in patients with unexplained syncope and negative or positive tilt response. Am J Cardiol 90:488–491
10. Dendi R, Goldstein DS (2002) Meta-analysis of nonselective versus beta-1 adrenoceptor-selective blockade in prevention of tilt-induced neurocardiogenic syncope. Am J Cardiol 89:1319–1321
11. Cox MM, Perlman BA, Mayor MR et al (1995) Acute and long-term beta-adrenergic blockade for patients with neurocardiogenic syncope. J Am Coll Cardiol 26:1293–1298
12. Sheldon RS, Rose S, Flanagan P et al (1996) Effect of beta-blockers on the time to first syncope recurrence in patients after a positive isoproterenol-tilt table test. Am J Cardiol 78:536–539
13. Alegria JR, Gersh BJ, Scott CG et al (2003) Comparison of frequency of recurrent syncope after beta-blocker therapy versus conservative management for patients with vasovagal syncope. Am J Cardiol 92: 82–84
14. Mahanonda N, Bhuripanyo K, Kangkagate C et al (1995) Randomized double-blind, placebo-controlled trial of oral atenolol in patients with unexplained syncope and positive upright tilt table test results. Am Heart J 130:1250–1253
15. Madrid AH, Ortega J, Rebollo JG et al (2001) Lack of efficacy of atenolol for the prevention of neurally mediated syncope in a highly symptomatic population: a prospective, double-blind, randomized and placebo-controlled study. J Am Coll Cardiol 37:554–559
16. Flevari P, Livanis EG, Theodorakis GN et al (2002) Vasovagal syncope: a prospective, randomized, crossover evaluation of the effect of propranolol, nadolol and placebo on syncope recurrence and patients' well-being. J Am Coll Cardiol 40:499–504
17. Ventura R, Maas R, Zeidler D et al (2002) A randomized and controlled pilot trial of beta-blockers for the treatment of recurrent syncope in patients with a positive or negative response to head-up tilt test. Pacing Clin Electrophysiol 25:816–821
18. Sheldon RS, Rose S, Connolly S on behalf of the POST Investigators (2003) Prevention of syncope trial (post): a randomized clinical trial of beta blockers in the prevention of vasovagal syncope. rationale and study design. Europace 5:71–75
19. Sheldon RS, Rose S, Flanagan P et al (1996) Risk factors for recurrent syncope following a positive tilt table test in patients with syncope. Circulation 93:973–981
20. Sheldon RS, Rose S (2001) Components of clinical trials for vasovagal syncope. Europace 3:233–240
21. Natale A, Newby KH, Dhala A et al (1996) Response to beta blockers in patients with neurocardiogenic syncope: How to predict beneficial effects. J Cardiovasc Electrophysiol 7:1154–1158
22. Leor J, Rotstein Z, Vered Z et al (1994) Absence of tachycardia during tilt test pre-

dicts failure of beta-blocker therapy in patients with neurocardiogenic syncope. Am Heart J 127:1539–1543

23. Klingenheben T, Kalusche D, Li Y et al (1996) Changes in plasma epinephrine concentration and in heart rate during head-up tilt testing in patients with neurocardiogenic syncope: correlation with successful therapy with β-receptor antagonists. J Cardiovasc Electrophysiol 7:802–805

Has Psychiatric Treatment Any Role in the Management of Vasovagal Syncope?

F. Giada[1], I. Silvestri[2], A. Rossillo[1], M. Madalosso[1], P.G. Nicotera[2], A. Raviele[1]

Introduction

Syncope is a very frequent clinical symptom. About 30% of the general population undergo one syncopal episode in their lifetime, while at least 3% faint more than once. In most cases, the aetiology of syncope is vasovagal [1].

Vasovagal syncope is generally a benign and isolated event which does not need specific interventions. However, some patients have frequent fainting fits, often associated with major trauma and severe impairment of quality of life. The treatment of vasovagal syncope involves behavioural measures for all patients, drug therapy for those who are most symptomatic, and pacemaker implantation in a very limited and selected group of patients. However, drug therapy has yielded disappointing results and, although pacemaker implantation seems to restore quality of life to a normal level and offer an attractive cost-effectiveness ratio, we have insufficiently compelling data on the real efficacy of cardiac pacing for the treatment of vasovagal syncope [1]. Thus, at the present time, treatment of patients with frequently recurrent vasovagal syncope still remains a controversial issue.

In this paper we will discuss the possible role of psychiatric and/or psychological interventions in the management of severe vasovagal fainters. We will analyse the relationship between vasovagal syncope and psychiatric disorders, how to perform psychiatric evaluation in subjects with syncope, and the data regarding the effects of psychiatric treatment on syncopal recurrence.

[1]Division of Cardiology, Cardiovascular Department, Umberto I Hospital, Mestre-Venice, Italy; [2]Division of Neurology, Umberto I Hospital, Mestre-Venice, Italy

Relationship Between Vasovagal Syncope and Psychiatric Disorders

Various factors seem to suggest an association between vasovagal syncope and psychological disturbances. Acute emotional stress or fear can facilitate and/or trigger vasovagal syncope [2, 3]; some psychiatric illnesses, such as anxiety and depression, may trigger vasovagal reactions [4]; after reassurance about the benign nature of their condition, vasovagal fainters have significantly fewer syncopal recurrences [5]; the only drug shown to be efficacious in preventing vasovagal syncope in placebo-controlled studies is paroxetine, an inhibitor of serotonin re-uptake commonly used as an antidepressant [6].

In the international literature, data about the prevalence of psychiatric disorders and the quality of life of patients suffering from vasovagal syncope are rather scanty and incomplete. Some studies have reported a high prevalence of psychiatric disorders such as anxiety, depression, somatisation disorders, and alcoholism in patients with unexplained syncope [7–13]. Moreover, some authors have found that patients with recurrent syncope of various aetiologies also suffered a significant reduction in their quality of life in both the physical and the psychosocial domains [14–16]. The above-mentioned studies, however, include some bias and confounding factors: poor homogeneity of the study population (enrolled patients had syncope of various origins, or were suffering from unexplained syncope); patients were very often affected by co-morbid conditions in addition to syncope (with the possibility that these concomitant illnesses may have affected the psychological profile and quality of life of the patients examined); lack a suitable control group that is representative of the general population.

In a recently published study, we compared the psychological profile and quality of life in patients with severe vasovagal syncope confirmed by positive tilt testing with full symptom reproduction and no concomitant associated diseases, with those obtained in a control group made up of healthy sex- and age-matched subjects without syncope [17]. In this study we observed a higher prevalence of mild or moderate psychiatric disorders in patients with vasovagal syncope than in controls, especially with regard to anxiety, mood, and somatisation disorders. Moreover, we observed a marked reduction in all the quality of life scales in patients with vasovagal syncope in comparison with controls, and in patients with psychiatric disorders versus those without. Finally, the presence of psychiatric disorders constituted a potent risk factor for recurrence during follow-up.

As all the above-mentioned studies were case-controlled observational studies, no conclusion can be drawn as to whether the psychiatric disorders were the cause or the result of the recurrent syncopal episodes, or represent only a co-morbidity without any role in the pathogenesis of syncope.

Vasovagal syncope and psychiatric disorders may be linked through the serotonin pathway or, most probably, through input coming from the cortex to the brainstem, the site where the vasovagal reflex develops.

How to Perform Psychiatric Evaluation in Patients with Vasovagal Syncope

In patients with syncope psychiatric evaluation is generally performed by mean of a structured interview with a psychologist and/or specific questionnaires. Among these, one of the most used is the Minnesota Multiphasic Personality Inventory-2 (MMPI-2) questionnaire. The MMPI-2 is a widely recognised instrument for assessing the psychological profile of adult subjects [18, 19]. Made up of over 500 items, the questionnaire uses specific scales to explore various aspects of the individual's personality. After psychiatric assessment, clinical diagnoses are formulated in accordance with the criteria of the Diagnostic and Statistical Manual of Mental Disorders-IV (DSM-IV) [4]. Assessment of quality of life is generally by means of specific questionnaires. The Short-Form Health Survey (SF-36) questionnaire is an international standardised instrument for assessing the general state of health [20, 21]. It is often employed to evaluate the impact of syncope on the patient's physical and psychological functions.

Effects of Psychiatric Treatment on Syncopal Recurrence

In the literature, data regarding the effects of psychiatric interventions in the treatment of patients with vasovagal syncope are rather limited, and consist mostly of single case reports or case series. In these small studies psychotherapy and/or pharmacotherapy were employed in patients with refractory vasovagal syncope and in those with blood/injury phobia.

Vasovagal Syncope

Cognitive behavioural therapy, like biofeedback and relaxation, is used to teach patients to apply realistic and reassuring thoughts to physical symptoms they see as alarming, with the aim of developing more adaptive beliefs about their ability to manage and cope with syncope, and to regain self-assurance in situations that provoke syncope. McGrady et al. undertook a randomised, controlled trial involving 22 patients with refractory vasovagal syncope [22]. They reported a significant reduction in syncopal recurrence in patients randomised to undergo biofeedback and relaxation therapy with respect to controls. The treatment was most effective in younger patients whose syncope was associated with a strong psycho-physiological response. Similar encouraging results were reported by Newton et al. in a case series of 9 patients with severe vasovagal syncope [23]. In this open label study, cognitive behavioural therapy resulted in a dramatic reduction of syncopal episodes.

Linzer et al. [8], in a open label study, used psychotherapy plus pharmacotherapy to treat 11 patients with syncope of unknown origin and psychiatric disorders, and obtained resolution of symptoms in the majority of patients. Kadri et al. [24] used clonazepam, a well-tolerated benzodiazepine, in 35 patients with refractory vasovagal syncope and anxiety or sleep disorders. In this non-randomised, non-placebo-controlled observational study, 83% of patients were free of syncopal recurrence during follow-up.

Blood/Injury Phobia

Blood/injury phobia is a common psychiatric disorder (2–4.5% of children and adults), in which fear can be triggered by seeing blood, by undergoing an invasive medical procedure, or by sustaining an injury. It is highly familial, and is usually associated with vasovagal reaction and syncope. Psychological deconditioning is considered the first choice therapy for this condition. During psychological deconditioning patients are exposed to phobic stimuli (such as the sight of blood) and taught to apply muscle tension. They are generally also treated with cognitive behavioural therapy. Ost et al. reported, during 1-year follow-up, an improvement in symptoms in 84–90% of patients after one to five sessions of psychological deconditioning [25]. Similar good results were also reported in case series by Van Dijk et al. [26], Hellstrom et al. [27], and Marks [28].

Conclusions

Patients with recurrent vasovagal syncope frequently display mild to moderate psychiatric disorders, and the presence of psychiatric illness seem to predict the risk of recurrence. Thus, in our opinion, psychiatric evaluation should be included in the clinical management of patients with severe vasovagal syncope, because it may be valuable in identifying which subjects are at high risk of recurrence and really need long-term treatment.

Psychiatric and psychological interventions seem to represent a promising treatment, at least in patients with refractory vasovagal syncope and in those with blood/injury phobia. However, before becoming a first-line therapy for most vasovagal fainters, the positive effects of psychiatric treatment need to be verified in larger, randomised and placebo-controlled trials.

References

1. Brignole M, Alboni P, Benditt DG et al (2004) Guidelines on management (diagnosis and treatment) of syncope – update 2004. Europace 6:467–537
2. Schmidt RT (1975) Personality and fainting. J Psychosom Res 19:21–25
3. Sledge WH (1978) Antecedent psychological factors in the onset of vasovagal syncope. Psychosom Med 40:568–579
4. American Psychiatric Association (1994) Diagnostic and Statistical Manual of Mental Disorders, 4th ed (DSM-IV). American Psychiatric Association, Washington DC, p 20
5. Sheldon R, Rose S, Flanagan P et al (1996) Risk factors for syncope recurrence after a positive tilt-table test in patients with syncope. Circulation 93:973–981
6. Di Girolamo E, Di Iorio C, Sabatini P et al (1999) Effects of paroxetine hydrochloride, a selective serotonin re-uptake inhibitor, on refractory vasovagal syncope: a randomized, double-blind, placebo-controlled study. J Am Coll Cardiol 33:1227–1230
7. Kapoor WN, Fortunato M, Hanusa BH et al (1995) Psychiatric illnesses in patients with syncope. Am J Med 99:505–512
8. Linzer M, Felder A, Hackel A et al (1990) Psychiatric syncope: a new look at an old disease. Psychosomatics 31:181–188
9. Koenig D, Linzer M, Pontinen M et al (1992) Syncope in young adults: evidence for combined medical and psychiatric approach. J Intern Med 232:169–176
10. Kouakam C, Lacroix D, Baux P et al (1996) Anxiety neurosis and unexplained syncope of presumed vaso-vagal origin. Arch Mal Coeur 89:1247–1254
11. Cohen TJ, Thayapran N, Ibrahim B et al (2000) An association between anxiety and neurocardiogenic syncope during head-up tilt table testing. Pacing Clin Electrophysiol 23:837–841
12. Ventura R, Maas R, Ruppel R et al (2001) Psychiatric conditions in patients with recurrent unexplained syncope. Europace 3:311–316
13. Kouakam C, Lacroix D, Klug D et al (2002) Prevalence and prognostic significance of psychiatric disorders in patients evaluated for recurrent unexplained syncope. Am J Cardiol 89:530–535
14. Linzer M, Pontinen M, Gold DT et al (1991) Impairment of physical and psychosocial function in recurrent syncope. J Clin Epidemiol 44:1037–1043
15. Linzer M, Gold DT, Pontinen M et al (1994) Recurrent syncope as a chronic disease: preliminary validation of a disease-specific measure of functional impairment. J Gen Intern Med 9:181–185
16. Rose MS, Koshman ML, Spreng S et al (2000) The relationship between health-related quality of life and frequency of spells in patients with syncope. J Clin Epidemiol 53:1209–1216
17. Giada F, Silvestri I, Rossillo A et al (2005) Psychiatric profile, quality of life and risk of syncopal recurrence in patients with tilt-induced vasovagal syncope. Europace (in press in press)
18. Butcher JN, Dahlstrom GW, Graham JR (1989) MMPI-2 manual for administration and scoring. University of Minnesota Press, Minneapolis, p 81
19. Pancheri P, Sirigatti S (1995) MMPI-2 Minnesota Multiphase Personality Inventory-2 manual. Italian adaptation. OS (Organizzazioni Speciali), Florence, Italy, p 34
20. Ware JE, Sherbourne CD (1992) The MOS 36-Item Short-Form Health Survey (SF-36): I. Conceptual framework and item selection. Med Care 30:473–483

21. Mc-Horney CA, Ware JE, Raczek AE (1993) The MOS 36-Item Short-Form Health Survey (SF-36): II. Psychometric and clinical tests of validity in measuring physical and mental health constructs. Med Care 31:247–263
22. McGrady AV, Kern-Buell C, Bush E et al (2003) Biofeedback-assisted relaxation therapy in neurocardiogenic syncope: a pilot study. Appl Psychophysiol Biofeedback 28:183–192
23. Newton JL, Kenny RA, Baker CR (2003) Cognitive behavioural therapy as potential treatment for vasovagal/neurocardiogenic syncope – a pilot study. Europace 5:299–301
24. Kadri NN, Hee TT, Rovang KS et al (1999) Efficacy and safety of clonazepam in refractory neurally mediated syncope. Pacing Clin Electrophysiol 22:307–314
25. Ost LG, Hellstrom K, Kaver A (1992) One versus five sessions of exposure in the treatment of injection phobia. Behav Res Ther 23:263–282
26. Van Dijk N, Velzeboer SCJM, Destree-Vonk A et al (2001) Psychological treatment of malignant vasovagal syncope due to blood phobia. Pacing Clin Electrophysiol 24:122–124
27. Hellstrom K, Fellenius J, Ost LG (1996) One versus five sessions of applied tension in the treatment of blood phobia. Behav Res Ther 34:101–112
28. Marks I (1988) Blood-injury phobia: a review. Am J Psychiatry 145:1207–1213

Familial Vasovagal Syncope: Clinical Characteristics and Potential Genetic Substrates

A. González-Hermosillo, M.F. Márquez, M. Vallejo, K.I. Urias, M. Cárdenas

Introduction

Vasovagal syncope (VVS) is a common clinical problem that has been the subject of extensive research in recent years. In this type of syncope, which affects all age groups, cerebral hypoperfusion develops as a consequence of abnormal autonomic control of the circulation, leading to hypotension with or without bradycardia. Estimates are that approximately 12–48% of healthy young adults and 6% of older individuals suffer from recurrent syncopal events, and the quality of life may be compromised by the condition [1]. Syncopal events that do not reach medical attention occur much more frequently. In fact, recently published results of a survey of students averaging 20 years of age demonstrated that about 20% of males and 50% of females had experienced at least one syncopal episode [2]. While the exact aetiology and pathophysiologic processes involved in VVS have yet to be fully elucidated, a basic understanding has begun to emerge. Studies have shown that the autonomic nervous system plays a fundamental role in the pathophysiology of VVS [3]. Several lines of evidence indicate the presence of central and peripheral abnormalities of sympathetic function. A better understanding of the pathophysiology of VVS could provide a more rational basis for therapy and help to optimise the resources currently used to obtain a diagnosis.

Under some circumstances, a diagnosis of VVS can be made based on the clinical history and is often confirmed by tilt testing. Therapy is aimed at preventing or reducing the recurrence of syncope.

Calkins et al. [4], in a study done at a tertiary-care centre, estimated that up to US $16 000 of unnecessary testing may be performed on patients who

Electrocardiology Department, Instituto Nacional de Cardiología 'Ignacio Chávez', Tlalpan, México ultimately receive a diagnosis of VVS, emphasising the difficulty of making the diagnosis.

Family History in Vasovagal Syncope

In VVS, especially when confirmed, there is frequently a positive family history, especially when the onset is below the age of 20. A case control study by Camfield and Camfield [5] showed that among children with VVS a significant proportion, 27/30 (90%), had a parent or sibling with syncope, an association not seen in control subjects. In this study, none of the patients' best friends fainted, although 33% (8/24) of their friends had a first-degree relative with syncope. Mathias et al. [6] reported a familial tendency for VVS in patients with an onset before the age of 20. A family history of VVS was found in 57% (33/58) of these patients compared with 18% (11/61) with a later onset. Of the 44 with a family history, 73% had a least one parent or child with a VVS. They included four patients with a family history over three generations, and one who had a twin sister with syncope. In 9%, a sibling was the only relative with VVS; 18% had a grandparent, aunt, uncle, or cousin with VVS. Most adult-onset patients with VVS did not have a family history. In those with a family history, 73% had a parent or child with a history of VVS, but only 27% ($n = 12$) had other relatives with syncope [6].

A study from Newcastle, UK, suggested that in at least 20% of patients with recurrent syncope, other members of the family had experienced syncopal symptoms, suggesting familial clustering of VVS and that this syndrome has a significant inheritable component [1]. From a data base of the Royal Victory Infirmary, researchers identified 603 individuals with a diagnosis of VVS. Of these, 441 (81%) answered a postal questionnaire, of whom 84 (19%) described a positive family history for faints and 75 (89%) supplied details of first-degree relatives. Overall, of the 389 first-degree relatives, 145 were affected (37.2%). The total number of siblings in affected families was 145, with 47 (32.4%) affected. The total number of offspring was 102, with 42 affected (41%) [1]. Further evidence for a genetic basis to this condition is provided by examining haemodynamic responses to head-up tilt in first-degree relatives of patients with VVS. Newton et al. [1] described a total of 11 first-degree relatives from six families who agreed to undergo the head-up tilt test with nitrates provocation. Seven were affected and four unaffected. All eleven individuals had abnormal responses to tilt testing: five out of the 11 subjects tested became hypotensive in association with symptoms, three of these were affected subjects who had full reproduction of presyncopal symptoms and the remaining two were unaffected subjects who experienced symptoms that clinically resembled those experienced by 'fainters.' Neither of the latter two subjects could recall a prior similar experience. Of the remaining six tested subjects, five became tachycardic (four previously affected subjects experienced presyncopal symptoms and one previously unaffected subject experienced new symptoms clinically consistent with presyncope). The remaining subject who was previously unaffected developed syncope in association with bradycardia, although he had never experienced these symptoms before. This finding suggests that first-degree relatives of those with VVS, even if they do not express the syncopal phenotype, still have a vasovagal reaction tendency. Intriguingly this raises the possibility of incomplete penetrance of a genetic disorder or 'genetic variability' in unaffected first-degree relatives of VVS patients. One alternative explanation is that VVS is a complex trait arising from the interaction between one or more alleles and the environment. Environmental factors may include infectious agents, medication, nutrition, toxins, and stress [1]. Therefore, the inherited tendency to faint may be multifactorial but requires an environmental stimulus for expression. Another alternative is that the disorder represents an autosomal recessive condition, but with a relatively common frequency of the recessive allele [7].

Recently [7], the findings from a family that showed VVS inheritance in at least three generations, in absence of any cardiac or autonomic abnormalities, were reported. The proband was a 10-year-old child with an 18-month history of recurrent syncopal episodes. The proband's sibling had developed syncopal episodes at the age of 12. Their father had suffered from occasional syncopal episodes, and the paternal uncle also had similar symptoms. A child of the proband's uncle also developed syncope at the age of 10. The other child provided no history of syncopal events, though one possible presyncopal event was noted. The paternal grandfather, and his brother and sister had all suffered presyncopal events during their early to late teens. Although it was not possible to ascertain whether the great-grandparents had experienced syncopal events, there was some suggestion that the great-grandfather may have experienced them, There was no evidence for syncope in the proband's mother's family. No family members had abnormal autonomic function or heart-rate variability when compared with age and sex controls. In the proband, the tilt test confirmed the diagnosis of VVS with hypotension and reproduction of syncope. In the seven family members originally described as affected or possibly affected, on clinical evaluation all had symptom reproduction during tilt testing. In the three unaffected family members who underwent tilt testing, two were normal (mother and maternal grandmother).The third (paternal grandmother) had hypotension in association with presyncope, which she had never experienced previously. The pedigree of this family suggests that familial VVS may be an autosomal dominant disorder with incomplete penetrance in some individuals.

Assessment of the phenotype of this common condition allows better characterisation of affected and unaffected family members and, using whole genome scanning and linkage analysis in suitable families, will potentially lead to identification of the responsible locus [7].

We have reported two groups of monozygotic twins, from different families, and a family with several members affected with VVS. One set of twins consisted of male patients with no history of syncope in their parents or relatives. The other set consisted of females with a history of syncopal attacks in their mother. Tilt testing was positive in all [8]. In another family, the proband was a 20-year-old woman referred to our unit with a 4-year history of recurrent syncopal episodes, the father, a brother, and two sisters were affected and all had a positive tilt test.

These data alone strongly indicate that genetic factors play a role in the aetiology of VVS. However, it is difficult, if not impossible to define whether familial syncopes have a genetic basis or are due to the high frequency of this symptom in the general population.

Mendelian Forms of Hypotension

Several genetic determinants that control blood pressure and cardiovascular responses are known, with some being possible candidates for a gene causing familial VVS.

Identification of the molecular basis of several autosomal-dominant forms of hypertension has permitted unambiguous identification of mutant gene carriers, allowing the spectrum of blood pressures in gene carriers to be assessed. Some family members who have inherited these mutations have normal or only minimally elevated blood pressures, which suggests that, just as there are alleles that raise blood pressure, there are likely to be alleles in the population that lower blood pressure [9].

One approach to this problem to determining the genetic basis of VVS is to identify mutations causing recessive forms of severe hypotension; heterozygous carriers of these same mutations, which will be much more prevalent than their homozygous counterparts, may be protected from the development of hypertension. Once relevant mutations are identified, the hypothesis that the heterozygous state lowers blood pressure can be tested [8]. Most of the patients with VVS have a long history of arterial hypotension during their youth. In 1996, the molecular causes of two inherited forms of hypotension were reported. Autosomal recessive pseudohypoaldosteronism type 1 (PHA-1) is characterised by life-threatening dehydration in the neonatal period, marked hypotension, salt-wasting, a high serum potassium level, metabolic acidosis, and marked elevation in plasma rennin activity and aldosterone levels. Genetic analysis of affected offspring of consanguineous unions demonstrated linkage of this disease to segments of either chromosome 12 or 16, each of which contains genes encoding different subunits of the epithelial sodium channel (ENaC). Examination of the ENaC subunit genes in families with PHA-1 revealed mutations that result in loss of function [8]. This was previously known from familial forms of defects in renal salt handling, such as Gitelman's syndrome, which is due to mutations and loss of function of the renal sodium-chloride cotransporter (NCCT) that increase salt clearance and lead to hypotension [10]. Gitelman's syndrome is an autosomal recessive trait characterised by low serum potassium and high serum bicarbonate levels, renal salt wasting, low urinary calcium excretion, low serum magnesium levels, and an activated renin-angiotensin system. Patients with this disorder have low blood pressure and neuromuscular abnormalities. The gene causing Gitelman's syndrome has been mapped to a region of chromosome 16 that contains the gene encoding the renal thiazide-sensitive NA-Cl co transporter, which mediates reabsorption of sodium and chloride [11].

Genetic Catecholamine Disorders

Many syndromes associated with orthostatic intolerance show similarities to VVS, suggesting a potential overlap and possible common aetiology [12]. Postural orthostatic tachycardia syndrome (POTS) is a disabling chronic disorder characterised by tachycardia, symptoms of cerebral hypoperfusion, and sympathetic activation. Most attempts to explain the hyperadrenergic state in these patients have focused on an increased release of norepinephrine (NE) in response to the change from supine to upright posture. An alternative explanation is an abnormality in the clearance of the NE from the synaptic cleft. Recently, a missense mutation (converting alanine to proline) in the human NE transporter (NET) gene A457P, located on chromosome 16q12.2, was identified in an individual and her identical twin suffering from POTS [13]. This mutation renders the transporter nonfunctional. In these subjects, the release of NE into the synapse is normal, but reduced amounts are taken back up into the sympathetic nerve terminal as a result of the decreased activity of NET. Spillover of NE into the circulation is increased, and more NE is available in the synapse to interact with adrenergic receptors. However, the A457P mutation does not explain all cases of POTS. The mutation was not present in any of 254 unrelated persons, including normal subjects, patients with hypertension, and other patients with orthostatic intolerance. Furthermore, although family members who had the mutation also had some of the physiologic and biochemical abnormalities detected in the proband and her twin sister, none had the full-blown syndrome.

Dopamine-β-hydroxylase (DBH) is the enzyme responsible for intraneural conversion of dopamine to NE. Its deficiency results in failure of NE synthesis, excessive dopamine release, orthostatic hypotension, and, sometimes, ptosis of the eyelids. Subjects with DBH deficiency syndrome have worsening symptoms in late adolescence, including reduced ability to exercise, nasal stuffiness, dyspnoea, nuchal discomfort, precordial pain, syncope, and frequent postural symptoms [15]. The DBH gene maps to chromosome 9q34, and several mutations of the DBH gene that cause this very rare syndrome have now been identified. Kim et al. [14] identified seven novel variants, including four potentially pathogenic mutations, in the human DBH gene of two unrelated DBH-deficient patients and their families. A sole finding of absent plasma DBH is insufficient, since about 4% of the population lacks DBH. Once the specific enzymatic defect for DBH deficiency had been elucidated, investigators were able to devise a better treatment. A favourable long-term result has been achieved with l-dihydroxyphenylserine (l-DOPS). This agent is a prodrug acted upon by endogenous dopa-decarboxylase to yield NE. The administration of DOPS to DBH-deficient patients resulted in dramatic increases in blood pressure and in restoration of plasma and urinary levels of NE to nearly normal [15]. The successful treatment of DBH deficiency encourages us to hope that other autonomic disorders may one day also yield to genuinely effective therapeutic intervention.

Streeten et al. [16] described a familial form of postural orthostatic hypotension with marked rise in heart rate, syncope, and associated cutaneous dilatation in the face and lower limbs. The findings have been attributed to excessive bradykinin levels. Recently, DeStefano et al. [17] showed linkage in these families to a 25cM region of chromosome 18q between 18S858 and 18S541. Whilst no specific mutations in any genes have been described in this particular syndrome, the renal urea transporters HUT1 and HUT2 are located in this region and polymorphism in the latter is known to be associated with reduced diastolic blood pressure in males [18].

There are other hereditary autonomic disorders associated with orthostatic hypotension. In the majority there are associated neurological deficits. It is far beyond the scope of this chapter to review every autonomic disorder. Interested readers are referred to an excellent text on the subject [19].

Conclusions

Disturbances in autonomic function can result in a wide variety of conditions that may ultimately culminate in the loss of consciousness. Success in identification of genes conferring susceptibility to hypotension and its clinical sequelae is expected to provide new insights into the pathophysiology of this condition and lead to development of highly accurate genetic tests, permitting identification of subjects with specific inherited susceptibility. These insights may permit intervention at preclinical stages with therapies tailored to underlying primary abnormalities, improving efficacy of treatment (nowadays, mostly empirical), and reducing morbidity from these diseases.

References

1. Newton JL (2003) Prevalence of family history in vasovagal syncope and haemodynamic response to head up tilt in first degree relatives. Preliminary data for the Newcastle cohort. Clin Auton Res 13:22–26
2. Wieling W, Ganzeboom KS, Philip SJ (2004) Reflex syncope in children and adolescents. Heart 90:1094–1100
3. Kochiadakis GE, Papadimitriou EA, Marketou ME et al (2004) Autonomic nervous system changes in vasovagal syncope: Is there any difference between young and older patients? PACE 27:1371–1377
4. Calkins H, Byrne M, el-Atassi R et al (1993) The economic burden of unrecognized vasodepressor syncope. Am J Med 95:473–479
5. Camfield PR, Camfield CS (1990) Syncope in childhood: A case control clinical study of the familial tendency to faint. Can J Neurol Sci 17:306–308
6. Mathias C, Deguchi K, Bleasdale-Barr K, Smith S (1998) Frequency of family history in vasovagal syncope. Lancet 352:33–34
7. Newton JL, Kerr S, Pairman J et al (2005) Familial neurocardiogenic (vasovagal) syncope. Am J of Med Genetics 133A:176–179
8. Márquez MF, Urias KI, Hermosillo AG et al (2005) Familial vasovagal syncope. Europace (in press)
9. Lifton RP (1996) Molecular genetics of human blood pressure variation. Science 272:676–680
10. Cruz DN, Simon DB, Nelson-Williams C et al (2001) Mutations in the Na-Cl co transporter reduce blood pressure in humans. Hypertension 37:1458–1464
11. Cruz DN, Shaer AJ, Bia MJ et al (2001) Yale Gitelman's and Bartter syndrome Collaborative Study Group. Gitelman's syndrome revisited: A reevaluation of the symptoms and health related quality of life. Kidney Int 59:710–717
12. Gonzalez-Hermosillo A, Márquez MF, Kostine A et al (2004) Vasovagal syncope, orthostatic hypotension and postural orthostatic tachycardia syndrome: Is there a connection? In: Raviele A (ed) Cardiac Arrhythmias 2003. Springer, Milan, pp 615–624
13. Shannon JR, Flattem NL, Jordan J (2000) Orthostatic intolerance and tachycardia associated with norepinephrine-transporter deficiency. N Engl J Med 342:541–549
14. Kim CH, Zabetian CP, Cubells JF (2001) Mutations in the dopamine ß-hydroxylase gene are associated with human norepinephrine deficiency. Am J Med Genet 108:140–147
15. Robertson D, Haile V, Perry SE et al (1991) Dopamine beta-hydroxylase deficiency. A genetic disorder of cardiovascular regulation. Hypertension 18:1–8
16. Streeten DHP, Kerr LP, Kerr CB et al (1972) Hyperbradykinism: A new orthostatic syndrome. Lancet II:1048–1053
17. DeStefano AL, Baldwin CT, Burzstyn M et al (1998) Autosomal dominant hypoten-

sive disorder maps to chromosome 18q. Am J Hum Genet 163:1425–1430
18. Ranade K, Wu KD, Hwu CM et al (2001) Genetic variation in the human urea transporter is associated with variation in blood pressure. Hum Mol Genet 10:2157–2164
19. Mathias CJ, Bannister R (1999) Dopamine ß-hydroxylase deficiency with a note on other genetically determined causes of autonomic failure. In: Mathias CJ, Bannister R (eds) Autonomic Failure. A Textbook of Clinical Disorders of the Autonomic Nervous System. Fourth edition. Oxford University Press, Oxford-New York, pp 387–401

Subject Index